P9-EEU-942

HEART DISEASE IS THE #1 KILLER IN AMERICA.

One in four Americans dies from heart disease, often with no warning signs. Prevention is the key. Food is the best medicine.

HOW CAN
THE FAT AND CHOLESTEROL COUNTER
HELP PROTECT YOUR HEALTH?

The scientific findings behind fat, cholesterol, and heart disease have changed drastically in recent years. It no longer matters *how much* fat you eat but *which* fats. And restricting cholesterol may not be the best preventative approach.

Nolan and Heslin explain exactly what all the latest research means for you. This comprehensive guide provides fat, cholesterol, trans fat, fiber, and sugar values for more than 10,000 of your favorite foods so that you can make the best choices for your heart at every meal.

Books by Karen J. Nolan and Jo-Ann Heslin

The Calorie Counter (Sixth Edition)

The Fat and Cholesterol Counter

The Complete Food Counter (Fourth Edition)

The Ultimate Carbohydrate Counter (Third Edition)

The Protein Counter (Third Edition)

The Diabetes Counter (Fifth Edition)

The Most Complete Food Counter (Third Edition)

Books by Annette B. Natow, Jo-Ann Heslin, and Karen J. Nolan

The Cholesterol Counter (Seventh Edition)

The Fat Counter (Seventh Edition)

The Healthy Wholefoods Counter

Books by Annette B. Natow and Jo-Ann Heslin

Eating Out Food Counter

The Healthy Heart Food Counter

The Vitamin and Mineral Food Counter

Ebooks by Karen J. Nolan, Jo-Ann Heslin, and Annette B. Natow

The Most Complete Food Counter (Second Edition)

Apps by Karen J. Nolan and Jo-Ann Heslin

Your Complete Food Counter
(http://itunes.apple.com/us/app/your-complete-food
-counter/id444558777?mt=8)

The
Fat and Cholesterol Counter

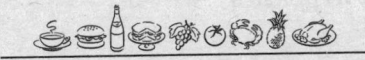

Karen J. Nolan, Ph.D.
and
Jo-Ann Heslin, M.A., R.D.

POCKET BOOKS

New York   London   Toronto   Sydney   New Delhi

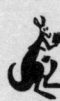

Pocket Books
A Division of Simon & Schuster, Inc.
1230 Avenue of the Americas
New York, NY 10020

Copyright © 2014 by Karen J. Nolan and
Jo-Ann Heslin

First Pocket Books paperback edition January 2014

POCKET and colophon are registered trademarks of Simon & Schuster, Inc.

For information about special discounts for bulk purchases, please contact Simon & Schuster Special Sales at 1-866-506-1949 or business@simonandschuster.com.

The Simon & Schuster Speakers Bureau can bring authors to your live event. For more information or to book an event contact the Simon & Schuster Speakers Bureau at 1-866-248-3049 or visit our website at www.simonspeakers.com.

Manufactured in the United States of America

10 9 8 7 6 5 4 3 2 1

ISBN 978-1-4516-2165-5

For
Our families,
who support us through every project.

ACKNOWLEDGMENTS

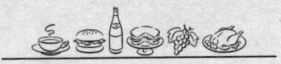

For all her continuous support and help, our agent, Nancy Trichter.

For her suggestions and editing skills, Sara Clemence.

For all her patience, comments, and questions—our favorite reviewer, Jean Schwarsin.

Without the tireless cooperation of Stephen Llano and the production department at Pocket Books, *The Fat and Cholesterol Counter* would never have been completed.

A special thank-you to our editor, Emilia Pisani.

We would also like to thank all of our readers for their suggestions and questions. Your input helps us provide you with the most useful information.

*. . . those who regard their own welfare . . .
are asking how to choose foods wisely . . .
how the science of nutrition can be made
to function most successfully in their daily
lives.*

Mary Swartz Rose, Ph.D.
Feeding the Family
The Macmillan Company, 1919

CONTENTS

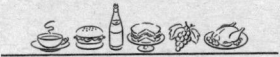

PART ONE
Brand Name, Nonbranded (Generic), and Take-Out Foods
65

PART TWO
Restaurant Chains
359

The
Fat and Cholesterol Counter

INTRODUCTION

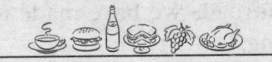

*Understanding how food impacts your
health should make you think about
what you choose to eat but should not
destroy your pleasure in eating.*

The most important thing you will learn from *The Fat
and Cholesterol Counter* is:

**The kind of fat you eat is far more important
than how much fat you eat.**

Hold on to your dinner plate—this could be a bumpy
ride! Modifying the amount of fat you eat to reduce
heart disease, the number 1 killer in the U.S. today, is a
worthy goal. But the way we have gone about this may
be all wrong.

For the last 40 years Americans have had a love/
hate relationship with fat. We adore it in premium ice
creams, crispy fried chicken, and butter-drenched popcorn. At the same time, we hate it because we've been
told it is not good for our waistlines or our hearts. So
we have dutifully stopped eating steak and stocked the
house with no fat cookies and lowfat cheese and tried
to convince ourselves that fat free baked potato chips
taste like the real thing. In an effort to enjoy food, we
drank gallons of soda and sweetened fruit drinks. Then

we turned around and gorged ourselves on no carb diets that allowed us to eat bacon and steak.

None of these approaches worked. In fact we have gotten fatter, there is a growing epidemic of type 2 diabetes, and the inroads we have made to prevent heart disease are fading.

The time has come to make friends with fat and to understand that food is truly your best friend and the best medicine you'll ever take.

The Fat and Cholesterol Counter is going to sort out the myths, explain the latest research, and help you form a healthy relationship with fat to reduce your risk for heart disease. It is easier than you think, and it will taste good, too.

Let's get started.

Players in the Healthy Heart Game

In addition to calories, *The Fat and Cholesterol Counter* gives you values for total fat, saturated fat, polyunsaturated fat, monounsaturated fat, trans fat, cholesterol, sugar, and fiber. Each is an important player to help you achieve a lower risk for heart disease. For some you need to eat more, for others you should eat less. We will help you sort all that out as the fat and cholesterol story unfolds.

WHY THE FAT AND CHOLESTEROL STORY HAS CHANGED

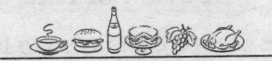

*When it comes to heart disease risk,
it is not about one bad actor—it is a
company of players gone awry.*

Science evolves, and in doing so it sometimes appears to contradict itself. A good example of this is the story of margarine. In an effort to reduce our intake of saturated fat, which is found in butter, we were told to switch to margarine, lower in saturated fat. The first margarine produced was in stick form. It was made with hydrogenated (hardened) vegetable oil. In the process of changing liquid oil to solid margarine, trans fats are formed. As research moved forward, it showed that trans fats might be more damaging to our health than the saturated fat found in butter. Researchers were not trying to mislead you; they making recommendations based on the evidence they had on hand at that time.

Most eating recommendations come from a balance of scientific evidence and scientific judgment. This is called an "evidence-based approach." Experts gather all the research available and use their trained judgment to make recommendations for you about what to eat, how to eat, and when to eat.

But science keeps moving ahead, and the evidence the experts look at often changes. The recommendations about fat and cholesterol are perfect examples of the evolution of scientific findings.

The Story of Fats

In the mid-1980s we were all urged to lower our fat intake. What the experts really meant was that we should eat fewer foods high in fat and substitute some of our high fat intake with more fruits, vegetables, and healthy, whole grain carbohydrates. Food companies viewed this as a marketing opportunity, and soon the supermarkets were flooded with nonfat or lowfat cookies, ice cream, salad dressing, cheese, and sour cream. Potato chips were baked, and numerous sweet snacks appeared to fill the gap for the fatty foods we gave up. The shift in diet did not achieve what the researchers had proposed. We were eating less fat, but we were also eating far more sugar and refined carbohydrate. We had swapped sugar and starch for fat. At the same time, very few people increased the amount of fruit, vegetables, or fiber they ate.

As the science of fats evolved, researchers learned that certain fats were healthy and others were less healthy. They recommended that people eat more polyunsaturated and monounsaturated fat (vegetable oils) and eat less saturated fat (animal fats). Today we are suggesting that eating a moderate amount of fat—not a low fat diet—may be the best approach, and that trans fat (solid fats used in baking and food processing like shortening) should be avoided.

Sadly, the only message that was heard loud and clear

by most consumers is that fat is bad for you. But we know now that simply isn't true.

The Cholesterol Story

More than 55 years ago, researchers began to monitor 5000 residents from Framingham, Massachusetts, to better understand why some people got heart disease and others did not. They were suspicious of cholesterol, a fat that could be measured in the blood.

The researchers discovered, by following all these people for many years, that there was a connection between the level of cholesterol in the blood and the risk for heart disease. This was important, groundbreaking news. From that point on, high levels of total cholesterol became a marker for the risk for heart disease and remains so today.

As time went on, researchers realized that cholesterol came in different forms, HDL and LDL. They realized that high levels of the HDL form appeared protective against heart disease, but high levels of the LDL form increased risk.

That may sound confusing, and it is. You want your total cholesterol to be low to reduce your risk for heart disease. But within that number, for example 201, you want your HDL cholesterol to be high and your LDL cholesterol to be low. That's why when you get a blood test done, your doctor looks at total cholesterol, HDL cholesterol and LDL cholesterol, to assess your risk.

Even though we currently know a lot about cholesterol, the story is still unfolding. Many experts question whether our current recommendations for the amount of cholesterol to eat daily are too low. Some experts believe that a certain amount of cholesterol has a positive effect on health and we should not aim to reduce our cholesterol so much. Other countries—Canada, Australia, the European Union, United Kingdom, Ireland, Korea, Japan, India, and New Zealand—no longer recommend an upper limit of cholesterol intake each day. The experts from these countries do not feel that restricting cholesterol provides heart health benefits.

And, if all that isn't confusing enough, we now know that there is a type of cholesterol experts are referring to as "ugly" or "ultra-bad" cholesterol. It is a remnant cholesterol form that may triple heart disease risk because it is more likely to stick to artery walls and build up fatty plaques. People who are older, overweight, or have type 2 diabetes are more likely to have higher levels of ugly cholesterol.

Why Sugar and Fiber Are Important

Americans eat far too much sugar and not enough fiber. How does this affect heart disease risk, you wonder? When the low fat eating craze took effect, experts hoped that people would lower their intake of high fat foods and substitute healthy carbohydrates instead—whole grains, beans, fruits, and vegetables. This did not happen. Instead we piled on refined carbohydrates with limited fiber and lots of sugar—white bread, cookies, cake, white rice, candy, soda, and sweetened fruit drinks.

We have tipped the carbohydrate pattern in this country away from whole grains and toward too much sugar. Whole grains, which provide fiber, boosts your immune system, reduces your risk for type 2 diabetes, and reduces inflammation, a major player in heart disease. Yet 96% of Americans don't eat enough fiber each day, and most of us eat far too much sugar, as much as 300 to 400 sugar calories each day. This equals 19 to 25 teaspoons of sugar a day!

FIBER TIP—

An easy way to add more fiber to your diet is to switch from white bread to whole wheat bread.

Americans have a love affair with sugar. As sugar intake goes up, the quality of the diet goes down—more calories, less fiber, fewer vitamins and minerals, and more unhealthy fats are eaten. This is the exact opposite of what you want to be eating to prevent heart disease.

Added sugars make up as much as 25% of our calories daily. Soda, candy, fruit drinks, cakes, cookies, ice cream, jelly, and syrup are full of added sugar. They offer little besides sweetness and calories. Simply cutting back on sweetened drinks would cut your added sugar intake a good deal.

Grains, fruits, vegetables, milk, and plain yogurt all contain sugars, as well, but these are *natural sugars* found in the food along with vitamins, minerals, and fiber. To make the healthiest food choices, choose foods with natural sugars more often and foods with added sugars less often.

We still have a lot to learn about the connection between sugar and heart disease. But we do know that eating too much sugar provides no health benefits; eating less will have a positive effect on your health.

YOU SHOULD KNOW—

Diet Protects Against Heart Disease

Those who eat a heart-healthy, moderate-fat diet reduce their risk of dying from heart disease, having a heart attack, or having a stroke by 30%.

RATING YOUR RISKS

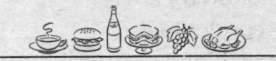

Heart disease often gives you no warning signs.
That's why prevention is so important.

How Inflammation Attacks Your Heart

When you get a splinter in your finger, the surrounding skin swells and gets red. You feel pain. This is inflammation—a sign that your body's immune system is mobilizing to repair the damage.

Heart disease has its roots in inflammation, too. The LDL form of cholesterol can burrow into an artery wall and trigger inflammation. To reduce the inflammation, the body sends white blood cells to gobble up the troublesome LDL cholesterol. The white blood cells become stuffed with LDL cholesterol, and the combination forms a fatty streak in the artery wall. Over time, debris in the blood gets caught and builds up on these fatty streaks, and they eventually turn into plaque that starts to block and harden the artery. If a piece of the plaque ruptures or breaks off, it can block the artery, and a heart attack or stroke occurs.

There are things you can do to prevent inflammation and lower your risk for heart disease. The following quiz will help you identify some of your risks.

RATE YOUR RISKS

Is your total cholesterol high?	Yes	No
Is your LDL cholesterol high?	Yes	No
Is your HDL cholesterol low?	Yes	No
Are your triglycerides high?	Yes	No
Do you have high blood pressure?	Yes	No
Do you have diabetes?	Yes	No
Do you do less than 30 minutes of exercise each day?	Yes	No
Are you overweight?	Yes	No
Men—is your waist measurement greater than 42 inches?	Yes	No
Women—is your waist measurement greater than 35 inches?	Yes	No
Do you drink 3 or more alcoholic drinks a day?	Yes	No
Are you frequently stressed?	Yes	No
Are you 55 or older?	Yes	No
Do you have a close relative with heart disease?	Yes	No
Do you get less than 7 to 8 hours sleep each night?	Yes	No
Do you smoke?	Yes	No

The more times you answered *yes*, the higher your risk for heart disease. Every *no* answer lowers your risk. Let's see what you can do to turn some of those *yes* answers to *no*.

Understanding Risks

The concept of risk factors related to disease is relatively new in medicine. Researchers didn't even think lifestyle—diet, exercise, smoking, weight—was a factor in heart disease until the 1960s. But now we know that many things you do can increase your risk. Everything you said yes to on the quiz is a risk for heart disease. And, unfortunately, risks tend to build on each other, creating an even more powerful negative effect on your health. If you have 2 or more risk factors, your chance of getting heart disease is quadrupled. Having three or more risk factors makes you 8 to 20 times more likely to get heart disease than if you had no risk factors at all.

YOU SHOULD KNOW—

Understanding % Risk

A 10% risk means for every 100 people, 10 people will be affected by a particular problem.
If 35% to 40% of all smoking-related deaths are from heart disease, that means for every 100 smokers who die, the cause of death for 35 to 40 of them will be heart disease.
Simply convert the % risk to that number out of 100 people.
(50% risk = 50 out of every 100 people)

While you can't do much about your relatives or your age, you can control other factors. Changing the way you live and eat can reduce your chances of developing heart disease, and simple changes can have surprisingly big effects. The sooner you know what puts you at greater risk, the sooner you can do something about it.

Levels of Fat in the Blood That Lead to Problems—Dyslipidemias

Dyslipidemia is a term that refers to levels of fat in the blood that can cause health problems—high levels of total cholesterol, high levels of LDL cholesterol, high levels of triglycerides, or low levels of HDL cholesterol. All increase the risk for heart disease. Exercising, losing weight, eating well, drinking moderate amounts of alcohol, and not smoking all help bring blood fats into the normal range.

YOU SHOULD KNOW—

> *Dyslipidemia—dys* (problematic)
> *lipid* (fat) *emia* (in blood)

High Blood Pressure

One out of 3 adults in the U.S. has high blood pressure. The higher your blood pressure, the greater your risk for heart disease. Blood pressure is measured by the top (systolic) number over the bottom (diastolic) number. For every 20 point rise in the top number or every 10 point rise in the bottom number over 115/75 your risk for heart disease doubles. People with high blood pressure also frequently have high cholesterol. All the lifestyle changes that lower troublesome blood fats will also lower high blood pressure.

Diabetes

More than 26 million Americans have diabetes, and 75% of all deaths related to diabetes are caused by heart disease. Of course, the best way to lower this risk is to avoid getting diabetes. Second best is to keep the condition under control by managing blood sugar, blood pressure, and blood fats. All three can be done with lifestyle changes and medication.

Exercise

Few Americans are as active as they should be—30% do no exercise at all, and very few of the rest meet the daily recommendation of 30 minutes of activity each day. Not exercising can increase your risk of heart disease substantially—as much as smoking a pack of cigarettes every day. Fortunately, it's easy to start moving; all you need to do is walk. Start with simple things like not using the drive-thru, parking at the end of the lot, or walking around the mall once before you start shopping. Exercise also makes you feel good, can help you lose weight, and lowers blood pressure.

Weight Loss

This one is the biggie—no pun intended. Over 70% of adults weigh too much, and being overweight increases your chances of having high cholesterol, high triglycerides, high blood pressure, diabetes, and heart disease. An overweight 45–year-old man will, on average, die 6 years before his lean counterpart and suffer from heart disease 3 years longer. An overweight 45–year-old woman will die almost 8.5 years before her lean counterpart and suffer from heart disease for an additional year and a half.

You're at even higher risk if you have the type of body that stores extra weight around the belly. Abdominal, or belly, fat has been linked to a higher risk for heart disease, diabetes, and hypertension. Belly fat is active and works like a mini-factory producing triglycerides, a type of fat in the blood. They are an important risk factor for heart disease, especially in older women.

The good news: When you lose weight cholesterol goes down, triglycerides go down, high blood pressure goes down, and HDL cholesterol goes up. Losing as little as 5% to10% of your current weight reduces your risk for heart disease. Lose more and your risk profile gets even better.

YOU SHOULD KNOW—

Though men may show symptoms 10 years earlier than women, heart disease is still the number one cause of death for both women and men.

Your Age and Your Relatives

You can't become younger or disown Uncle Sol or Aunt Bessie, no matter how hard you try. But it is important to know what diseases your close relatives currently have or what they died from: the information can help your doctor make judgments about your care. Remember that brothers, sisters, and parents count more heavily than more distant relatives like aunts and cousins.

Alcohol

The question isn't, Do you drink? It's, How much? Studies have shown that 1 to 2 drinks a day can reduce the risk for heart disease by raising HDLs. But more than that—3 or more drinks a day and up—increases the risk for high blood pressure and heart disease. Moderation is the key.

YOU SHOULD KNOW—

One drink equals a 5-ounce glass of wine, 12-ounces of beer, or a shot (1.5 ounces) of hard alcohol such as gin, whiskey, scotch, or vodka.

Stress

We once thought that people who were overachievers, type A personalities, were more prone to heart disease. But the evidence is inconclusive. Many ambitious, hard-working, busy people are perfectly healthy. Still, it does appear that people who experience a good deal of anger may be at higher risk of developing heart disease. Some of the things experts suggest to lower stress—exercising and drinking less, for example—are good for your heart, too.

Sleep

Americans are chronically sleep-deprived. Our bodies run on a 24-hour cycle, and for part of that cycle, at least 7 to 8 hours a day, we should be resting. This allows the body a chance to recharge, rest, and heal. Without rest, the body is stressed and more susceptible to illness and fatigue.

Getting enough sleep helps regulate the heart and blood vessels that move blood through the body. Chronically disrupting your normal sleeping patterns could increase the risk for heart disease.

YOU SHOULD KNOW—

High fat diets appear to disrupt our normal day/night cycle, promoting weight gain and increasing the risk for type 2 diabetes and heart disease.

Smoking

This is a risk factor you can reduce to zero. If you smoke, try to quit. If you don't smoke, don't start. Heart disease is the cause of 35% to 40% of all smoking-related deaths. And heart disease causes 8% of all deaths related to secondhand smoke.

12 STEPS TO PROTECT YOUR HEART

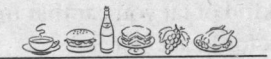

*A healthy lifestyle trumps genes when it comes
to reducing your risk for heart disease.*

You've heard it over and over again. Make unhealthy
choices—eat poorly, get little or no exercise, smoke,
drink too much, or gain weight—and your risk for heart
disease goes up dramatically.

Initiating 12 healthy lifestyle strategies could reduce
your risk for heart disease by up to 50%. Maybe you
can't change everything about the way you live, but if
you strive for small changes, over time, the results will
add up. You'll feel better, you'll have more energy, and
you will be healthier.

1. **Eat less saturated fat and trans fat.**
   - Reduce the amount of animal fat you
     regularly eat—meat, butter, bacon, cheese.
   - Try to eliminate as much trans fat as
     possible—fried foods and solid shortening
     found in some baked sweets, such as cookies,
     pastries, and cakes.
   - The good news is that there are less trans fat
     foods on the market today.

2. Eat more monounsaturated and polyunsaturated fat.

- Eat more olive, avocado, walnut, grapeseed, sunflower, safflower, canola, corn, and soybean oil.
- We now understand it isn't how much fat but the kind of fat you eat that increases your risk for heart disease.

3. Eat more omega-3 fat.

- Eat fish often—at least twice a week.
- Eat foods rich in omega-3, including flaxseed, walnuts, purslane, soy, and pumpkin seeds.
- Try some omega-3 enriched foods—orange juice, soymilk, and eggs.
- A number of large population studies showed that high omega-3 intakes reduced the risk for heart disease by 46% to 70%.

4. Eat more nuts and seeds.

- Rich in healthy fats, eating 2 servings a week can reduce your risk of dying of heart disease by 11%.
- Regularly eating nuts helps lower total cholesterol.
- Nuts are rich in polyunsaturated and monounsaturated fats.
- Walnuts are rich in omega-3 fats.

5. Eat more whole grains and fiber and less sugar and refined carbohydrates.

- Choose whole grains whenever possible— aim for at least 3 servings a day.
- A food that is a good source of fiber has

3 grams of fiber per serving; an excellent
source has 5 or more grams per serving.

- People who eat whole grain cereal every
  day have a 28% lower risk for heart disease.
- Switch from white bread to whole grain
  bread, white rice to brown rice.
- Select whole grain cereal and pasta most
  of the time.
- Eat less sugar, but you don't need to cut it
  out completely.
- Reduce the amount of soda and
  sweetened drinks you use regularly. Dilute
  presweetened drinks with sparkling water
  and drink more sugar-free, calorie-free water.

6. **Eat more veggies and fruits.**
   - There is no denying it, fruits and vegetables
     (including beans) are nature's superfoods—
     aim for at least 5 servings a day.
   - Berries—blueberries, strawberries,
     cranberries, raspberries—may boost HDL
     cholesterol.
   - Eat whole fruits and vegetables rather than
     drinking juice.
   - For each additional serving you eat daily, you
     decrease your risk for heart disease by 4%.

7. **Think outside the box when it comes to
   protein.**
   - Replace some of the animal protein in your
     diet with vegetable protein—try having at
     least 1 meatless meal each week.
   - Use meat to flavor dishes rather than
     dominate your plate.

- Keep portions of meat reasonable, to about 4 ounces.
- Areas of the world that eat the most animal foods have the highest rates of heart disease.

8. Eat regularly; don't fast then feast.
- People who eat 6 small meals a day have lower cholesterol levels than those who eat 1 to 2 big meals each day.
- Eating small, frequent meals also helps regulate blood sugar and triglyceride levels and promotes more reasonable portion sizes.

9. Don't drink. If you do, keep your intake moderate.
- 1 drink a day for women and 2 drinks a day for men should be max.
- A drink a day has been shown to protect your heart, but for some people it can raise triglycerides.

10. Exercise
- Activity increases the blood flow through your blood vessels, stimulating them to elongate, widen, and form new connections which keeps them healthy.
- Try to be active every day, aiming for 30 minutes of exercise. Vacuuming the rugs, mowing the lawn, or window shopping during lunch counts.
- Exercise lowers triglycerides and boosts HDL cholesterol.

11. Don't smoke
- Smoking isn't good for triglyceride levels— or anything else.
- Less is better, none is best.

12. Get enough sleep.
- Sleep-deprived people are at greater risk for heart disease.
- Sleep-deprived people weigh more.
- Sleeping helps your body heal and restore itself.
- Aim for 7 to 8 hours a night.

DO YOU KNOW
YOUR NUMBERS?

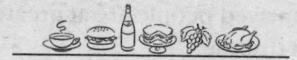

The numbers on your blood test are a window into your future heart health.

You go to the doctor, get blood drawn, and get a report. Do you know what these numbers really mean? You should, because they will help you understand your risk for heart disease.

Total Cholesterol
   Desirable: less than 200 mg/dl
   Borderline high: 200 to 239 mg/dl
   High: 240 mg/dl or higher

Total cholesterol is just that—the amount of cholesterol in a given volume of blood. It is measured as the number of milligrams (mg) of cholesterol in about a half cup of blood, or 1 deciliter (dl) of blood. For example, 222 mg/dl = 222 milligrams of cholesterol per deciliter of blood. To make things simpler, your doctor may give you just the number, 222, rather than the complete measurement.

YOU SHOULD KNOW—

*Cholesterol levels change with the season
and are highest in the winter.*

Blood is mainly made up of water. To travel through the blood, cholesterol, a fatlike substance, is coated with a protein. The combination of fat and protein is called a *lipoprotein.* If your total cholesterol values are high, your doctor will want to know the amount of LDL (low density lipoprotein) cholesterol and HDL (high density lipoprotein) cholesterol as well, because each form of cholesterol is part of your total risk package for heart disease.

A high total cholesterol value tells your doctor to look further. A complete lipid profile measures the amounts of total cholesterol, LDL cholesterol, HDL cholesterol, and triglycerides.

YOU SHOULD KNOW—

*Though you may be advised not to eat
for 9 to 12 hours before your blood test,
fasting may not be necessary.
Research studies have shown little difference
between the values for fasting and non-fasting blood
tests that are used to evaluate heart disease risk.*

LDL Cholesterol—the lower the number, the better
Normal: less than 100 mg/dl
Near or slightly above optimal: 100 to 129 mg/dl
Borderline high: 130 to 159 mg/dl
High: 160 to 189 mg/dl
Very high: 190 mg/dl and above

LDL is the major carrier of cholesterol in your bloodstream. If too much LDL cholesterol circulates in the blood, it can stick to the walls of arteries that lead to the heart and brain, eventually forming plaque. A blocked artery to the heart can cause a heart attack. A blocked artery to the brain can cause a stroke. That's why LDL cholesterol is often referred to as "bad" cholesterol. The lower your levels of LDL, the lower your risk of heart disease.

HDL Cholesterol—the higher the number the better
High: 60 mg/dl or higher
Average for women: 50 to 60 mg/dl
Average for men: 40 to 50 mg/dl
Low: less than 40 mg/dl

About one-third of the blood's cholesterol is carried by HDLs. Experts believe HDL cholesterol carries cholesterol away from the arteries and back to the liver, where it is broken down and removed from the body, helping to prevent plaque. For this reason, HDL is referred to as "good" cholesterol.

YOU SHOULD KNOW—

For every 1 point increase in HDLs, there is a 2% decrease in heart attacks and strokes for men, and a 3% decrease for women.

Cholesterol Ratio
TC/HDL: total cholesterol to HDL cholesterol
Good: 5:1
Optimum: 3.5:1

Your "ratio" is found by dividing HDL cholesterol into total cholesterol (TC). Some experts believe your total cholesterol to HDL ratio (TC/HDL) may be more important than cholesterol alone for monitoring your risk for heart disease.

Triglycerides
    Normal: less than 150 mg/dl
    Borderline high: 150 to 199 mg/dl
    High: 200 to 499 mg/dl
    Very high: 500 mg/dl or higher

Triglycerides are the main type of fat found in food, and the major storage form of fat in your body. High levels in the blood can be a risk factor for heart disease. Your triglycerides go up if you are overweight, do little exercise, drink too much alcohol, eat too much sugar and too little fiber, smoke, or have type 2 diabetes. Triglycerides can be lowered by making healthy lifestyle choices.

It is important to know your blood values. Abnormal blood fats can be used to identify those at risk for heart disease before they have symptoms.

Other Blood Tests Your Doctor May Order

If your family history, blood cholesterol levels, or triglyceride values put you at moderate to high risk for heart disease, your doctor may evaluate two other blood values, homocysteine and C-reactive protein.

Homocysteine
    Normal: values less than 12
    Increased risk: values above 12

Homocysteine is an amino acid, a building block of protein found in meat and other high protein foods. High levels in the blood are a marker for heart disease. Experts are not sure why homocysteine increases the risk for heart disease, but there appears to be a link between high homocysteine levels and hardening of the arteries and the formation of blood clots.

Usually, levels below 7 are associated with the lowest risk—but not always. Some studies have shown a reduction in heart disease when homocysteine levels go down, but in other studies this same positive effect has not been seen. Obviously, we still have more to learn.

C-reactive Protein (CRP)

Low risk: levels below 1
Average risk: levels between 1 and 3
High risk: levels over 3

Elevated levels of C-reactive protein (CRP) can triple your risk for heart disease. For postmenopausal women, CRP levels may be more accurate than cholesterol in predicting heart disease risk.

CRP is an indication of inflammation in the body. Almost all healthy lifestyle changes are helpful in lowering inflammation and CRP levels—weight loss, exercise, smoking cessation, blood pressure control, reduced alcohol intake, and eating a heart-healthy diet rich in fiber and lower in sugar.

Knowing your numbers and working to get them to healthy levels is an important step to protect your health and lower your risk for heart disease.

SORTING OUT FATS

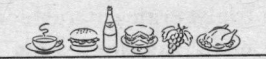

*The type of fat you eat may be more important
to your health than the amount you eat.
Eating moderate amounts of the
right fat can be healthy, possibly even
healthier than low fat eating plans.*

Fat gets no respect. Fat in food is considered bad for you. Fat on your body is considered unattractive. But you need fat—both in your food and on your body.

Fats mystify people. They have big-sounding names that are hard to wrap your tongue around and even harder to understand—triglycerides, saturated, mono-unsaturated, polyunsaturated, and cholesterol. But the information doesn't have to be hard to understand, and we'll help you make sense of it all.

Basic Fat Facts

Fats are also called *lipids*. The structure of all fats is similar. Both the fat on your body and the fat you eat look the same. That is why it is so easy for your body to either use or store the fats you eat in food.

Triglycerides are the most typical fat found in food. They are made up of smaller fat fragments called *fatty* *acids.* The triglycerides we eat in food can be in solid (butters) or liquid (oils). Triglycerides in your body come from the fat you eat. They can also be made from excess calories that are eaten and stored as fat for future use.

High levels of triglycerides in the blood usually result from eating too many calories, eating too much sugar and refined carbs (white bread, white flour, sweetened drinks, cakes, cookies, pastries, and candy), and drinking too much alcohol. High triglycerides can put you at risk for:

- Blocked arteries
- Abnormal blood clotting
- Lower HDL (good) cholesterol
- Higher levels of the most damaging type of LDL cholesterol
- Poorly controlled diabetes
- Heart attack or stroke

Fatty acids are the building blocks that make up triglycerides. There are different types of fatty acids—saturated, monounsaturated, and polyunsaturated. Each type of fat that we eat affects our bodies differently. Some have a good effect, others do not.

Every food with fat you eat actually contains a mixture of different fatty acids, but we classify the food by the predominant fatty acid. For example: butter contains all three types of fatty acids, but it is especially high in saturated fatty acids, so we call it a saturated fat. Olives contain a lot of monounsaturated fatty acids. Corn oil is high in polyunsaturated fatty acids.

Saturated fats are animal fats high in saturated fats and are usually solid at room temperature. You can't eliminate all saturated fats from your diet, and you really don't have to, but it is important to limit them because this type of fat:

- Raises total cholesterol levels
- Raises LDL (bad) cholesterol
- Raises triglyceride levels
- Increases the risk for stroke
- Increases the risk for heart disease

FOODS HIGH IN SATURATED FATS

Bacon	Meat
Butter	Poultry
Cheese	Palm oil
Cocoa butter	Palm kernel oil
Coconut and coconut oil	Pies
Cream	Pastries
Ice cream	Sour cream
Lard	Whole milk

There are good reasons to include some saturated fat in your diet. Many of the foods with saturated fats—milk, meat, and poultry—contain important nutrients we all need for good health. In addition, not all saturated fats are bad for you. A good example is a saturated fat called stearic acid, found in beef and chocolate, which does not raise cholesterol levels.

YOU SHOULD KNOW—

A study showed that your body burns more
polyunsaturated fats than saturated fats
after exercising.
Saturated fats were more likely to be stored;
just another reason to eat them in moderation.

Monounsaturated fats are fats found mainly in plant foods. All monounsaturated vegetable oils are liquid at room temperature. They should be used to replace some saturated fats in your diet because monounsaturated fats:

- Reduce total cholesterol levels
- Reduce triglyceride levels
- Reduce LDL (bad) cholesterol
- Maintain or raise HDL (good) cholesterol
- May help lower blood pressure
- Reduce the risk for type 2 diabetes, which increases the risk for heart disease

FOODS HIGH IN MONOUNSATURATED FATS

Almonds and almond oil	Grapeseed oil
Avocado and avocado oil	Macadamia nuts
Canola oil	Olives and olive oil
Cashews	Peanuts and peanut oil
Chicken fat	Pistachios
Hazelnuts	Pinenuts

A Handful, Not a Canful

*Nuts have gone from high fat
forbidden foods to heart healthy choices.
A small serving of nuts daily is a healthy habit
because they are rich in monounsaturated fats.*

Polyunsaturated fats are fats found mainly in plant foods. Most of the oils we eat are rich in polyunsaturated fats.

> **YOU SHOULD KNOW—**
>
> *Soft, whipped and squeeze margarines
> have more polyunsaturated fats.
> Stick margarines have more saturated fats.*

There are two main groups of polyunsaturated fats: omega-6 and omega-3. Just think of them as two different strands of beads, similar in shape but different in color sequence. Each is important to good health, so eating foods with both is important.

Omega-6 rich polyunsaturated fats should be eaten regularly because they:

- Reduce cholesterol levels
- Reduce LDL (bad) cholesterol
- Improve blood pressure
- Reduce blood clots
- Reduce heart disease risk

FOODS HIGH IN OMEGA-6 FATS

Avocado and avocado oil	Safflower oil
Canola oil	Sesame oil
Corn oil	Soft margarine
Eggs	Soybeans and soybean oil
Nuts, nut butters, and nut oils	Sunflower oil
	Wheat germ
Pumpkin seeds	

YOU SHOULD KNOW—

*More than 80% of the vegetable oil used in the U.S.
is soybean oil rich in omega-6 fat.
It is the preferred oil used by food manufacturers
and restaurants.
Based on that, it is wise to select another type of
vegetable oil at home to vary the types of fatty
acids you eat—all have benefits.*

Omega-3 rich polyunsaturated fats are in shorter supply in our diets. Some experts feel it is important to balance our intake of omega-6 to omega-3 fat because early humans evolved on a diet that provided about equal amounts of the two types of fat. Others feel we should not focus on the ratio between the two fats and simply substitute omega-6 fats for some of the saturated fat we eat and try to regularly eat more omega-3 rich foods.

Omega-3 rich polyunsaturated fats should be eaten regularly because they:

- Reduce triglyceride levels
- Protect against sudden cardiac death, which causes half of all heart disease deaths
- Reduce inflammation
- Reduce formation of plaque in arteries
- Reduce blood clots
- Reduce blood pressure

YOU SHOULD KNOW—

> *Experts agree that low-dose aspirin and omega-3 fats reduce inflammation, but until recently they did not know why.*
> *Aspirin helps trigger the production of resolvins, substances made in the body from omega-3 fats. Resolvins shut off, or resolve, inflammation, which is the underlying destructive action in lung disease, arthritis, and heart disease.*

FOODS HIGH IN OMEGA-3 FATS

Bluefish	Mackerel
Canola oil	Olives and olive oil
Catfish	Oysters
Chia seeds	Pecans
Cod	Salmon
Flaxseeds and flaxseed oil	Sardines
Halibut	Trout
Hazelnuts	Tuna
Hempseeds	Walnuts and walnut oil
Herring	

YOU SHOULD KNOW—

> *Eating as little as 2 servings of fish, a rich source of omega-3 fats, every week can lower your risk for heart disease.*

Trans fats may be a greater health risk than eating foods rich in saturated fats, according to some experts.

Almost all the trans fat found in our foods is created artificially by passing hydrogen gas through vegetable oil, a process called *hydrogenation,* which turns liquid oil into a solid fat—think stick margarine or shortening.

Hydrogenated fats, high in trans fatty acids, were used initially to replace saturated fats such as lard and butter. As our knowledge about fats expanded, we learned that eating trans fat was as bad for our health.

You'll be seeing more and more trans fat free food as time goes on. Restaurants and food companies are working to reformulate recipes and products to cut down or eliminate trans fats. Food consumption surveys are already showing a steady decline in the amount we eat. Cutting down on or eliminating foods with trans fats will not eliminate any important nutrients from your diet. In fact, it may help you cut back on less healthy choices like French fries and cakes.

Trans fats should be avoided because they:

- Raise cholesterol levels
- Lower HDL (good) cholesterol
- Raise LDL (bad) cholesterol
- Raise triglyceride levels
- Trigger inflammation
- May increase the risk for blood clots
- Increase the risk for type 2 diabetes, which increases the risk for heart disease

---

YOU SHOULD KNOW—

Trans fats raise your risk of heart disease more than any other fat.
For every 2% increase in trans fats, your heart disease risk jumps by more than 20%.

FOODS HIGH IN TRANS FATS*

Cookies	Doughnuts
Crackers	Muffins
Cakes	Pastries
Breaded and deep-fried fish and chicken nuggets	Partially hydrogenated oil
	Processed cheese foods
	Shortening
Deep-fried foods	Stick margarine

*Brands of some of these foods may no longer contain trans fat due to product reformulation.

As with most scientific findings, the story of trans fat is not all bad. There are small amounts of naturally occurring trans fat in meat, butter, milk, cheese, and cabbage. But these natural trans fats have a different structure than those artificially produced, and they may have health benefits. One natural trans fat, CLA (conjugated linoleic acid), may play a role in preventing cancer, heart disease, and diabetes.

YOU SHOULD KNOW—

*You do not have to limit
naturally occurring trans fat.
Just avoid trans fat that is artificially produced
and found in fried and processed foods.*

The amount of CLA we eat from natural sources is very low, but CLA is now being sold as a weight loss supplement with recommended daily doses of up to 6 grams a day. Some experts believe that these higher amounts of CLA in supplement form could increase the risk for heart disease. Unfortunately, right now we simply don't know enough to make a recommendation.

YOU SHOULD KNOW—

Finding Fats on the Nutrition Facts Label

Companies are required to list total fat, cholesterol, saturated fat, and trans fat on the nutrition label. Values for polyunsaturated and monounsaturated fats are not required, but more and more companies are voluntarily listing these values.

Summing Up Fats: Choose Wisely

- Saturated fats—eat less of this type of fat. Keep portions small.
- Polyunsaturated fats—use these fats to replace some saturated fat.
- Monounsaturated fats—eat more of these fats.
- Trans fats—eat as little as possible of these fats.

UNDERSTANDING CHOLESTEROL

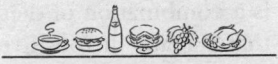

Good for you? Bad for you? The jury is still out.

Say the word *cholesterol* and people automatically think of some poisonous substance that will cause a heart attack. Foods high in cholesterol have been shunned for decades, and 1 in 4 people over the age of 45 are taking medication to lower their cholesterol.

For decades we have been told having too much cholesterol in the blood is unhealthy. The extra cholesterol can be deposited in your artery walls, narrowing them and interfering with normal blood flow. This is true, but the cholesterol message has become more complicated as we learn more.

What Is Cholesterol?

Cholesterol is a white, waxy, fatlike substance that is part of every cell in your body. It insulates nerve cells and helps skin cells retain moisture. Cholesterol makes up a major part of your brain and is the main building block for vitamin D and essential hormones such as cortisone, estrogen, progesterone, and testosterone.

You get cholesterol every time you eat animal foods—

meat, poultry, fish, eggs, milk, yogurt, cheese, and butter. This type of cholesterol is called *dietary cholesterol*. There is no cholesterol in any food that grows in the ground—vegetables, fruits, nuts, seeds, cereals, and grains.

Serum cholesterol is the type that travels in your bloodstream. It is a combination of dietary cholesterol and cholesterol that is made in your liver. In fact, most people make 3 times more cholesterol in their body than they eat in food.

YOU SHOULD KNOW—

Making Coffee—Use Paper Filters

Coffee raises serum cholesterol because it contains cafestol, a potent cholesterol-elevating agent.
If you brew coffee through a paper filter, it removes the coffee oils that contain cafestol.

There are different types of cholesterol. HDL cholesterol does not accumulate in arteries and in fact delivers cholesterol back to the liver to be broken down and removed from the body. It also appears to play a role in boosting your immune system and preventing inflammation and clot formation. All of these are important to prevent heart disease.

LDL cholesterol is the type that is more likely to build up plaque in the arteries. Over time, this buildup can cause arteries to harden, a process called *atherosclerosis*. If arteries stiffen and narrow, blood flow to the heart muscle is slowed down and may even be blocked. A blocked artery to the heart can cause a heart attack. A blocked artery to the brain can cause a stroke.

As with all things bad, there is always some good.

We need cholesterol to form every cell in the body, and LDL is the main carrier of cholesterol to cells. LDL cholesterol helps repair and build muscles after you exercise. LDL works on repair, and HDL cleans up after the repair is done. Some researchers have suggested that cholesterol-lowering medications may be contributing to loss of muscle as we age, because older adults with low cholesterol build less muscle after exercising.

Bottom Line: What Does All This Mean?

We still have a lot to learn about cholesterol. There is no question that high total cholesterol and high LDL cholesterol indicate a greater risk for heart disease. Both provide warning signs that something is wrong. Does the person exercise too little? Do they eat poorly? Do they smoke and weigh too much?

Heart disease—its causes and prevention are complex, and we need to focus on all the players in the game. Cholesterol may be just one.

WHAT IS FIBER'S ROLE IN HEART HEALTH?

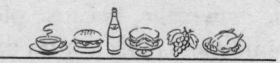

*Eating foods high in fiber gives
good bacteria a fighting chance.*

Fiber is a type of carbohydrate that cannot be broken down in your body for energy. It prevents constipation, helps with weight control, helps control diabetes, reduces cholesterol, and reduces your risk for heart disease.

YOU SHOULD KNOW—

*Foods naturally high in fiber are almost always
naturally low in cholesterol and saturated fat.*

   Living in your digestive track are trillions of friendly microbes (probiotics) that use fiber as their main source of food. Amazingly, there are 10 times more bacterial cells than human cells in your body. These friendly bacteria have been with you since birth. They help protect you against unfriendly bacteria that could make you sick. When you eat enough fiber, your friendly bacteria are well fed and can put up a good fight against harmful bacteria. When you eat too little fiber, the unfriendly bacteria can start to take over.

GOOD SOURCES OF FIBER

Apples

Barley

Beans

Berries—blueberries, blackberries, raspberries, and strawberries

Brown rice

Carrots

Citrus fruits

Cracked wheat

Dried fruits

Fig Newtons

Fruit, especially with peels

Graham crackers

Lentils

Nuts

Oatmeal and oat bran

Peas

Popcorn

Raisins

Rye

Seeds—pumpkin, sunflower, flaxseed

Shredded wheat

Soybeans in every form—soynuts, tempeh, edamame

Vegetables, especially unpeeled

Whole wheat bread, crackers, cereal, pasta

Your intestinal tract is like a war zone where the good guys are constantly fighting the bad guys. By eating enough whole grain foods and fruits and vegetables rich in fiber you are building up your army of good bacteria so they can squash the bad guys. Imbalances in the gut bacteria, where the bad guys are winning, can lead to chronic inflammation and heart disease. We now realize that the root of much of the damage caused by heart disease is unchecked inflammation in your body.

Consuming food rich in probiotics—yogurt, sauerkraut, kimchi, miso, kefir, pickles, and probiotic-supplemented foods (soymilk, cereal, and snack bars)—which contain "live friendly bacteria and yeasts" are the best way to boost the population of friendly microbes in your gut. Fiber-rich foods (prebiotics) feed the friendly microbes so they can grow and multiply.

Friendly bacteria have the ability to unlock powerful, protective nutrients in your food. Though humans lack the enzymes to digest fiber, bacteria can break down this same fiber and use it for energy. In the process the bacteria produce gases and acids that are healthy for you. One of the acids prevents colon cancer cells from forming. Another blocks the production of cholesterol, lowering blood cholesterol and decreasing your risk for heart disease. Friendly bacteria also release phytochemicals trapped in fibers that have anti-inflammatory properties.

The interaction of your intestinal bacteria and your body is anything but simple. But when the system works well, it protects you and safeguards your health.

Prebiotics (fiber) and probiotics (friendly organisms living in your digestive tract) work together to boost your health from the inside out and protect you from heart disease.

Are You a Floater or a Sinker?

*Simply looking at your bowel movements is one way
to gauge the health of the microbes in your gut.
Floaters suggest healthy fermentation
and production of gas, which is trapped
and expelled in feces.
Sinkers show poor fermentation with little trapped
gas and poorer health for your friendly gut warriors.*

THE ROLE OF SUGAR IN HEART DISEASE IS CONTROVERSIAL, BUT—

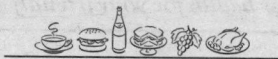

*The country's big low-fat message backfired.
The overemphasis on reducing fat caused
the consumption of carbohydrates
and sugar in our diets to soar.*

Dr. Frank Hu, Harvard School of Public Health

Eating too much sugar may increase the risk for:

- Obesity, which increases the risk for heart disease
- High triglyceride levels
- Low HDL cholesterol
- High blood pressure
- Inflammation, which is an underlying cause of heart disease
- Low fiber intake, which increases the risk for heart disease

Though the evidence is still inconclusive, most health professionals agree that a diet high in refined carbs—white bread, white rice, white flour—and high in sugar, including soda, candy, desserts, cakes, cookies, fruit drinks, ice cream, and sugar in alcoholic drinks, is not a recipe for good health.

This is a good example of correlation and causation. We can correlate—in other words, connect—sugar and poorer health and being overweight, but the scientific evidence has yet to draw conclusions about causation (one thing resulting from another). The American Heart Association has estimated that we eat more than 22 teaspoons of sugar a day (355 calories). Others estimate daily intake at 475 sugar calories a day, equal to 30 teaspoons of sugar. Almost a third of these sugar calories come from soda, and an additional 10% come from sweetened fruit drinks. Together those are the number one source of added sugar in our diets.

Liquid sugar calories are different from the calories in solid food because they do not give us the same feeling of fullness and satisfaction. If you are offered more, you drink more. Think about the endless drink refills offered at restaurants. Studies have shown that adults eat the same amount of food at a meal whether they drink soda (with calories) or water (with no calories). But adding soda or a sweetened fruit drink to a meal will dramatically increase the amount of calories eaten.

Added sugar was not a significant part of our diets until modern food processing began in the last 75 years. Since then, sugar intake has risen steadily because of the continuous stream of food products—cookies, cakes, candy, ice cream, soda, and bottled drinks—readily available in stores at relatively low prices. There has been a 500% increase in soda consumption over the last 50 years, as the sweet stuff has displaced healthier drinks. In the U.S., we now drink more soda per person per year than we drink milk. That's a sad and unhealthy commentary on our diet.

From the perspective of health, sugar can be divided into 2 main groups—natural sugars and added sugars. Grains, fruits, vegetables, milk, and plain yogurt all contain *natural sugars*. These sugars come packaged along with the vitamins, minerals, and fiber also found in these foods. Soda, candy, fruit drinks, cakes, cookies, ice cream, jelly, and syrup offer little more than sweetness and calories. These foods are loaded with *added sugar*. We should aim to eat foods with natural sugars more often and those foods with added sugars less often.

Nutrition Label Confusion

On nutrition labels, all sugars are lumped together, making it hard for you to determine if the sugar is added or natural. The nutrition label on a quart of milk will tell you that one cup has 14 grams of sugar. The label on fruit punch tells you that one cup has 30 grams of sugar. But the difference is significant. All of the sugar in milk comes from naturally occurring *lactose,* or milk sugar, but almost all the sugar in the fruit punch is added.

How can you tell natural sugars from added sugars? Check the ingredient listing on food labels for the terms below—if any appear, it means sugar has been added to the food. Ingredients on labels are listed in descending order by volume, so the closer sugar is to the beginning of the list, the more sugar is in each serving of food.

SUGAR BY ANY OTHER NAME

Agave syrup or nectar	Fruit juice concentrate
Barley malt syrup	High fructose corn syrup
Beet juice	Honey
Brown rice syrup	Invert sugar
Brown sugar	Jaggery
Cane syrup	Maltodextrin
Confectioners	Maple sugar
(powdered) sugar	Maple syrup
Corn sweetener	Molasses
Corn syrup	Muscavado
Crystalline fructose	Raw sugar
Demarara sugar	Rice syrup
Dextrose	Sorghum
Evaporated cane juice	Sucrose
Fructose	Sugar in the raw
Fruit juice	Turbinado

If a food contains little or no milk or fruit, the sugar number listed on the nutrition label will be a good estimate of the amount of added sugar in each serving.

Even though the connection between sugar and heart disease is not conclusive at this time, eating too much sugar has no positive impact on your health. Everyone should aim to eat less.

YOU SHOULD KNOW—

Sorting Out Sugar on Labels

*On the nutrition facts panel, you will see a value
for total carbohydrate and right beneath it
a value for sugars.*

*Sugar is part of the total carbohydrate value.
If a food has 30 g (grams) of carb and
28 g of sugar, it is high in sugar.*

HOW MUCH
SHOULD YOU EAT?

Fat, Cholesterol, Fiber, Sugar

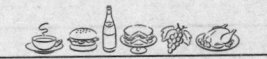

*Grocery shopping data show that
Americans buy too many refined grains,
fats, sugar, and sweets, and they buy too
few fruits, vegetables, and whole grains.*

5 Heart Healthy Eating Goals:
- **Eat a moderate amount of fat, divided
  between foods with saturated,
  polyunsaturated, and monounsaturated
  fats.**
- **Avoid foods with trans fats.**
- **Eat 200 to 400 milligrams of cholesterol
  a day is a safe range, depending on your
  individual risks.**
- **Eat more whole grains and fiber-rich
  foods.**
- **Eat less foods with added sugar.**

In the past, the prescription for a heart healthy diet
was very specific. You might have been told exactly

how much cholesterol or fat to eat daily. For some, this may still be the case. Others may just need more of an awareness of what to eat—the foods to select more often and those to eat less often. Regardless of what your specific goals are, *The Fat and Cholesterol Counter* will serve as a useful guide.

We offer recommendations that are backed up by expert opinion. You can modify these recommendations to meet your individual goals.

YOU SHOULD KNOW—

When people look at nutrition labels, they are most concerned with the amount of calories in food; they look at the amount of fat next, and over one-third of grocery shoppers are concerned about sugar.

How much fat should you eat each day?

About 33% of the total calories Americans eat each day come from fat. Eating between 25% and 40% is a healthy range. If you aim for 25% to 30%, you will have a low fat intake; 30% to 40% would be considered a moderate fat diet.

You might be surprised that a diet that is 40% fat can be considered healthy. If you are choosing healthy fats, making good overall food choices, and you do not currently have heart disease, this range is safe.

YOU SHOULD KNOW—

Going Too Low Is Not Healthy

Very low fat diets with total fat intakes below 15% to 20% lower good HDL cholesterol.

That means if you regularly eat 1800 calories a day, you should eat less than 2 grams (1%) of trans fat each day.

$$1\% \times 1800 \text{ calories} = 18 \text{ trans fat calories a day}$$

To convert trans fat calories into grams of fat, all you need to know is that 1 gram of any type of fat = 9 calories.

$$18 \text{ trans fat calories } (1\%) \div 9 = 2 \text{ grams of trans fat}$$

Trans fat intake has significantly decreased in the U.S. as restaurants and food companies have made efforts to reformulate foods. Yet Americans on average still eat about 1.3 grams (0.6% of calories each day) of artificial trans fat each day, and some eat much more. Foods with the most trans fat include fried foods, microwave popcorn, frozen pizzas, cake, cookies, pie, margarines, ready-to-use frosting, and coffee creamers. (See page 35.)

Trans Fat Free Labeling Loophole

Labeling regulations allow food companies to state 0 grams trans fat on nutrition labels when a serving of food contains 0.49 grams or less. If you ate 3 servings of a food you believed to be trans fat free but that actually contained 0.49 grams per serving, you would be eating 1.47 grams of trans fat. That may not sound like much, but research shows that increasing the amount of trans fat you eat every day by just small amounts, from 2 grams to 5 grams, can increase your risk for heart disease by 30%. Many are calling on the Food & Drug Administration (FDA), which oversees nutrition labeling, to amend the regulations for labeling trans fat to provide more accurate information to consumers.

How do you decide what amount of cholesterol is right for you?

The National Cholesterol Education Program recommends eating no more than 200 milligrams of cholesterol a day. The American Heart Association (AHA) recommends that you limit cholesterol to less than 300 milligrams a day, or 200 milligrams if you already have heart disease.

If you are healthy and you are not overweight, up to 400 milligrams of cholesterol each day is considered to be a safe amount.

YOU SHOULD KNOW—

It's simple.
If a food grows in the ground, it has no cholesterol.
If the food comes from a source that has a face
(example: an egg, milk, or a steak), it has cholesterol.

How much fiber should you eat?

We all eat too little fiber, about 15 grams a day. With fiber it is easy to figure out how much to eat—no calculations are needed. Just check the following chart to find your daily fiber recommendation.

DAILY FIBER RECOMMENDATIONS

Men

19–50 years	38 grams of fiber
51 and older	30 grams of fiber

Women

19–50 years	25 grams of fiber
51–70 years	21 grams of fiber
71 and older	20 grams of fiber
Pregnant	28 grams of fiber

YOU SHOULD KNOW—

Chew on This

*Eating fiber-rich foods is smarter
than popping fiber supplements.
Fiber-rich foods are also rich in
antioxidants, vitamins, and minerals.
Supplements are not.*

How much sugar should you eat?

Most experts agree that we should all be eating less sugar. But, right now, there is no specific recommendation on how much to eat every day.

The U.S. Dietary Reference Intakes (from the National Academy of Sciences, Institute of Medicine) suggest 25% of daily calories from added sugar as the maximum. The World Health Organization (WHO) has suggested limiting added sugars to 10% or less of total calories. The American Heart Association recommends that women eat no more than 100 calories a day (25 grams, or slightly over 6 teaspoons) of added sugar, and that men should not eat more than 150 sugar calories daily (38 grams, or slightly more than 9 teaspoons).

All these recommendations are for added sugar, not for sugars found naturally in fruits, milk, grains, and vegetables. As we discussed earlier, it is very hard to sort out natural and added sugars in foods because the nutrition label lumps the two types together. We've provided sugar values so you can easily find food choices that are very high in sugar and those that are low in sugar.

Rather than get caught up in grams of sugar per day, it might be wiser to simply try these easy tips to reduce your sugar intake.

- Stop drinking regular soda.
- Drink 100% fruit juice, not presweetened fruit drinks and other highly sweetened drinks— orange juice instead of fruit punch.
- Eat more naturally sweet fruit.
- Keep portion sizes of sweets moderate— ½ cup of ice cream instead of a soup bowl full, 2 cookies rather than a box, or a snack-size candy bar.
- Eat unsweetened or mildly sweetened cereals; aim for options with 6 or less grams of sugar per serving.
- Eat plain yogurt and drink plain, unsweetened milk.

If you wish to track the amount of sugar you eat daily, first decide what your daily target is. For example:

If you eat 1800 calories a day and want to keep sugar calories to 10%, the WHO recommendation, simply:

$$10\% \times 1800 \text{ calories} = 180 \text{ sugar calories each day}$$

To convert those sugar calories into grams of sugar, all you need to know is that 1 gram of any type of sugar = 4 calories.

180 sugar calories (10%) ÷ 4 = 45 grams of sugar

If you eat 1800 calories a day and want to keep sugar calories to no more than 25%, the U.S. Dietary Reference Intakes recommendation, simply:

25% × 1800 calories = 450 sugar calories each day

To convert those sugar calories into grams of sugar, all you need to know is that 1 gram of any type of sugar = 4 calories.

450 sugar calories (25%) ÷ 4 = 113 grams of sugar

Keep in mind as you track your sugar intake that currently the sugar values available for foods do not separate natural sugars and added sugar. For this reason you may wish to give yourself a higher percentage daily, to take into consideration the natural sugars you will be eating from milk, grains, fruits, and vegetables.

YOU SHOULD KNOW—

According to the American Heart Association, our progress against heart disease is slowing. Americans' poor eating and exercise habits could literally be the death of us.

USING YOUR FAT AND CHOLESTEROL COUNTER

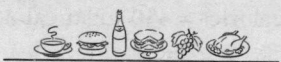

The Fat and Cholesterol Counter lists the portion size, calories, total fat, cholesterol, saturated fat, polyunsaturated fat, monounsaturated fat, trans fat, fiber, and sugar values for more than 10,000 foods. These are the key nutrients to consider when evaluating and lowering your risk for heart disease. Now you can compare the values in your favorite foods and, when necessary, choose substitutes before you go out to shop or eat. This will save you time and help you decide what to buy.

The counter section of the book is divided into two parts: Part One: Brand Name, Nonbranded (Generic), and Take-Out Foods (page 65); and Part Two: Restaurant Chains (page 359). Each part lists foods or restaurant chains alphabetically.

In Part One, for each category you will find nonbranded (generic) foods listed first in alphabetical order, followed by an alphabetical listing of brand name foods. The nonbranded listings will help you estimate calorie, fat, cholesterol, fiber, and sugar values when you don't see your favorite brands. They can also help you evaluate store brands. Large categories are divided into subcategories, such as canned, fresh, frozen, and ready-to-eat, to make it easier to find what you're looking for. Some categories have "see" and "see also" references, to help you find related items.

Because we eat out so often, more than 900 take-out foods are listed in Part One. These are found in the take-out subcategory in many categories throughout Part One. Foods you take out or order in are rarely nutrition labeled.

Most foods are listed alphabetically. In some cases, though, foods are grouped by category. For example, a tuna sandwich is found in the sandwich category. Other group categories include:

ALCOHOL DRINKS: Page 66
    Includes all alcoholic beverages
    and mixed drinks except
    beer, champagne, and wine,
    which have their own separate
    categories.

ASIAN FOOD: Page 75
    Includes all types of Asian
    foods except egg rolls and
    sushi, which are found in the
    egg rolls and sushi categories.

DELI MEATS/COLD CUTS: Page 169
    Includes all sandwich meats
    except chicken, ham, and
    turkey, which have their own
    separate categories.

DINNER: Page 170
    Includes all prepared dinners
    listed by brand name, except
    pasta dinners, which are found
    in the pasta dinners category.

NUTRITION SUPPLEMENTS: Page 239
Includes all dieting aids, meal
replacements, and drinks,
except energy bars and energy
drinks, which have their own
separate categories.

SANDWICHES: Page 297
Includes popular sandwich,
calzone, and panini choices.

SNACKS: Page 310
Includes a variety of snack
items, such as cheese puffs.

SPANISH FOOD: Page 323
Includes all types of Spanish
and Mexican foods except salsa
and tortillas, which have their
own separate categories.

In Part Two, Restaurant Chains, 35 national and regional restaurant, coffee, doughnut, frozen yogurt, ice cream, pizza, sandwich, and soup chains are listed. Brand name foods are required by federal law to have nutrition information on labels, but restaurants are different. In most areas of the country, restaurants provide this information voluntarily.

With *The Fat and Cholesterol Counter* as your guide, you can count on a healthy heart.

DEFINITIONS

as prep (as prepared): refers to food that has been prepared according to package directions

lean and fat: describes meat with some fat on its edges that is not cut away before cooking, or poultry prepared with skin and fat as purchased

lean only: refers to lean meat that is trimmed of all visible fat, or poultry without skin

not prep (not prepared): refers to food that has not been cooked and may require the addition of other ingredients to prepare

shelf-stable: refers to prepared products found on the supermarket shelf that are not canned or frozen but are packaged and ready-to-eat or are ready to be heated and do not require refrigeration

take-out: describes prepared dishes that you purchase ready-to-eat; those included serve as a guide to the calories, fat, cholesterol, fiber, and sugar in products you may buy

ABBREVIATIONS

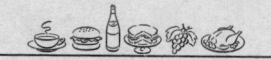

avg	=	average
diam	=	diameter
fl	=	fluid
frzn	=	frozen
g	=	gram
in	=	inch
lb	=	pound
lg	=	large
med	=	medium
mg	=	milligram
oz	=	ounce
pkg	=	package
pt	=	pint
prep	=	prepared
qt	=	quart
reg	=	regular
sec	=	second
serv	=	serving
sm	=	small
sq	=	square
tbsp	=	tablespoon
tr	=	trace
tsp	=	teaspoon
w/	=	with
w/o	=	without
<	=	less than

NOTES

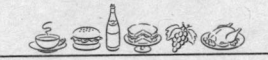

cals = calories
total fat = total fat
chol = cholesterol
sat fat = saturated fat
poly fat = polyunsaturated fat
mono fat = monounsaturated fat
trans fat = trans fat
fiber = fiber
sugar = sugar
All total fat, saturated fat, polyunsaturated fat,
    monounsaturated fat, trans fat, fiber, and sugar
    values are given in grams.
All cholesterol values are given in milligrams.
– (dash) indicates that values are not available
tr (trace) = less than 1 gram of total fat, saturated fat,
    polyunsaturated fat, monounsaturated fat, trans fat, fi-
    ber, or sugar, and less than 1 milligram of cholesterol
0 (zero) indicates there are no calories, total fat, cho-
    lesterol, saturated fat, polyunsaturated fat, mono-
    unsaturated fat, trans fat, fiber, or sugar in that food

Discrepancies in figures are due to rounding of values,
product reformulation, and reevaluation. The current
labeling law allows rounding. Some of the data listed is
analysis data, obtained directly from manufacturers, not
from labels; therefore, some values may differ slightly
from labels because the values have not been rounded.

PART ONE

Brand Name, Nonbranded (Generic), and Take-Out Foods

DISHING UP MYPLATE

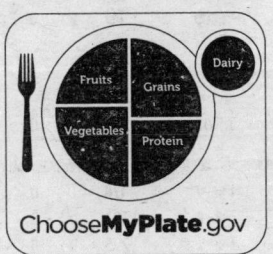

MyPlate offers a quick visual guide to heart-healthy eating based on the recommendation from the 2010 Dietary Guidelines. It helps you make the best choices when you choose your next meal. We have a long way to go before most dinner plates resemble MyPlate. It is estimated that only 2% of Americans meet the recommendations.

FOOD	PORTION	CALS	TOTAL FAT	CHOL	SAT FAT	POLY FAT	MONO FAT	TRANS FAT	FIBER	SUGAR
ABALONE										
breaded & fried	1 serv (3 oz)	162	6	80	1	tr	2	–	tr	tr
steamed	1 serv (3 oz)	127	3	84	1	1	1	0	0	tr
ACAI										
Amafruits										
Acai Berry Puree frzn	1 pkg (3.5 oz)	80	6	0	2	–	–	0	3	0
ACAI JUICE										
Naked										
Acai Machine	8 oz	160	3	0	1	–	–	0	3	24
Ultra Lo-Gly										
Acai-Blue	1 bottle (10 oz)	45	0	0	0	0	0	0	0	10
ACEROLA										
fresh	1 (5 g)	2	tr	0	tr	tr	tr	–	tr	–
ACEROLA JUICE										
juice	1 cup	56	1	0	tr	tr	tr	–	1	11
ADZUKI BEANS										
canned sweetened	½ cup	351	tr	0	tr	–	–	–	–	–
dried cooked w/o salt	½ cup	147	tr	0	tr	–	–	–	8	–
AGAVE (see SYRUP)										
AKEE										
fresh	3.5 oz	223	20	0	–	–	–	–	–	–
ALCOHOL DRINKS (see also BEER AND ALE, CHAMPAGNE, MALT, WINE)										
7&7	1 serv	178	0	0	0	0	0	0	0	–
alabama slammer	1 serv	103	tr	0	0	–	–	–	tr	–
amaretto sour	1 serv	295	tr	0	tr	–	–	–	4	–
angel's kiss	1 serv	85	1	5	1	–	–	–	0	–
anisette	1 oz	111	0	0	0	–	–	0	0	–
antifreeze cocktail	1 serv	177	tr	0	tr	–	–	–	tr	–
apricot brandy	1 oz	96	0	0	0	–	–	0	0	–
apricot sour	1 serv	164	tr	0	0	–	–	–	tr	–
b 52	1 serv	247	4	0	2	–	–	–	0	–
b&b	1 serv	75	0	0	0	0	0	0	0	0
bahama breeze	1 serv	70	tr	0	tr	–	–	–	tr	–
bahama mama	1 serv	153	tr	0	tr	–	–	–	tr	–
bailey's & amaretto	1 serv	184	5	0	3	–	–	–	0	–
banana colada	1 serv	376	1	0	tr	–	–	–	3	–

FOOD	PORTION	CALS	TOTAL FAT	CHOL	SAT FAT	POLY FAT	MONO FAT	TRANS FAT	FIBER	SUGAR
bay breeze	1 serv	173	tr	0	tr	–	–	–	tr	–
bend me over	1 serv	242	tr	0	tr	–	–	–	tr	–
benedictine	1 oz	104	0	0	0	–	–	0	0	–
betsy ross	1 serv	206	0	0	0	0	0	0	0	–
black devil	1 serv	220	tr	0	tr	–	–	–	tr	–
black russian	1 serv	184	tr	0	tr	–	–	–	0	–
bloody mary	1 serv	150	tr	0	tr	–	–	–	1	–
blue whale	1 serv	222	tr	0	0	–	–	–	0	–
bourbon & soda	1 serv (4 oz)	105	0	0	0	0	0	0	0	0
bourbon sour	1 serv	166	tr	0	0	–	–	–	tr	–
brandy alexander	1 serv	266	6	20	4	–	–	–	0	–
brandy sour	1 serv	164	tr	0	0	–	–	–	tr	–
bushwacker	1 serv	286	5	0	2	–	–	–	tr	–
coffee liqueur	1 serv (1.5 oz)	175	tr	0	tr	tr	tr	–	0	24
cognac	1 oz	67	0	0	0	0	0	0	0	0
cosmopolitan martini	1 serv	126	tr	0	0	–	–	–	tr	–
creme de menthe	1 serv (1.5 oz)	186	tr	0	tr	tr	tr	–	0	21
curacao liqueur	1 oz	81	0	0	0	–	–	0	0	–
daiquiri	1 serv (2 oz)	112	tr	0	tr	tr	tr	–	tr	3
daiquiri banana	1 serv	277	tr	0	tr	–	–	–	1	–
daiquiri frozen pineapple	1 serv	186	tr	0	tr	–	–	–	2	–
dark & stormy	1 serv	64	0	0	0	0	0	0	0	0
doctor pepper	1 serv	95	0	0	0	0	0	0	0	–
fuzzy navel	1 serv	247	tr	0	tr	–	–	–	tr	–
gin	1 serv (1.5 oz)	110	0	0	0	0	0	0	0	0
gin & tonic	1 serv (7.5 oz)	171	0	0	0	0	0	0	–	–
gin ricky	1 serv	114	tr	0	0	–	–	–	tr	–
grasshopper	1 serv	275	5	15	3	–	–	–	0	–
happy hawaiian	1 serv	434	8	0	5	–	–	–	tr	–
harvey wallbanger	1 serv	198	tr	0	tr	–	–	–	tr	–
head banger	1 serv	165	0	0	0	0	0	0	0	–
hot buttered rum	1 serv (8.8 oz)	316	12	30	8	tr	3	–	tr	4
hot toddy	1 serv	188	1	0	tr	–	–	–	5	–
hurricane	1 serv	205	tr	0	0	–	–	–	tr	–
kamikaze	1 serv	136	0	0	0	0	0	0	0	–
long island iced tea	1 serv	292	tr	0	0	–	–	–	0	–
lynchburg lemonade	1 serv	465	tr	0	tr	–	–	–	1	–
mai tai	1 serv	165	tr	0	tr	–	–	–	tr	–
manhattan	1 serv	171	tr	0	0	–	–	–	tr	–
margarita	1 serv	173	0	0	0	0	0	0	0	–

FOOD	PORTION	CALS	TOTAL FAT	CHOL	SAT FAT	POLY FAT	MONO FAT	TRANS FAT	FIBER	SUGAR
margarita strawberry	1 serv	106	tr	0	tr	–	–	–	1	–
martini	1 serv (3 oz)	206	0	0	0	0	0	0	0	tr
martini apple	1 serv	147	tr	0	tr	–	–	–	tr	–
martini rum	1 serv	131	0	0	0	0	0	0	tr	–
mellow yellow	1 serv	95	0	0	0	0	0	0	0	–
mexican grasshopper	1 serv	638	19	66	12	–	–	–	0	–
mint julep	1 serv	136	tr	0	tr	–	–	–	tr	–
mississippi mud	1 serv	496	12	45	7	–	–	–	0	–
mudslide	1 serv	566	10	0	6	–	–	–	0	–
narragansett	1 serv	168	0	0	0	0	0	0	0	–
nutcracker	1 serv	730	10	0	6	–	–	–	0	–
old fashioned	1 serv	223	tr	0	0	–	–	–	tr	–
orange crush	1 serv	461	tr	0	tr	–	–	–	tr	–
pain killer	1 serv	277	tr	0	tr	–	–	–	tr	–
peppermint pattie	1 serv	344	tr	0	tr	–	–	–	0	–
pina colada	1 serv (4.5 oz)	245	3	0	2	tr	tr	–	tr	31
planter's cocktail	1 serv	105	0	0	0	0	0	0	tr	–
planter's punch	1 serv	233	tr	0	tr	–	–	–	4	–
presbyterian	1 serv	170	0	0	0	0	0	0	tr	–
purple passion	1 serv	215	tr	0	tr	–	–	–	0	–
rob roy	1 serv	171	0	0	0	0	0	0	tr	–
rum	1 serv (1.5 oz)	97	0	0	0	0	0	0	0	0
rum boogie	1 serv	134	tr	0	0	–	–	–	tr	–
rum cola	1 serv	209	tr	0	0	–	–	–	tr	–
rum highball	1 serv	170	0	0	0	0	0	0	0	–
rum punch	1 serv	448	1	0	tr	–	–	–	1	–
rum screwdriver	1 serv	166	tr	0	tr	–	–	–	tr	–
rum sour	1 serv	156	tr	0	0	–	–	–	tr	–
rum swizzle	1 serv	187	0	0	0	0	0	0	0	–
rusty nail	1 serv	159	0	0	0	0	0	0	0	–
sake	1 serv (1 oz)	39	0	0	0	0	0	0	0	0
salty dog	1 serv	210	tr	0	tr	–	–	–	tr	–
scotch & soda	1 serv	104	0	0	0	0	0	0	tr	–
sea breeze	1 serv	207	tr	0	tr	–	–	–	tr	–
sex on the beach	1 serv	190	tr	0	tr	–	–	–	tr	–
slippery nipple	1 serv	142	2	0	2	–	–	–	0	–
sloe gin fizz	1 serv (2.5 oz)	132	0	0	0	0	0	0	0	–
snake bite	1 serv	362	0	0	0	0	0	0	0	–
tequila frozen screwdriver	1 serv	159	tr	0	tr	–	–	–	1	–
tequila gimlet	1 serv	150	tr	0	0	–	–	–	1	–

FOOD	PORTION	CALS	TOTAL FAT	CHOL	SAT FAT	POLY FAT	MONO FAT	TRANS FAT	FIBER	SUGAR
tequila sour	1 serv	156	tr	0	0	–	–	–	tr	–
tequila stinger	1 serv	221	tr	0	0	–	–	–	0	–
tequila sunrise	1 serv (6.8 oz)	232	tr	0	tr	tr	tr	–	0	–
tom collins	1 serv (7.5 oz)	121	0	0	0	0	0	0	–	–
vermouth cassis	1 serv	97	tr	0	0	–	–	–	tr	–
vodka	1 serv (1.5 oz)	97	0	0	0	0	0	0	0	0
vodka gimlet	1 serv	150	tr	0	0	–	–	–	1	–
vodka sour	1 serv	138	tr	0	0	–	–	–	tr	–
vodka stinger	1 serv	378	tr	0	tr	–	–	–	0	–
whiskey	1 serv (1.5 oz)	105	0	0	0	0	0	0	0	–
whiskey 86 proof	1 jigger (1.5 oz)	105	0	0	0	0	0	0	0	tr
whiskey sour	1 serv (3.5 oz)	162	tr	0	tr	tr	tr	–	0	14
white russian	1 serv	290	8	31	5	–	–	–	0	–
zombie	1 serv	235	tr	0	tr	–	–	–	tr	–

ALE (see BEER AND ALE)

ALFALFA

FOOD	PORTION	CALS	TOTAL FAT	CHOL	SAT FAT	POLY FAT	MONO FAT	TRANS FAT	FIBER	SUGAR
sprouts	½ cup	40	tr	0	tr	tr	tr	–	tr	tr

ALLIGATOR

FOOD	PORTION	CALS	TOTAL FAT	CHOL	SAT FAT	POLY FAT	MONO FAT	TRANS FAT	FIBER	SUGAR
cooked	3 oz	126	2	57	–	–	–	–	0	0

ALLSPICE

FOOD	PORTION	CALS	TOTAL FAT	CHOL	SAT FAT	POLY FAT	MONO FAT	TRANS FAT	FIBER	SUGAR
ground	1 tsp	5	tr	0	tr	tr	tr	0	tr	–

ALMONDS

FOOD	PORTION	CALS	TOTAL FAT	CHOL	SAT FAT	POLY FAT	MONO FAT	TRANS FAT	FIBER	SUGAR
almond butter w/ salt	2 tbsp	203	19	0	2	4	2	–	1	2
almond butter w/o salt	2 tbsp	203	19	0	2	4	12	–	1	–
almond extract	1 tsp	38	tr	0	–	–	–	–	0	–
almond paste	¼ cup	260	16	0	1	3	10	–	3	21
chocolate covered	6 pieces (0.6 oz)	102	8	1	1	2	5	–	2	3
dry roasted w/ salt	¼ cup	206	18	0	1	4	12	–	4	2
dry roasted w/o salt	¼ cup	206	18	0	1	4	12	–	4	2
honey roasted	¼ cup	214	18	0	2	4	12	–	5	–
jordan almonds	6 (0.7 oz)	99	4	0	tr	1	3	–	1	13
oil roasted w/ salt	¼ cup	238	22	0	2	5	14	–	4	2
oil roasted w/o salt	¼ cup	238	22	0	2	5	14	–	4	2
praline	17 pieces (1.4 oz)	210	12	0	1	–	–	–	3	17

FOOD	PORTION	CALS	TOTAL FAT	CHOL	SAT FAT	POLY FAT	MONO FAT	TRANS FAT	FIBER	SUGAR
yogurt covered	6 pieces (0.8 oz)	122	8	0	3	1	3	–	1	8
Blue Diamond										
Thin-Shell Hint Of Salt Shelled	24 (1 oz)	170	15	0	1	–	–	0	3	1
Thin-Shell Unsalted Shelled	24 (1 oz)	170	15	0	1	–	–	0	3	1
Frito Lay										
Roasted Salted	3 tbsp (1 oz)	190	16	0	2	–	–	0	3	1
Kettle Brand										
Butter Salted	2 tbsp (1 oz)	180	17	0	2	4	11	0	2	0
Nut Harvest										
Lightly Roasted	2 tbsp	180	15	0	2	–	–	0	3	1
Planters										
Chocolate Lovers Dark Chocolate	11 pieces (1.4 oz)	220	17	5	6	–	–	0	3	13
Flavor Grove Chili Lime	1 oz	170	15	0	1	–	9	0	3	2
Flavor Grove Sea Salt & Olive Oil	1 oz	170	15	0	2	9	–	0	3	1
Slivered	1 pkg (2 oz)	330	28	0	2	–	–	0	7	3
Smoked	1 pkg (1.5 oz)	250	22	0	2	–	14	0	5	2
Sante										
Chipotle	¼ cup (1 oz)	190	16	0	2	6	8	0	1	3
Wild Squirrel										
Almond Butter Chocolate Sunflower Seed	2 tbsp (1.1 oz)	200	17	0	2	–	–	0	4	2
Almond Butter Vanilla Espresso	2 tbsp (1.1 oz)	190	16	0	1	–	–	0	4	2

AMARANTH

FOOD	PORTION	CALS	TOTAL FAT	CHOL	SAT FAT	POLY FAT	MONO FAT	TRANS FAT	FIBER	SUGAR
grain cooked w/o salt	½ cup (4.6 oz)	125	2	0	–	–	–	0	3	–
grain uncooked	½ cup (3.4 oz)	358	7	0	1	3	2	0	7	2
leaves cooked w/o salt	1 cup (4.6 oz)	28	tr	0	tr	tr	tr	0	–	–
leaves raw	1 cup (1 oz)	6	tr	0	tr	tr	tr	0	–	–

ANCHOVY

FOOD	PORTION	CALS	TOTAL FAT	CHOL	SAT FAT	POLY FAT	MONO FAT	TRANS FAT	FIBER	SUGAR
boneless	1 oz	60	3	24	1	1	1	–	0	0
canned in oil drained	1 can (2 oz)	94	4	38	1	1	2	–	0	0
fresh	1 (4 g)	8	tr	3	tr	tr	tr	–	0	0
Arroyabe										
In Olive Oil	1 oz	60	3	25	1	–	–	0	0	0

FOOD	PORTION	CALS	TOTAL FAT	CHOL	SAT FAT	POLY FAT	MONO FAT	TRANS FAT	FIBER	SUGAR
King Oscar										
Fillet In Olive Oil	⅓ can (0.6 oz)	25	2	15	0	–	–	0	0	0
ANISE										
seed	1 tsp	7	tr	0	tr	tr	tr	0	tr	–
ANTELOPE										
roasted	4 oz	215	4	127	2	tr	1	–	0	0
APPLE										
CANNED										
sliced sweetened	½ cup	68	1	0	tr	tr	tr	–	2	15
Dole										
Squish'ems	1 pkg	80	0	0	0	0	0	0	1	17
Jake & Amos										
Red Spiced Rings	1 (1 oz)	35	0	0	0	0	0	0	0	8
DRIED										
chopped	½ cup	104	tr	0	tr	tr	tr	–	4	24
cooked w/o sugar	½ cup	73	tr	0	tr	tr	tr	–	3	17
rings	5	78	tr	0	tr	tr	tr	–	3	18
Del Monte										
Dried Apples	¼ cup (1.4 oz)	100	0	0	0	0	0	0	5	24
FRESH										
apple	1 lg	110	tr	0	tr	tr	tr	–	5	22
apple	1 sm	55	tr	0	tr	tr	tr	–	3	11
apple	1 med	72	tr	0	tr	tr	tr	–	3	14
candied	1 sm (4.9 oz)	179	3	0	2	tr	tr	–	3	32
candied	1 med (6.5 oz)	234	4	0	3	tr	tr	–	4	42
candied	1 lg (9.8 oz)	357	6	6	4	tr	1	–	6	64
golden delicious	1 med (6 oz)	96	tr	0	–	–	–	0	4	22
golden delicious w/ skin sliced	1 med (3.7 oz)	62	tr	0	–	–	–	0	3	11
w/ skin sliced	1 cup	57	tr	0	tr	tr	tr	–	3	11
w/o skin sliced	1 cup	53	tr	0	tr	tr	tr	–	1	11
Chiquita										
Apple Slices	1 pkg (2.2 oz)	30	0	0	0	0	0	0	2	5
Crunch Pak										
DipperZ Sweet Apples w/ Chocolate Dip	1 pkg (2.75 oz)	70	1	0	0	–	–	0	2	12
DipperZ Sweet Apples w/ Low Fat Caramel Dip	1 pkg (2.75 oz)	80	1	0	0	–	–	0	1	14

FOOD	PORTION	CALS	TOTAL FAT	CHOL	SAT FAT	POLY FAT	MONO FAT	TRANS FAT	FIBER	SUGAR
DipperZ Sweet Apples w/ Peanut Butter	1 pkg (2.75 oz)	150	11	0	2	–	–	0	2	8
DipperZ Sweet Apples w/ Yogurt Dip	1 pkg (2.75 oz)	150	11	0	2	–	–	0	2	8
DipperZ Tart Apples w/ Low Fat Caramel Dip	1 pkg (2.75 oz)	80	1	0	0	–	–	0	1	14
FlavorZ Grape	1 pkg (2 oz)	30	0	0	0	0	0	0	tr	5
FlavorZ Peach Mango	1 pkg (2 oz)	35	0	0	0	0	0	0	tr	5
FlavorZ Strawberry Vanilla Cream	1 pkg (2 oz)	35	0	0	0	0	0	0	tr	5
Foodles Apples Granola & Yogurt	1 pkg (5 oz)	230	6	0	1	–	–	0	3	18
Snackers Apples w/ Caramel Dip & Chocolate	1 pkg (4.7 oz)	260	10	<5	5	–	–	0	2	31
Snackers Apples w/ Grapes & Caramel	1 pkg (4.7 oz)	140	2	0	0	–	–	0	1	19
Snackers Apples w/ Pretzels & Cheese	1 pkg (4.7 oz)	240	10	30	6	–	–	0	2	9
Snackers Apples w/ Raisins & Pretzels	1 pkg (4.7 oz)	210	2	0	0	–	–	0	3	23
Dole										
Apple	1 med (5.4 oz)	80	0	0	0	0	0	0	4	16
Grapple										
Grape Flavored	1 med (6.4 oz)	95	0	0	0	0	0	0	4	19
Ready Pac										
Apples w/ Caramel Dip	1 pkg (6 oz)	200	0	0	0	0	0	0	2	34
Apples w/ Peanut Butter Dip	1 pkg (5.7 oz)	340	24	0	5	–	–	0	6	17
FROZEN										
sliced w/o sugar	½ cup	42	tr	0	tr	tr	tr	–	2	–
REFRIGERATED										
Dole										
Fruit Crisp Apple Cinnamon	1 pkg (4 oz)	160	4	0	0	–	–	0	3	20
Parfait Apples & Creme	1 pkg (4.3 oz)	130	3	0	2	–	–	0	1	20
TAKE-OUT										
baked no sugar added	1 (5.6 oz)	90	tr	0	tr	tr	tr	0	4	18
baked w/ sugar	1 (6 oz)	162	tr	0	tr	tr	tr	0	4	37
fried apple rings	1 serv (2.7 oz)	91	4	0	1	1	2	–	2	12
scalloped	½ cup (3.3 oz)	90	tr	0	tr	tr	tr	–	2	20

FOOD	PORTION	CALS	TOTAL FAT	CHOL	SAT FAT	POLY FAT	MONO FAT	TRANS FAT	FIBER	SUGAR
APPLE JUICE										
cider	1 cup	117	tr	0	tr	tr	tr	–	tr	27
juice + vitamin C & calcium	1 cup	117	tr	0	tr	tr	tr	–	tr	27
mulled cider	1 serv	265	1	0	tr	–	–	–	6	–
unsweetened w/o vitamin C	1 cup	117	tr	0	tr	tr	tr	–	tr	27
Apple & Eve										
100% Juice	8 oz	110	0	0	0	0	0	0	–	22
Kedem										
100% Juice	8 oz	100	0	0	0	0	0	0	–	21
Minute Maid										
100% Juice	8 oz	100	0	0	0	0	0	0	–	26
Old Orchard										
100% Juice Apple Cider	8 oz	130	0	0	0	0	0	0	–	29
R.W. Knudsen										
Organic 100% Juice	8 oz	120	0	0	0	0	0	0	0	30
Smart Juice										
Organic 100% Juice	8 oz	117	0	0	0	0	0	0	tr	27
TreeTop										
100% Juice	8 oz	120	0	0	0	0	0	0	–	26
Fiber Rich	8 oz	150	0	0	0	0	0	0	6	29
Grower's Best Apple Cider	8 oz	120	0	0	0	0	0	0	–	27
Tropicana										
Trop50 Farmstand Apple	8 oz	50	0	0	0	0	0	0	0	12
APPLESAUCE										
sweetened	½ cup	97	tr	0	tr	tr	tr	–	2	21
unsweetened	½ cup	52	tr	0	tr	tr	tr	–	2	12
GoGo Squeeze										
Apple	1 pkg (3.2 oz)	60	1	0	0	–	–	0	1	13
Apple Banana	1 pkg (3.2 oz)	60	tr	0	0	–	–	0	1	11
Apple Cinnamon	1 pkg (3.2 oz)	50	tr	0	0	–	–	0	1	9
Apple Peach	1 pkg (3.2 oz)	60	tr	0	0	–	–	0	1	12
Seneca										
Apple Sauce	1 pkg (4 oz)	70	0	0	0	0	0	0	2	15
TreeTop										
Apple Sauce	1 pkg (4 oz)	70	0	0	0	0	0	0	2	15
APRICOT JUICE										
nectar	6 oz	106	tr	0	tr	tr	tr	–	1	26

FOOD	PORTION	CALS	TOTAL FAT	CHOL	SAT FAT	POLY FAT	MONO FAT	TRANS FAT	FIBER	SUGAR
APRICOTS										
canned in heavy syrup	½ cup	91	tr	0	tr	tr	tr	0	3	20
canned in juice	½ cup	59	tr	0	tr	tr	tr	0	2	13
canned in light syrup	½ cup	80	tr	0	tr	tr	tr	0	2	19
canned in water	½ cup	33	tr	0	tr	tr	tr	0	2	6
dried halves	6	51	tr	0	tr	tr	tr	0	2	11
dried halves cooked w/o sugar	½ cup	106	tr	0	tr	tr	tr	0	3	24
fresh	1	17	tr	0	tr	tr	tr	0	1	3
fresh sliced	½ cup	40	tr	0	tr	tr	tr	0	2	8
frozen sweetened	½ cup	119	tr	0	tr	tr	tr	0	3	–
Del Monte										
Halves Lite	½ cup (4.3 oz)	60	0	0	0	0	0	0	1	15
Mediterranean Dried	5 (1.4 oz)	100	0	0	0	0	0	0	4	18
Dole										
Fresh	3 (4 oz)	60	1	0	0	–	–	0	1	11
Fruit Bliss										
Soft Dried	1 pkg (1.76 oz)	135	0	0	0	0	0	0	3	18
ARROWHEAD										
corm boiled	1 med	9	tr	0	–	–	–	–	–	–
ARROWROOT										
raw	1 root (1.2 oz)	21	tr	0	tr	tr	tr	–	tr	–
raw root sliced	1 cup	78	tr	0	tr	tr	tr	–	2	–
ARTICHOKE										
CANNED										
hearts in oil	1 serv (3 oz)	100	7	0	1	1	5	–	4	1
Progresso										
Hearts	2	30	0	0	0	0	0	0	2	2
Hearts Marinated	2 (1.1 oz)	60	5	0	1	–	–	1	0	7
Reese										
Cocktail Artichokes Original	½ jar (5 oz)	50	0	0	0	0	0	0	2	2
Victoria										
Hearts	1 oz	25	1	0	–	–	–	0	0	0
FRESH										
cooked	1 med	60	tr	0	tr	tr	tr	–	7	1
hearts cooked	½ cup	42	tr	0	tr	tr	tr	–	5	1
FROZEN										
cooked	1 cup	42	tr	0	tr	tr	tr	–	5	1
cooked w/o salt	1 pkg (9 oz)	108	1	0	0	1	0	–	11	2

FOOD	PORTION	CALS	TOTAL FAT	CHOL	SAT FAT	POLY FAT	MONO FAT	TRANS FAT	FIBER	SUGAR
TAKE-OUT										
stuffed	1 (8.8 oz)	397	14	8	3	2	8	–	10	6

ASIAN FOOD (see also CURRY, DINNER, EGG ROLLS, SAUCE, SOY SAUCE, SUSHI)

FOOD	PORTION	CALS	TOTAL FAT	CHOL	SAT FAT	POLY FAT	MONO FAT	TRANS FAT	FIBER	SUGAR
CANNED										
chow mein chicken w/o noodles	1 cup	194	8	51	2	3	3	–	2	6
FRESH										
wonton wrapper	1 (0.3 oz)	23	tr	1	tr	tr	tr	0	tr	–
Nasoya										
Won Ton Wraps	8 (2.1 oz)	160	1	10	0	–	–	0	1	1
FROZEN										
Crazy Cuizine										
Korean Inspired BBQ Chicken	¼ pkg (5 oz)	240	10	55	2	–	–	0	0	16
Mandarin Orange Chicken	1 cup (5 oz)	260	7	30	1	–	–	0	0	14
Tangerine Beef	1 cup (5 oz)	360	18	30	6	–	–	0	1	18
Healthy Choice										
Sweet & Sour Chicken	1 pkg (11.9 oz)	420	9	20	2	5	3	0	6	25
Lean Cuisine										
Cafe Cuisine Chow Fun Beef	1 pkg (9 oz)	320	5	20	2	1	2	0	3	18
Cafe Cuisine Sweet & Sour Chicken	1 pkg (10 oz)	300	3	30	1	1	1	0	2	16
Cafe Cuisine Thai-Style Chicken	1 pkg (9 oz)	260	4	35	1	2	1	0	0	9
Simple Favorites Chicken Chow Mein	1 pkg (9 oz)	240	4	25	1	2	1	0	3	3
Newman's Own										
Skillet Meal General Paul's Chicken	½ pkg (10.9 oz)	400	16	40	3	–	–	0	5	20
Purely Asian Brand										
Broccoli Beef	½ pkg (11 oz)	400	22	20	5	–	–	0	8	8
Mandarin Orange Chicken	½ pkg (12 oz)	450	10	35	3	–	–	0	7	47
Sweet & Sour Chicken	½ pkg (12 oz)	380	11	25	4	–	–	0	5	39
Quorn										
Kung Pao Chik'n	1 pkg (8.9 oz)	240	2	0	0	–	–	0	5	19
Vegetarian Plus										
Vegan Kung Pao Chicken	¼ pkg (2.5 oz)	205	7	0	2	–	–	0	6	4
Weight Watchers										
Chicken Teriyaki Stir Fry	1 pkg (11.8 oz)	340	6	45	1	2	2	0	5	13

FOOD	PORTION	CALS	TOTAL FAT	CHOL	SAT FAT	POLY FAT	MONO FAT	TRANS FAT	FIBER	SUGAR
SHELF-STABLE										
Dr. McDougall's										
Asian Entree Pad Thai Noodle Gluten Free as prep	1 pkg (2 oz)	200	2	0	0	–	–	0	2	2
Asian Entree Spicy Kung Pao Noodle as prep	1 pkg (2 oz)	220	2	0	0	–	–	0	2	5
Asian Entree Teriyaki Noodle as prep	1 pkg (2 oz)	200	1	0	0	–	–	0	3	8
Asian Entree Thai Peanut Noodles as prep	1 pkg (2 oz)	220	3	0	0	–	–	0	4	4
TAKE-OUT										
beef & broccoli	1 cup	221	12	54	3	3	5	–	3	3
beef w/ black bean sauce	1 serv (7 oz)	288	14	85	5	4	5	–	1	5
bo bia roll shrimp	1 (2.5 oz)	82	2	15	1	tr	1	–	2	1
buddha's delight w/ cellophane noodles fat choi jai	1 serv (7.6 oz)	211	4	tr	1	–	–	–	2	3
bun baked red bean	1 (1.1 oz)	102	3	8	2	tr	1	–	1	–
cha siu bao steamed buns w/ chicken filling	1 (2.3 oz)	160	3	15	1	–	–	–	tr	4
chicken masala	1 serv (8 oz)	430	25	128	9	6	9	–	0	–
chicken tandoori	1 serv (4 oz)	156	8	49	3	1	3	–	0	–
chicken tikka	1 serv (2.5 oz)	173	8	60	3	2	3	–	1	–
chinese garlic chicken	1 cup (5.7 oz)	290	19	83	5	5	8	–	1	3
chinese style fried egg noodles w/ seafood & lettuce	1 serv (14 oz)	694	37	257	14	5	16	–	8	1
chow mein beef w/o noodles	1 cup	271	15	51	4	3	7	–	3	4
chow mein chicken w/ noodles	1 cup (7.7 oz)	273	14	44	2	6	4	–	2	5
chow mein noodles	1 cup	237	14	0	2	8	3	–	2	tr
chow mein pork w/o noodles	1 cup	284	16	55	4	4	8	–	3	4
chow mein shrimp w/ noodles	1 cup (7.7 oz)	262	12	119	2	7	3	–	3	6
chow mein shrimp w/o noodles	1 cup	154	5	92	1	3	1	–	2	6

FOOD	PORTION	CALS	TOTAL FAT	CHOL	SAT FAT	POLY FAT	MONO FAT	TRANS FAT	FIBER	SUGAR
chow mein vegetable w/o noodles	1 cup	224	15	0	2	8	5	0	4	8
dim sum deep fried beancurd w/ shrimp	1 (1.1 oz)	77	6	9	2	1	2	–	1	–
dim sum deep fried yam	1 (2.4 oz)	201	12	3	5	1	5	0	2	–
dim sum meat filled	3 pieces (4 oz)	124	3	54	1	1	1	–	1	1
dim sum pork hash	1 (1.1 oz)	59	3	3	1	1	1	–	0	–
dim sum shrimp	3 (4 oz)	307	16	14	4	4	7	–	2	6
dim sum steamed chives & prawns	1 (1.2 oz)	48	2	10	1	tr	1	–	1	–
egg foo yung beef	1 patty (6 oz)	243	16	336	4	4	6	–	1	3
egg foo yung chicken	1 patty (3 oz)	121	8	166	2	2	3	–	1	2
egg foo yung pork	1 patty (3 oz)	125	8	166	2	2	3	–	1	2
egg foo yung shrimp	1 patty (3 oz)	153	12	184	3	3	5	–	1	2
filipino chicken adobo	1 serv (15 oz)	555	26	116	7	–	–	–	1	tr
foochow fish ball	1 (1 oz)	36	2	6	1	–	–	–	1	0
fried rice	1 cup	333	12	103	2	6	3	–	1	2
fried rice beef	1 cup	346	14	107	3	4	6	–	1	1
fried rice chicken	1 cup	329	12	105	2	3	5	0	1	1
fried rice pork	1 cup	335	13	103	3	3	6	–	1	1
fried rice shrimp	1 cup	323	12	115	2	6	3	–	1	2
general tsao's chicken	1 cup (5 oz)	296	17	66	4	5	6	–	1	5
green beans szechuan style	1 cup	176	12	0	2	6	4	–	6	3
indian style fried egg noodles w/ eggs tomato sauce & lime	1 serv (15 oz)	721	31	377	13	4	14	–	8	2
korean spicy shredded chicken	1 serv (5 oz)	258	16	30	5	3	7	–	2	5
kung pao beef	1 cup	410	30	62	8	6	13	–	2	2
kung pao chicken	1 cup (5.7 oz)	434	31	65	5	10	14	–	2	4
kung pao pork	1 cup	460	34	60	7	9	16	–	2	4
kung pao shrimp	1 cup (5.7 oz)	345	20	191	3	7	9	–	2	3
lemon chicken w/o vegetables	1 serv (6.6 oz)	503	28	127	7	7	11	–	1	3
lo mein beef	1 cup	286	11	26	3	3	5	–	3	3
lo mein chicken	1 cup (7 oz)	280	9	26	2	3	4	–	3	3
lo mein meatless	1 cup	234	6	0	1	2	2	–	3	3
lo mein pork	1 cup	314	14	22	4	3	6	–	3	3
lo mein shrimp	1 cup	236	7	48	1	2	3	–	4	2
moo goo gai pan chicken	1 cup (7.6 oz)	272	19	35	4	7	7	–	3	5

FOOD	PORTION	CALS	TOTAL FAT	CHOL	SAT FAT	POLY FAT	MONO FAT	TRANS FAT	FIBER	SUGAR
moo shu pork w/o pancake	1 cup	512	46	172	7	21	16	–	1	2
pad thai w/ chicken	1 cup (7 oz)	358	15	64	3	5	6	–	2	5
pad thai w/ shrimp	1 cup (7 oz)	314	11	186	2	4	4	–	1	6
pakhoras	1 (2.5 oz)	163	8	0	3	2	3	–	4	–
paneer pakhora	1 (2.2 oz)	183	13	16	6	2	–	–	2	–
peking duck w/ pancakes & seafood sauce	1 serv (14 oz)	1871	121	189	39	20	55	–	5	39
pork w/ chinese cabbage	1 serv (4 oz)	120	8	25	3	2	3	–	1	0
sesame seed paste bun	1 (2.5 oz)	220	6	0	1	–	–	–	2	12
shrimp chips banh phong tom	6 med	214	14	21	2	7	4	–	tr	1
shrimp w/ lobster sauce	1 cup	298	12	259	2	5	4	–	1	2
shu mai chicken & vegetable dumplings	6 (3.6 oz)	160	5	35	1	–	–	–	1	6
sukiyaki beef	1 cup	165	7	130	3	1	3	–	1	4
sukiyaki chicken	1 serv (18 oz)	436	8	175	2	–	–	–	4	7
sweet & sour chicken w/o rice	1 cup	670	37	169	9	9	15	–	2	4
sweet & sour pork w/ rice	1 cup	268	6	29	2	2	2	–	2	10
sweet & sour pork w/o rice	1 cup	231	8	38	2	2	3	–	2	15
sweet & sour shrimp	1 cup	480	30	70	4	15	10	–	1	40
szechuan chicken	1 cup (5.7 oz)	180	9	42	2	3	3	–	2	2
szechuan shrimp & vegetables	1 cup	159	7	94	1	3	2	–	2	3
tempura hawaiian fish tofu vegetable	2 cups	285	22	200	4	9	7	–	2	9
tempura vegetable	8 pieces	90	6	36	1	2	2	–	1	1
teriyaki beef	1 cup	454	19	149	6	3	7	–	tr	9
teriyaki chicken	¾ cup	399	27	92	6	11	7	–	–	–
teriyaki chicken w/ rice	1 serv (11 oz)	430	6	25	1	–	–	–	1	10
teriyaki shrimp	1 cup	271	3	269	1	1	tr	–	1	6
thai style pineapple rice w/ ham & pork floss	1 serv (7.7 oz)	408	14	63	6	1	6	–	6	22
wonton fried meat filled	1 (0.7 oz)	54	3	20	1	tr	1	–	tr	tr
wonton meat & shrimp boiled	1 (0.5 oz)	19	1	3	tr	tr	tr	–	tr	–

ASPARAGUS
CANNED

FOOD	PORTION	CALS	TOTAL FAT	CHOL	SAT FAT	POLY FAT	MONO FAT	TRANS FAT	FIBER	SUGAR
spears	1	3	tr	0	tr	tr	tr	0	tr	tr
spears	1 cup	46	2	0	tr	1	tr	–	4	3

FOOD	PORTION	CALS	TOTAL FAT	CHOL	SAT FAT	POLY FAT	MONO FAT	TRANS FAT	FIBER	SUGAR
Del Monte										
Spears Tender Young	½ cup (4.3 oz)	20	0	0	0	0	0	0	1	0
Tips	½ cup (4.2 oz)	20	0	0	0	0	0	0	1	0
FRESH										
cooked	½ cup	20	tr	0	tr	tr	tr	–	2	1
spears cooked	4	13	tr	0	tr	tr	tr	0	1	1
spears raw	4	10	tr	0	tr	tr	tr	–	1	1
Dole										
Spears	5 med (2.8 oz)	15	0	0	0	0	0	0	2	2
FROZEN										
cooked	1 pkg (10 oz)	53	1	0	tr	1	tr	–	5	1
spears cooked	4	11	tr	0	tr	tr	tr	0	1	tr
AVOCADO										
california mashed	¼ cup	96	9	0	1	1	6	–	4	tr
california peeled & pitted	1	289	27	0	4	3	17	–	12	1
florida mashed	¼ cup	69	6	0	1	1	3	–	1	0
florida peeled & pitted	1	365	31	0	6	5	17	–	17	7
Dole										
Fresh	⅕ med (1 oz)	50	5	0	1	–	–	0	2	0
Margaritaville										
Guacamole Zesty Island Garlic	1 oz	40	4	0	1	–	–	0	2	0
Wholly Guacamole										
Classic	2 tbsp (1 oz)	60	5	0	1	1	4	0	2	0
Guacamole Snack Packs	1 pkg (2 oz)	100	10	0	2	1	7	0	3	0
TAKE-OUT										
guacamole	1 serv (2.2 oz)	105	10	0	1	–	–	–	2	1
BACON										
bacon grease	1 tbsp	116	13	12	5	1	6	–	0	0
beef breakfast strips cooked	3 strips	153	12	40	5	1	6	–	0	0
pan fried	2 strips (0.8 oz)	108	8	23	3	1	4	tr	0	0
turkey	2 (0.8 oz)	84	6	22	6	–	–		0	0
Hormel										
Black Label Lower Sodium	2 slices (0.5 oz)	80	7	15	3	–	–	0	0	0
Oscar Mayer										
Bacon Bits	1 tbsp (7 g)	25	2	5	1	–	–	0	0	0
Fully Cooked	3 slices (0.5 oz)	70	5	15	2	–	–	0	0	0

FOOD	PORTION	CALS	TOTAL FAT	CHOL	SAT FAT	POLY FAT	MONO FAT	TRANS FAT	FIBER	SUG
Hardwood Smoked	2 slices (0.5 oz)	70	6	15	2	–	–	0	0	0
Lower Sodium	3 slices (0.5 oz)	70	6	10	3	–	–	0	0	0
Super Thick Applewood Smoked	0.6 oz	90	7	15	3	–	–	0	–	0
Turkey	0.5 oz	35	3	15	1	–	–	0	0	0
Turkey Lower Sodium	0.5 oz	35	3	15	1	–	–	0	0	0

BACON SUBSTITUTES

FOOD	PORTION	CALS	TOTAL FAT	CHOL	SAT FAT	POLY FAT	MONO FAT	TRANS FAT	FIBER	SUG
bacon bits meatless	1 tbsp	33	2	0	tr	1	tr	–	1	0
meatless	1 strip	16	1	0	tr	1	tr	–	tr	0
McCormick										
Bac'n Pieces	1 tbsp (7 g)	30	1	0	–	–	–	0	0	–

BAGEL

FOOD	PORTION	CALS	TOTAL FAT	CHOL	SAT FAT	POLY FAT	MONO FAT	TRANS FAT	FIBER	SUG
cinnamon raisin	1 lg (4 in)	244	2	0	tr	1	tr	–	2	5
cinnamon raisin mini	1	71	tr	0	tr	tr	tr	–	1	2
egg	1 lg (4.5 in)	364	3	31	1	1	1	–	3	–
low carb	1 (4 oz)	216	0	10	0	0	0	0	14	0
oat bran	1 lg (4 in)	227	1	0	tr	tr	tr	–	3	1
onion mini	1 (1.4 oz)	100	0	0	0	0	0	0	1	1
plain	1 sm (3 in)	190	1	0	tr	tr	tr	–	2	–
plain	1 med (3.5 in)	289	2	0	tr	1	tr	–	2	–
plain	1 lg (4.5 in)	360	2	0	tr	1	tr	–	3	–
Nature's Own										
Original	1 (3.7 oz)	270	1	0	0	0	0	0	2	5
Thin Sliced 100% Whole Wheat	1 (1.6 oz)	110	1	0	0	1	0	0	5	4
Pepperidge Farm										
Bagel Flats Plain	1	100	1	0	0	0	0	0	5	3

BAKING POWDER

FOOD	PORTION	CALS	TOTAL FAT	CHOL	SAT FAT	POLY FAT	MONO FAT	TRANS FAT	FIBER	SUG
baking powder	1 tsp	2	0	0	0	0	0	0	0	0
low sodium	1 tsp	5	tr	0	tr	tr	0	0	tr	0

BAKING SODA

FOOD	PORTION	CALS	TOTAL FAT	CHOL	SAT FAT	POLY FAT	MONO FAT	TRANS FAT	FIBER	SUG
baking soda	1 tsp	0	0	0	0	0	0	0	0	0
Arm & Hammer										
Baking Soda	¼ tsp	0	0	0	0	0	0	0	0	0

BALSAM PEAR (BITTER GOURD)

FOOD	PORTION	CALS	TOTAL FAT	CHOL	SAT FAT	POLY FAT	MONO FAT	TRANS FAT	FIBER	SUG
leafy tips cooked w/o salt	1 cup	20	tr	0	tr	tr	tr	–	1	1
leafy tips raw	1 cup	14	tr	0	–	–	–	–	–	–

FOOD	PORTION	CALS	TOTAL FAT	CHOL	SAT FAT	POLY FAT	MONO FAT	TRANS FAT	FIBER	SUGAR
pods raw sliced	1 cup	16	tr	0	–	–	–	–	3	–
pods sliced cooked w/ salt	1 cup	24	tr	0	–	–	–	–	3	2

BAMBOO SHOOTS

canned sliced	½ cup	12	tr	0	tr	tr	tr	–	1	1
fresh sliced cooked w/ salt	½ cup	7	tr	0	tr	tr	tr	–	1	–
raw sliced	½ cup	20	tr	0	tr	tr	tr	–	2	2

BANANA

banana chips	1 oz	147	10	0	8	tr	1	–	2	–
fresh	1 sm (6 in)	90	tr	0	tr	tr	tr	–	3	12
fresh	1 lg (8 in)	121	tr	0	tr	tr	tr	–	4	17
fresh	1 med (7 in)	105	tr	0	tr	tr	tr	–	3	14
fresh baby	1 extra sm (<6 in)	72	tr	0	tr	tr	tr	0	2	10
fresh mashed	½ cup	100	tr	0	tr	tr	tr	–	3	14
fresh sliced	1 cup	134	1	0	tr	tr	tr	–	4	18
green fried	1 (3.1 oz)	152	8	0	1	3	4	–	2	11
green pickled	½ cup	240	22	0	3	2	16	–	1	6
green sliced fried	1 cup	323	18	0	2	8	7	–	5	24
powder	1 tbsp	21	tr	0	tr	tr	tr	–	1	3
red ripe	1 (7 in)	93	tr	0	tr	tr	tr	0	3	13
red ripe sliced	1 cup	134	1	0	tr	tr	tr	–	4	18
whole dried	1 piece (1.2 oz)	130	1	0	0	–	–	–	2	22

Crunchies
Freeze Dried Organic	¼ cup (0.3 oz)	32	0	0	0	0	0	0	1	7

Crunchy N'Yummy
Organic Freeze Dried	1 pkg (1 oz)	110	0	0	0	0	0	0	tr	0

Dole
Fresh	1 med (4.4 oz)	110	0	0	0	0	0	0	3	15

TAKE-OUT
batter dipped fried	1 sm (4 oz)	266	15	17	2	7	5	–	3	9
batter dipped fried sliced	1 cup	335	19	22	3	9	6	–	3	12
fried dwarf w/ cheese	1 (1.4 oz)	84	5	4	1	2	2	–	1	5
fritter	1 (2.3 oz)	197	5	0	3	tr	1	1	2	14

BANANA JUICE
R.W. Knudsen
Sensible Sippers Organic	1 box (4.23 oz)	35	0	0	0	0	0	0	–	8

FOOD	PORTION	CALS	TOTAL FAT	CHOL	SAT FAT	POLY FAT	MONO FAT	TRANS FAT	FIBER	SUGAR
BARBECUE SAUCE										
barbecue	2 tbsp	52	tr	0	0	tr	tr	0	tr	9
low sodium	2 tbsp	52	tr	0	0	tr	tr	0	tr	9
Ali's All Natural										
Homestyle	2 tbsp	10	0	0	0	0	0	0	–	1
Raspberry Chipotle	2 tbsp	10	0	0	0	0	0	0	–	1
David's Unforgettables										
Balsamic Spicy	2 tbsp (1 oz)	70	5	0	0	–	–	0	0	5
Jake & Amos										
Apple Butter Barbecue Sauce	2 tbsp (0.5 oz)	30	0	0	0	0	0	0	0	7
OrganicVille										
Original No Added Sugar	2 tbsp (1 oz)	50	0	0	0	0	0	0	tr	11
BARLEY										
flour	1 cup	511	2	0	tr	1	tr	–	15	1
pearled cooked	1 cup (5.5 oz)	193	1	0	tr	tr	tr	–	6	tr
pearled uncooked	¼ cup	176	1	0	tr	tr	tr	–	8	tr
BARRACUDA										
broiled	4 oz	239	14	62	4	4	5	–	0	tr
cooked flaked	1 cup	287	16	75	4	4	6	–	0	tr
poached	4 oz	227	11	67	3	3	4	–	0	0
TAKE-OUT										
breaded & fried	4 oz	282	17	59	4	5	6	–	tr	tr
BARRAMUNDI										
Australis										
Barramundi fresh or frzn	6 oz	140	2	70	0	–	–	0	0	0
Crispy Asian Sesame Panko	1 piece (4 oz)	240	11	30	2	–	–	0	1	2
Fast & Delicious Mediterranean Seafood	½ pkg (6 oz)	230	9	45	2	–	–	0	2	1
Fast & Delicious Rosemary Parmesan	½ pkg (6 oz)	230	11	40	3	–	–	0	2	2
Fast & Delicious Seafood Penne	½ pkg (6 oz)	250	11	50	5	–	–	0	1	3
Fast & Delicious Seafood Pomodoro	½ pkg (6 oz)	230	12	50	3	–	–	0	1	1
Fast & Delicious Seafood Risotto	½ pkg (6 oz)	250	15	80	7	–	–	0	1	1

FOOD	PORTION	CALS	TOTAL FAT	CHOL	SAT FAT	POLY FAT	MONO FAT	TRANS FAT	FIBER	SUGAR
Fast & Delicious Seafood Teriyaki	½ pkg (6 oz)	180	4	30	1	–	–	0	1	7
Fast & Delicious Seafood Veracruz	½ pkg (6 oz)	150	3	40	0	–	–	0	2	2
Lemon Herb Butter	1 piece (4.5 oz)	131	6	43	2	–	–	0	0	1

BASIL

FOOD	PORTION	CALS	TOTAL FAT	CHOL	SAT FAT	POLY FAT	MONO FAT	TRANS FAT	FIBER	SUGAR
fresh chopped	2 tbsp	1	tr	0	tr	tr	tr	0	tr	tr
ground	1 tsp	4	tr	0	tr	tr	tr	0	1	tr
leaves fresh	5	1	tr	0	tr	tr	tr	0	tr	tr

BASS

FOOD	PORTION	CALS	TOTAL FAT	CHOL	SAT FAT	POLY FAT	MONO FAT	TRANS FAT	FIBER	SUGAR
breaded baked	4 oz	205	7	129	1	2	3	0	1	1
pickled mero en escabeche	2 oz	156	14	16	2	2	10	0	tr	tr
striped baked	3 oz	105	3	88	1	1	1	0	0	0
striped bass farm raised	4 oz	110	3	90	1	–	–	–	0	0

BAY LEAF

FOOD	PORTION	CALS	TOTAL FAT	CHOL	SAT FAT	POLY FAT	MONO FAT	TRANS FAT	FIBER	SUGAR
crumbled	1 tsp	2	tr	0	tr	tr	tr	0	tr	tr

BEANS (see also individual names)

CANNED

FOOD	PORTION	CALS	TOTAL FAT	CHOL	SAT FAT	POLY FAT	MONO FAT	TRANS FAT	FIBER	SUGAR
baked beans plain	½ cup	119	tr	0	tr	tr	tr	–	5	–
baked beans vegetarian	½ cup	119	tr	0	tr	tr	tr	–	5	–
baked beans w/ franks	½ cup	184	9	8	3	1	4	–	9	–
baked beans w/ pork	½ cup	134	2	9	1	tr	1	–	7	–
baked beans w/ pork & tomato sauce	½ cup	119	1	9	tr	tr	1	–	5	7

Bush's

FOOD	PORTION	CALS	TOTAL FAT	CHOL	SAT FAT	POLY FAT	MONO FAT	TRANS FAT	FIBER	SUGAR
Boston Recipe	½ cup (4.6 oz)	150	1	0	0	–	–	0	5	11
Cocina Latina Frijoles A La Mexicana	½ cup (4.6 oz)	100	2	0	1	–	–	0	4	1
Cocina Latina Frijoles Charros Machacados	½ cup (4.6 oz)	130	3	0	1	–	–	0	5	1
Country Style	½ cup (4.6 oz)	160	1	0	0	–	–	0	5	16
Grillin' Beans Bourbon & Brown Sugar	½ cup (4.6 oz)	170	1	0	0	–	–	0	6	15
Grillin' Beans Steakhouse Recipe	½ cup (4.6 oz)	180	1	0	0	–	–	0	5	21
Grillin' Beans Sweet Mesquite	½ cup (4.6 oz)	160	1	0	0	–	–	0	5	13

FOOD	PORTION	CALS	TOTAL FAT	CHOL	SAT FAT	POLY FAT	MONO FAT	TRANS FAT	FIBER	SUG
Honey Baked	½ cup (4.6 oz)	160	1	0	0	–	–	0	6	14
Maple Cured Bacon	½ cup (4.6 oz)	140	1	0	0	–	–	0	5	11
Onion Baked	½ cup (4.6 oz)	140	1	0	0	–	–	0	5	12
Original	½ cup (4.6 oz)	140	1	0	0	–	–	0	5	12
Refried Fat Free	½ cup (4.4 oz)	130	0	0	0	0	0	0	7	0
Refried Traditional	½ cup (4.4 oz)	150	3	0	1	–	–	0	7	0
Vegetarian Fat Free	½ cup (4.6 oz)	130	0	0	0	0	0	0	5	12
Goya										
Fiesta Baked Beans Original	½ cup (4.6 oz)	200	1	0	0	–	–	0	9	18
Jake & Amos										
Four Bean Salad	2 tbsp	32	0	0	0	0	0	0	0	6
Van Camp's										
Beanee Weenee Original	1 can (7.75 oz)	240	8	40	3	–	–	0	8	8
FROZEN										
Lean Cuisine										
Simple Favorites Sante Fe Rice & Beans	1 pkg (10.4 oz)	290	5	15	2	1	1	0	4	8
TAKE-OUT										
baked beans	½ cup	191	7	6	2	1	3	–	7	–
barbecue beans	3.5 oz	120	tr	0	tr	tr	tr	–	–	–
frijoles a la charra w/ pork tomatoes & chili peppers	1 cup	341	22	27	8	3	10	–	5	2
refried beans	½ cup	43	2	2	1	tr	1	–	–	–
three bean salad	1 cup	114	5	0	1	2	1	–	5	2

BEAN SPROUTS (see ALFALFA, SPROUTS)

BEAR
simmered	3 oz	220	11	83	3	2	5	0	0	0

BEAVER
roasted	4 oz	240	8	132	2	2	2	0	0	0

BEE POLLEN
bee pollen	1 tsp (5 g)	16	tr	0	tr	tr	tr	0	tr	2

BEECHNUTS
dried	1 oz	163	14	0	2	6	6	0	–	–

BEEF (see also BEEF DISHES, JERKY, MEATBALLS, VEAL)
CANNED
corned beef	1 oz	71	4	24	2	tr	2	–	0	0

FOOD	PORTION	CALS	TOTAL FAT	CHOL	SAT FAT	POLY FAT	MONO FAT	TRANS FAT	FIBER	SUGAR
FRESH										
arm pot roast trim 0 fat braised	3.5 oz	297	19	95	8	1	8	–	0	0
arm pot roast trim ⅛ in fat braised	3.5 oz	302	19	79	8	1	8	–	0	0
australian waygu tenderloin steak not prep	1 (6 oz)	429	33	12	13	1	15	1	0	0
beef crumbles 70% lean pan browned	3 oz	230	15	75	6	tr	7	–	0	0
bottom round roast trim 0 fat braised	4 oz	253	10	112	4	tr	4	–	0	0
bottom round roast trim 0 fat roasted	3.5 oz	187	8	86	3	tr	3	–	0	0
bottom round roast trim ½ in fat braised	4 oz	337	22	109	8	1	10	–	0	0
bottom round roast trim ⅛ in fat braised	4 oz	280	13	86	5	1	6	–	0	0
bottom round roast trim ⅛ in fat roasted	4 oz	247	13	85	5	1	6	–	0	0
bottom sirloin butt roast trim 0 fat roasted	3.5 oz	182	8	71	3	tr	4	–	0	0
brisket flat half trim ⅛ in fat braised	3.5 oz	298	19	80	8	1	8	–	0	0
brisket flat trim 0 fat braised	3.5 oz	221	9	46	4	tr	4	–	0	0
brisket point half trim 0 fat braised	3.5 oz	358	29	92	11	1	13	–	0	0
brisket point half trim ¼ in fat braised	3.5 oz	404	22	92	14	1	15	–	0	0
brisket point half trim ⅛ in fat braised	3.5 oz	349	27	92	11	1	12	–	0	0
chuck boston cut roast trim 0 fat roasted	3.5 oz	207	11	69	4	tr	5	–	0	0
chuck boston cut roast trim ¼ in fat roasted	3.5 oz	242	15	75	6	1	7	–	0	0
chuck bottom roast trim 0 fat braised	3.5 oz	334	24	104	10	1	10	–	0	0
chuck bottom roast trim ¼ in fat braised	3.5 oz	345	26	104	10	1	11	–	0	0
chuck fillet steak trim 0 fat broiled	4 oz	181	6	71	2	tr	3	–	0	0

FOOD	PORTION	CALS	TOTAL FAT	CHOL	SAT FAT	POLY FAT	MONO FAT	TRANS FAT	FIBER	SUGAR
chuck top roast trim 0 fat broiled	4 oz	245	13	69	4	tr	6	–	0	0
club steak trim ½ in fat broiled	4 oz	384	29	91	12	1	13	–	0	0
corned beef brisket cooked	3 oz	213	16	83	5	1	8	–	0	0
crosscut shank trim ¼ in fat stewed	1 serv (6.8 oz)	510	28	155	11	1	13	–	0	0
delmonico steak trim ¼ in fat broiled	4 oz	409	33	95	13	1	14	–	0	0
entrecote steak trim ½ in fat broiled	4 oz	413	33	95	14	1	15	–	0	0
eye round roast trim 0 fat roasted	4 oz	190	5	61	2	tr	2	–	0	0
eye round roast trim ¼ in fat roasted	4 oz	283	17	82	7	1	8	–	0	0
filet mignon roast trim ¼ in fat roasted	4 oz	376	29	97	11	1	12	–	0	0
filet mignon roast trim ⅛ in fat roasted	4 oz	367	28	96	11	1	12	–	0	0
filet mignon trim 0 fat broiled	4 oz	247	13	95	5	tr	5	–	0	0
filet mignon trim ⅛ in fat broiled	4 oz	303	19	102	8	1	8	–	0	0
ground 70% lean broiled	3.5 oz	273	18	82	7	tr	9	–	0	0
ground 75% lean broiled	2.5 oz	195	13	62	5	tr	6	–	0	0
ground 80% lean broiled	3 oz	234	15	77	6	tr	7	–	0	0
ground 85% lean pan fried	3 oz	197	12	73	5	tr	5	–	0	0
ground 90% lean pan fried	3 oz	173	9	70	4	tr	4	–	0	0
ground 95% lean pan fried	3 oz	139	5	65	2	tr	2	–	0	0
ground 97% lean irradiated	4 oz	160	8	70	3	–	–	–	0	0
ground lowfat w/ carrageenan raw	4 oz	160	7	53	4	–	–	–	–	–
london broil trim 0 fat broiled	3.5 oz	188	8	45	3	tr	3	–	0	0
london broil trim ¼ in fat broiled	4 oz	260	12	95	4	1	5	–	0	0
new york strip steak trim 0 fat broiled	4 oz	219	9	66	3	tr	4	–	0	0
oxtails cooked	6 pieces (6.3 oz)	472	26	191	10	1	11	0	0	0

FOOD	PORTION	CALS	TOTAL FAT	CHOL	SAT FAT	POLY FAT	MONO FAT	TRANS FAT	FIBER	SUGAR
porterhouse steak trim 0 fat broiled	1 lb	1252	87	304	33	3	39	–	0	0
porterhouse steak trim ¼ in fat broiled	1 lb	1492	117	327	46	5	52	–	0	0
porterhouse steak trim ⅛ in fat broiled	4 oz	337	25	80	10	1	11	–	0	0
porterhouse steak trim ⅛ in fat broiled	1 lb	1324	99	322	38	3	43	–	0	0
rib roast trim ¼ in fat roasted	4 oz	406	33	95	13	1	14	–	0	0
rib steak trim ¼ in fat broiled	4 oz	388	31	93	13	1	13	–	0	0
ribeye roast trim ¼ in fat roasted	3.5 oz	365	30	85	12	1	13	–	0	0
ribeye steak boneless 0 fat grilled	1 (7.3 oz)	514	33	159	12	1	14	1	0	0
round tip roast trim 0 fat roasted	4 oz	213	9	105	3	tr	4	–	0	0
sandwich steaks thinly sliced	1 serv (2 oz)	173	15	40	6	tr	6	–	0	0
shell steak trim ¼ in fat broiled	4 oz	366	27	90	11	1	11	–	0	0
shortribs lean & fat braised	1 serv (7.8 oz)	1060	94	212	40	3	42	–	0	0
skirt steak trim 0 fat grilled	1 (6 oz)	508	36	177	13	2	14	2	0	0
t-bone steak trim 0 fat broiled	4 oz	280	18	68	7	1	8	–	0	0
t-bone steak trim ¼ in fat broiled	1 lb	1388	103	295	40	4	46	–	0	0
t-bone steak trim ⅛ in fat broiled	1 lb	804	56	178	22	2	25	–	0	0
tip round roast trim ⅛ in fat roasted	4 oz	248	13	93	5	tr	5	–	0	0
top loin filet boneless trim ⅛ in fat grilled	1 (4.7 oz)	263	12	116	4	tr	5	tr	0	0
top round roast trim 0 fat braised	4 oz	237	7	102	3	tr	3	–	0	0
top round roast trim ¼ in fat braised	4 oz	281	13	102	5	1	5	–	0	0
top round roast trim ¼ in fat roasted	4 oz	265	15	93	6	1	6	–	0	0

FOOD	PORTION	CALS	TOTAL FAT	CHOL	SAT FAT	POLY FAT	MONO FAT	TRANS FAT	FIBER	SUGAR
top round steak trim ¼ in fat pan fried	4 oz	314	17	110	6	2	7	–	0	0
top sirloin steak trim ⅛ in fat broiled	4 oz	275	16	85	6	1	7	–	0	0
top sirloin steak trim ⅛ in fat pan fried	4 oz	355	24	111	9	2	10	–	0	0
tri-tip roast trim 0 fat roasted	3.5 oz	218	12	94	5	tr	6	–	0	0
tri-tip steak trim 0 fat broiled	4 oz	300	17	77	6	1	9	–	0	0
READY-TO-EAT										
dried beef smoked chopped	1 oz	37	1	13	1	tr	1	–	0	–
roast beef spread	¼ cup	127	9	40	4	tr	3	–	tr	tr
TAKE-OUT										
roast beef rare	2 oz	70	2	30	1	–	–	–	0	0

BEEF DISHES
CANNED
Dinty Moore

FOOD	PORTION	CALS	TOTAL FAT	CHOL	SAT FAT	POLY FAT	MONO FAT	TRANS FAT	FIBER	SUGAR
Beef Stew	½ can	200	10	30	4	–	–	–	1	3
Hormel										
Corned Beef Hash 50% Reduced Fat	1 cup (8.3 oz)	290	12	60	6	–	–	1	2	2
TAKE-OUT										
beef bourguignonne	1 cup	339	12	85	3	2	5	–	1	3
beef satay + peanut sauce	2 skewers	253	16	62	8	–	–	0	1	4
bool kogi korean grilled beef	1 serv (5.2 oz)	256	15	67	5	–	–	–	tr	3
bool kogi korean marinated beef ribs	4 oz	190	10	55	4	–	–	–	0	4
bracciola	1 roll (4.7 oz)	276	14	76	5	1	6	–	1	1
chipped beef on toast	1 slice (5 oz)	226	10	22	3	3	4	–	1	7
goulash w/ potatoes	1 cup	298	12	66	4	1	6	–	2	3
greek moussaka	1 serv (8.5 oz)	450	33	179	14	–	–	–	1	4
meatloaf	1 lg slice (5 oz)	294	17	114	6	1	8	–	1	2
pepper steak	1 cup	317	20	69	4	8	7	–	1	2
pot roast w/ gravy	1 serv (6 oz)	320	10	110	4	–	–	–	0	0
shepherds pie	1 serv (7 oz)	282	16	70	6	1	7	–	2	–
sloppy joes	1 serv (9 oz)	398	6	67	2	–	–	–	12	5
stew w/ potatoes & vegetables	1 cup	199	5	30	1	1	2	–	3	3
stroganoff	1 cup	394	25	69	10	5	8	–	1	2
swiss steak w/ sauce	1 serv (8 oz)	234	10	66	2	3	4	–	1	3

FOOD	PORTION	CALS	TOTAL FAT	CHOL	SAT FAT	POLY FAT	MONO FAT	TRANS FAT	FIBER	SUGAR
BEEFALO										
ground	3.5 oz	171	18	20	–	–	–	–	0	0
roasted	3.5 oz	188	6	58	3	tr	3	–	0	0
t-bone steak	3.5 oz	111	3	13	–	–	–	–	0	0
BEER AND ALE										
ale brown	10 oz	77	0	0	0	0	0	0	0	–
ale pale	10 oz	88	0	0	0	0	0	0	0	–
beer cooler	1 (16 oz)	194	0	0	0	0	0	0	1	–
beer light	12 oz can	103	0	0	0	0	0	0	0	tr
beer regular	12 oz can	153	0	0	0	0	0	0	0	0
black & tan	1 serv (12 oz)	146	0	0	0	0	0	0	1	–
black velvet	1 (10 oz)	160	0	0	0	0	0	0	1	–
boilermaker	1 serv	216	0	0	0	0	0	0	1	–
lager	10 oz	80	0	0	0	0	0	0	0	–
lager & black	1 (14 oz)	241	0	0	0	0	0	0	–	–
mead	1 serv	250	0	0	0	0	0	0	1	–
shandy	1 serv	125	0	0	0	0	0	0	1	–
stout	10 oz	102	0	0	0	0	0	0	0	–
trojan horse	1 (16 oz)	189	0	0	0	0	0	0	–	–
Budweiser										
Beer	1 bottle (12 oz)	146	0	0	0	0	0	0	0	0
Bud Light	1 bottle (12 oz)	110	0	0	0	0	0	0	0	0
Select	1 bottle (12 oz)	99	0	0	0	0	0	0	0	0
Michelob										
Ultra	1 bottle (12 oz)	96	0	0	0	0	0	0	0	0
BEET JUICE										
juice	7 oz	72	0	0	0	0	0	0	–	–
BEETS										
CANNED										
harvard	½ cup	90	tr	0	tr	tr	tr	–	3	–
pickled	½ cup	74	tr	0	tr	tr	tr	–	3	–
sliced	½ cup	37	tr	0	tr	tr	tr	–	2	8
Butter Kernel										
Sliced	½ cup (4.2 oz)	40	0	0	0	0	0	0	1	6
Del Monte										
Pickled Sliced	½ cup (4.5 oz)	80	0	0	0	0	0	0	2	16
Sliced	½ cup (4.3 oz)	45	0	0	0	0	0	0	2	8
Jake & Amos										
Harvard	1 serv (4 oz)	90	0	0	0	0	0	0	1	20

FOOD	PORTION	CALS	TOTAL FAT	CHOL	SAT FAT	POLY FAT	MONO FAT	TRANS FAT	FIBER	SUGAR
FRESH										
greens cooked w/o salt	½ cup	19	tr	0	tr	tr	tr	–	2	tr
sliced cooked	½ cup	37	tr	0	tr	tr	tr	–	2	7
whole cooked	2 med (3.5 oz)	44	tr	0	tr	tr	tr	–	2	8

BEVERAGES (see ALCOHOL DRINKS, BEER AND ALE, CHAMPAGNE, COFFEE, DRINK MIXERS, ENERGY DRINKS, FRUIT DRINKS, ICED TEA, MALT, MILKSHAKE, SMOOTHIES, SODA, TEA/HERBAL TEA, WATER, WINE, YOGURT DRINKS)

BISCUIT

FOOD	PORTION	CALS	TOTAL FAT	CHOL	SAT FAT	POLY FAT	MONO FAT	TRANS FAT	FIBER	SUGAR
MIX										
plain as prep	1 (2 oz)	190	7	2	2	2	2	–	1	–
Bisquick										
Heart Smart	⅓ cup (1.4 oz)	140	3	0	0	1	2	0	tr	3
REFRIGERATED										
plain baked	1 (1 oz)	93	4	0	1	1	2	–	tr	tr
Immaculate Baking Co.										
Buttermilk	1 (2 oz)	170	7	0	5	–	–	0	0	4
TAKE-OUT										
buttermilk	1 lg (2.7 oz)	280	13	1	2	5	5	–	1	1
plain	1 sm (1.2 oz)	127	6	0	1	2	2	–	1	tr
tea biscuit	1 (3 oz)	210	3	0	2	–	–	–	1	12
w/ egg	1 (4.8 oz)	373	22	245	5	6	9	–	1	–
w/ egg & bacon	1 (5.3 oz)	458	31	353	8	7	13	–	1	1
w/ egg & ham	1 (6.7 oz)	442	27	300	6	8	11	–	1	2
w/ egg & sausage	1 (6.3 oz)	581	39	302	15	4	16	–	1	1
w/ egg & steak	1 (5.2 oz)	410	28	272	9	6	12	–	–	–
w/ egg cheese & bacon	1 (5.1 oz)	477	31	261	11	3	14	–	–	–
w/ ham	1 (4 oz)	386	18	25	11	1	5	–	1	1
w/ sausage	1 (4.4 oz)	485	32	35	14	3	13	–	1	1

BISON (see BUFFALO)

BLACK BEANS

FOOD	PORTION	CALS	TOTAL FAT	CHOL	SAT FAT	POLY FAT	MONO FAT	TRANS FAT	FIBER	SUGAR
dried cooked w/o salt	1 cup (6 oz)	227	1	0	tr	tr	tr	–	15	–
Bush's										
Black Beans	½ cup (4.6 oz)	105	1	0	0	–	–	0	6	1
Reduced Sodium	½ cup (4.6 oz)	105	1	0	0	–	–	0	6	1

BLACKBERRIES

FOOD	PORTION	CALS	TOTAL FAT	CHOL	SAT FAT	POLY FAT	MONO FAT	TRANS FAT	FIBER	SUGAR
canned in heavy syrup	½ cup	118	tr	0	tr	tr	tr	–	4	25
fresh	½ cup	31	tr	0	tr	tr	tr	–	4	4
unsweetened frzn	½ cup	48	tr	0	tr	tr	tr	–	4	8

FOOD	PORTION	CALS	TOTAL FAT	CHOL	SAT FAT	POLY FAT	MONO FAT	TRANS FAT	FIBER	SUGAR
Dole										
Fresh	1 cup (5.1 oz)	60	1	0	0	–	–	0	8	7
Marion frzn	1 cup (4.9 oz)	90	0	0	0	0	0	0	7	15
BLACKBERRY JUICE										
canned	6 oz	65	1	0	tr	1	tr	–	tr	13
BLACKEYE PEAS										
CANNED										
cowpeas	1 cup (8.4 oz)	185	1	0	tr	1	tr	–	8	–
w/pork	1 cup (8.4 oz)	199	4	17	1	1	2	–	8	–
Bush's										
Blackeye Peas	½ cup (4.6 oz)	75	0	0	0	0	0	0	3	0
Blackeye Peas w/ Bacon	½ cup (4.6 oz)	95	2	0	0	–	–	0	3	0
DRIED										
catjang cooked w/o salt	1 cup (6 oz)	200	1	0	tr	1	tr	–	6	–
cooked w/o salt	1 cup (5.8 oz)	160	1	0	tr	tr	tr	–	8	5
FRESH										
cowpeas leafy tips chopped cooked w/o salt	1 cup (1.9 oz)	12	tr	0	tr	tr	tr	–	–	–
TAKE-OUT										
blackeye peas & pork	1 cup (6.3 oz)	236	5	27	2	1	2	–	8	4
frijol de ojo negro guisados	1 cup (9.1 oz)	289	3	0	1	1	1	–	9	6
hopping john	1 cup (7.9 oz)	419	20	20	7	3	9	–	6	3
BLINTZE										
Golden										
Cheese	1 (2.1 oz)	80	2	15	1	–	–	0	2	5
Tofutti										
Mintz's Blintzes Dairy Free	1 (2 oz)	140	5	0	1	–	–	0	2	16
TAKE-OUT										
cheese	1 (2.7 oz)	160	9	65	4	–	–	–	tr	4
BLUEBERRIES										
canned in heavy syrup	½ cup	113	tr	0	tr	tr	tr	–	2	26
fresh	½ cup	41	tr	0	tr	tr	tr	–	2	7
fresh	1 pt	229	1	0	tr	1	tr	–	10	40
frzn unsweetened	½ cup	40	1	0	tr	tr	tr	–	2	7
Dole										
Blueberries frzn	1 pkg (3 oz)	50	1	0	0	–	–	0	2	7
Blueberries frzn	1 cup (4.9 oz)	70	1	0	0	–	–	0	4	12

FOOD	PORTION	CALS	TOTAL FAT	CHOL	SAT FAT	POLY FAT	MONO FAT	TRANS FAT	FIBER	SUGAR
Top Crop										
Fresh	1 cup (4.9 oz)	80	0	0	0	0	0	0	5	9
BLUEFIN										
fillet baked	4.1 oz	186	6	88	1	2	3	–	0	0
BLUEFISH										
fresh baked	3 oz	135	5	64	1	1	2	–	0	0
BOK CHOY (see CABBAGE)										
BONITO										
dried	1 oz	50	2	13	tr	1	1	0	0	0
BORAGE										
fresh chopped	1 cup	19	tr	0	tr	tr	tr	–	–	–
BOTTLED WATER (see WATER)										
BOYSENBERRIES										
frzn unsweetened	½ cup	33	tr	0	tr	tr	tr	–	4	5
in heavy syrup	½ cup	113	tr	0	tr	tr	tr	–	3	–
BRAINS										
beef pan fried	3 oz	167	13	1696	3	2	3	–	0	0
beef simmered	3 oz	123	9	2635	3	tr	2	–	0	0
lamb braised	3 oz	123	9	1737	2	1	2	0	0	0
lamb fried	3 oz	232	19	2128	5	2	3	0	0	0
pork braised	3 oz	117	8	2169	2	1	1	–	0	0
veal braised	3 oz	116	8	2635	2	1	1	0	0	0
veal fried	3 oz	181	14	1802	3	2	4	0	0	0
BRAN										
corn	1 cup (2.7 oz)	170	1	0	tr	tr	tr	–	65	–
oat	½ cup (1.6 oz)	116	3	0	1	1	1	–	7	–
oat cooked	½ cup (3.8 oz)	44	1	0	tr	tr	tr	–	3	–
rice	½ cup (2.1 oz)	187	12	0	2	4	4	–	12	–
wheat	½ cup (2 oz)	63	1	0	tr	1	tr	–	12	–
Mother's										
Oat Bran not prep	½ cup (1.4 oz)	150	3	0	1	1	1	0	6	1
BRAZIL NUTS										
dried unblanched	1 oz	186	19	0	5	7	7	–	–	–

FOOD	PORTION	CALS	TOTAL FAT	CHOL.	SAT FAT	POLY FAT	MONO FAT	TRANS FAT	FIBER	SUGAR
BREAD										
CANNED										
boston brown	1 slice (1.6 oz)	88	1	0	tr	tr	tr	–	2	5
FROZEN										
Kineret										
Challah Pull Apart	1 piece	140	3	0	0	–	–	0	3	2
Pepperidge Farm										
Garlic Toast	1 slice	150	7	0	3	–	–	0	1	2
Texas Toast Five Cheese	1 slice	150	7	5	2	–	–	0	2	1
Texas Toast Garlic	1 slice	140	7	0	2	–	–	0	tr	2
Tuscan Sourdough	2 in slice	170	7	0	3	–	–	0	1	1
Soul										
Naan Garlic	1 (3 oz)	340	6	10	3	–	–	0	2	0
Naan Tandoori	1 (3 oz)	320	6	10	3	–	–	0	2	0
Tandoor Chef										
Tandoori Naan	1 piece (3 oz)	182	2	0	1	–	–	0	3	0
MIX										
cornbread	1 piece (2 oz)	188	6	37	2	1	3	–	1	–
READY-TO-EAT										
anadama	1 piece (1.1 oz)	87	1	1	tr	tr	1	–	1	3
baguette whole wheat	2 oz	140	0	0	0	0	0	0	1	tr
cassava	1 piece (3.5 oz)	299	1	0	tr	tr	tr	–	3	3
challah	1 slice (1.4 oz)	115	2	20	1	tr	1	–	1	1
cinnamon	1 slice (0.9 oz)	69	1	0	tr	tr	tr	–	1	1
cracked wheat	1 slice (1.1 oz)	78	1	0	tr	tr	1	–	2	–
cuban bread	1 slice (1.1 oz)	83	1	0	tr	tr	tr	–	1	1
french	1 slice (1.1 oz)	88	1	0	tr	tr	tr	–	1	tr
italian	1 loaf (1 lb)	1255	4	0	1	tr	2	–	–	–
navajo fry	1 piece	281	10	6	4	1	4	–	–	2
oat bran	1 slice (1.1 oz)	71	1	0	tr	1	tr	–	1	2
oatmeal	1 slice (0.9 oz)	73	1	0	tr	tr	tr	–	1	2
pan criollo	1 piece (0.9 oz)	69	1	0	tr	tr	tr	–	tr	tr
panettone	1 slice (0.9 oz)	86	2	18	1	tr	1	–	1	5
pita	1 sm (1 oz)	77	tr	0	tr	tr	tr	–	1	tr
pita	1 lg (2 oz)	165	1	0	tr	tr	tr	–	1	1
pita whole wheat	1 sm (1 oz)	74	1	0	tr	tr	tr	–	2	tr
pita whole wheat	1 lg (2.2 oz)	170	2	0	tr	1	tr	–	5	1
pumpernickel	1 slice (0.9 oz)	65	1	0	tr	tr	tr	–	2	tr
raisin	1 slice (1.1 oz)	88	1	0	tr	tr	1	–	1	2

FOOD	PORTION	CALS	TOTAL FAT	CHOL	SAT FAT	POLY FAT	MONO FAT	TRANS FAT	FIBER	SUGAR
rye	1 slice (1.1 oz)	83	1	0	tr	tr	tr	–	2	tr
seven grain	1 slice (1.1 oz)	80	1	0	tr	tr	tr	–	2	3
wheat berry	1 slice (0.9 oz)	65	1	0	tr	tr	tr	–	1	1
wheat bran	1 slice (1.3 oz)	89	1	0	tr	tr	1	–	1	3
wheat germ	1 slice (1 oz)	73	1	0	tr	tr	tr	–	1	1
white cubed	1 cup	93	1	0	tr	tr	tr	–	1	2
whole wheat	1 slice (1 oz)	69	1	0	tr	tr	tr	–	2	6
Arnold										
Pocket Thins Flatbread 100% Whole Wheat	½ (1.5 oz)	100	2	0	0	1	0	0	5	2
Farm To Market Bread										
100% Whole Wheat	1 slice	110	0	0	0	0	0	0	3	3
Grains Galore	1 slice (2 oz)	140	4	0	0	2	1	0	3	4
San Francisco Sour Dough	1 slice (1.4 oz)	90	0	0	0	0	0	0	1	0
Food For Life										
Ezekiel 4:9 Flax Sprouted Grain Organic	1 slice (1.2 oz)	80	1	0	0	–	–	0	4	0
Garden Of Eatin'										
Pita Organic Bible Bread Original	1 (2 oz)	145	1	0	0	–	–	0	1	1
Kontos										
Pocket-Less Pita Whole Wheat	1 (2.8 oz)	210	2	0	1	–	–	0	4	4
La Tortilla Factory										
Smart & Delicious Soft Wraps Multi Grain	1 (2.2 oz)	100	4	0	1	0	2	0	12	1
Smart & Delicious Soft Wraps Tomato Basil	1 (2.2 oz)	100	3	0	0	0	2	0	12	1
Smart & Delicious Soft Wraps Traditional	1 (2.2 oz)	90	3	0	0	0	2	0	13	tr
Smart & Delicious Soft Wraps Whole Grain	1 (2.2 oz)	170	4	0	1	0	2	0	5	1
Smart & Delicious Soft Wraps Whole Grain White	1 (2.2 oz)	100	3	0	0	0	2	0	13	0
Levy's										
Real Jewish Rye Everything	1 slice (1.1 oz)	90	2	0	0	–	–	0	tr	1
Manna Organics										
Banana Walnut Hemp	1 slice (2 oz)	140	3	0	0	2	1	0	2	12
Carrot Raisin	1 slice (2 oz)	130	0	0	0	0	0	–	5	10
Fig Fennel Flax	1 slice (2 oz)	120	2	0	0	1	0	0	5	8

FOOD	PORTION	CALS	TOTAL FAT	CHOL	SAT FAT	POLY FAT	MONO FAT	TRANS FAT	FIBER	SUGAR
Millet Rice	1 slice (2 oz)	130	0	0	0	0	0	0	5	9
Whole Rye	1 slice (2 oz)	150	0	0	0	0	0	0	5	7
Matthew's										
Golden White	1 slice (1.1 oz)	90	1	0	0	0	0	0	tr	2
Honey 12 Grain	1 slice (1.1 oz)	80	2	0	0	1	0	0	1	3
Nature's Own										
100% Whole Grain	1 slice (0.9 oz)	70	2	0	0	1	0	0	2	2
100% Whole Grain Sugar Free	1 slice (0.9 oz)	50	1	0	0	0	0	0	2	0
12 Grain	1 slice (1.5 oz)	100	2	0	0	1	0	0	3	3
40 Calorie 9 Grain	1 slice (0.8 oz)	40	1	0	0	tr	0	0	3	1
Cinnamon Raisin Swirl	2 slices (2 oz)	160	3	0	1	1	1	0	2	13
Double Fiber	1 slice (1 oz)	50	1	0	0	–	–	0	5	tr
Honey Wheat	1 slice (0.9 oz)	70	1	0	0	0	0	0	tr	2
Oatmeal Toasters Cinnamon Raisin	1 (2.3 oz)	170	2	0	0	1	0	0	4	9
Oatmeal Toasters Cranberry Orange	1 (2.3 oz)	160	2	0	0	1	0	0	4	9
Thin Sandwich Rounds 100% Whole Wheat	1 (1.5 oz)	100	1	0	0	1	0	0	5	3
Pepperidge Farm										
100% Whole Wheat	1 slice	100	2	0	1	1	0	0	4	3
15 Grain Whole Grain	1 slice	100	2	0	1	1	1	0	4	3
Ancient Grains	1 slice	100	2	0	0	1	0	0	4	3
Cinnamon Swirl	1 slice	80	2	0	0	1	0	0	tr	4
Cinnamon Swirl Raisin	1 slice	80	2	0	0	1	0	0	tr	5
Deli Swirl	1 slice	80	1	0	0	1	0	0	1	tr
Farmhouse Hearty White	1 slice	120	2	0	1	1	0	0	1	4
Farmhouse Honey Wheat	1 slice (1.5 oz)	120	2	0	1	1	0	0	2	5
Farmhouse Oatmeal	1 slice (1.5 oz)	120	2	0	1	0	1	0	1	3
Farmhouse Sourdough	1 slice	120	2	0	1	1	0	0	1	2
Farmhouse Whole Grain White	1 slice	110	2	0	1	1	0	0	3	4
German Dark Wheat	1 slice	100	2	0	0	1	1	0	3	2
Goldfish 100% Whole Wheat	2 slices	100	2	0	1	1	0	0	4	3
Goldfish Soft White	2 slices	100	1	0	1	0	0	0	4	4
Hearty Oatmeal	1 slice	100	2	0	0	1	0	0	4	3
Italian w/ Sesame Seeds	1 slice	90	1	0	0	1	0	0	tr	1
Jewish Rye Party	5 slices	130	2	0	0	1	0	0	2	1
Jewish Rye Seeded	1 slice	80	1	0	0	0	0	0	2	1

FOOD	PORTION	CALS	TOTAL FAT	CHOL	SAT FAT	POLY FAT	MONO FAT	TRANS FAT	FIBER	SUGAR
Light Style Extra Fiber Wheat	1 slice	120	1	0	0	0	0	0	6	3
Pumpernickel	1 slice	80	1	0	0	1	0	0	1	1
Swirl Cinnamon Raisin 100% Whole Wheat	1 slice (1 oz)	80	1	0	0	1	0	0	2	4
Swirled White & Wheat	1 slice (1.5 oz)	110	2	0	0	1	0	0	2	4
Stonefire										
Naan Original	½ (2.2 oz)	190	5	5	2	–	–	0	1	2
Naan Whole Grain	½ (2.2 oz)	180	5	5	2	–	–	0	4	3
Pita Original	½ (1.6 oz)	120	1	0	0	–	–	0	1	2
Pita Whole Grain	½ (1.6 oz)	120	1	0	0	–	–	0	3	3
Tandoori Roti White	½ (1.6 oz)	150	6	0	1	–	–	0	1	2
Tandoori Roti Whole Grain	½ (1.6 oz)	150	6	0	1	–	–	0	3	2
Tumaro's										
Deli Style Wraps Cracked Pepper	1 (2.1 oz)	100	3	0	1	–	–	0	12	1
Deli Style Wraps Everything	1 (2.1 oz)	80	3	0	0	–	–	0	10	1
Deli Style Wraps Pumpernickel	1 (2.1 oz)	80	2	0	0	–	–	0	9	1
Deli Style Wraps Rye	1 (2.1 oz)	80	2	0	0	–	–	0	9	1
Deli Style Wraps Sour Dough	1 (2.1 oz)	80	2	0	0	–	–	0	9	1
Wonder										
100% Whole Wheat Soft	2 slices (1.6 oz)	110	2	0	0	–	–	0	3	3
Classic White	1 slice (1 oz)	70	1	0	0	0	0	0	0	2
Light White	1 slice (0.8 oz)	40	0	0	0	0	0	0	2	2
Smart White	1 slice (0.9 oz)	50	1	0	0	0	0	0	2	2
Texas Toast	1 slice (1.4 oz)	100	1	0	0	0	0	0	tr	2
Whole Grain White	2 slices (2 oz)	140	2	0	1	1	0	0	3	5
TAKE-OUT										
banana	1 slice (2 oz)	196	6	26	1	2	3	–	1	–
chapati as prep w/ fat	1 (1.6 oz)	95	2	3	1	–	–	–	3	1
cornbread	1 piece (2.3 oz)	183	6	26	1	3	2	–	2	4
cornstick	1 (1.4 oz)	118	4	17	1	2	1	–	1	3
focaccia onion	1 piece (4.6 oz)	282	10	0	1	1	7	–	2	2
focaccia rosemary	1 piece (3.5 oz)	251	7	0	1	1	5	–	2	1
focaccia tomato olive	1 piece (4.7 oz)	270	8	0	1	1	6	–	2	1
garlic bread	1 slice (1 oz)	96	4	0	1	1	2	–	1	tr

FOOD	PORTION	CALS	TOTAL FAT	CHOL.	SAT FAT	POLY FAT	MONO FAT	TRANS FAT	FIBER	SUGAR
irish soda bread	1 slice (3 oz)	247	4	15	1	1	2	–	2	–
italian garlic	1 loaf (11 oz)	990	38	0	7	11	18	–	8	1
naan	1 bread (3.5 oz)	286	9	46	5	–	–	–	2	3
papadum fried	1 (6 g)	30	2	0	1	tr	1	–	tr	–
paratha plain	1 (1.6 oz)	136	5	19	3	tr	2	–	2	–
poori indian puffed bread	1 piece (1.3 oz)	112	4	0	2	1	1	–	2	tr
zucchini	1 slice (1.4 oz)	150	7	26	1	4	2	–	1	10

BREADCRUMBS

dry seasoned	¼ cup	115	2	0	tr	1	tr	–	2	2
fresh	¼ cup	30	tr	0	tr	tr	tr	–	tr	tr
plain	¼ cup	107	1	0	tr	1	tr	–	1	2

Progresso

Italian Style	¼ cup (1 oz)	110	2	0	1	–	–	0	1	2
Panko Lemon Pepper	¼ cup (1 oz)	120	5	0	0	–	–	0	tr	0
Panko Plain	¼ cup (1 oz)	110	3	0	0	–	–	0	0	1
Plain	¼ cup (1 oz)	110	2	0	1	–	–	0	1	2

BREADFRUIT

fresh	1 sm (13.5 oz)	396	1	0	tr	tr	tr	–	19	42
fried	1 cup	379	21	0	3	10	7	–	9	21
raw	1 cup	227	1	0	tr	tr	tr	–	11	24

BREADNUTTREE SEEDS

dried	1 oz	104	tr	0	tr	tr	tr	–	–	–

BREADSTICKS

plain	1 lg	41	1	0	tr	tr	tr	–	tr	tr
plain	1 sm	21	tr	0	tr	tr	tr	–	tr	tr

BREAKFAST BARS (see CEREAL BARS, ENERGY BARS)

BREAKFAST DRINKS

Carnation

Breakfast Essentials Classic French Vanilla	1 bottle (11.4 oz)	250	5	10	2	–	–	0	0	31
Breakfast Essentials Classic French Vanilla as prep w/ fat free milk	1 serv	220	0	9	0	–	–	0	0	18
Breakfast Essentials Rich Chocolate Milk as prep w/ fat free milk	1 serv	220	1	9	tr	–	–	0	tr	19

FOOD	PORTION	CALS	TOTAL FAT	CHOL	SAT FAT	POLY FAT	MONO FAT	TRANS FAT	FIBER	SUGAR
Breakfast Essentials Rich Milk Chocolate	1 bottle (11.4 oz)	260	5	10	2	–	–	0	1	39
Breakfast Essentials Vanilla No Sugar Added as prep w/ fat free milk	1 serv	150	0	9	0	–	–	0	3	8

BROCCOFLOWER

FOOD	PORTION	CALS	TOTAL FAT	CHOL	SAT FAT	POLY FAT	MONO FAT	TRANS FAT	FIBER	SUGAR
fresh flowerets cooked	1 cup (2.9 oz)	26	tr	0	tr	tr	tr	–	3	3
fresh raw	1 cup (2.2 oz)	20	tr	0	tr	tr	tr	–	2	2
head fresh raw	1 lg (18 oz)	158	2	0	tr	1	tr	–	16	15

BROCCOLI
FRESH

FOOD	PORTION	CALS	TOTAL FAT	CHOL	SAT FAT	POLY FAT	MONO FAT	TRANS FAT	FIBER	SUGAR
chinese broccoli (gai lan) cooked	1 cup (3 oz)	19	1	0	tr	tr	tr	–	2	1
cooked w/o salt chopped	½ cup (2.7 oz)	27	tr	0	tr	tr	tr	–	3	1
cooked w/o salt spear 5 in	1 (1.3 oz)	13	tr	0	tr	tr	tr	–	1	1
raab cooked	½ cup (3 oz)	28	tr	0	tr	tr	tr	0	2	1
raw	1 bunch (1.3 lbs)	207	2	0	tr	tr	tr	–	16	10
raw floweret	1 (0.4 oz)	3	tr	0	tr	tr	tr	–	–	–
raw flowers	1 cup (2.5 oz)	20	tr	0	tr	tr	tr	–	–	–
raw spear 5 in long	1 (1.1 oz)	11	tr	0	tr	tr	tr	–	1	1
Dole										
Broccoli	1 stalk (5.2 oz)	50	1	0	0	–	–	0	4	3
Broccoli Slaw	1 cup (3 oz)	25	0	0	0	0	0	0	2	2
Eat Smart										
Beneforte	1 serv (3 oz)	25	0	0	0	0	0	0	2	2
Florets	1 serv (3 oz)	25	0	0	0	0	0	0	2	2
Mann's										
Broccoli Wokly	1 serv (3 oz)	25	0	0	0	0	0	0	2	2
Broccolini	8 stalks (3 oz)	35	0	0	0	0	0	0	1	2
Ready Pac										
Microwave Broccoli Rabe as prep	½ cup (3 oz)	30	0	0	0	0	0	0	2	0
River Ranch										
Florets	¼ pkg (3 oz)	25	0	0	0	0	0	0	2	1
FROZEN										
chopped cooked w/o salt	1 cup (6.5 oz)	52	tr	0	tr	tr	tr	–	6	3
spears cooked w/o salt	1 cup (6.5 oz)	52	tr	0	tr	tr	tr	–	6	3

FOOD	PORTION	CALS	TOTAL FAT	CHOL	SAT FAT	POLY FAT	MONO FAT	TRANS FAT	FIBER	SUGAR
Lisa's Organics										
Florets In Gorgonzola Bleu Cheese Sauce	½ pkg (4 oz)	60	3	0	1	–	–	0	2	1
TAKE-OUT										
batter dipped & fried	3 pieces (1.4 oz)	58	4	7	1	1	2	–	1	1
w/ cheese sauce	1 cup (8 oz)	242	15	32	7	2	5	–	5	5
BROWNIE										
brownie	1 (2 oz)	227	9	10	2	1	5	–	1	21
butterscotch	1 (1.2 oz)	151	8	20	1	3	3	–	tr	12
Fiber One										
Chocolate Peanut Butter	1 (0.89 oz)	90	35	0	2	–	–	0	5	7
Chocolate Fudge	1 (0.89 oz)	90	3	0	2	–	–	0	5	8
French Meadow Bakery										
Gluten Free Fudge	1 (2.82 oz)	350	16	55	2	–	–	0	2	34
Jiffy										
Fudge Mix as prep	⅛ pkg	160	7	21	2	–	–	1	tr	15
No Pudge!										
All Flavors as prep	1/12 pkg	120	0	0	0	0	0	0	1	22
Sans Sucre										
Blondie Mix as prep	⅛ pkg	130	0	3	0	–	–	0	0	0
Chocolate Fudge Mix as prep	⅛ pkg	130	3	0	0	–	–	0	tr	0
Milk Chocolate Mix as prep	⅛ pkg	130	3	0	0	–	–	0	0	1
Sheila G's										
Brownie Brittle Chocolate Chip	6 pieces (1 oz)	120	4	0	1	–	–	0	tr	14
Brownie Brittle Toffee Crunch	6 pieces (1 oz)	120	4	0	1	–	–	0	tr	14
Brownie Brittle Traditional Walnut	6 pieces (1 oz)	120	4	0	1	–	–	0	tr	13
BRUSSELS SPROUTS										
CANNED										
Jake & Amos										
Pickled Dill Brussels Sprouts	2 tbsp	10	0	0	0	0	0	0	0	0
FRESH										
cooked	6 pieces	45	1	0	tr	tr	tr	–	3	2
Dole										
Brussels Sprouts	4 (2.9 oz)	30	0	0	0	0	0	0	3	1

FOOD	PORTION	CALS	TOTAL FAT	CHOL	SAT FAT	POLY FAT	MONO FAT	TRANS FAT	FIBER	SUGAR
Eat Smart										
Brussels Sprouts	1 serv (3 oz)	35	0	0	0	0	0	0	3	2
FROZEN										
cooked	1 cup	65	1	0	tr	tr	tr	–	6	3
Green Giant										
Seasoned Steamers w/ Sea Salt & Black Pepper as prep	½ cup	70	3	0	0	–	–	0	3	2
BUCKWHEAT										
groats roasted cooked	1 cup (6 oz)	155	1	0	tr	tr	tr	0	5	2
groats roasted uncooked	½ cup	292	3	0	1	1	1	–	9	–
Wolff's										
Kasha not prep	¼ cup (1.6 oz)	170	1	0	0	–	–	0	2	0
BUFFALO (see also HOT DOG, JERKY, SAUSAGE)										
burger	3 oz	202	13	71	5	1	5	0	0	0
chuck braised	4 oz	205	6	118	2	tr	2	0	0	0
top round steak broiled	3 oz	313	9	153	4	tr	3	0	0	0
water buffalo roasted	3 oz	111	2	52	1	tr	tr	–	0	0
BULGUR										
cooked	½ cup	76	tr	0	tr	tr	tr	0	4	tr
uncooked	½ cup	239	1	0	tr	tr	tr	0	13	tr
TAKE-OUT										
tabbouleh	1 cup	198	15	0	2	2	11	–	4	2
BURBOT (FISH)										
fresh baked	3 oz	98	1	65	tr	tr	tr	–	0	0
BURDOCK ROOT										
cooked w/o salt	1 root (5.8 oz)	146	tr	0	tr	tr	tr	–	3	6
cooked w/o salt	1 cup	110	tr	0	tr	tr	tr	–	2	4
BUTTER										
clarified butter	1 tbsp (0.4 oz)	112	13	33	8	tr	4	–	0	0
clarified butter	¼ cup (1.8 oz)	449	51	131	32	2	15	0	0	0
ghee cow's milk	1 tbsp	126	14	39	–	–	–	–	0	–
ghee vegetable oil	1 tbsp	126	14	0	–	–	–	–	0	–
honey butter	¼ cup (2.5 oz)	338	23	62	15	1	6	–	tr	35
honey butter	1 tbsp (0.6 oz)	85	6	15	4	tr	2	–	0	9
light butter whipped salted	1 tbsp (0.3 oz)	48	5	10	3	tr	2	–	0	0
stick salted	1 tbsp (0.5 oz)	102	12	31	7	tr	3	–	0	tr
stick salted	1 (4 oz)	810	92	243	58	3	24	–	0	tr

FOOD	PORTION	CALS	TOTAL FAT	CHOL	SAT FAT	POLY FAT	MONO FAT	TRANS FAT	FIBER	SUGAR
stick salted	¼ cup (2 oz)	407	46	122	29	2	12	–	0	tr
stick unsalted	1 (4 oz)	810	92	243	58	3	24	–	0	tr
stick unsalted	¼ cup (2 oz)	407	46	122	29	2	12	–	0	tr
stick unsalted	1 tbsp (0.5 oz)	102	12	31	7	tr	3	–	0	tr
whipped salted	¼ cup (1.3 oz)	271	31	83	19	1	9	–	0	tr
whipped salted	1 tbsp (0.3 oz)	67	8	21	5	2	tr	–	0	tr
Breakstone's										
Salted	1 tbsp (0.5 oz)	100	11	30	7	–	–	0	0	0
Epicurean										
Scampi Butter	1 tbsp (0.5 oz)	90	10	25	6	–	–	0	–	–
Gopi										
Pure Ghee	1 tsp (5 g)	35	5	12	3	–	–	0	0	0
Karoun										
Unsalted	1 tbsp (0.5 oz)	100	11	30	7	tr	3	0	–	0
Land O Lakes										
Butter Spread Cinnamon Sugar	1 tbsp (0.5 oz)	70	6	10	3	–	–	0	0	4
Honey	1 tbsp (0.5 oz)	90	8	15	4	–	–	0	0	3
Roasted Garlic w/ Oil	1 tbsp (0.5 oz)	90	10	20	5	–	–	0	0	0
Plugra										
European Style Unsalted	1 tbsp (0.5 oz)	100	11	30	7	–	–	0	0	0
Straus										
Organic European Style Lightly Salted	1 tbsp (0.5 oz)	110	12	30	8	–	–	0	0	0
Organic European Style Sweet Butter	1 tbsp (0.5 oz)	110	12	30	8	–	–	0	0	0
BUTTER SUBSTITUTES										
stick	1 stick	811	91	99	32	18	37	–	–	–
Melt										
Rich & Creamy Organic	1 tbsp (0.5 oz)	80	9	0	4	1	4	0	0	0
BUTTERBUR										
canned fuki chopped	1 cup	3	tr	0	–	–	–	–	–	–
fresh fuki	1 cup	13	tr	0	–	–	–	–	–	–
BUTTERNUTS										
dried	1 oz	174	16	0	tr	12	3	–	–	–

BUTTERSCOTCH (see CANDY)

FOOD	PORTION	CALS	TOTAL FAT	CHOL	SAT FAT	POLY FAT	MONO FAT	TRANS FAT	FIBER	SUGAR
CABBAGE (see also COLESLAW)										
chinese bok choy shredded cooked w/o salt	1 cup	20	tr	0	tr	tr	tr	0	2	1
chinese pe-tsai shredded cooked w/o salt	1 cup	17	tr	0	tr	tr	tr	0	2	–
green raw shredded	1 cup	19	tr	0	tr	tr	tr	0	2	2
green shredded cooked w/o salt	1 cup	34	tr	0	tr	tr	tr	0	3	4
japanese pickled	½ cup	22	tr	0	tr	tr	tr	0	2	1
red raw shredded	1 cup	22	tr	0	tr	tr	tr	0	2	3
red shredded cooked w/o salt	1 cup	44	tr	0	tr	tr	tr	0	4	5
savoy shredded cooked w/o salt	1 cup	35	tr	0	tr	tr	tr	0	4	–
Dole										
Shredded Red Fresh	1½ cups (3 oz)	25	0	0	0	0	0	0	2	3
Ready Pac										
Ready Fixin's Shredded Red	2 cups (3 oz)	25	0	0	0	0	0	0	2	3
River Ranch										
Angel Hair	1½ cups (3 oz)	25	0	0	0	0	0	0	2	3
TAKE-OUT										
coleslaw w/ pineapple & dressing	1 cup (4.6 oz)	194	16	8	2	8	4	–	2	10
creamed	1 cup	158	10	6	3	3	4	–	2	7
kimchee	1 cup	32	tr	0	tr	tr	tr	0	2	2
stuffed cabbage w/ rice & beef	1 (3.6 oz)	117	5	42	2	tr	2	–	1	4
CACTUS										
fresh cooked w/ fat	1 pad (1 oz)	11	1	0	tr	tr	tr	0	1	tr
fresh cooked w/o fat	1 cup (5.2 oz)	22	tr	0	tr	tr	tr	0	3	2
pricklypear fresh	1 cup (5.2 oz)	61	1	0	tr	tr	tr	0	5	–
pricklypear fresh	1 (3.6 oz)	42	1	0	tr	tr	tr	0	4	–
CAKE (see also CAKE MIX)										
cream puff shell	1 (2.3 oz)	239	17	129	4	5	7	–	–	–
crumpet	1 (2.3 oz)	131	1	0	–	–	–	–	2	–
dutch honey cake	1 slice (0.8 oz)	70	0	0	0	0	0	0	0	8
sponge	1 piece (1.3 oz)	110	1	39	tr	tr	tr	0	tr	14
sponge cake dessert shell	1 (0.8 oz)	70	2	20	1	–	–	–	0	7
turnover guava	1 (2.7 oz)	239	13	0	3	4	5	–	3	12

FOOD	PORTION	CALS	TOTAL FAT	CHOL	SAT FAT	POLY FAT	MONO FAT	TRANS FAT	FIBER	SUGAR
Athens										
Baklava	2 pieces (2 oz)	230	11	0	2	–	–	2	1	17
Balocco										
Il Panettone	1 (3.5 oz)	380	15	120	9	–	–	tr	2	30
Coppenrath										
Mousse Cake Chocolate	⅛ cake (1.8 oz)	140	7	40	4	–	–	0	2	12
Mousse Cake Coconut	⅛ cake (1.8 oz)	140	8	45	5	–	–	0	2	11
Mousse Duets Chocolate	1 (3.2 oz)	290	15	35	9	–	–	0	2	25
Mousse Duets Lemon Chiffon	1 (3.2 oz)	280	16	35	9	–	–	0	tr	23
Entenmann's										
Apple Puffs	1 (3 oz)	290	13	0	6	–	–	0	1	21
Blackout Iced	⅛ cake (2.2 oz)	210	8	30	3	–	–	0	1	23
Cheese Buns	1 (3 oz)	320	15	40	6	–	–	0	1	22
Chocolate Chip Iced	⅛ cake (2.5 oz)	330	18	25	7	–	–	0	tr	31
Chocolate Fudge	⅛ cake (2.2 oz)	240	10	25	4	–	–	0	2	28
Cinnamon Swirl Buns	1 (3 oz)	320	14	35	5	–	–	0	2	21
Coffee Cake Cheese Filled Crumb	⅛ cake (2 oz)	210	10	25	4	–	–	0	tr	13
Danish Twist Cheese	⅛ cake (1.9 oz)	220	11	20	4	–	–	0	tr	14
Danish Twist Raspberry	⅛ cake (1.8 oz)	210	10	15	4	–	–	0	tr	14
Devil's Food Marshmallow Iced	⅛ cake (2.2 oz)	260	12	20	5	–	–	0	tr	30
Fudge Iced Golden Cake	⅛ cake (2.2 oz)	260	11	25	4	–	–	0	1	28
Lemon Crunch	⅛ cake (3 oz)	320	13	45	4	–	–	0	tr	35
Lemon Loaf	⅙ cake (2 oz)	210	10	40	2	–	–	0	0	17
Louisiana Crunch	⅛ cake (2.7 oz)	310	13	45	4	–	–	0	tr	33
Utlimate Super Cinnamons	½ bun (2.5 oz)	280	10	25	4	–	–	0	1	19
Vanilla Bean Iced	⅛ cake (2.2 oz)	290	17	25	7	–	–	0	0	28
Kineret										
Babka Chocolate	1 piece (1 oz)	100	3	10	1	–	–	0	1	9

FOOD	PORTION	CALS	TOTAL FAT	CHOL	SAT FAT	POLY FAT	MONO FAT	TRANS FAT	FIBER	SUGAR
Nature's Path										
Toaster Pastries Blueberry Organic	1 (1.8 oz)	210	5	0	2	–	–	0	1	18
Toaster Pastries Frosted Brown Sugar Maple Cinnamon Organic	1 (1.8 oz)	210	5	0	3	–	–	0	1	20
Toaster Pastries Frosted Chocolate Organic	1 (1.8 oz)	210	5	0	3	–	–	0	1	18
Toaster Pastries Frosted Strawberry	1 (1.8 oz)	210	4	0	2	–	–	0	1	19
Pepperidge Farm										
Coconut 3 Layer	⅛ cake	240	10	20	3	–	–	2	tr	25
German Chocolate 3 Layer	⅛ cake	240	10	15	3	–	–	2	1	23
Red Velvet 3 Layer	⅛ cake	230	11	20	3	–	–	2	0	25
Turnover Apple	1	260	13	0	7	–	–	0	1	11
Turnover Cherry	1	260	13	0	7	–	–	0	1	10
Weight Watchers										
Lemon Creme	1 (0.9 oz)	80	3	25	1	–	–	0	4	8
TAKE-OUT										
angelfood	1 slice (2 oz)	143	tr	0	tr	tr	tr	0	tr	17
apple crisp	1 serv (8.6 oz)	384	8	0	1	3	3	0	4	49
apple turnover	1 (6.6 oz)	661	34	0	7	11	15	–	3	30
baklava	1 piece (2.7 oz)	334	23	35	10	4	8	0	2	10
basbousa namoura	1 piece (1 oz)	60	3	0	0	–	–	–	2	10
bean cake	1 cake (1.1 oz)	130	7	0	1	3	3	0	1	7
black forest chocolate cherry	1 piece (2.5 oz)	187	9	30	4	2	3	0	1	23
boston cream pie	1 slice (3.2 oz)	232	8	34	2	1	4	0	1	33
carrot w/ icing	1 slice (4.7 oz)	543	28	80	5	12	9	0	2	52
cheesecake	1 slice (4.5 oz)	410	25	86	10	4	9	0	tr	28
cheesecake chocolate	1 slice (4.5 oz)	489	32	118	15	4	11	0	2	29
chinese moon cake	1 (4.8 oz)	458	6	69	1	2	1	0	4	49
cobbler pineapple	1 cup (7.6 oz)	414	10	2	3	3	4	–	2	45
coconut mochiko filipino cake	1 piece (2.7 oz)	252	12	0	10	tr	1	0	2	11
coffeecake iced	1 piece (1.6 oz)	175	8	31	1	4	2	0	1	15
cream puff custard filled chocolate frosted	1 (3.9 oz)	293	18	142	5	4	7	0	1	7

FOOD	PORTION	CALS	TOTAL FAT	CHOL	SAT FAT	POLY FAT	MONO FAT	TRANS FAT	FIBER	SUGAR
eclair	1 (3.5 oz)	262	16	127	4	4	6	0	1	7
french apple tart	1 (3.5 oz)	302	15	60	9	1	4	–	2	15
fruitcake	1 slice (1.5 oz)	139	4	2	tr	1	2	0	2	13
funnel cake	1 (3.2 oz)	276	14	62	3	6	5	0	1	4
gingerbread	1 piece (2.4 oz)	213	7	24	2	1	4	0	1	22
jelly roll	1 slice (1.8 oz)	146	2	93	1	tr	1	0	tr	20
jelly roll lemon filled	1 slice (3 oz)	210	2	35	1	1	1	–	tr	29
napoleon	1 (3 oz)	348	25	39	7	11	6	0	1	4
napoleon	1 mini (1 oz)	123	9	14	2	4	2	0	tr	1
panettone	1/12 cake (2.9 oz)	300	12	90	9	–	–	–	2	21
petit fours	2 (0.9 oz)	120	7	0	3	–	–	–	0	12
pineapple upside down	1 piece (4.2 oz)	387	15	27	4	4	6	0	1	41
pound	1 slice (1 oz)	120	5	32	1	2	2	–	–	–
pound fat free	1 slice (2 oz)	160	1	0	tr	tr	tr	0	1	19
pumpkin bread w/ raisins	1 slice (2.1 oz)	178	4	26	1	2	2	–	1	22
red velvet cupcake w/ cream cheese frosting	1 sm	272	12	63	–	–	–	–	1	–
red velvet w/ cream cheese frosting	1/16 cake	520	24	117	–	–	–	–	1	–
sacher torte	1 slice (2.2 oz)	240	11	50	5	–	–	–	4	11
strawberry shortcake	1 serv (4.1 oz)	211	5	109	2	tr	2	0	1	35
strudel apple	1 piece (2.2 oz)	175	7	4	1	3	2	0	1	16
strudel cheese	1 piece (2.2 oz)	195	8	42	4	1	3	0	tr	14
strudel cherry	1 piece (2.2 oz)	179	6	9	1	3	2	0	1	18
strudel pineapple	1 piece (2.2 oz)	159	4	10	1	1	2	–	1	22
sweet potato w/ glaze	1 piece (2.7 oz)	275	12	40	2	7	3	–	1	26
tiramisu	1 piece (5.1 oz)	409	30	171	15	–	–	–	tr	17
tiramisu	1 cake (4.4 lbs)	5732	421	2395	217	–	–	–	3	234
torte chocolate ganache	1 slice (3.5 oz)	400	26	90	10	–	–	–	6	24

FOOD	PORTION	CALS	TOTAL FAT	CHOL	SAT FAT	POLY FAT	MONO FAT	TRANS FAT	FIBER	SUGAR
white w/ coconut icing	1 slice (3.9 oz)	399	12	1	4	2	4	–	1	64
zucchini bread	1 slice (1.4 oz)	150	7	26	1	3	3	0	1	10
CAKE ICING										
chocolate	¼ cup	269	7	1	2	2	3	0	1	51
vanilla	¼ cup	322	8	0	2	2	4	0	0	62
Pillsbury										
Chocolate Fudge Sugar Free	2 tbsp (1 oz)	100	6	0	2	–	–	2	3	0
Creamy Supreme Buttercream	2 tbsp (1.2 oz)	150	6	0	2	–	–	2	0	22
Creamy Supreme Classic White	2 tbsp (1.2 oz)	150	6	6	2	–	–	2	0	0
Creamy Supreme Coconut Pecan	2 tbsp (1.2 oz)	160	10	0	4	–	–	2	tr	16
Creamy Supreme Milk Chocolate	2 tbsp (1.2 oz)	140	6	0	2	–	–	2	tr	19
Creamy Supreme Vanilla	2 tbsp (1.2 oz)	150	6	0	2	–	–	2	0	22
Easy Frost Chocolate Fudge	2 tbsp (1.2 oz)	140	6	0	2	–	–	2	tr	19
Easy Frost Cream Cheese	2 tbsp (1.2 oz)	150	6	0	2	–	–	2	0	22
Easy Frost Vanilla	2 tbsp (1.2 oz)	150	6	0	2	–	–	2	0	22
Funfetti Pink Vanilla	2 tbsp (1.2 oz)	140	5	0	2	–	–	2	0	22
Vanilla Sugar Free	2 tbsp (1 oz)	100	6	0	2	–	–	2	3	0
Whipped Supreme Cream Cheese	1 tbsp (0.8 oz)	100	5	0	2	–	–	2	0	14
Whipped Supreme Strawberry	2 tbsp (0.8 oz)	110	5	0	2	–	–	2	0	14
CAKE MIX										
Bisquick										
Heart Smart	⅓ cup (1.4 oz)	140	3	0	0	1	2	0	tr	3
Jell-O										
No Bake Peanut Butter as prep	⅛ cake	360	21	3	9	–	–	0	0	27
No Bake Real Cheesecake as prep	⅛ cake	360	21	3	9	–	–	0	0	27
Jiffy										
Devil's Food as prep	⅕ cake	220	5	42	2	–	–	0	1	23

FOOD	PORTION	CALS	TOTAL FAT	CHOL	SAT FAT	POLY FAT	MONO FAT	TRANS FAT	FIBER	SUGAR
Krusteaz										
Honey Cornbread as prep	1 piece (2x2 in)	140	6	15	3	–	–	0	tr	8
Sans Sucre										
Apple Cinnamon Coffee Cake as prep	½ pkg	150	4	0	0	–	–	0	tr	3

CALZONE (see SANDWICHES)

CANADIAN BACON

FOOD	PORTION	CALS	TOTAL FAT	CHOL	SAT FAT	POLY FAT	MONO FAT	TRANS FAT	FIBER	SUGAR
grilled	2 slices (1.6 oz)	87	4	27	1	tr	2	0	0	0
Oscar Mayer										
Fully Cooked	3 slices (1.9 oz)	60	2	30	1	–	–	0	0	1

CANDY

FOOD	PORTION	CALS	TOTAL FAT	CHOL	SAT FAT	POLY FAT	MONO FAT	TRANS FAT	FIBER	SUGAR
butterscotch	1 piece (6 g)	24	tr	1	tr	0	tr	–	–	–
candied cherries	1 (4 g)	12	tr	0	tr	–	–	–	–	–
candied citron	1 oz	89	tr	0	–	–	–	–	–	–
candied lemon peel	1 oz	90	tr	0	–	–	–	–	–	–
candied orange peel	1 oz	90	tr	0	–	–	–	–	–	–
candied pineapple slice	1 slice (2 oz)	179	tr	0	tr	–	–	–	–	–
candy corn	1 oz	105	0	0	0	0	0	0	–	–
caramels	1 piece (8 g)	31	1	1	1	tr	tr	–	–	–
caramels chocolate	1 piece (6 g)	22	tr	0	tr	tr	tr	–	–	–
dark chocolate	1 oz	150	10	0	6	tr	3	–	–	–
fondant	1 piece (0.6 oz)	57	0	0	–	–	–	0	–	–
fondant chocolate coated	1 piece (0.4 oz)	40	1	0	1	tr	tr	–	–	–
fondant mint	1 oz	105	0	0	0	0	0	0	–	–
fudge brown sugar w/ nuts	1 piece (0.5 oz)	56	1	1	tr	1	tr	–	–	–
fudge chocolate marshmallow	1 piece (0.7 oz)	84	3	5	2	tr	1	–	–	–
fudge chocolate marshmallow w/ nuts	1 piece (0.8 oz)	96	4	5	2	1	1	–	–	–
fudge chocolate w/ nuts	1 piece (0.7 oz)	81	3	3	1	1	1	–	–	–
fudge peanut butter	1 piece (0.6 oz)	59	1	1	tr	tr	tr	–	–	–
fudge vanilla w/ nuts	1 piece (0.5 oz)	62	2	2	1	1	1	–	–	–
gumdrops	10 lg (3.8 oz)	420	0	0	0	0	0	0	–	–
gumdrops	10 sm (0.4 oz)	135	0	0	0	0	0	0	–	–
hard candy	1 oz	106	0	0	0	0	0	0	–	–
jelly beans	10 lg (1 oz)	104	tr	0	–	–	–	–	–	–
jelly beans	10 sm (0.4 oz)	40	tr	0	–	–	–	–	–	–

FOOD	PORTION	CALS	TOTAL FAT	CHOL	SAT FAT	POLY FAT	MONO FAT	TRANS FAT	FIBER	SUGAR
lollipop	1 (6 g)	22	0	0	0	0	0	0	–	–
marzipan	1 oz	128	7	0	1	1	5	–	2	–
milk chocolate	1 bar (1.55 oz)	226	14	10	8	tr	4	–	–	–
milk chocolate crisp	1 bar (1.45 oz)	203	11	8	7	tr	4	–	–	–
milk chocolate w/ almonds	1 bar (1.45 oz)	215	14	8	7	1	6	–	–	20
peanut brittle	1 oz	128	5	4	1	1	2	–	–	–
peanuts chocolate covered	10 (1.4 oz)	208	13	4	6	2	5	–	–	–
peanuts chocolate covered	1 cup (5.2 oz)	773	50	13	22	6	19	–	–	–
praline	1 piece (1.4 oz)	177	10	0	1	2	6	–	–	–
sesame crunch	20 pieces (1.2 oz)	181	12	0	2	5	4	–	–	–
taffy	1 piece (0.5 oz)	56	1	1	tr	tr	tr	–	–	–
toffee	1 piece (0.4 oz)	65	4	13	2	tr	1	–	–	–
truffles	1 piece (0.4 oz)	59	4	6	3	tr	1	–	–	–
3 Musketeers										
Bar	1 (2.1 oz)	260	8	5	5	–	–	0	1	40
Fun Size	3 (1.6 oz)	190	6	5	4	–	–	0	1	30
Minis	7 (1.4 oz)	170	5	5	4	–	–	0	1	27
Mint	1 pkg (1.5 oz)	190	6	5	4	–	–	0	1	26
Altoids										
Cinnamon	3 (2 g)	10	0	0	0	0	0	0	–	2
Azature Chocolates										
Black Diamond Wild Treasure Cocoa	1 pkg (1 oz)	143	10	0	5	–	–	0	2	8
Green Diamond Poire William	1 pkg (1 oz)	130	7	5	5	–	–	0	1	11
Purple Diamond Chai	1 pkg (1 oz)	155	12	0	7	–	–	0	3	9
Brach's										
Bridge Mix	15 pieces (1.4 oz)	190	10	0	5	–	–	0	1	21
Candy Corn	19 (1.4 oz)	140	0	0	0	0	0	0	–	32
Hard Candy Cinnamon	3 (0.6 oz)	70	0	0	0	0	0	0	–	14
Hard Candy Cinnamon Sugar Free	3 (0.6 oz)	35	0	0	0	0	0	0	–	0
Hard Candy Lemon Drops	4 (0.6 oz)	70	0	0	0	0	0	0	–	11
Hard Candy Lemon Drops Sugar Free	4 (0.6 oz)	35	0	0	0	0	0	0	–	0
Mandarin Orange Slices	3 (1.6 oz)	150	0	0	0	0	0	0	–	28
Milk Chocolate Stars	10 (1.3 oz)	190	10	5	7	–	–	0	1	22
Milk Maid Caramels	4 (1.3 oz)	150	4	0	3	–	–	0	0	15

FOOD	PORTION	CALS	TOTAL FAT	CHOL	SAT FAT	POLY FAT	MONO FAT	TRANS FAT	FIBER	SUGAR
Peanut Clusters	3 (1.4 oz)	210	15	5	6	–	–	0	2	16
Sour Gummi Bears	5 (1.3 oz)	120	0	0	0	0	0	0	–	24
Star Brites Peppermints	3 (0.5 oz)	60	0	0	0	0	0	0	–	11
Butterfinger										
Crisp Bar	1 (2.1 oz)	270	11	0	6	–	–	0	1	29
Original Bar	1 (2.1 oz)	270	11	0	6	–	–	0	1	29
Snackerz	1 pkg (1.3 oz)	170	8	0	4	–	–	0	2	15
Coco										
Brain Truffles Orange	1 (0.5 oz)	56	3	2	2	–	–	0	1	5
Preggers Truffles Dark Chocolate	1 (0.5 oz)	56	3	2	2	–	–	0	1	5
Dots										
Gumdrops Fruit	11 (1.4 oz)	130	0	0	0	0	0	0	–	21
Dove										
Cookies & Creme Silky Smooth	1 bar (1.3 oz)	210	12	10	7	–	–	0	0	20
Dark Chocolate & Raspberry Swirl Promises Silky Smooth	1 bar (1.4 oz)	220	14	5	8	–	–	0	2	21
Dark Chocolate Silky Smooth	1 bar (1.4 oz)	220	13	5	8	–	–	0	3	19
Milk Chocolate Almond Promises Silky Smooth	1 bar (1.4 oz)	210	13	5	7	–	–	0	2	19
Milk Chocolate Covered Raisins & Peanuts Silky Smooth	22 pieces (1.4 oz)	210	12	5	6	–	–	0	2	20
Milk Chocolate Peanut Butter Promises Silky Smooth	1 bar (1.4 oz)	220	14	5	8	–	–	0	1	18
Milk Chocolate Silky Smooth	1 bar (1.4 oz)	220	13	15	8	–	–	0	1	22
Droste										
Pastilles Bittersweet Chocolate	8 (1.4 oz)	220	13	<5	8	–	–	0	2	19
Elmer Chocolates										
Assorted	5 (2 oz)	240	10	0	6	–	–	0	1	35
Frankford										
Gold Coins Milk Chocolate	1 pkg (1.5 oz)	220	13	5	8	–	–	0	tr	25
Ginger People										
Ginger Chews Peanut	2 (0.4 oz)	40	1	0	0	–	–	0	0	8
Ginger Chews Spicy Apple	2 (0.4 oz)	40	0	0	0	0	0	0	0	10
Gin-Gins	3 (0.3 oz)	35	0	0	0	0	0	0	0	7
Godiva										
Gems Truffles Milk Chocolate	4 (1.5 oz)	200	13	15	8	–	–	0	tr	18

FOOD	PORTION	CALS	TOTAL FAT	CHOL	SAT FAT	POLY FAT	MONO FAT	TRANS FAT	FIBER	SUGAR
Guylian										
Twists Original Praline	2 (0.8 oz)	130	8	5	4	–	–	0	1	12
Hershey's										
Pot Of Gold Assorted Milk & Dark Chocolate	4 (1.4 oz)	200	12	5	7	–	–	0	1	22
Jelly Belly										
Peas & Carrots	49 (1.4 oz)	140	0	0	0	0	0	0	–	29
KitKat										
Bar Snack Size	3 (1.5 oz)	210	11	<5	7	–	–	0	tr	21
Life Savers										
Gummies 5 Flavors	1 pkg (1.5 oz)	130	0	0	0	0	0	0	–	25
Variety	4 (0.5 oz)	45	0	0	0	0	0	0	–	9
Lindt										
Lindor Truffles Extra Dark Chocolate	3 pieces (1.3 oz)	230	19	<5	13	–	–	0	2	11
M&M's										
Pretzel Fun Size	3 pkg (1.4 oz)	180	6	5	4	–	–	0	1	21
Manischewitz										
Fruit Slices	2 (1.3 oz)	90	0	0	0	0	0	0	0	23
Maple Grove Farms										
Maple	5 pieces (1.5 oz)	160	0	0	0	0	0	0	–	37
Milky Way										
Bar	1 (2 oz)	260	10	5	7	–	–	0	1	35
Fun Size	2 (1.2 oz)	150	6	5	4	–	–	0	0	20
Midnight Bar	1 (1.76)	220	8	5	5	–	–	0	1	29
Midnight Minis	5 (1.4 oz)	180	7	5	4	–	–	0	1	24
Minis	5 (1.5 oz)	190	7	5	4	–	–	0	0	25
Simply Caramel Bar	1 (1.9 oz)	250	11	5	8	–	–	0	0	31
Mounds										
Bar Snack Size	1 (0.6 oz)	80	5	0	4	–	–	0	1	7
Peeps										
Marshmallow Chicks	5 (1.5 oz)	140	0	0	0	0	0	0	–	34
Raisinets										
Candy	¼ cup (1.6 oz)	190	8	5	5	–	–	0	1	28
Red Vines										
Licorice Black Sugar Free	1 bar (2.5 oz)	90	0	0	0	0	0	0	–	8
Licorice Black Twists	1 bar (2.5 oz)	140	0	0	0	0	0	0	–	16
Licorice Red Twists	1 bar (2.5 oz)	140	0	0	0	0	0	0	–	16

FOOD	PORTION	CALS	TOTAL FAT	CHOL	SAT FAT	POLY FAT	MONO FAT	TRANS FAT	FIBER	SUGAR
Russell Stover										
All Dark Assorted	2 pieces (1.2 oz)	150	7	<5	4	–	–	0	1	18
Assorted Chocolates	2 pieces (1.1 oz)	160	7	5	4	–	–	0	1	18
Sadaf										
Halva Pistachio	1 oz	150	8	0	1	–	–	0	1	15
Skinny Cow										
Heavenly Crisp Bar	1 (0.8 oz)	110	4	0	0	–	–	0	1	9
Skittles										
Original	1 pkg (2.2 oz)	250	3	0	3	–	–	0	0	47
Snap Infusion										
Supercandy Bean Multi-Berry	1 pkg (1 oz)	90	0	0	0	0	0	0	0	18
Snickers										
Bar	1 bar (2 oz)	280	14	5	5	–	–	0	1	30
Fun Size	2 (1.2 oz)	160	8	5	3	–	–	0	1	17
Miniatures	4 (1.3 oz)	170	8	5	3	–	–	0	1	18
Sour Jacks										
Original	15 (1.3 oz)	140	0	0	0	0	0	0	0	26
Watermelon	15 (1.4 oz)	140	0	0	0	0	0	0	0	18
Starburst										
Jellybeans	¼ cup (1.5 oz)	150	0	0	0	0	0	0	0	29
Original	8 (1.4 oz)	160	4	0	3	–	–	0	0	23
SunRidge Farms										
Rainbow Drops Milk Chocolate	¼ cup (1.4 oz)	170	10	5	6	–	–	0	1	19
Twix										
Caramel Cookie	1 (1.8 oz)	250	12	5	7	–	–	0	1	24
Fun Size	1 (0.6 oz)	80	4	0	2	–	–	0	0	8
Unreal										
#41 Candy Coated Chocolates	50 (1.5 oz)	190	10	5	6	–	–	0	3	19
#45 Candy Coated Chocolates w/Peanuts	19 (1.5 oz)	200	11	0	5	–	–	0	3	16
#5 Chocolate Caramel Nougat Bar	1 (1.6 oz)	170	7	5	4	–	–	0	5	19
#77 Peanut Butter Cups	2 (1.3 oz)	190	12	5	6	–	–	0	3	11
#8 Chocolate Caramel Peanut Nougat Bar	1 (1.7 oz)	200	12	5	5	–	–	0	5	17

FOOD	PORTION	CALS	TOTAL FAT	CHOL	SAT FAT	POLY FAT	MONO FAT	TRANS FAT	FIBER	SUGAR
Welch's										
Licorice All Flavors	1 pkg (1.8 oz)	170	0	0	0	0	0	0	0	26
Licorice Filled All Flavors	½ pkg (1.8 oz)	170	9	0	0	0	0	0	0	26
Whitman's										
Assorted Chocolates	4 pieces (1.5 oz)	210	10	5	6	–	–	0	1	23
CANTALOUPE										
balls frzn	10 (4.7 oz)	46	tr	0	tr	tr	tr	0	1	11
dried	3.5 pieces (1.4 oz)	140	0	0	0	0	0	0	1	32
fresh cubed	1 cup (5.6 oz)	54	tr	0	tr	tr	tr	0	1	13
melon large	⅛ (3.6 oz)	35	1	0	tr	tr	tr	0	1	8
melon med	⅛ (2.4 oz)	23	tr	0	tr	tr	tr	0	1	5
melon sm	⅛ (1.9 oz)	19	tr	0	tr	tr	tr	0	1	4
Crispy Green										
Freeze-dried	1 pkg (0.35 oz)	40	0	0	0	0	0	0	1	7
Dole										
Fresh	¼ med (4.7 oz)	45	0	0	0	0	0	0	1	11
CANTALOUPE JUICE										
nectar	1 cup (8.8 oz)	155	tr	0	tr	tr	tr	0	1	39
CAPERS										
capers canned	1 tbsp (0.3 oz)	2	tr	0	tr	tr	tr	0	tr	tr
Victoria										
Capers	2 tbsp (1 oz)	100	0	0	0	0	0	0	0	0
CARAWAY										
seed	1 tbsp	22	1	0	tr	tr	tr	0	3	tr
CARDAMOM										
ground	1 tsp	6	tr	0	tr	tr	tr	0	1	–
CARDOON										
fresh cooked w/o salt	1 serv (3.5 oz)	22	tr	0	tr	tr	tr	0	2	–
fresh shredded	1 cup (6.2 oz)	30	tr	0	tr	tr	tr	0	3	–
CARIBOU										
roasted	3 oz	142	4	93	1	1	1	–	0	0
CARISSA										
fresh	1	12	tr	0	–	–	–	–	–	–

FOOD	PORTION	CALS	TOTAL FAT	CHOL	SAT FAT	POLY FAT	MONO FAT	TRANS FAT	FIBER	SUGAR
CAROB										
carob mix	3 tsp	45	0	0	0	0	0	0	–	–
carob mix as prep w/ whole milk	9 oz	195	8	33	5	tr	2	–	–	–
flour	1 tbsp	14	tr	0	tr	tr	tr	–	–	–
flour	1 cup	185	1	0	tr	tr	tr	–	–	–
CARP										
fresh cooked	1 fillet (6 oz)	276	12	143	2	3	5	–	0	0
fresh cooked	3 oz	138	6	72	1	2	3	–	0	0
fresh raw	3 oz	108	5	56	1	1	2	–	0	0
roe raw	1 oz	37	tr	103	–	–	–	–	–	–
CARROT JUICE										
canned	1 cup (8.3 oz)	210	tr	0	tr	tr	tr	–	2	9
CARROTS										
CANNED										
Allens										
Tiny Sliced	½ cup (4.5 oz)	45	0	0	0	0	0	0	3	3
Butter Kernel										
Sliced	½ cup (4.3 oz)	35	0	0	0	0	0	0	3	5
DRIED										
dehydrated	¼ cup (0.6 oz)	63	tr	0	tr	tr	tr	–	4	7
FRESH										
baby raw	1 (0.5 oz)	6	tr	0	tr	tr	tr	–	–	–
diced	½ cup (2.2 oz)	26	tr	0	tr	tr	tr	–	2	3
large raw	1 (2.5 oz)	30	tr	0	tr	tr	tr	–	2	3
medium raw	1 (2.1 oz)	25	tr	0	tr	tr	tr	–	2	3
raw shredded	½ cup (1.9 oz)	23	tr	0	tr	tr	tr	–	2	3
slices cooked w/o salt	½ cup (2.7 oz)	27	tr	0	tr	tr	tr	–	2	3
small raw	1 (1.8 oz)	20	tr	0	tr	tr	tr	–	1	2
Crunch Pak										
Baby Carrots w/ Ranch Dressing	⅕ pkg	50	3	<5	0	–	–	0	2	5
DipperZ Carrot Sticks w/ Ranch Dip	1 pkg (2.75 oz)	50	2	0	0	–	–	0	2	4
Foodles Carrots Cheese & Pretzels	1 pkg (5 oz)	200	10	30	6	–	–	0	4	5
Dole										
Mini Cut	11 (3 oz)	30	0	0	0	0	0	0	2	4

FOOD	PORTION	CALS	TOTAL FAT	CHOL	SAT FAT	POLY FAT	MONO FAT	TRANS FAT	FIBER	SUGAR
Grimmway Farms										
Baby	3 oz	35	0	0	0	0	0	0	2	5
Carrot Chips	3 oz	35	0	0	0	0	0	0	2	5
Carrot Creations Honey Brown Sugar & Cinnamon	¼ pkg (3 oz)	70	3	10	2	–	–	0	2	7
Carrot Creations Roasted Garlic & Savory Herbs	¼ pkg (3 oz)	70	5	10	3	–	–	0	2	5
Carrot Dippers	1 pkg (2.2 oz)	110	9	10	2	–	–	0	1	4
Shredded	3 oz	35	0	0	0	0	0	0	2	5
Ready Pac										
Baby Carrots	7 (3 oz)	40	0	0	0	0	0	0	2	5
FROZEN										
slices cooked w/o salt	1 cup (5.1 oz)	54	1	0	tr	tr	tr	–	5	6
CASABA										
cubed	1 cup (6 oz)	46	tr	0	tr	tr	tr	0	2	10
melon fresh	¼ (14 oz)	115	tr	0	tr	tr	tr	0	4	23
CASHEWS										
butter w/ salt	1 tbsp (0.5 oz)	94	8	0	2	1	5	–	tr	1
butter w/o salt	1 tbsp (0.5 oz)	94	8	0	2	1	5	–	tr	–
dry roasted w/o salt	¼ cup (1.2 oz)	197	16	0	3	3	9	–	1	2
oil roasted w/o salt	¼ cup (1.1 oz)	187	15	0	3	3	8	–	1	2
raw	1 oz	157	12	0	2	2	7	–	1	2
Frito Lay										
Whole Salted	3 tbsp	180	15	0	3	3	9	0	1	2
Kettle Brand										
Butter Unsalted	2 tbsp (1 oz)	160	14	0	3	3	8	0	1	0
Nut Harvest										
Whole Sea Salted	2 tbsp (1 oz)	170	13	0	3	–	–	0	1	2
Planters										
Chocolate Lovers Milk Chocolate	10 pieces (1.5 oz)	230	16	5	7	–	–	0	1	15
Halves & Pieces	1 oz	160	13	0	3	–	7	0	1	2
Halves & Pieces Lightly Salted	1 oz	160	13	0	3	–	7	0	1	2
Whole Honey Roasted	1 oz	150	11	0	2	–	6	0	1	5
Sante										
Cardamon Cashews	¼ cup (1 oz)	220	17	0	3	5	9	0	1	7

FOOD	PORTION	CALS	TOTAL FAT	CHOL	SAT FAT	POLY FAT	MONO FAT	TRANS FAT	FIBER	SUGAR
CASSAVA										
diced cooked w/o fat	1 cup (4.6 oz)	213	tr	0	tr	tr	tr	0	2	2
root raw	1 (14.3 oz)	653	1	0	tr	tr	tr	0	7	7
TAKE-OUT										
fritter crab meat stuffed	1 (4.4 oz)	341	16	45	4	2	9	–	2	7
CATFISH										
channel breaded & fried	3 oz	194	11	69	3	3	5	–	–	–
wolffish atlantic baked	3 oz	105	3	50	tr	1	1	–	0	0
CAULIFLOWER										
flowerets fresh	1 (0.5 oz)	3	tr	0	tr	tr	tr	0	tr	tr
flowerets fresh cooked w/o salt	3 (2 oz)	12	tr	0	tr	tr	tr	0	1	1
fresh	1 cup	25	tr	0	tr	tr	tr	0	3	2
fresh cooked w/o salt	1 cup	29	1	0	tr	tr	tr	0	3	3
fresh head small	1 (9.2 oz)	66	tr	0	tr	tr	tr	0	7	6
frzn cooked w/o salt	1 cup	34	tr	0	tr	tr	tr	0	5	2
green fresh	1 cup	20	tr	0	tr	tr	tr	0	2	2
green fresh small head	1 (11.4 oz)	101	1	0	tr	tr	tr	0	10	10
pickled	¼ cup	14	tr	0	tr	tr	tr	0	1	2
pickled chow chow	¼ cup	74	1	0	tr	tr	tr	0	1	15
Dole										
Fresh	1 cup (3.4 oz)	25	0	0	0	0	0	0	2	2
Jake & Amos										
Sweet Pickled Hot Cauliflower	1 tbsp	40	0	0	0	0	0	0	0	8
Mann's										
Cauliettes Fresh	1 serv (3 oz)	20	0	0	0	0	0	0	2	2
River Ranch										
Florets Fresh	1 cup (3 oz)	20	0	0	0	0	0	0	2	2
Victoria										
Tangy	¼ cup (1 oz)	5	0	0	0	0	0	0	0	0
TAKE-OUT										
batter dipped fried	1 cup	178	13	14	3	4	5	–	2	1
batter dipped fried	1 piece (0.9 oz)	55	4	4	1	1	2	–	1	tr
w/ cheese sauce	1 cup	249	18	36	8	2	6	–	3	6
CAVIAR										
black or red	2 tbsp	81	6	188	1	2	1	0	0	0

FOOD	PORTION	CALS	TOTAL FAT	CHOL	SAT FAT	POLY FAT	MONO FAT	TRANS FAT	FIBER	SUGAR
CELERY										
fresh	1 lg stalk (2.2 oz)	9	tr	0	tr	tr	tr	0	1	1
pickled	½ cup	10	tr	0	tr	tr	tr	0	1	1
raw diced	½ cup	8	tr	0	tr	tr	tr	0	1	1
seed	1 tsp	1	tr	0	tr	tr	tr	0	tr	–
strips	1 cup	17	tr	0	tr	tr	tr	0	2	2
Dole										
Hearts	2 stalks (4 oz)	15	0	0	0	0	0	0	2	0
Ready Pac										
Sticks	5 (3 oz)	10	0	0	0	0	0	0	1	1
TAKE-OUT										
creamed	½ cup	87	6	3	1	2	2	–	1	4
stir fried	½ cup	30	2	0	tr	1	1	–	1	2
stuffed w/ cheese	1 (5 inch)	38	3	10	2	tr	1	–	tr	tr
CELERY JUICE										
juice	1 cup	42	tr	0	tr	tr	tr	0	4	6
CELERY ROOT										
fresh cooked w/o salt	1 cup (5.4 oz)	42	tr	0	–	–	–	0	2	–
fresh cut up	1 cup (5.5 oz)	66	tr	0	tr	tr	tr	0	3	3
CELTUCE										
raw	3.5 oz	22	tr	0	–	–	–	–	–	–
CEREAL										
bran flakes	¾ cup	90	1	0	tr	tr	tr	–	–	–
corn flakes	1¼ cups	110	tr	0	tr	tr	tr	–	–	–
farina as prep w/ water	¾ cup	88	tr	0	tr	tr	tr	–	2	–
granola	½ cup	285	15	0	3	6	5	–	6	–
oatmeal instant as prep w/ water	1 cup (8.2 oz)	138	2	0	tr	1	1	–	4	–
oatmeal regular & quick as prep w/ water	¾ cup (6.1 oz)	149	2	0	tr	1	1	–	3	–
oatmeal regular & quick not prep	⅓ cup (0.9 oz)	104	2	0	tr	1	1	–	3	–
puffed rice	1 cup	56	tr	0	tr	–	–	–	tr	–
puffed wheat	1 cup	44	tr	0	tr	–	–	–	1	–
shredded mini wheats	1 cup	107	1	0	tr	tr	tr	–	3	–
shredded wheat rectangular	1 biscuit (0.8 oz)	85	tr	0	tr	tr	tr	–	2	–

FOOD	PORTION	CALS	TOTAL FAT	CHOL	SAT FAT	POLY FAT	MONO FAT	TRANS FAT	FIBER	SUGAR
Annie's Homegrown										
Bunny O's Honey	¾ cup (1 oz)	110	1	0	0	–	–	0	1	7
Bunny O's Organic	¾ cup (1 oz)	120	2	0	0	–	–	0	1	2
Barbara's Bakery										
Organic Brown Rice Crisps Fruit Juice Sweetened	1 cup (1 oz)	120	1	0	0	–	–	0	1	1
Puffins Honey Rice Gluten Free	¾ cup (1 oz)	120	1	0	0	–	–	0	3	6
Puffins Multigrain Gluten Free	¾ cup (1 oz)	110	0	0	0	–	–	0	3	6
BetterOats										
Abundance Apple & Cinnamon	1 pkg (1.5 oz)	160	3	0	0	2	1	0	3	9
Good'N Hearty Maple & Brown Sugar	1 pkg (1.5 oz)	160	3	0	0	1	1	0	3	9
Lavish Dark Chocolate	1 pkg (1.5 oz)	160	3	0	1	1	1	0	3	12
MMM...Muffins Oatmeal Raisin Cookie	1 pkg (1.4 oz)	150	2	0	0	1	1	0	3	14
Oat Fit Cinnamon Roll	1 pkg (1 oz)	100	2	0	0	1	1	0	3	0
Oat Revolution! Cinnamon & Spice	1 pkg (1.6 oz)	170	3	0	0	1	1	0	3	15
Oat Revolution! Peaches & Cream	1 pkg (1.2 oz)	130	2	0	0	1	0	0	2	12
Oat Revolution! Thick & Hearty Classic	1 pkg (1.2 oz)	130	3	0	0	2	1	0	4	0
Cascadian Farm										
Organic Granola Berry Cobbler	⅔ cup (2.1 oz)	230	4	0	1	1	2	0	3	15
Cheerios										
Chocolate	¾ cup (1 oz)	100	2	0	0	1	1	0	2	9
MultiGrain	1 cup (1 oz)	110	1	0	0	1	0	0	3	6
Cinnamon Toast Crunch										
Cinnamon Sugar	¾ cup (1.1 oz)	130	3	0	1	1	2	0	2	9
CoCo Wheats										
Hot Cereal as prep w/ skim milk	1 serv	160	tr	3	0	0	0	0	1	0
Dr. McDougall's										
Organic Instant Oatmeal	1 pkg (1 oz)	120	2	0	0	–	–	0	3	0
Organic Maple 4 Grain	1 pkg (2.6 oz)	260	3	0	0	–	–	0	6	16

FOOD	PORTION	CALS	TOTAL FAT	CHOL	SAT FAT	POLY FAT	MONO FAT	TRANS FAT	FIBER	SUG
EnviroKidz										
Amazon Frosted Flakes Organic	⅔ cup (1.1 oz)	120	0	0	0	0	0	0	2	6
Gorilla Munch Organic	¾ cup (1 oz)	120	0	0	0	0	0	0	2	8
Koala Crisp Organic	¾ cup (1.1 oz)	110	1	0	0	–	–	0	2	11
Panda Puffs Organic	¾ cup (1.1 oz)	130	3	0	0	–	–	0	2	7
Erin Baker's										
Granola Fruit & Nut	½ cup (1.6 oz)	190	8	0	2	–	–	0	4	10
Fiber One										
Nutty Clusters & Almonds	1 cup (1.9 oz)	180	3	0	0	1	2	0	11	12
Giddy Up & Go										
Granola Notoriously Nutty	¾ cup (2 oz)	250	11	1	1	3	4	0	5	11
Granola Seriously Seedy	¾ cup (2 oz)	230	10	0	2	5	5	0	5	11
Kaia Foods										
Organic Granola Buckwheat Cinnamon Raisin	½ cup (2 oz)	230	10	0	2	–	–	0	6	12
Organic Granola Buckwheat Cocoa Bliss	½ cup (2 oz)	220	8	0	2	–	–	0	5	14
Kellogg's										
All-Bran Bran Buds	⅓ cup (1 oz)	80	1	0	0	0	0	0	13	8
All-Bran Complete Wheat Flakes	¾ cup (1 oz)	90	1	0	0	0	0	0	5	5
All-Bran Original	½ cup (1.1 oz)	80	1	0	0	1	0	0	10	6
Apple Jacks	1 cup (1 oz)	110	1	0	1	0	0	0	3	12
Corn Flakes	1 cup (1 oz)	100	0	0	0	0	0	0	1	3
Corn Pops	1 cup (1 oz)	120	0	0	0	0	0	0	3	9
Cracklin' Oat Bran	¾ cup (1.7 oz)	200	7	0	3	2	3	0	6	14
Crispix	1 cup (1 oz)	110	0	0	0	0	0	0	tr	4
Crunchmania Cinnamon Bun	1 pkg (1.8 oz)	220	7	0	2	–	–	0	2	12
Crunchy Nut Golden Honey Nut	⅓ cup (1.1 oz)	120	1	0	0	0	1	0	tr	10
Fiber Plus Antioxidants Cinnamon Oat Crunch	¾ cup (1.1 oz)	110	2	0	0	1	0	0	9	7
Froot Loops	1 cup (1 oz)	110	1	0	1	0	0	0	3	12
Frosted Flakes	¾ cup (1 oz)	110	0	0	0	0	0	0	tr	11
Frosted Mini-Wheat Crunch Brown Sugar	1 cup (2 oz)	200	2	0	0	1	1	0	5	12
Frosted Mini-Wheats Little Bites Original	1 cup (2 oz)	200	1	0	0	1	0	0	6	11

FOOD	PORTION	CALS	TOTAL FAT	CHOL	SAT FAT	POLY FAT	MONO FAT	TRANS FAT	FIBER	SUGAR
Frosted Mini-Wheats Maple Brown Sugar	25 (2 oz)	190	1	0	0	1	0	0	6	12
Frosted Mini-Wheats Strawberry	25 (2 oz)	190	1	0	0	1	0	0	6	12
Granola Low Fat	½ cup (1.7 oz)	190	3	0	1	1	1	0	3	14
Honey Smacks	¾ cup (1 oz)	100	1	0	0	0	0	0	1	15
Krave Chocolate	¾ cup (1.1 oz)	120	4	0	1	2	1	0	3	11
Mueslix	⅔ cup (2 oz)	200	3	0	0	1	2	0	5	14
Product 19	1 cup (1 oz)	110	0	0	0	0	0	0	tr	4
Raisin Bran	1 cup (2 oz)	190	1	0	0	0	0	0	7	18
Raisin Bran Crunch	1 cup (1.9 oz)	190	1	0	0	0	0	0	4	19
Smart Start Original Antioxidants	1 cup (1.8 oz)	190	1	0	0	0	0	0	3	14
Smorz	1 cup (1.1 oz)	120	2	0	1	0	1	0	tr	13
Love Crunch										
Carrot Cake Organic	¼ cup (1.1 oz)	130	4	0	1	2	1	0	2	8
Dark Chocolate & Red Berries Organic	¼ cup (1.1 oz)	140	6	0	1	3	2	0	2	6
Malt-O-Meal										
Apple Zings	1 cup (1.2 oz)	130	1	0	0	0	0	0	1	16
Chocolate not prep	3 tbsp (1.2 oz)	130	0	0	0	0	0	0	1	7
Coco Roos	¾ cup (1 oz)	120	2	0	0	0	0	0	tr	15
Crispy Rice	1¼ cups (1.2 oz)	130	0	0	0	0	0	0	0	3
Golden Puffs	¾ cup (1 oz)	110	0	0	0	0	0	0	0	15
Honey Nut Scooters	1 cup (1 oz)	110	2	0	0	1	1	0	2	10
Mateys Marshmallow	1 cup (1 oz)	120	1	0	0	1	1	0	1	13
Original Cream Hot Wheat not prep	3 tbsp (1.2 oz)	130	0	0	0	0	0	0	1	0
Original not prep	3 tbsp (1.2 oz)	130	1	0	0	0	0	0	1	0
Tootie Fruities	1 cup (1.1 oz)	130	1	0	0	0	0	0	1	15
Mom's Best Naturals										
Blue Pom Wheat-fuls	1 cup (1.9 oz)	210	1	0	0	1	0	0	6	11
Honey Grahams	¾ cup (1 oz)	130	3	0	1	1	1	0	1	10
Mallow Oats	1 cup (1 oz)	120	1	0	0	1	1	0	1	13
Raisin Bran	1 cup (2.1 oz)	230	2	0	0	1	0	0	6	20
Mother's										
Barley Hot Cereal not prep	⅓ cup (1.7 oz)	160	1	0	0	0	0	0	5	0
Peanut Butter Bumpers	1 cup (1.2 oz)	130	3	0	1	1	1	0	1	10
Rolled Oats not prep	½ cup (1.4 oz)	150	3	0	1	1	1	0	4	1
Toasted Oat Bran	¾ cup (1.1 oz)	120	2	0	0	1	1	0	3	5

FOOD	PORTION	CALS	TOTAL FAT	CHOL	SAT FAT	POLY FAT	MONO FAT	TRANS FAT	FIBER	SUGAR
Naked Granola										
Taste Of Seattle Nights	½ pkg (1.2 oz)	110	6	0	2	–	–	0	5	5
Nature's Path										
Corn Flakes Organic	¾ cup (1.1 oz)	110	0	0	0	0	0	0	2	3
Granola Hemp Plus Organic	¾ cup (1.9 oz)	260	10	0	2	6	3	0	5	10
Granola Peanut Butter Organic	¾ cup (1.9 oz)	260	11	0	2	–	–	0	4	9
Granola Pumpkin Flax Plus Organic	¾ cup (1.9 oz)	260	10	0	2	5	3	0	5	10
Heritage Crunch Organic	¾ cup (1.9 oz)	230	3	0	1	–	–	0	6	6
Instant Oatmeal Flax Plus Organic	1 pkg (1.8 oz)	210	3	0	1	–	–	0	5	10
Instant Oatmeal Hemp Plus Organic	1 pkg (1.4 oz)	160	3	0	0	2	1	0	4	6
Instant Oatmeal Maple Nut Organic	1 pkg (1.8 oz)	210	4	0	1	–	–	0	4	11
Instant Oatmeal Optimum Cranberry Ginger Organic	1 pkg (1.4 oz)	150	2	0	0	–	–	0	3	10
Instant Oatmeal Original Organic	1 pkg (1.8 oz)	210	4	0	1	–	–	0	6	0
Kamut Puffs Organic	1 cup (0.5 oz)	50	0	0	0	0	0	0	2	0
Maple Pecan Crunch Flax Plus Organic	¾ cup (1.9 oz)	220	7	0	1	3	2	0	5	10
Millet Rice Flakes Organic	¾ cup (1.1 oz)	120	2	0	0	–	–	0	3	4
Optimum Blueberry Cinnamon Organic	1 cup (1.9 oz)	200	3	0	0	2	0	0	7	9
Optimum Cranberry Ginger Organic	¾ cup (1.9 oz)	190	3	0	0	–	–	0	8	13
Red Berry Crunch Flax Plus Organic	¾ cup (1.9 oz)	210	4	0	1	3	1	0	5	10
Rice Puffs Organic	1 cup (0.5 oz)	50	0	0	0	0	0	0	1	0
Shredded Oaty Bites Organic	¾ cup (1.1 oz)	110	2	0	0	–	–	0	2	5
Post										
Grape-Nuts	½ cup (2 oz)	200	1	0	0	1	0	0	7	5
Great Grains Raisins Dates & Pecans	¾ cup (2 oz)	200	4	0	0	1	2	0	5	14
Honey Bunches Of Oats	1 cup (1.8 oz)	200	2	0	0	1	1	0	2	14
Honey Bunches Of Oats Almonds	¾ cup (1.1 oz)	120	3	0	0	1	2	0	2	6

FOOD	PORTION	CALS	TOTAL FAT	CHOL	SAT FAT	POLY FAT	MONO FAT	TRANS FAT	FIBER	SUGAR
Selects Cranberry Almond Crunch	¾ cup (1.8 oz)	200	3	0	0	1	2	0	3	14
Shredded Wheat Spoon Size	1 cup (1.7 oz)	170	1	0	0	1	0	0	6	0
Quaker										
Oatmeal	1 pkg (2.6 oz)	290	8	0	1	5	2	0	5	22
Oatmeal Cherry Pistachio as prep	1 pkg (2.6 oz)	290	8	0	1	3	4	0	5	19
Oatmeal Peach Almond	1 pkg (2.6 oz)	290	7	0	1	2	4	0	6	19
Oatmeal Summer Berry	1 pkg (2.5 oz)	250	3	0	1	1	1	0	7	14
Oatmeal Squares	1 cup (2 oz)	210	3	0	1	1	1	0	5	9
Ralston										
Enriched Wheat Bran Flakes	¾ cup (1 oz)	90	1	0	0	0	0	0	5	5
Shredded Wheat Frosted Bite Size	1¼ cups (1.9 oz)	190	1	0	0	1	0	0	5	11
Reese's										
Puffs	¾ cup (1 oz)	120	3	0	1	1	2	0	1	10
Rice Krispies										
Cereal	1¼ cups (1.2 oz)	130	0	0	0	0	0	0	tr	4
Simpli										
Instant Oatmeal Apricot Gluten Free	1 pkg (1.7 oz)	170	3	0	0	–	–	0	4	10
Instant Oatmeal Plain Gluten Free	1 pkg (1.4 oz)	150	3	0	0	–	–	0	4	0
Skinner's										
Raisin Bran	1 cup (1.9 oz)	190	1	0	0	–	–	0	6	8
Special K										
Original	1 cup (1.1 oz)	120	1	0	0	0	0	0	0	4
Protein Plus	¾ cup (1.1 oz)	120	1	0	0	1	0	0	3	7
Red Berries	1 cup (1.1 oz)	110	0	0	0	0	0	0	3	9
Uncle Sam										
Honey Almond	¾ cup (1.9 oz)	230	6	0	0	–	–	0	6	5
Original	¾ cup (1.9 oz)	190	5	0	1	–	–	0	10	tr
Strawberry	¾ cup (2.1 oz)	240	5	0	0	–	–	0	8	7

CEREAL BARS (see also ENERGY BARS, FRUIT AND NUT BARS)

FOOD	PORTION	CALS	TOTAL FAT	CHOL	SAT FAT	POLY FAT	MONO FAT	TRANS FAT	FIBER	SUGAR
Annie's Homegrown										
Organic Peanut Butter	1 (1 oz)	120	5	0	1	–	–	0	1	5
Cascadian Farms										
Organic Granola Oats & Cocoa	2 (1.4 oz)	190	8	0	2	–	–	0	3	9

FOOD	PORTION	CALS	TOTAL FAT	CHOL	SAT FAT	POLY FAT	MONO FAT	TRANS FAT	FIBER	SUGAR
Organic Granola Oats & Honey	2 (1.4 oz)	180	7	0	1	–	–	0	3	9
Organic Granola Peanut Butter	2 (1.4 oz)	190	8	0	1	–	–	0	3	9
Earnest Eats										
Almond Trail Mix	1 (1.94 oz)	210	9	0	1	3	5	0	1	14
Choco Peanut Butter	1 (1.94 oz)	230	10	0	2	3	4	0	4	14
Cran Lemon Zest	1 (1.94 oz)	210	9	0	1	3	5	0	4	14
EnviroKidz										
Crispy Rice Cheetah Berry Organic	1 (1 oz)	110	3	0	0	–	–	0	1	7
Crispy Rice Lemur Peanut Choco Drizzle Organic	1 (1 oz)	120	5	0	1	–	–	0	1	8
Crispy Rice Panda Peanut Butter	1 (1 oz)	110	3	0	0	–	–	0	1	7
Fiber One										
Chewy Chocolate	1 (1 oz)	100	3	0	2	–	–	0	5	8
Chewy Strawberry PB&J	1 (1 oz)	110	4	0	2	–	–	0	5	7
Chocolate Caramel & Pretzel	1 (0.8 oz)	90	2	0	2	–	–	0	5	5
Oats & Caramel	1 (1.4 oz)	140	4	0	2	–	–	0	9	9
Oats & Chocolate	1 (1.4 oz)	140	4	0	2	–	–	0	9	10
Oats & Peanut Butter	1 (1.4 oz)	150	5	0	2	–	–	0	9	9
Fruition										
Blueberry	1 (1.7 oz)	160	2	0	0	1	1	0	4	21
Cran-Raspberry	1 (1.7 oz)	160	2	0	0	1	1	0	4	22
Lemon	1 (1.7 oz)	160	3	0	0	0	1	0	4	19
Gnu										
Flavor & Fiber Banana Walnut	1 (1.6 oz)	140	4	0	0	–	–	0	12	8
Flavor & Fiber Chocolate Brownie Bar	1 (1.6 oz)	140	4	0	1	–	–	0	12	9
Flavor & Fiber Cinnamon Raisin	1 (1.6 oz)	130	3	0	0	–	–	0	12	11
Flavor & Fiber Expresso Chip	1 (1.6 oz)	140	4	0	1	–	–	0	12	8
Flavor & Fiber Lemon Ginger	1 (1.6 oz)	130	4	0	0	–	–	0	12	10
Flavor & Fiber Orange Cranberry	1 (1.6 oz)	130	3	0	0	–	–	0	12	11
Flavor & Fiber Peanut Butter	1 (1.6 oz)	140	5	0	1	–	–	0	12	7

FOOD	PORTION	CALS	TOTAL FAT	CHOL	SAT FAT	POLY FAT	MONO FAT	TRANS FAT	FIBER	SUGAR
JK Gourmet										
Granola Bar Nuts & Cranberries	1 (1.6 oz)	230	18	0	5	–	–	0	3	10
Granola Bar Roasted Nuts & Blueberries	1 (1.6 oz)	240	19	0	5	–	–	0	3	10
Granola Bar Roasted Nuts & Dates	1 (1.6 oz)	240	19	0	5	–	–	0	3	11
Kashi										
Granola Chewy Trail Mix	1 (1.2 oz)	140	5	0	1	2	3	0	4	6
Kellogg's										
FiberPlus Antioxidants Berry Yogurt Crunch	1 cup (1.9 oz)	180	1	0	0	0	0	0	10	12
Kraft										
MilkBite Chocolate	1 (1.2 oz)	140	6	10	3	–	–	0	3	10
MilkBite Mixed Berry	1 (1.2 oz)	140	5	15	3	–	–	0	3	10
MilkBite Oatmeal Raisin	1 (1.2 oz)	130	5	15	3	–	–	0	3	10
MilkBite Peanut Butter	1 (1.2 oz)	140	6	10	3	–	–	0	3	8
MilkBite Strawberry	1 (1.2 oz)	140	5	15	3	–	–	0	3	10
Kudos										
Dove	1 (0.8 oz)	100	3	0	2	–	–	0	1	8
Snickers	1 (0.8 oz)	100	4	0	2	–	–	0	1	8
w/ M&Ms	1 (0.8 oz)	100	3	0	2	–	–	0	1	9
Nature Valley										
Crunchy Granola Peanut Butter	2 (1.5 oz)	190	7	0	1	–	–	0	2	11
Oats 'N Honey	2 (1.5 oz)	190	6	0	1	–	–	0	2	12
Protein Chewy Peanut Almond & Dark Chocolate	1 (1.4 oz)	190	12	0	4	2	6	0	5	6
Protein Chewy Peanut Butter Dark Chocolate	1 (1.4 oz)	190	12	0	4	1	7	0	5	6
Sweet & Salty Granola Almond	1 (1.2 oz)	160	7	0	2	–	–	0	2	12
Nature's Path										
Granola Bar Apple Pie Crunch Chia Plus Organic	2 (1.4 oz)	190	8	0	1	2	6	0	3	8
Granola Bar Honey Oat Crunch Flax Plus Organic	2 (1.4 oz)	190	7	0	1	2	5	0	3	9
Granola Bar Peanut Choco Organic	1 (1.2 oz)	150	6	0	2	–	–	0	2	11

FOOD	PORTION	CALS	TOTAL FAT	CHOL	SAT FAT	POLY FAT	MONO FAT	TRANS FAT	FIBER	SUGAR
Granola Bar Pumpkin-N-Spice Organic	1 (1.2 oz)	140	4	0	1	2	1	0	2	10
Granola Bar Sunny Hemp Organic	1 (1.2 oz)	140	4	0	1	2	1	0	3	11
Nutri-Grain										
Apple Cinnamon	1 (1.3 oz)	120	3	0	1	–	–	0	3	12
Mixed Berry	1 (1.3 oz)	120	3	0	1	–	–	0	3	11
Planters										
Nut-rition Antioxidant Almonds Blueberries & Dark Chocolate	1 (1.2 oz)	160	8	0	2	–	4	0	2	9
Nut-rition Bone Health Honey Roasted Peanuts Cashews & Almonds	1 (1.2 oz)	160	9	0	2	4	–	0	2	8
Nut-rition Energy Honey Roasted Peanuts Almonds & Chocolate	1 (1.2 oz)	170	9	0	2	–	5	0	2	10
Nut-rition Heart Healthy Cranberry Almond Peanut	1 (1.2 oz)	160	8	0	1	–	4	0	3	9
ProBar										
Cran-Lemon Twister	1 (3 oz)	360	16	0	2	–	–	0	7	28
Kettle Corn	1 (3 oz)	390	20	0	4	–	–	0	8	17
Koka Moka	1 (3 oz)	360	18	0	4	–	–	0	7	21
Old School PB&J	1 (3 oz)	370	17	0	2	–	–	0	6	20
Superfood Slam	1 (3 oz)	380	19	0	5	–	–	0	7	17
Quaker										
Chewy Granola Chocolate Chip	1 (0.84 oz)	100	3	0	1	1	1	0	1	7
Soft Baked Banana Nut Bread	1 (1.5 oz)	140	4	10	1	1	2	0	5	11
Soft Baked Cinnamon Pecan Bread	1 (1.5 oz)	140	4	10	1	1	2	0	5	11
Rice Krispies										
Treats	1 (0.8 oz)	90	2	0	1	–	–	0	0	8
Rickland Orchards										
Greek Yogurt Granola Apple & Honey	1 (1.4 oz)	160	6	0	3	–	–	0	5	12
Greek Yogurt Granola Blueberri Acai	1 (1.4 oz)	160	6	0	3	–	–	0	5	11
Greek Yogurt Granola Cranberry Almond	1 (1.4 oz)	160	6	0	3	–	–	0	5	12

FOOD	PORTION	CALS	TOTAL FAT	CHOL	SAT FAT	POLY FAT	MONO FAT	TRANS FAT	FIBER	SUGAR
Greek Yogurt Granola Orchard Peach	1 (1.4 oz)	160	6	0	3	–	–	0	5	8
Greek Yogurt Granola Peanut Butter	1 (1.4 oz)	170	8	0	3	–	–	0	5	8
Greek Yogurt Granola Strawberry	1 (1.4 oz)	150	4	0	2	–	–	0	5	8
Greek Yogurt Granola Toasted Coconut	1 (1.4 oz)	170	10	0	3	–	–	0	5	8
Rise Bar										
Breakfast Crunchy Cashew Almond	1 (1.4 oz)	190	12	0	2	–	–	0	3	11
Breakfast Crunchy Cranberry Apple	1 (1.4 oz)	160	7	0	1	–	–	0	3	19
South Beach										
Fiber Bar Granola Fudge Graham	1 (1.23 oz)	120	4	0	2	–	–	0	9	6
Protein Fit Cinnamon Raisin	1 (1.2 oz)	130	3	<5	2	–	–	0	3	8
Snack Bar Fudgy Chocolate Mint	1 (0.98 oz)	100	4	0	2	–	–	0	6	5
Special K										
Granola Chocolatey Peanut Butter	1 (0.95 oz)	110	3	0	2	0	1	0	4	7
Lemon Twist	1 (1.6 oz)	160	4	5	2	–	–	0	5	11
Protein & Fiber Chocolatey Peanut Butter	1 (0.9 oz)	110	3	0	2	0	1	0	4	7
Raspberry Cheesecake	1 (0.8 oz)	90	2	0	2	–	–	0	3	7
Sweet & Savory										
Cocoa Pistachio	1 (3 oz)	390	22	0	5	–	–	0	7	17
Tasty										
Carrot Cake	1 (1.2 oz)	110	2	0	0	–	–	0	3	14
Pumpkin Pie	1 (1.2 oz)	120	3	0	0	–	–	0	3	15
Zone Perfect										
Cookie Dough Chocolate Chip	1 (1.58 oz)	180	5	30	3	–	–	0	tr	18
Cookie Dough Oatmeal Raisin	1 (1.58 oz)	170	4	20	2	–	–	0	tr	16
Cookie Dough Peanut Butter	1 (1.58 oz)	190	7	20	3	–	–	0	1	16
Sweet & Salty Cashew Pretzel	1 (1.58 oz)	200	7	<5	3	–	–	0	1	14
Sweet & Salty Trail Mix	1 (1.58 oz)	200	8	<5	3	–	–	0	1	12

FOOD	PORTION	CALS	TOTAL FAT	CHOL	SAT FAT	POLY FAT	MONO FAT	TRANS FAT	FIBER	SUGAR
CHAMPAGNE										
champagne	1 serv (3.5 oz)	84	0	0	0	0	0	0	0	1
mimosa	1 serv	117	tr	0	tr	–	–	–	tr	–
punch	1 serv (4 oz)	73	tr	0	tr	tr	tr	0	0	6
sekt german champagne	1 serv (3.5 oz)	84	0	0	0	0	0	0	–	–
CHAYOTE										
fresh cooked	1 cup	38	1	0	–	–	–	–	–	–
raw	1 (7 oz)	49	1	0	–	–	–	–	–	–
raw cut up	1 cup	32	tr	0	–	–	–	–	–	–
Dole										
Fresh cooked	½ cup (2.8 oz)	17	0	0	0	0	0	0	2	0
CHEESE *(see also* CHEESE DISHES, CHEESE SUBSTITUTES, COTTAGE CHEESE, CREAM CHEESE, CREAM CHEESE SUBSTITUTES, NEUFCHATEL)										
american	1 oz	93	7	18	4	tr	2	–	–	–
american cheese spread	1 oz	82	6	16	4	tr	2	–	–	–
beaufort	1 oz	115	9	34	6	tr	3	–	0	tr
blue	1 oz	100	8	21	6	tr	2	–	–	–
blue crumbled	1 cup (4.7 oz)	477	39	102	25	1	11	–	–	–
bocconcini smoked	1 oz	90	6	25	4	–	–	0	0	0
brick	1 oz	105	8	27	5	tr	2	–	–	–
brie	1 oz	95	8	28	–	–	–	–	–	–
cacio di roma sheep's milk cheese	1 oz	130	10	30	6	–	–	–	0	0
camembert	1 oz	85	7	20	4	tr	2	–	–	–
cantal	1 oz	105	9	26	6	tr	3	–	0	tr
chabichou	1 oz	95	8	23	5	tr	2	–	0	tr
chaource	1 oz	83	7	20	4	tr	2	–	0	tr
cheddar	1 oz	114	9	30	6	tr	3	–	–	–
cheddar low sodium	1 oz	113	9	28	6	tr	3	–	–	–
cheddar lowfat	1 oz	49	2	6	1	tr	1	–	–	–
cheddar shredded	1 cup	455	37	119	24	1	11	–	–	–
cheshire	1 oz	110	9	29	–	–	–	–	–	–
colby	1 oz	112	9	27	6	tr	3	–	–	–
colby low sodium	1 oz	113	9	28	6	tr	3	–	–	–
colby lowfat	1 oz	49	2	6	1	tr	1	–	–	–
comte	1 oz	114	9	34	5	tr	2	–	0	tr
coulommiers	1 oz	88	7	23	5	tr	2	–	0	tr
crottin	1 oz	105	9	23	6	tr	2	–	0	tr
emmentaler	1 oz	115	9	26	–	–	–	–	–	–

FOOD	PORTION	CALS	TOTAL FAT	CHOL	SAT FAT	POLY FAT	MONO FAT	TRANS FAT	FIBER	SUGAR
feta	1 oz	75	6	25	4	tr	1	–	–	–
fontina	1 oz	110	9	33	5	tr	2	–	–	–
goat fresh	1 oz	23	2	5	1	tr	tr	–	0	tr
goat hard	1 oz	128	10	30	7	tr	2	–	–	–
gouda	1 oz	101	8	32	5	tr	2	–	–	–
grana padano parmesan shaved	1 tbsp	20	2	5	1	–	–	0	0	0
gruyere	1 oz	117	9	31	5	tr	3	–	–	–
limburger	1 oz	93	8	26	5	tr	2	–	–	–
maroilles	1 oz	97	8	26	5	tr	2	–	0	tr
morbier	1 oz	99	8	23	5	tr	2	–	0	tr
mozzarella	1 oz	80	6	22	4	tr	2	–	–	–
mozzarella fresh	1 oz	80	6	20	4	–	–	–	0	0
mozzarella part skim	1 oz	72	5	16	3	tr	1	–	–	–
muenster	1 oz	104	9	27	5	tr	2	–	–	–
parmesan grated	1 tbsp	23	2	4	1	tr	tr	–	–	–
parmesan hard	1 oz	111	7	19	5	tr	2	–	–	–
picodon	1 oz	99	8	23	5	tr	2	–	0	tr
pimento	1 oz	106	9	27	6	tr	3	–	–	–
pont l'eveque	1 oz	86	7	20	4	tr	2	–	0	tr
port du salut	1 oz	100	8	35	5	tr	3	–	–	–
provolone	1 oz	100	8	20	5	tr	2	–	–	–
pyrenees	1 oz	101	8	26	5	tr	2	–	0	tr
quark 20% fat	1 oz	33	1	5	–	–	–	–	–	–
quark 40% fat	1 oz	48	3	11	–	–	–	–	–	–
quark made w/ skim milk	1 oz	22	tr	tr	–	–	–	–	–	–
queso anejo	1 oz	106	9	30	5	tr	2	–	–	–
queso asadero	1 oz	101	8	30	5	tr	2	–	–	–
queso chihuahua	1 oz	106	8	30	5	tr	2	–	–	–
queso manchego	1 oz	107	8	27	–	–	–	–	0	–
raclette	1 oz	102	8	26	5	tr	2	–	0	tr
reblochon	1 oz	88	7	23	5	tr	2	–	0	tr
ricotta part skim	½ cup (4.4 oz)	171	10	38	6	tr	3	–	–	–
ricotta whole milk	½ cup (4.4 oz)	216	16	63	10	tr	5	–	–	–
romano	1 oz	110	8	29	–	–	–	–	–	–
roquefort	1 oz	105	9	26	5	tr	2	–	–	–
rouy	1 oz	95	8	23	5	tr	2	–	0	tr
saint marcellin	1 oz	94	8	23	5	tr	3	–	0	tr
saint nectaire	1 oz	97	8	23	5	tr	2	–	0	tr
saint paulin	1 oz	85	6	20	4	tr	2	–	0	tr

FOOD	PORTION	CALS	TOTAL FAT	CHOL	SAT FAT	POLY FAT	MONO FAT	TRANS FAT	FIBER	SUGAR
sainte maure	1 oz	99	8	23	5	tr	2	–	0	tr
selles sur cher	1 oz	93	8	20	5	tr	2	–	0	tr
swiss	1 oz	107	8	26	5	tr	2	–	–	–
swiss processed	1 oz	95	7	24	5	tr	2	–	–	–
tilsit	1 oz	96	7	29	5	tr	2	–	–	–
tome	1 oz	92	7	23	5	tr	2	–	0	tr
triple creme	1 oz	113	11	34	7	tr	3	–	0	tr
vacherin	1 oz	92	8	23	5	tr	2	–	0	tr
yogurt cheese	1 oz	80	7	15	3	–	–	–	0	0
Athenos										
Blue Crumbled	¼ pkg (1.1 oz)	110	9	30	6	–	–	0	1	0
Feta Black Peppercorn	1 oz	80	6	20	4	–	–	0	0	0
Feta Crumbled Garlic & Herb	⅕ pkg (1.2 oz)	90	7	25	4	–	–	0	1	0
Gorgonzola Crumbled	2 tbsp (1.1 oz)	110	9	30	6	–	–	0	1	0
Boar's Head										
Colby Jack	1 oz	110	9	25	6	3	0	0	0	0
Cabot										
Cheddar Extra Sharp	1 oz	110	9	30	6	–	–	0	0	0
Cracker Barrel										
Baby Swiss	1 oz	110	9	25	6	–	–	0	0	0
Cheddar Extra Sharp 2% Milk	1 oz	90	6	20	4	–	–	0	0	0
Cheddar Sharp	1 oz	120	10	30	7	–	–	0	0	0
Cheddar Sharp Shredded	1 oz	110	9	25	6	–	–	0	0	0
Cheddar Extra Extra Sharp Shredded 2% Milk	1 oz	80	6	20	4	–	–	0	0	0
White Cheddar Reduced Fat	1 oz	90	6	20	4	–	–	0	0	0
Easy Cheese										
American	2 tbsp (1.1 oz)	90	6	15	2	–	–	0	0	2
Cheddar	2 tbsp (1.1 oz)	90	6	15	3	–	–	0	0	2
Finlandia										
Baby Muenster	1 oz	100	8	20	5	–	–	0	0	0
Double Gloucester Deli Slices	1 slice (0.8 oz)	83	7	23	4	–	–	0	0	0
Gouda Deli Slices	1 slice (0.8 oz)	79	6	15	4	–	–	0	0	0
Havarti Deli Slices	1 slice (0.8 oz)	86	7	18	4	–	–	0	0	0
Muenster Deli Slices	1 slice (0.8 oz)	86	7	19	4	–	–	0	0	0
Swiss Deli Slices	1 slice (0.8 oz)	86	7	16	4	–	–	0	0	0
Swiss Light Deli Slices	1 slice (0.8 oz)	57	3	8	2	–	–	0	0	0
Viola	2 tbsp (1 oz)	87	8	19	5	–	–	0	0	1

FOOD	PORTION	CALS	TOTAL FAT	CHOL	SAT FAT	POLY FAT	MONO FAT	TRANS FAT	FIBER	SUGAR
Galbani										
Precious Fresh Mozzarella Sliced	1 oz	90	6	30	4	–	–	0	0	0
Precious Sticksters Cheddar	1 (1 oz)	110	9	30	5	–	–	0	0	0
Precious Stringsters Mozzarella Part Skim	1 (1 oz)	80	6	15	3	–	–	0	0	0
Grana Padano										
PDO Cheese	1 oz	120	8	12	5	–	–	–	0	0
Hans All Natural										
Spread Cheddar & Jalapeno	2 tbsp (1 oz)	90	7	20	4	–	–	0	0	3
Spread Swiss Cheese & Almonds	2 tbsp (1 oz)	90	7	20	4	–	–	0	0	3
Karoun										
Ackawi	1 oz	110	8	10	5	–	–	0	0	0
Ani	1 in cube (1 oz)	110	8	10	5	–	–	0	0	0
Labne Kefir	2 tbsp (1 oz)	80	5	20	3	–	–	0	0	1
Paneer	1 oz	90	7	25	5	–	–	0	0	1
Kraft										
Big Slice Swiss	1 (0.8 oz)	90	7	25	5	–	–	0	0	0
Cheese Spread Pimento	2 tbsp	80	6	20	4	–	–	0	0	2
Cheese Spread Roka Blue	2 tbsp	80	7	20	5	–	–	0	0	1
Cheese Spread Sharp Old English	2 tbsp (1.1 oz)	90	8	25	5	–	–	0	0	0
Fresh Take Cheese Breadcrumb Mix Italian Parmesan	1 oz	100	5	15	3	–	–	0	0	0
Fresh Take Cheese Breadcrumb Mix Southwest Three Cheese	1 oz	100	6	15	3	–	–	0	0	1
Grated 100% Parmesan	1 tsp (5 g)	20	2	5	1	–	–	0	0	0
Grated 100% Romano	1 tsp (5 g)	20	2	5	1	–	–	0	0	0
Grated Parmesan Reduced Fat	1 tsp (5 g)	20	1	5	1	–	–	0	0	0
Shredded Cheddar Fat Free	1 oz	45	0	5	0	0	0	0	0	0
Shredded Mexican Style Taco 2% Milk	1 serv (1 oz)	80	5	15	3	–	–	0	0	0
Shredded Mozzarella 2% Milk + Calcium	1 oz	70	5	15	3	–	–	0	0	0
Singles American	1 (0.7 oz)	60	4	15	3	–	–	0	0	1

FOOD	PORTION	CALS	TOTAL FAT	CHOL	SAT FAT	POLY FAT	MONO FAT	TRANS FAT	FIBER	SUGAR
Singles American 2% Milk	1 (0.7 oz)	45	3	10	2	–	–	0	0	2
Singles Pepper Jack	1 slice (0.7 oz)	80	6	20	4	–	–	0	0	0
Slices Havarti	1 (0.7 oz)	80	7	20	4	–	–	0	0	0
Slices Monterey Jack	1 (0.7 oz)	80	6	20	4	–	–	0	0	0
Laughing Cow										
Cinnamon Cream ⅓ Less Fat	1 wedge (0.7 oz)	45	4	10	3	–	–	0	0	1
Classic Cream ⅓ Less Fat	1 wedge (0.7 oz)	45	4	10	3	–	–	0	0	tr
Creamy Swiss Light	1 wedge (0.7 oz)	35	2	<5	1	–	–	0	0	1
Creamy Swiss Original	1 wedge (0.7 oz)	50	4	10	3	–	–	0	0	1
Garden Vegetable ⅓ Less Fat	1 wedge (0.7 oz)	45	4	10	3	–	–	0	0	1
Strawberries & Cream ⅓ Less Fat	1 wedge (0.7 oz)	45	4	10	3	–	–	0	0	1
Lifeway										
Farmer	2 tbsp (1.1 oz)	40	2	6	1	–	–	–	–	4
Farmer Lite	2 tbsp (1.1 oz)	25	1	<5	1	–	–	–	–	1
Sweet Kiss Spread Peach	1 oz	50	2	<5	1	–	–	–	–	6
Sweet Kiss Spread Plain	1 oz	50	2	<5	1	–	–	0	–	5
Sweet Kiss Spread Raisins	1 oz	45	1	<5	1	–	–	–	–	6
Organic Valley										
American Singles Unprocessed Organic	1 slice (0.7 oz)	70	6	20	4	–	–	0	0	tr
Polly-O										
Mozzarella Shredded Fat Free	1 oz	40	0	5	0	0	0	0	1	1
Mozzarella Shredded Part Skim	1 oz	80	5	15	4	–	–	0	0	0
Mozzarella Shredded Whole Milk	1 oz	90	7	20	4	–	–	0	0	0
String-Ums Mozzarella Part Skim	1 (1 oz)	80	6	20	4	–	–	0	0	0
Sara Lee										
Colby & Monterey Jack	3 slices (1.2 oz)	130	11	35	6	–	–	0	0	0
Sartori										
BellaVitano Chai	1 oz	120	10	30	5	–	–	0	0	0

FOOD	PORTION	CALS	TOTAL FAT	CHOL	SAT FAT	POLY FAT	MONO FAT	TRANS FAT	FIBER	SUGAR
BellaVitano Espresso	1 oz	120	10	30	5	–	–	0	0	0
Goat Extra Aged	1 oz	100	8	30	5	–	–	0	0	0
Parmesan SarVecchio	1 oz	102	7	23	4	–	–	0	0	0
Pastorale Blend	1 oz	110	8	25	6	–	–	0	0	0
Sorrento										
Mozzarella Fresh	1 oz	90	6	30	4	–	–	0	0	0
Yanni										
Grilling Cheese Original	1 oz	80	7	25	5	–	–	0	0	0

CHEESE DISHES
Alexia

FOOD	PORTION	CALS	TOTAL FAT	CHOL	SAT FAT	POLY FAT	MONO FAT	TRANS FAT	FIBER	SUGAR
Mozzarella Stix w/ Olive Oil & Italian Herbs	2 (1.3 oz)	120	6	10	3	2	2	0	1	1
Farm Rich										
Cheese Sticks	2 (2 oz)	170	9	15	4	–	–	0	0	1
Mozzarella Sticks Marinara Stuffed	2 (2.3 oz)	160	8	10	3	–	–	0	1	2
Mozzarella Bites	4 (1.8 oz)	150	6	10	3	–	–	0	1	4
TAKE-OUT										
fondue	½ cup (3.8 oz)	247	15	49	9	1	4	–	–	–
fried mozzarella sticks	3 (4.6 oz)	503	32	107	16	2	11	–	1	2
souffle	1 serv (7 oz)	504	38	370	17	5	14	–	1	5

CHEESE SUBSTITUTES

FOOD	PORTION	CALS	TOTAL FAT	CHOL	SAT FAT	POLY FAT	MONO FAT	TRANS FAT	FIBER	SUGAR
mozzarella	1 oz	70	3	0	1	tr	2	–	–	–
Daiya										
Cheddar Style Shreds	¼ cup (1 oz)	90	6	0	2	–	–	0	1	0
Mozzarella Style Shreds	¼ cup (1 oz)	90	6	0	2	–	–	0	1	0
Follow Your Heart										
Vegan Cheddar	1 oz	70	7	0	0	–	–	0	1	0
Vegan Mozzarella	1 oz	70	7	0	1	–	–	0	1	0
Go Veggie!										
American Slices Dairy Free Vegan	1 (0.7 oz)	40	2	0	0	1	1	0	0	0
American Slices Lactose Free	1 (0.6 oz)	40	3	0	0	1	2	0	0	0
Tofutti										
Better Ricotta Milk Free	¼ cup (2.2 oz)	100	7	0	4	–	–	0	1	0
Soy American	1 slice (0.7 oz)	80	6	0	3	–	–	0	0	–
Soy Mozzarella	1 slice (0.7 oz)	80	6	0	3	–	–	0	0	–

FOOD	PORTION	CALS	TOTAL FAT	CHOL	SAT FAT	POLY FAT	MONO FAT	TRANS FAT	FIBER	SUGAR
CHERIMOYA										
fresh	1	515	2	0	–	–	–	–	–	–
CHERRIES										
CANNED										
maraschino	¼ cup (1.4 oz)	66	tr	0	tr	tr	tr	0	1	16
maraschino	1 (4 g)	7	tr	0	tr	tr	tr	0	tr	2
sour in heavy syrup	½ cup	116	tr	0	tr	tr	tr	0	1	28
sour in light syrup	½ cup	94	tr	0	tr	tr	tr	0	1	–
sour water packed	½ cup	44	tr	0	tr	tr	tr	0	1	9
sweet juice pack	½ cup	68	tr	0	tr	tr	tr	0	2	15
sweet pitted in heavy syrup	½ cup	105	tr	0	tr	tr	tr	0	2	25
sweet water pack	½ cup	57	tr	0	tr	tr	tr	0	2	13
Del Monte										
Sweet Dark Pitted In Heavy Syrup	½ cup (4.2 oz)	100	0	0	0	0	0	0	tr	24
Jake & Amos										
Brandied Sweet	½ cup (4.4 oz)	90	0	0	0	0	0	0	2	10
DRIED										
bing unsulfured	¼ cup	130	0	0	0	0	0	0	2	21
montmorency tart pitted	⅓ cup	160	1	0	0	–	–	–	2	24
rainier unsulfured	⅓ cup	140	1	0	0	–	–	–	2	30
tart	½ cup	200	1	0	0	–	–	0	2	41
yogurt covered	¼ cup	170	6	0	6	–	–	–	5	22
FRESH										
sour	1 cup	52	tr	0	tr	tr	tr	0	2	9
sour pitted	1 cup	78	tr	0	tr	tr	tr	0	3	13
sweet	20	86	1	0	tr	tr	tr	0	3	17
Dole										
Cherries	1 cup (4.9 oz)	90	0	0	0	0	0	0	3	18
Domex Superfresh Growers										
Rainier	21 (5 oz)	90	0	0	0	0	0	0	3	16
FROZEN										
sour unsweetened	½ cup	36	tr	0	tr	tr	tr	0	1	7
sweet sweetened	½ cup	115	tr	0	tr	tr	tr	0	3	26
Dole										
Dark Sweet	1 cup (4.9 oz)	90	0	0	0	0	0	0	3	18
CHERRY JUICE										
tart cherry concentrate	1 cup	140	0	0	0	0	0	0	0	27

FOOD	PORTION	CALS	TOTAL FAT	CHOL	SAT FAT	POLY FAT	MONO FAT	TRANS FAT	FIBER	SUGAR
Cheribundi										
Tart Cherry	8 oz	130	0	0	0	0	0	0	–	28
Froose										
Cheerful Cherry	1 box (4.2 oz)	80	0	0	0	0	0	0	3	8
Old Orchard										
Very Cherre 100% Tart Cherry Juice	8 oz	130	0	0	0	0	0	0	–	21
Smart Juice										
Organic 100% Juice Tart Cherry	8 oz	140	0	0	0	0	0	0	1	24
CHERVIL										
seed	1 tsp	1	tr	0	–	–	–	–	–	–
CHESTNUTS										
chinese steamed	3 (1 oz)	43	tr	0	tr	tr	tr	–	–	–
creme de marrons	1 oz	73	tr	0	tr	tr	tr	–	1	10
japanese roasted	1 oz	57	tr	0	tr	tr	tr	–	–	–
ready-to-eat vacuum packed	5 (1 oz)	40	0	0	0	0	0	0	0	0
roasted	3 (1 oz)	70	1	0	tr	tr	tr	–	1	3
Matiz										
Organic	7–8	86	1	0	0	–	–	0	5	12
CHEWING GUM										
bubble gum	1 block	20	tr	0	tr	tr	tr	0	tr	5
stick	1 piece	7	tr	0	tr	tr	tr	0	tr	2
sugarless	1 piece	5	tr	0	tr	tr	tr	0	0	0
5 Gum										
Cobalt	1 piece	5	0	0	0	0	0	0	–	0
Big Red										
Gum	1 stick	10	0	0	0	0	0	0	–	2
Doublemint										
Gum	1 piece	10	0	0	0	0	0	0	–	2
Freedent										
Gum	1 piece	10	0	0	0	0	0	0	–	2
Hubba Bubba										
Ouch! Bubble Gum	1 piece	5	0	0	0	0	0	0	–	0
Orbit										
Spearmint	1 piece	<5	0	0	0	0	0	0	0	0
Snap Infusion										
Citrus	1 piece (2.5 g)	5	0	0	0	0	0	0	0	0

FOOD	PORTION	CALS	TOTAL FAT	CHOL	SAT FAT	POLY FAT	MONO FAT	TRANS FAT	FIBER	SUGAR
Stride										
All Flavors	1 piece (1.9 g)	<5	0	0	0	0	0	0	–	0
Spark	1 piece (1.9 g)	5	0	0	0	0	0	0	–	0
Trident										
White Peppermint	2 pieces (3 g)	5	0	0	0	0	0	0	–	0
Vitamingum										
Fresh Sugar Free All Flavors	1 piece (3 g)	5	0	0	0	0	0	0	–	0
Sport Bubblegum	1 piece (6 g)	15	0	0	0	0	0	0	–	4

CHIA SEEDS

FOOD	PORTION	CALS	TOTAL FAT	CHOL	SAT FAT	POLY FAT	MONO FAT	TRANS FAT	FIBER	SUGAR
dried	1 oz	134	7	0	3	2	2	–	–	–
Dole										
Chia & Fruit Clusters Cranberry Apple	12 (1 oz)	120	3	0	0	–	–	0	4	8
Chia & Fruit Clusters Mixed Berry	12 (1 oz)	120	3	0	0	–	–	0	4	8
Milled Seeds	5 tbsp (1 oz)	150	9	0	1	–	–	0	11	0
Whole Seeds	3 tbsp (1 oz)	150	9	0	1	–	–	0	11	0
Health Warrior										
Chia Bar Peanut Butter Chocolate	1 (0.9 oz)	100	5	0	1	2	1	0	3	4
TruRoots										
Chia	1 tbsp (0.4 oz)	55	9	0	0	–	–	0	6	–

CHICKEN (see also CHICKEN DISHES, CHICKEN SUBSTITUTES, DINNER, HOT DOG, MEATBALLS)

FOOD	PORTION	CALS	TOTAL FAT	CHOL	SAT FAT	POLY FAT	MONO FAT	TRANS FAT	FIBER	SUGAR
CANNED										
chicken spread	1 serv (2 oz)	88	10	31	2	1	3	–	tr	tr
meat drained	1 can (5 oz)	230	10	62	3	2	4	–	0	0
FRESH										
back w/ skin roasted bones removed	1 (3.7 oz)	318	22	93	6	5	9	–	0	0
back w/o skin roasted bones removed	1 (2.8 oz)	191	11	72	3	2	4	–	0	0
breast roasted diced	1 cup (5 oz)	231	5	119	1	1	2	–	0	0
breast w/ skin battered fried bones removed	½ breast (4.9 oz)	364	18	119	5	4	8	–	tr	0
breast w/ skin floured fried bones removed	1 (3.4 oz)	218	9	87	2	2	3	–	tr	–
breast w/ skin roasted bones removed	½ breast (3.4 oz)	193	8	82	2	2	3	–	0	0

FOOD	PORTION	CALS	TOTAL FAT	CHOL	SAT FAT	POLY FAT	MONO FAT	TRANS FAT	FIBER	SUGAR
breast w/ skin stewed bones removed	½ breast (3.9 oz)	202	8	82	2	2	3	–	0	0
breast w/o skin fried bones removed	½ breast (3 oz)	161	4	78	1	1	1	–	0	0
breast w/o skin roasted bones removed	½ breast (3 oz)	142	3	73	1	1	1	–	0	0
breast w/o skin stewed bones removed	1 (3.3 oz)	143	3	73	1	1	1	–	0	0
broiler/fryer w/ skin roasted bones removed	½ (10.5 oz)	715	41	263	11	9	16	–	0	0
capon meat & skin roasted bones removed	½ (1.4 lbs)	1459	74	548	21	16	30	–	0	0
cornish hen w/ skin roasted	1 (9 oz)	668	47	337	13	9	21	–	0	0
cornish hen w/ skin roasted	½ (4.5 oz)	335	23	169	7	5	10	–	0	0
cornish hen w/o skin roasted	½ (4 oz)	147	4	117	1	1	1	–	0	0
cornish hen w/o skin roasted	1 (7.7 oz)	295	9	233	2	2	3	–	0	0
dark meat w/o skin roasted diced	1 cup (5 oz)	287	14	130	4	3	5	–	0	0
drumstick w/ skin battered floured & fried bones removed	1 (1.7 oz)	120	7	44	2	2	3	–	0	–
drumstick w/ skin battered fried bones removed	1 (2.5 oz)	193	11	62	3	3	5	–	tr	–
drumstick w/ skin roasted bones removed	1 (1.8 oz)	112	6	47	2	1	2	–	0	0
drumstick w/ skin stewed bones removed	1 (2 oz)	116	6	47	2	1	2	–	0	0
drumstick w/o skin fried bones removed	1 (1.5 oz)	82	3	39	1	1	1	–	0	0
drumstick w/o skin roasted bones removed	1 (1.5 oz)	76	2	41	1	1	1	–	0	0
drumstick w/o skin stewed bones removed	1 (1.6 oz)	78	3	40	1	1	1	–	0	0
feet cooked	1 (1.2 oz)	73	5	29	1	1	2	–	0	0
ground crumbled fried	3 oz	161	9	91	3	2	4	tr	0	0
ground patty cooked	1 lg (2.8 oz)	190	11	70	3	2	4	–	0	0
ground patty cooked	1 med (2.1 oz)	142	8	52	2	2	3	–	0	0
ground patty cooked	1 sm (1.7 oz)	114	6	42	2	1	3	–	0	0
meat & skin stewed bones removed	¼ chicken (4.6 oz)	372	25	103	7	6	9	–	0	0

FOOD	PORTION	CALS	TOTAL FAT	CHOL	SAT FAT	POLY FAT	MONO FAT	TRANS FAT	FIBER	SUGAR
neck w/ skin battered fried	1 (1.8 oz)	172	12	47	3	3	5	–	–	–
neck w/ skin fried	1 (1.3 oz)	120	9	34	2	2	3	–	–	–
neck w/ skin simmered	1 (1.3 oz)	94	7	27	2	1	3	–	0	0
roaster meat & skin roasted bones removed	¼ chicken (8.4 oz)	535	32	182	9	7	13	–	0	0
skin battered fried from ½ chicken	6.7 oz	749	55	141	14	13	23	–	–	–
skin floured fried from ½ chicken	2 oz	281	24	41	7	5	10	–	–	–
skin roasted	1 oz	131	12	37	3	2	5	tr	0	0
skin stewed from ½ chicken	2.5 oz	261	24	45	7	5	10	–	0	0
tail cooked	1 (1 oz)	84	5	25	1	1	2	–	tr	0
thigh w/ skin battered & fried bones removed	1 (3 oz)	238	14	80	4	3	6	–	tr	–
thigh w/ skin floured fried bones removed	1 (2.2 oz)	162	9	60	3	2	4	–	tr	–
thigh w/ skin roasted bones removed	1 (2.2 oz)	153	10	58	3	2	4	–	0	0
thigh w/ skin stewed bones removed	1 (2.4 oz)	158	10	57	3	2	4	–	0	0
thigh w/o skin fried bones removed	1 (1.8 oz)	113	5	53	1	1	2	–	0	0
thigh w/o skin roasted bones removed	1 (1.8 oz)	109	6	49	2	1	2	–	0	0
thigh w/o skin stewed bones removed	1 (1.9 oz)	107	5	50	1	1	2	–	0	0
wing w/ skin battered fried bones removed	1 (1.7 oz)	159	11	39	3	2	4	–	tr	–
wing w/ skin floured fried bones removed	1 (1.1 oz)	103	7	26	2	2	3	–	0	–
wing w/ skin roasted bones removed	1 (1.4 oz)	100	7	28	2	1	3	–	0	0
wing w/o skin fried bones removed	1 (0.7 oz)	42	2	17	1	tr	1	–	0	0
wing w/o skin roasted bones removed	1 (0.7 oz)	43	2	18	tr	tr	1	–	0	0
wing w/o skin stewed bones removed	1 (0.8 oz)	43	2	18	tr	tr	1	–	0	0
Coleman										
Organic Breast Boneless Skinless	4 oz	120	2	65	0	–	–	0	0	0

FOOD	PORTION	CALS	TOTAL FAT	CHOL	SAT FAT	POLY FAT	MONO FAT	TRANS FAT	FIBER	SUGAR
Organic Drumsticks	4 oz	180	10	90	3	–	–	0	0	0
Foster Farms										
Back & Necks	4 oz	340	31	100	–	–	–	0	0	0
Breast Skinless Boneless	4 oz	120	2	65	–	–	–	0	0	0
Drumsticks not prep	1 (2.8 oz)	130	7	65	–	–	–	0	0	0
Ground not prep	4 oz	210	14	93	–	–	–	0	0	0
Party Wings	5 (3.8 oz)	230	17	80	–	–	–	0	0	0
Thighs	1 (4.6 oz)	270	20	110	–	–	–	0	0	0
Rocky										
The Range Chicken Whole	4 oz	240	17	100	5	–	–	0	0	0
Rosie										
Organic Breast Boneless Skinless	4 oz	120	2	65	0	–	–	0	0	0
FROZEN										
breast roll roasted	2 oz	75	4	22	1	1	2	–	0	tr
fajita strips	1 (0.3 oz)	13	1	8	tr	tr	tr	–	0	0
patty cooked	1 (3.5 oz)	287	20	43	4	5	8	–	tr	0
Coleman										
Breast Nuggets Gluten Free	6 (2.7 oz)	130	6	30	1	–	–	0	0	1
Breast Strips	6 (2.7 oz)	130	3	30	0	–	–	0	1	1
Perdue										
Simply Smart Grilled Chicken Strips	3 oz	110	3	55	1	–	–	0	–	0
Simply Smart Lightly Breaded Chicken Strips	3 oz	140	5	40	1	–	–	0	–	0
Simply Smart Roasted Chicken Chunks	3 oz	120	2	45	0	–	–	0	–	1
Weaver										
Breast Nuggets	4 (2.8 oz)	190	11	20	2	4	5	0	1	0
Breast Strips	2 (2.7 oz)	190	12	15	3	5	5	0	0	0
Patties Breast	1 (2.9 oz)	200	11	20	3	5	5	0	1	0
Popcorn Chicken	12 pieces (2.9 oz)	200	10	20	2	4	4	0	1	0
Wings Buffalo Style	3 (2.9 oz)	160	10	90	2	3	5	0	0	0
READY-TO-EAT										
Foster Farms										
Breast Strips Grilled	3 oz	110	3	45	–	–	–	0	0	0
Cutlets Breaded	3 oz	180	8	35	2	–	–	0	0	tr
Perdue										
Short Cuts Chicken Breast Grilled Italian	½ cup (2.5 oz)	100	2	75	1	–	–	0	–	1

FOOD	PORTION	CALS	TOTAL FAT	CHOL	SAT FAT	POLY FAT	MONO FAT	TRANS FAT	FIBER	SUGAR
TAKE-OUT										
chicken tenders	4 (2.2 oz)	180	10	31	2	2	6	–	tr	1

CHICKEN DISHES
CANNED
Dinty Moore

FOOD	PORTION	CALS	TOTAL FAT	CHOL	SAT FAT	POLY FAT	MONO FAT	TRANS FAT	FIBER	SUGAR
Chicken & Dumplings Big Bowl	½ pkg	220	7	35	2	–	–	–	1	1
Chicken & Noodles	1 can (7.5 oz)	190	9	35	3	–	–	–	1	2
Chicken Stew	½ can	220	11	35	4	–	–	–	2	3
Swanson										
Chicken A La King	1 can (10.5 oz)	320	19	40	6	4	8	1	2	3
FROZEN										
Crazy Cuizine										
Teriyaki Chicken	1 cup (5 oz)	240	8	45	2	–	–	0	3	21
Tandoor Chef										
Chicken Biryani (9.9 oz)	1 pkg	480	15	115	5	–	–	0	0	0
Samosa Tandoori	2 (2 oz)	130	7	10	1	–	–	0	0	0
TAKE-OUT										
arroz con pollo	1 serv (16 oz)	579	14	126	7	–	–	–	2	3
barbecued pulled chicken	1 serv (9 oz)	312	2	147	1	–	–	–	2	27
boneless breast w/ apple stuffing	1 serv (5 oz)	260	9	80	2	–	–	–	1	2
breast & wing breaded & fried	2 pieces (5.7 oz)	494	30	148	8	7	12	–	–	–
buffalo wing + sauce	2 (1.7 oz)	147	10	39	3	3	4	–	0	tr
cacciatore breast + sauce	1 serv (5.9 oz)	323	18	88	4	5	7	–	1	3
cacciatore drumstick + sauce	1 serv (3.2 oz)	172	9	47	2	3	4	0	1	2
cacciatore thigh + sauce	1 serv (3.8 oz)	204	11	56	3	3	4	–	1	2
cacciatore wing + sauce	1 serv (2.1 oz)	113	6	31	2	2	2	–	tr	1
chicharrones de pollo	3 (2.6 oz)	289	18	58	4	6	7	–	1	tr
chicken & dumplings	1 cup (8.6 oz)	368	19	88	5	4	8	–	1	1
chicken & noodles in cream sauce	1 cup (8 oz)	323	11	76	3	3	4	–	1	5
chicken a la king	1 cup (8.5 oz)	465	34	190	12	7	13	–	1	4
chicken cordon bleu + sauce	1 roll (8 oz)	504	29	188	15	2	9	–	1	1
chicken meatloaf	1 lg slice (5 oz)	243	9	122	3	2	3	–	1	3
chicken paprikash	1½ cups	296	10	90	–	–	–	–	–	–

FOOD	PORTION	CALS	TOTAL FAT	CHOL	SAT FAT	POLY FAT	MONO FAT	TRANS FAT	FIBER	SUGAR
chicken satay + peanut sauce	2 skewers	239	12	64	6	–	–	0	1	4
chicken breast parmigiana	1 serv (5.8 oz)	278	14	119	5	3	4	–	1	3
chicken creole w/o rice	1 cup (8.6 oz)	187	4	69	1	1	2	–	2	5
chicken kiev breast meat	1 serv (9 oz)	653	34	276	16	4	10	–	1	1
chicken salad white meat	1 serv (4 oz)	300	21	85	2	–	–	0	0	0
creamed chicken	1 cup (8.5 oz)	388	23	87	6	6	10	–	tr	8
croquette	1 (2.2 oz)	159	9	28	2	2	4	–	tr	2
curry	1 cup (8.3 oz)	288	16	83	3	5	7	–	2	5
curry breast half + sauce	1 (7 oz)	244	14	70	3	4	6	–	2	4
curry drumstick + sauce	1 (3.7 oz)	129	7	37	1	2	3	–	1	2
curry thigh + sauce	1 (4.4 oz)	154	9	44	2	2	4	–	1	3
curry wing + sauce	1 (2.4 oz)	84	5	24	1	1	2	–	1	1
drumstick & thigh breaded & fried	2 pieces (5.2 oz)	431	27	166	7	6	11	–	–	–
fricassee	1 cup (8.6 oz)	322	18	85	5	4	8	–	tr	tr
groundnut stew hkatenkwan	1 serv (15.7 oz)	576	40	116	10	–	–	–	4	3
jamaican jerk wings	4 wings (9.9 oz)	709	51	172	14	–	–	–	tr	tr
jambalaya w/ sausage & rice	1 cup (8.6 oz)	393	21	98	6	4	9	–	1	2
kobete turkish chicken w/ pastry	1 serv	513	13	71	4	–	–	–	–	–
rotisserie seasoned breast w/ skin	1 serv (3.5 oz)	184	8	96	2	1	4	tr	0	0
rotisserie seasoned breast w/o skin	1 serv (3.5 oz)	148	3	89	1	tr	1	tr	0	0
rotisserie seasoned thigh w/o skin	1 serv (3.5 oz)	233	16	132	4	2	7	tr	0	0
rotisserie seasoned thigh w/o skin	1 serv (3.5 oz)	196	11	130	3	2	5	tr	0	0
sancocho de pollo dominican chicken stew	1 serv	702	30	195	8	–	–	–	1	4
stew	1 cup (8.8 oz)	176	5	43	1	2	1	–	3	4
tetrazzini	1 cup (8.6 oz)	369	18	49	6	4	6	–	2	2

CHICKEN SUBSTITUTES
Quorn

FOOD	PORTION	CALS	TOTAL FAT	CHOL	SAT FAT	POLY FAT	MONO FAT	TRANS FAT	FIBER	SUGAR
Chik'n Nuggets	3-4 (3 oz)	180	8	0	1	2	5	0	2	4
Chik'n Patties	1 (2.6 oz)	150	6	0	1	2	4	0	2	4

FOOD	PORTION	CALS	TOTAL FAT	CHOL	SAT FAT	POLY FAT	MONO FAT	TRANS FAT	FIBER	SUGAR
Gruyere Chik'n Cutlet	1 (4 oz)	260	15	20	4	7	4	0	3	3
Naked Chik'n Cutlet	1 (2.4 oz)	80	3	5	1	1	2	0	2	1
Vegetarian Plus										
Vegan Half Chicken	¼ pkg (3 oz)	180	10	0	2	–	–	0	3	0

CHICKPEAS
CANNED
chickpeas	1 cup	285	3	0	tr	1	1	–	–	–
Progresso										
Chick Peas	½ cup (4.6 oz)	120	3	0	0	–	–	0	5	3
DRIED										
cooked	1 cup	269	4	0	tr	2	1	–	–	–

CHICORY
endive fresh chopped	½ cup	4	tr	0	tr	tr	tr	–	–	–
greens raw chopped	½ cup	21	tr	0	tr	tr	tr	–	–	–
root raw	1 (2.1 oz)	44	tr	0	tr	tr	tr	–	–	–
roots raw cut up	½ cup (1.6 oz)	33	tr	0	tr	tr	tr	–	–	–
witloof head raw	1 (1.9 oz)	9	tr	0	tr	tr	tr	–	–	–
witloof raw	½ cup (1.6 oz)	8	tr	0	tr	tr	tr	–	–	–

CHILI
powder	1 tbsp	24	1	0	tr	tr	1	0	3	1
Bush's										
ChiliMagic Chili Starter Texas Recipe	½ cup (4.6 oz)	110	1	0	0	–	–	0	5	2
ChiliMagic Chili Starter Traditional Mild	½ cup (4.6 oz)	100	0	0	0	0	0	0	4	2
Frontera										
Chili Mix Chipotle Black Bean	½ cup (4.2 oz)	60	1	0	0	0	0	0	3	3
Chili Starter Green Chile White Bean	½ cup (4.4 oz)	80	2	0	0	–	–	0	4	2
Quorn										
Chili	1 pkg (8.9 oz)	160	3	0	0	–	–	0	7	7
Ro-Tel										
Chili Fixin's	½ cup (4.4 oz)	35	1	0	0	–	–	0	3	5
Stagg										
Chunkero	½ can	320	16	40	6	–	–	–	6	6
Classic	½ can	290	13	35	5	–	–	–	6	7
Ranch House Chicken	½ can	240	8	55	2	–	–	–	7	5

FOOD	PORTION	CALS	TOTAL FAT	CHOL	SAT FAT	POLY FAT	MONO FAT	TRANS FAT	FIBER	SUGAR
Silverado Beef	½ can	260	8	30	4	–	–	–	6	6
Turkey Ranchero	½ can	250	5	35	2	–	–	–	9	7
Vegetable Garden	½ can	200	1	0	0	–	–	–	8	9
TAKE-OUT										
chiles rellenos cheese filled	1 (5 oz)	365	30	167	13	2	13	0	1	5
chili con carne w/ beans	1 cup	264	11	53	4	1	5	–	7	6
chili con carne w/ beans & chicken	1 cup (8.9 oz)	218	7	53	2	2	3	–	6	6
chili con carne w/ beans & rice	1 cup	298	9	28	4	1	4	–	7	2
vegetarian	1 cup	272	7	0	1	3	2	–	11	7

CHILI PEPPER (see PEPPERS)

CHINESE FOOD (see ASIAN FOOD)

CHINESE PRESERVING MELON

FOOD	PORTION	CALS	TOTAL FAT	CHOL	SAT FAT	POLY FAT	MONO FAT	TRANS FAT	FIBER	SUGAR
cooked	½ cup	11	tr	0	tr	tr	tr	–	–	–

CHIPS (see also SNACKS)

FOOD	PORTION	CALS	TOTAL FAT	CHOL	SAT FAT	POLY FAT	MONO FAT	TRANS FAT	FIBER	SUGAR
apple chips	10 (0.8 oz)	101	5	0	tr	1	3	–	2	14
banana	1 oz	147	10	0	8	tr	1	–	2	10
carrot	28 (1 oz)	95	tr	0	tr	tr	tr	–	7	11
corn	1 oz	147	8	0	1	4	2	tr	2	tr
potato salted	1 oz	155	11	0	3	3	3	–	1	tr
potato sticks	½ cup (0.6 oz)	94	6	0	2	3	1	–	1	tr
potato sticks	1 pkg (1 oz)	148	10	0	3	5	2	–	1	tr
potato unsalted	1 oz	152	10	0	3	3	3	–	1	tr
potato unsalted reduced fat	1 oz	138	6	0	1	3	1	–	2	tr
shrimp	4 sm (0.4 oz)	56	4	8	1	tr	2	–	tr	tr
shrimp	4 med (0.9 oz)	141	9	21	2	1	5	–	tr	tr
shrimp	4 lg (1.4 oz)	219	14	33	4	2	8	–	tr	1
soy	1 oz	107	2	0	0	1	tr	0	1	1
sweet potato	1 oz	141	7	0	1	3	3	–	1	2
taro	10 (0.8 oz)	115	6	0	1	3	1	–	2	1
tortilla lowfat baked	1 oz	118	2	0	tr	1	tr	–	2	tr
tortilla lowfat unsalted	1 oz	118	2	0	tr	1	tr	–	2	tr
tortilla white corn	1 oz	139	7	0	1	3	2	tr	2	tr
tortilla yellow corn	1 oz	139	6	0	1	2	3	tr	1	tr
Bachman										
Corn Jumbo Chipitos	16 (1 oz)	150	8	0	2	–	–	0	2	0
Potato Golden Ridges	22 (1 oz)	160	10	<5	3	–	–	0	0	–

FOOD	PORTION	CALS	TOTAL FAT	CHOL.	SAT FAT	POLY FAT	MONO FAT	TRANS FAT	FIBER	SUG*
Tortilla Black Bean	1 oz	140	7	0	1	–	–	0	3	–
Tortilla Restaurant Style	11 (1 oz)	140	6	0	1	–	–	0	2	0
Tortilla Toasted Sweet Potato	11 (1 oz)	130	5	0	1	–	–	0	3	2
Beanfields										
Bean & Rice Naturally Unsalted	⅙ pkg (1 oz)	140	6	0	0	–	–	0	3	0
Bean & Rice Pico De Gallo	⅙ pkg (1 oz)	140	6	0	0	–	–	0	4	0
Bean & Rice Sea Salt	⅙ pkg (1 oz)	140	6	0	0	–	–	0	4	0
Bean & Rice Sea Salt & Pepper	⅙ pkg (1 oz)	140	6	0	0	–	–	0	4	0
Boulder Canyon										
Potato Honey Bar-B-Que	14 (1 oz)	140	7	0	1	1	5	0	1	2
Potato Sour Cream & Chive	14 (1 oz)	140	7	0	1	1	5	0	1	1
Potato Totally Natural	14 (1 oz)	140	8	0	1	1	5	0	1	0
Buffalo Nickel Wingers										
Potato Level 1: No Bull Barbecue	25 (1 oz)	120	4	0	0	–	–	0	1	2
Potato Level 3: Nacho Chiliehanga	25 (1 oz)	120	4	0	0	–	–	0	1	1
Potato Level 5: Fiery Buffalo Bleu	25 (1 oz)	120	4	0	0	–	–	0	1	1
Cape Cod										
Potato Chef's Recipe Feta & Rosemary	18 (1 oz)	140	7	0	1	–	–	0	1	0
Potato 40% Less Fat Aged Cheddar & Sour Cream	18 (1 oz)	140	6	0	1	–	–	0	1	0
Potato Original	19 (1 oz)	140	8	0	1	–	–	0	tr	0
Potato Original 40% Reduced Fat	19 (1 oz)	140	6	0	1	–	–	0	2	0
Potato Sea Salt & Cracked Pepper	18 (1 oz)	140	7	0	1	–	–	0	2	0
Potato Sour Cream & Green Onion	18 (1 oz)	140	8	0	1	–	–	0	1	tr
Potato Waffle Cut Sea Salt	17 (1 oz)	140	7	0	1	–	–	0	1	0
Whole Grain Toasted	10 (1 oz)	130	6	0	1	–	–	0	3	2
Doritos										
Tortilla Flamas	11 (1 oz)	140	8	0	1	–	–	0	1	0
Tortilla Nacho Cheese	11 (1 oz)	150	8	0	2	–	–	0	1	1
Tortilla Spicy Nacho	12 (1 oz)	140	7	0	1	–	–	0	1	1
Tortilla Toasted Corn	13 (1 oz)	140	7	0	1	–	–	0	1	0

FOOD	PORTION	CALS	TOTAL FAT	CHOL	SAT FAT	POLY FAT	MONO FAT	TRANS FAT	FIBER	SUGAR
Fritos										
Corn Lightly Salted	1 oz	160	10	0	2	5	3	0	1	0
Corn Original	32 (1 oz)	160	10	0	2	–	–	0	1	tr
Corn Scoops	10 (1 oz)	160	10	0	2	–	–	0	1	0
Frontera										
Tortilla Blue Corn	⅑ pkg (1 oz)	130	5	0	1	0	0	0	2	0
Tortilla Thick & Crunchy	⅑ pkg (1 oz)	130	5	0	1	0	0	0	2	0
Garden Of Eatin'										
Corn White Strips Mini	18 (1 oz)	140	6	0	1	1	5	0	2	0
Pita w/ Whole Grain Sea Salt	9 (1 oz)	120	3	0	0	–	–	0	2	1
Tortilla Blue Corn No Salt Added	16 (1 oz)	140	7	0	1	1	5	0	2	0
Tortilla Corn Sprouted Blues	11 (1 oz)	130	7	0	1	–	–	0	3	tr
Tortilla Guac-A-Mole	9 (1 oz)	140	6	0	1	1	5	0	2	tr
Tortilla Key Lime Jalapeno	15 (1 oz)	140	7	0	1	–	–	0	3	0
Tortilla Little Soy Blues	13 (1 oz)	140	7	0	1	1	5	0	2	0
Tortilla Multi Grain Everything	16 (1 oz)	140	7	0	1	–	–	0	3	1
Tortilla Popped Sea Salt	20 (1 oz)	110	3	0	0	–	–	0	3	1
Tortilla Red	15 (1 oz)	140	7	0	1	1	5	0	1	0
Tortilla Salsa Red	15 (1 oz)	140	7	0	1	1	5	0	3	0
Tortilla Sweet Potato Corn	9 (1 oz)	140	7	0	1	–	–	0	1	1
Tortilla Tamari	8 (1 oz)	140	7	0	1	1	5	0	3	0
Tortilla Yellow	13 (1 oz)	140	7	0	1	1	5	0	2	0
Veggie Salt & Garlic	17 (1 oz)	140	6	0	1	–	–	0	2	1
Hawaiian Snacks										
Potato Kettle Style	13 (1 oz)	140	9	0	3	–	–	0	1	0
Potato Luau BBQ	13 (1 oz)	140	9	0	2	–	–	0	1	1
Potato Mango Habanero	13 (1 oz)	140	9	0	2	–	–	0	1	1
Kettle Brand										
Potato Baked Fully Loaded	13 (1 oz)	150	9	0	1	1	7	0	1	1
Potato Baked Sea Salt & Vinegar	20 (1 oz)	120	3	0	1	1	2	0	2	0
Potato Baked Sour Cream And Onion	1 oz	120	4	0	0	0	2	0	2	1
Potato Krinkle Cut Buffalo Bleu	9 (1 oz)	150	9	0	1	1	7	0	1	1
Potato Krinkle Cut Salt & Fresh Ground Pepper	9 (1 oz)	140	9	0	1	1	7	0	1	0

FOOD	PORTION	CALS	TOTAL FAT	CHOL	SAT FAT	POLY FAT	MONO FAT	TRANS FAT	FIBER	SUG
Potato Krinkle Cut Sweet Chili Garlic	9 (1 oz)	150	9	0	1	1	7	0	1	1
Potato Krinkle Cut Zesty Ranch	9 (1 oz)	150	9	0	1	1	7	0	1	1
Potato New York Cheddar	13 (1 oz)	150	9	0	1	1	7	0	1	1
Potato Organic Country Style Barbeque	13 (1 oz)	150	9	0	1	1	7	0	2	1
Potato Reduced Fat Salt & Fresh Ground Pepper	13 (1 oz)	130	6	0	1	1	5	0	1	0
Potato Reduced Fat Sea Salt	13 (1 oz)	130	6	0	1	1	5	0	1	0
Potato Spicy Thai	13 (1 oz)	150	9	0	1	1	7	0	1	1
Potato Sweet Onion	13 (1 oz)	150	9	0	1	1	7	0	1	1
Potato Unsalted	13 (1 oz)	150	9	0	1	1	7	0	2	0
Tortilla Tias! Nacho Cheddar	12 (1 oz)	150	8	0	1	1	6	0	1	1
Tortilla Tias! Salsa Picante	12 (1 oz)	140	8	0	1	1	6	0	1	1
Tortilla Tias! Sweet Baja Barbeque	12 (1 oz)	140	8	0	1	1	6	0	1	1
Lay's										
Potato Balsamic Sweet Onion	15 (1 oz)	160	10	0	1	3	5	0	1	2
Potato Chipotle Ranch	15 (1 oz)	160	10	0	1	3	5	0	1	1
Potato Classic	15 (1 oz)	160	10	0	1	3	5	0	1	tr
Potato Garden Tomato & Basil	15 (1 oz)	160	10	0	1	5	5	0	1	2
Potato Kettle Cooked Crinkle Cut Spice Rubbed BBQ	15 (1 oz)	140	8	0	1	2	5	0	1	2
Potato Kettle Cooked Original	16 (1 oz)	160	9	0	1	3	5	0	1	tr
Potato Kettle Cooked Spicy Cayenne & Cheese	16 (1 oz)	150	9	0	1	2	5	0	1	1
Potato Lightly Salted	15 (1 oz)	160	10	0	1	3	5	0	1	tr
Potato Original Baked	15 (1 oz)	120	2	0	0	–	–	0	2	2
Potato Stax Sour Cream & Onion	12 (1 oz)	150	9	0	3	4	2	0	1	1
Potato Sweet Southern Heat Barbecue	15 (1 oz)	160	10	0	1	3	5	0	1	2
Potato Wavy Original	11 (1 oz)	160	10	0	1	3	5	0	1	tr
LesserEvil										
Chia Crisps Crunchy Dill Pickle	22 (1 oz)	110	4	0	0	1	2	0	3	1

FOOD	PORTION	CALS	TOTAL FAT	CHOL	SAT FAT	POLY FAT	MONO FAT	TRANS FAT	FIBER	SUGAR
Chia Crisps Feta And Black Olive	22 (1 oz)	110	4	0	0	1	2	0	3	1
Potato Krinkle Sticks Sea Salt	35 (1 oz)	120	5	0	0	–	–	0	1	0
Veggie Krinkle Sticks	35 (1 oz)	120	5	0	0	–	–	0	1	0
Lundberg										
Organic Black Bean Rice Spicy	9 (1 oz)	140	6	0	1	–	–	0	1	1
Rice Chips Honey Dijon	9 (1 oz)	140	6	0	1	–	–	0	1	1
Rice Chips Original Sea Salt	9 (1 oz)	140	6	0	1	–	–	0	1	0
Rice Chips Sesame	9 (1 oz)	140	6	0	1	–	–	0	1	1
Margaritaville										
Tortilla Sea Salt	1 oz	140	7	0	1	–	–	0	0	0
Maui Style										
Potato	14 (1 oz)	150	9	0	1	3	5	0	1	tr
Shrimp Chips	1 oz	150	8	0	1	5	3	0	tr	0
Mediterranean Snacks										
Baked Lentil Cucumber Dill	22 (1 oz)	110	3	0	0	–	–	0	3	1
Baked Lentil Roasted Pepper	22 (1 oz)	110	3	0	0	–	–	0	3	2
Baked Lentil Rosemary	22 (1 oz)	110	3	0	0	–	–	0	3	1
Baked Lentil Sea Salt	22 (1 oz)	110	3	0	0	–	–	0	3	0
Lentil Fiery Tomato	22 (1 oz)	105	3	0	0	–	–	0	3	2
Multi Grain Original	16 (1 oz)	130	6	0	1	2	4	0	1	2
Veggie Medley	28 (1 oz)	130	7	0	1	2	4	0	1	1
Michael Season's										
Popped Black Bean Nacho	17 (1 oz)	120	4	0	0	–	–	0	3	1
Popped Black Bean Red Pepper	17 (1 oz)	120	4	0	0	–	–	0	3	1
Popped Black Bean Sea Salt	17 (1 oz)	120	4	0	0	–	–	0	3	1
Mrs. Cubbison's										
Tortilla Strips Southwest	1½ tbsp (0.2 oz)	30	2	0	0	–	–	0	0	0
Popchips										
Tortilla Chili Limon	1 pkg (1 oz)	120	4	0	0	1	3	0	2	1
Tortilla Nacho Cheese	1 pkg (1 oz)	120	4	0	1	1	3	0	2	1
Tortilla Ranch	1 pkg (1 oz)	120	4	0	1	1	3	0	2	1
Rhythm										
Crispy Kale Bombay Curry	½ pkg (1 oz)	101	2	0	0	–	–	0	2	2
Crispy Kale Kool Ranch	½ pkg (1 oz)	100	5	0	1	–	–	0	2	1
Crispy Kale Zesty Nacho	½ pkg (1 oz)	106	5	0	1	–	–	0	2	2

FOOD	PORTION	CALS	TOTAL FAT	CHOL	SAT FAT	POLY FAT	MONO FAT	TRANS FAT	FIBER	SUG
Ruffles										
Baked Original Potato	9 (1 oz)	120	3	0	0	2	1	0	2	1
Original Potato	12 (1 oz)	160	10	0	1	3	5	0	1	tr
Reduced Fat Potato	13 (1 oz)	140	7	0	1	2	4	0	1	0
Reduced Fat Sea Salted Potato	1 oz	140	7	0	1	–	–	0	1	0
Santitas										
Tortilla Triangles White Corn	9 (1 oz)	140	6	0	1	4	2	0	2	0
Tortilla Triangles Yellow Corn	9 (1 oz)	140	6	0	1	4	2	0	2	0
Simply 7										
Hummus Chips Sea Salt	30 (1 oz)	130	5	0	1	–	–	0	tr	2
Lentil Chips Sea Salt	31 (1 oz)	140	6	0	0	–	–	0	tr	0
Special K										
Popcorn Butter	28 (1 oz)	120	2	0	0	0	1	0	tr	tr
Popcorn Sweet & Salty	28 (1 oz)	120	3	0	0	1	2	0	tr	2
Stacy's										
Bagel Chips Everything	12 (1 oz)	130	4	0	1	1	3	0	1	1
Pita Chips Cinnamon Sugar	1 oz	140	5	0	1	1	4	0	1	6
SunChips										
Multigrain French Onion	15 (1 oz)	140	6	0	1	1	4	0	3	3
Multigrain Original	16 (1 oz)	140	6	0	1	1	4	0	3	2
The Whole Earth										
Tortilla Really Seedy Multigrain	9 (1 oz)	140	9	0	1	–	–	0	2	1
Tostitos										
Tortilla Baked Scoops	14 (1 oz)	120	3	0	1	2	1	0	2	0
Tortilla Bite Size Rounds	24 (1 oz)	140	7	0	1	3	2	0	2	0
Tortilla Multigrain	8 (1 oz)	150	7	0	1	3	2	0	2	tr
Tortilla Scoops	12 (1 oz)	140	7	0	1	3	2	0	2	0
Umpqua Indian Foods										
Nana Crisps	⅕ pkg (1 oz)	120	6	0	0	–	–	0	tr	3
Veggie	¼ pkg (1 oz)	120	6	0	0	–	–	0	2	2
Want'ems										
Wonton Asian BBQ	16 (1 oz)	140	8	0	1	–	–	0	1	tr
Wonton Original	16 (1 oz)	140	8	0	1	–	–	0	1	0
Way Better Snacks										
Tortilla Black Bean Sprouted	11 (1 oz)	130	6	0	1	2	4	0	3	0
Tortilla Multi-Grain Sprouted	14 (1.25 oz)	170	9	0	1	2	6	0	4	0
Tortilla No Salt Naked Blues	11 (1 oz)	130	7	0	1	2	5	0	2	0

FOOD	PORTION	CALS	TOTAL FAT	CHOL.	SAT FAT	POLY FAT	MONO FAT	TRANS FAT	FIBER	SUGAR
Tortilla Sweet Potato Sprouted	11 (1 oz)	130	7	0	1	2	5	0	2	0
Unbeatable Blues Sprouted	11 (1 oz)	130	7	0	1	2	5	0	2	0
Willamette Valley										
Granola Chips Honey Nut	⅙ pkg (1 oz)	110	2	0	0	1	1	0	3	5

CHITTERLINGS

FOOD	PORTION	CALS	TOTAL FAT	CHOL.	SAT FAT	POLY FAT	MONO FAT	TRANS FAT	FIBER	SUGAR
pork cooked	3 oz	258	24	122	9	6	8	–	0	0

CHIVES

FOOD	PORTION	CALS	TOTAL FAT	CHOL.	SAT FAT	POLY FAT	MONO FAT	TRANS FAT	FIBER	SUGAR
freeze-dried	1 tbsp	1	tr	0	tr	tr	tr	–	–	–
fresh chopped	1 tsp	0	tr	0	tr	tr	tr	–	–	–
fresh chopped	1 tbsp	1	tr	0	tr	tr	tr	–	–	–

CHOCOLATE (see also CANDY, CHOCOLATE SYRUP, COCOA, HOT CHOCOLATE, ICE CREAM TOPPINGS, MILK DRINKS)

BAKING

FOOD	PORTION	CALS	TOTAL FAT	CHOL.	SAT FAT	POLY FAT	MONO FAT	TRANS FAT	FIBER	SUGAR
baking	1 oz	145	15	0	9	1	5	–	–	–
grated unsweetened	¼ cup	165	17	0	11	1	5	–	6	tr
liquid unsweetened	1 oz	134	14	0	7	3	3	–	5	0
mexican baking	1 sq (0.7 oz)	85	3	0	2	tr	1	–	1	14
squares unsweetened	1 sq (1 oz)	145	15	0	9	tr	5	–	5	tr
Baker's										
Semi-Sweet	0.5 oz	70	5	0	3	–	–	0	1	6
Unsweetened	0.5 oz	70	7	0	5	–	–	0	2	0
White	0.5 oz	80	5	0	3	–	–	0	0	9
CHIPS										
milk chocolate	1 cup (6 oz)	862	52	38	31	2	17	–	–	–
semisweet	1 cup (6 oz)	804	50	0	30	2	17	–	–	–
semisweet	60 pieces (1 oz)	136	9	0	5	tr	3	–	–	–
Ghirardelli										
Semi-Sweet	32 (0.5 oz)	70	5	0	3	–	–	0	tr	8
MIX										
drink mix powder	2–3 heaping tsp	75	1	0	tr	tr	tr	–	–	–
drink mix powder as prep w/ whole milk	9 oz	226	9	33	5	tr	3	–	–	–

CHOCOLATE MILK (see MILK DRINKS)

CHOCOLATE SYRUP

FOOD	PORTION	CALS	TOTAL FAT	CHOL.	SAT FAT	POLY FAT	MONO FAT	TRANS FAT	FIBER	SUGAR
syrup	2 tbsp	82	tr	0	tr	tr	tr	–	–	–

FOOD	PORTION	CALS	TOTAL FAT	CHOL	SAT FAT	POLY FAT	MONO FAT	TRANS FAT	FIBER	SU
syrup	1 cup	653	3	0	2	tr	1	–	–	–
syrup as prep w/ whole milk	1 cup (9.9 oz)	254	8	25	5	tr	2	–	1	32
CHUTNEY										
coconut	2 oz	87	9	0	7	tr	1	–	3	1
fresh mint	2 oz	18	0	0	0	0	0	–	1	3
mango	¼ cup (2 oz)	227	5	0	1	2	2	–	10	16
tomato	1 oz	90	7	6	1	3	2	–	2	6
CILANTRO										
fresh	¼ cup	1	tr	0	tr	tr	tr	0	tr	tr
fresh	1 tsp (2 g)	<1	tr	0	0	0	0	–	tr	–
fresh sprigs	5 (5 g)	1	tr	0	tr	tr	tr	0	tr	tr
CINNAMON										
cinnamon sugar	1 tsp	16	tr	0	tr	tr	tr	–	tr	4
ground	1 tsp (2.6 g)	6	tr	0	tr	tr	tr	0	1	tr
McCormick										
Grinder Cinnamon Sugar	1 tsp (3.5 g)	10	0	0	0	0	0	0	0	–
CISCO										
smoked	1 oz	50	3	9	tr	1	2	–	0	0
CLAMS										
CANNED										
drained meat only	1 cup (5.6 oz)	227	3	80	tr	1	tr	tr	0	0
liquid only	½ cup (4.2 oz)	2	tr	4	tr	tr	tr	–	0	0
smoked in oil	1 lg (2.1 oz)	113	7	20	2	2	3	–	0	0
Chicken Of The Sea										
Chopped	¼ cup	30	0	12	0	0	0	0	0	0
Whole Baby	¼ cup	30	0	10	0	0	0	0	0	0
FRESH										
meat + liquid	1 cup (8 oz)	195	2	68	tr	tr	tr	tr	0	0
raw	1 med (0.5 oz)	12	tr	4	tr	tr	tr	tr	0	0
raw	1 sm (0.3 oz)	8	tr	3	tr	tr	tr	tr	0	0
raw	1 lg (0.7 oz)	17	tr	6	tr	tr	tr	tr	0	0
raw	3 oz	73	1	26	tr	tr	tr	tr	0	0
steamed	20 sm (3.3 oz)	141	2	64	tr	1	tr	–	0	0
TAKE-OUT										
breaded & fried	10 sm (3.3 oz)	190	10	57	3	3	4	–	–	–
breaded & fried	12 med (5.3 oz)	286	12	75	2	4	4	–	1	1

OD	PORTION	CALS	TOTAL FAT	CHOL	SAT FAT	POLY FAT	MONO FAT	TRANS FAT	FIBER	SUGAR
sino	3 (3.2 oz)	108	4	14	1	1	2	–	1	2
ffed	1 lg (1.8 oz)	104	6	10	1	2	3	–	1	1

LEMENTINES

uties
| esh | 2 (6 oz) | 80 | 1 | 0 | 0 | – | – | 0 | 4 | 13 |

unkist
| esh | 2 (6 oz) | 80 | 1 | 0 | 0 | – | – | 0 | 5 | 15 |

LOVES
| ound | 1 tsp | 7 | tr | 0 | tr | tr | tr | 0 | 1 | tr |

OCOA (see also HOT CHOCOLATE)
| coa butter | 1 tbsp | 120 | 14 | 0 | 8 | tr | 4 | – | 0 | 0 |
| wder unsweetened | 1 tbsp | 12 | 1 | 0 | tr | tr | tr | – | 2 | tr |

ocoaVia
| pplement Mix Summer Citrus | 1 pkg (0.24 oz) | 20 | 0 | 0 | 0 | 0 | 0 | 0 | – | – |

onest CocoaNova
| erry Cacao | 8 oz | 50 | 0 | 0 | 0 | 0 | 0 | 0 | – | 13 |

OCONUT
ied sweetened shredded	¼ cup	116	8	0	7	tr	tr	0	1	10
ied toasted	1 oz	168	13	0	12	tr	1	0	–	–
ied unsweetened	1 oz	187	18	0	16	tr	1	0	5	2
esh from 1 coconut	14 oz	1405	133	0	118	1	6	0	36	25
esh shredded	¼ cup	71	7	0	6	tr	tr	0	2	1

aker's
| ngel Flake Sweetened | 0.5 oz | 70 | 5 | 0 | 5 | – | – | – | 1 | 5 |

OCONUT JUICE
coconut water fresh	½ cup	23	tr	0	tr	tr	tr	0	1	3
eamed sweetened canned	½ cup	264	12	0	11	tr	1	0	tr	38
ilk canned	½ cup	276	29	0	25	tr	1	0	3	4

oco King
| oasted w/ Pulp (11.75 oz) | 1 can (11.75 oz) | 130 | 0 | 0 | 0 | 0 | 0 | 0 | 1 | 26 |
| / Pulp | 1 can (11.85 oz) | 130 | 2 | 0 | 1 | – | – | 0 | – | 28 |

ocoZona
| oconut Water | 1 bottle (14.5 oz) | 70 | 0 | 0 | 0 | 0 | 0 | 0 | 0 | 16 |

FOOD	PORTION	CALS	TOTAL FAT	CHOL	SAT FAT	POLY FAT	MONO FAT	TRANS FAT	FIBER
KeVita									
Sparkling Probiotic Drink Organic	8 oz	5	0	0	0	0	0	0	–
Naked									
Coconut Water	1 box (11.2 oz)	60	0	0	0	0	0	0	0
Nature's Guru									
Instant Coconut Water Powder	1 pkg (0.5 oz)	50	0	0	0	0	0	0	0
Thai Kitchen									
Coconut Milk	⅓ cup (2.8 oz)	140	14	0	12	–	–	0	0
Vita Coco									
Coconut Water	½ box (8.5 oz)	45	0	0	0	0	0	0	1
Coconut Water w/ Peach & Mango	½ box (8.5 oz)	60	0	0	0	0	0	0	1
COD									
atlantic canned	3 oz	89	1	47	tr	tr	tr	–	0
atlantic canned	1 can (11 oz)	327	3	171	1	1	tr	–	0
atlantic dried	3 oz	246	2	129	tr	1	tr	–	0
atlantic fresh cooked	3 oz	89	1	47	tr	tr	tr	–	0
atlantic fresh cooked	1 fillet (6.3 oz)	189	2	99	tr	1	tr	–	0
atlantic fresh raw	3 oz	70	1	37	tr	tr	tr	–	0
pacific fresh baked	3 oz	95	1	43	tr	tr	tr	–	0
COFFEE (see also COFFEE BEVERAGES)									
INSTANT									
decaffeinated as prep	8 oz	2	0	0	0	0	0	0	0
decaffeinated powder	1 rounded tsp	4	0	0	0	0	0	0	0
regular powder	1 rounded tsp	4	tr	0	tr	tr	tr	0	0
REGULAR									
brewed	8 oz	2	tr	0	tr	tr	tr	0	0
COFFEE BEVERAGES									
Bean & Body									
Coffee Anti-OX	1 can (8 oz)	100	2	5	1	–	–	0	0
Coffee Energy	1 can (8 oz)	100	2	5	1	–	–	0	0
Coffee MarTeani	1 can (8 oz)	100	2	5	1	–	–	0	0
Coffee Rescue	1 can (8 oz)	100	2	5	1	–	–	0	0
Emmi									
Caffe Latte Cappuccino	1 pkg (7.7 oz)	140	4	15	2	–	–	0	0
Caffe Latte Vanilla	1 pkg (7.7 oz)	140	4	15	2	–	–	0	0

FOOD	PORTION	CALS	TOTAL FAT	CHOL	SAT FAT	POLY FAT	MONO FAT	TRANS FAT	FIBER	SUGAR
Health Is Wealth										
Nutriccino Vitamin Infused All Flavors	1 bottle (9.5 oz)	190	3	10	2	–	–	0	0	31
Vitamin Coffee Ener-G Infused Vanilla Latte	1 bottle (9.5 oz)	190	3	10	2	–	–	0	0	31
International Delight										
Iced Coffee All Flavors	8 oz	150	3	10	2	–	–	0	0	23
Seattle's Best Coffee										
Iced Latte	1 can (9.5 oz)	130	2	10	2	–	–	0	0	23
Iced Latte Vanilla	1 can (9.5 oz)	130	2	0	2	–	–	0	0	24
Iced Mocha	1 can (9.5 oz)	130	2	10	2	–	–	0	0	24
TAKE-OUT										
cafe amaretto w/ alcohol	1 serv	192	9	33	6	–	–	–	0	–
cafe au lait	1 cup (8 oz)	77	4	17	3	tr	1	–	–	7
cafe brulot	1 cup	48	0	0	0	0	0	0	–	3
cafe brulot w/ alcohol	1 serv	130	tr	0	tr	–	–	–	3	–
cappuccino	1 cup (8 oz)	77	4	17	3	tr	1	0	–	7
coffee con leche	1 cup (6 oz)	104	4	10	2	tr	1	0	0	17
dutch coffee w/ gin	1 (7 oz)	181	10	29	–	–	–	0	0	5
espresso	1 cup (4 oz)	2	tr	0	tr	tr	tr	0	0	0
french coffee w/ orange liqueur & kahlua	1 (8 oz)	232	10	29	–	–	–	0	0	–
irish coffee	1 serv (8 oz)	209	11	38	6	tr	3	0	0	4
latte w/ skim milk	1 serv (13 oz)	88	tr	4	tr	–	–	–	0	11
latte w/ whole milk	1 serv (14 oz)	143	6	20	3	tr	1	0	0	14
mocha	1 serv (17 oz)	403	9	29	5	1	2	0	2	54
puerto rican coffee w/ rum & kahlua	1 (8 oz)	166	10	29	–	–	–	0	0	–
turkish	1 cup (4 oz)	50	1	0	0	0	0	0	0	12
COFFEE WHITENERS										
Coffee-Mate										
Caramel Macchiato Liquid	1 tbsp (0.5 oz)	35	2	0	0	–	–	0	–	5
Natural Bliss Vanilla Liquid	1 tbsp (0.5 oz)	35	2	10	1	–	–	0	–	5
Original Liquid	1 tbsp (0.5 oz)	20	1	0	0	0	0	0	–	tr
Original Powder	1 tsp (2 g)	10	1	0	0	0	0	0	–	0
COLESLAW										
Dole										
Classic Coleslaw	1½ cups (3 oz)	20	0	0	0	0	0	0	2	3

FOOD	PORTION	CALS	TOTAL FAT	CHOL	SAT FAT	POLY FAT	MONO FAT	TRANS FAT	FIBER	SUGAR
Kit Creamy Coleslaw as prep	1½ cups (3.5 oz)	100	6	20	1	–	–	0	2	9
Eat Smart										
Broccoli Slaw	1 serv (3 oz)	25	0	0	0	0	0	0	3	2
Confetti Slaw	1 serv (3 oz)	25	0	0	0	0	0	0	2	2
Sunrise Slaw	1 serv (3 oz)	35	0	0	0	0	0	0	2	5
Mann's										
Broccoli Cole Slaw w/o Dressing	1 serv (3 oz)	25	0	0	0	0	0	0	3	2
Ready Pac										
Coleslaw	1½ cups (3 oz)	20	0	0	0	0	0	0	2	3
Coleslaw Mix as prep	1 cup (3.5 oz)	130	9	5	2	–	–	0	2	11
River Ranch										
Broccoli Slaw	1 cup (3 oz)	25	0	0	0	0	0	0	2	2
Three-Color Cole Slaw	1¼ cups (3 oz)	25	0	0	0	0	0	0	2	3
TAKE-OUT										
coleslaw w/ dressing	¾ cup	147	11	5	2	6	2	–	–	–
vinegar & oil coleslaw	3.5 oz	150	9	0	1	–	–	–	–	–

COLLARDS

fresh cooked	½ cup	17	tr	0	–	–	–	–	–	–
frzn chopped cooked	½ cup	31	tr	0	–	–	–	–	–	–
raw chopped	½ cup	6	tr	0	–	–	–	–	–	–

COOKIES
MIX

chocolate chip	1 (0.56 oz)	79	4	7	1	tr	2	–	–	–
oatmeal	1 (0.6 oz)	74	3	7	1	tr	2	–	tr	–
oatmeal raisin	1 (0.6 oz)	74	3	7	1	tr	2	–	tr	–

READY-TO-EAT

animal crackers	1 box (2.4 oz)	299	9	11	4	1	4	–	–	–
australian anzac biscuit	1	98	3	0	1	1	1	–	1	–
chocolate chip	1 box (1.9 oz)	233	12	12	5	1	5	–	–	–
chocolate chip low sugar low sodium	1 (0.24 oz)	31	1	0	1	tr	tr	–	–	–
chocolate chip lowfat	1 (0.25 oz)	45	2	0	tr	tr	1	–	–	–
chocolate chip soft-type	1 (0.5 oz)	69	4	0	1	tr	2	–	tr	–
chocolate wafer	1 (0.2 oz)	26	1	0	tr	tr	tr	–	–	–
cream cheese	1 (1.1 oz)	141	9	25	6	–	–	–	tr	6
gingersnaps	1 (0.24 oz)	29	1	0	tr	tr	tr	–	–	–
graham	1 sq (0.24 oz)	30	1	0	tr	tr	tr	–	–	–

FOOD	PORTION	CALS	TOTAL FAT	CHOL.	SAT FAT	POLY FAT	MONO FAT	TRANS FAT	FIBER	SUGAR
graham chocolate covered	1 (0.49 oz)	68	3	0	2	tr	1	–	–	–
graham honey	1 (0.24 oz)	30	1	0	tr	tr	tr	–	tr	–
hermits	1 (1 oz)	117	5	23	2	–	–	–	1	10
jumbles coconut	1 (1 oz)	121	7	26	5	–	–	–	1	7
ladyfingers	1 (0.38 oz)	40	1	40	tr	tr	tr	–	–	–
macaroons	1 (0.8 oz)	97	3	0	3	tr	tr	–	–	–
madeleines	1 (0.8 oz)	86	5	46	3	–	–	–	tr	5
molasses	1 (0.5 oz)	65	2	0	tr	tr	1	–	–	–
neapolitan tri-color cookie	1 (0.6 oz)	79	5	17	2	–	–	–	tr	5
oatmeal	1 (0.6 oz)	81	3	0	1	tr	2	–	1	–
oatmeal raisin	1 (0.6 oz)	81	3	0	1	tr	2	–	1	–
oatmeal raisin low sugar no sodium	1 (0.24 oz)	31	1	0	1	tr	1	–	–	–
peanut butter sandwich	1 (0.5 oz)	67	3	0	1	1	2	–	–	–
peanut butter soft-type	1 (0.5 oz)	69	4	0	1	1	2	–	tr	–
pinenut cookies	1 (1.1 oz)	134	9	0	1	–	–	–	1	8
raisin soft-type	1 (0.5 oz)	60	2	0	1	tr	1	–	–	–
reginette queen's biscuit	1 (0.8 oz)	86	3	tr	1	–	–	–	tr	4
shortbread	1 (0.28 oz)	40	2	2	1	tr	1	–	–	–
shortbread pecan	1 (0.49 oz)	79	5	5	1	1	3	–	tr	–
spritz	1 (0.4 oz)	42	2	6	1	–	–	–	tr	3
sugar	1 (0.52 oz)	72	3	8	1	tr	2	–	–	–
sugar low sugar sodium free	1 (0.24 oz)	30	1	0	tr	tr	1	–	–	–
sugar wafers w/ creme filling	1 (0.12 oz)	18	1	0	tr	tr	1	–	–	–
sugar wafers w/ creme filling sugar free sodium free	1 (0.14 oz)	20	1	0	tr	tr	tr	–	–	–
toll house original	1 (0.8 oz)	105	6	15	2	–	–	–	tr	9
vanilla sandwich	1 (0.35 oz)	48	2	0	tr	tr	1	–	tr	–
zeppole	1 (0.8 oz)	78	6	24	2	–	–	–	tr	4
6 Hour Energy										
Almond Cranberry Chocolate Chunk	½ (1.25 oz)	100	6	0	2	–	–	0	5	5
Anna's										
Chocolate Mint	6 (1 oz)	140	5	0	2	–	–	0	1	14
Vanilla Chocolate Chip	6 (1 oz)	140	6	0	2	–	–	0	0	8
Annie's Homegrown										
Bunny Ginger Gluten Free	29 (1 oz)	130	4	0	2	–	–	0	1	8
Bunny Gluten Free	27 (1 oz)	120	4	0	2	–	–	0	1	9
Bunny Grahams Chocolate	27 (1 oz)	130	5	0	0	–	–	0	2	9
Bunny Grahams Honey	28 (1 oz)	140	5	0	0	–	–	0	2	7

FOOD	PORTION	CALS	TOTAL FAT	CHOL	SAT FAT	POLY FAT	MONO FAT	TRANS FAT	FIBER	SUGAR
Bahlsen										
Deloba	5 (1.2 oz)	170	8	<5	5	–	–	0	tr	12
Hannover Waffeln	6 (1.1 oz)	180	10	0	6	–	–	0	0	7
Hit Cocoa Creme Filling	2 (1 oz)	150	8	<5	4	–	–	0	1	8
Hit Creme Filling	2 (1 oz)	140	7	<5	4	–	–	0	1	9
Nuss Dessert	3 (1 oz)	170	11	20	6	–	–	0	1	8
Barbara's Bakery										
Snackimals Chocolate Chip	10 (1 oz)	120	4	0	0	–	–	0	0	8
Bauducco										
Wafer Chocolate	4 (1.2 oz)	160	9	0	5	–	–	0	0	11
Wafer Vanilla	4 (1.2 oz)	140	8	0	4	–	–	0	0	11
BelVita										
Breakfast Biscuits Blueberry	1 pkg (1.8 oz)	230	8	0	1	2	5	0	3	13
Breakfast Biscuits Chocolate	1 pkg (1.8 oz)	230	8	2	2	2	5	0	3	11
Breakfast Biscuits Cinnamon Brown Sugar	1 pkg (1.8 oz)	230	8	0	1	2	5	0	3	10
Breakfast Biscuits Golden Oat	1 pkg (1.8 oz)	230	8	0	1	3	5	0	3	11
Brent & Sam's										
Chocolate Chip	2 (0.8 oz)	110	6	5	3	–	–	0	1	10
Caveman Cookies										
Alpine	2 (1 oz)	150	9	0	1	2	6	0	2	14
Original	2 (1 oz)	130	7	0	1	3	4	0	1	13
Tropical	2 (1 oz)	140	10	0	3	2	5	0	2	10
Erin Baker's										
Breakfast Banana Walnut	1 (3 oz)	300	8	0	1	–	–	0	5	17
Breakfast Caramel Apple	1 (3 oz)	280	4	0	1	–	–	0	5	21
Breakfast Double Chocolate Chunk	1 (3 oz)	300	6	0	1	–	–	0	6	19
Breakfast Oatmeal Raisin	1 (3 oz)	290	5	0	0	–	–	0	5	22
Breakfast Mini Fruit & Nut	1 (1 oz)	100	3	0	0	–	–	0	2	7
Fiber One										
Chocolate Chip	1 (0.89 oz)	90	3	0	2	–	–	0	5	8
Gamesa										
Animalitos	14 (1 oz)	110	1	0	0	–	–	0	tr	7
Emperador Vanilla Creme Sandwich	2 (0.9 oz)	120	4	<5	1	–	–	1	0	9
Hawaianas Coconut	3 (1 oz)	130	4	0	1	–	–	–	tr	9
Sugar Wafers Chocolate	3 (1.2 oz)	160	7	0	2	–	–	2	0	15

FOOD	PORTION	CALS	TOTAL FAT	CHOL	SAT FAT	POLY FAT	MONO FAT	TRANS FAT	FIBER	SUGAR
Girl Scout										
Do-si-dos	2 (0.8 oz)	110	5	0	2	–	–	0	tr	7
Dulce De Leche	4 (1 oz)	160	8	0	4	–	–	0	0	9
Peanut Butter Sandwich	3 (1.2 oz)	160	6	0	3	–	–	0	tr	8
Samoas	2 (1 oz)	140	7	0	5	–	–	0	1	10
Savannah Smiles	5 (1 oz)	140	5	0	2	–	–	0	0	10
Shout Outs!	4 (0.9 oz)	130	5	0	2	–	–	0	tr	8
Tagalongs	2 (0.9 oz)	140	9	0	5	–	–	0	tr	8
Thank U Berry Munch	2 (0.9 oz)	120	5	0	2	–	–	0	tr	7
Thin Mints	4 (1.1 oz)	160	8	0	5	–	–	0	tr	10
Trefoils	5 (1.2 oz)	160	8	0	3	–	–	0	tr	7
Grandma's										
Chocolate Brownie	1 (1.4 oz)	190	8	<5	3	1	4	0	2	14
Peanut Butter	1 (1.2 oz)	170	9	<5	3	–	–	0	2	10
Vanilla Creme Sandwich	5 (1.4 oz)	190	9	<5	3	1	4	0	tr	12
JK Gourmet										
Biscotti Almond Raisin	2 (1.1 oz)	150	11	20	1	–	–	0	2	6
Biscotti Dried Peach & Pistachio	3 (1.1 oz)	160	12	45	1	–	–	0	3	6
Jovial										
Checkerboard Organic	2 (0.9 oz)	120	6	20	3	–	–	0	1	6
Chocolate Cream Filled Organic	2 (1.1 oz)	160	7	15	3	–	–	0	1	9
Crispy Cocoa Organic	3 (1 oz)	140	6	0	3	–	–	0	1	6
Fig Fruit Filled Organic	2 (1.1 oz)	130	4	5	2	–	–	0	1	12
Ginger Spice Organic	2 (1.1 oz)	150	6	25	3	–	–	0	1	7
Vanilla Cream Filled Organic	2 (1.1 oz)	160	7	15	3	–	–	0	1	10
Jules Destrooper										
Butter Crisp	2 (0.9 oz)	120	4	15	3	–	–	0	tr	11
Chocolate Thins	3 (1 oz)	150	7	15	4	–	–	0	tr	14
Keebler										
Vienna Fingers Reduced Fat	2 (1.1 oz)	140	5	0	2	–	–	0	tr	12
Lotus										
Biscoff	4 (1.1 oz)	150	6	0	3	–	–	0	tr	12
LU										
Le Petit Beurre	4 (1.2 oz)	140	4	5	2	–	–	0	tr	8
Petit Ecolier Dark Chocolate	2 (0.9 oz)	130	6	5	4	–	–	0	1	9
Pim's Orange	2 (0.9 oz)	100	3	10	2	–	–	0	0	14
Mallomars										
Cookies	2 (0.9 oz)	120	5	0	3	0	2	0	1	12

FOOD	PORTION	CALS	TOTAL FAT	CHOL	SAT FAT	POLY FAT	MONO FAT	TRANS FAT	FIBER	SUGAR
Mary's Gone Crackers										
Chocolate Chip Gluten Free Organic	2 (0.9 oz)	130	6	0	3	1	2	0	2	9
Ginger Snaps Gluten Free Organic	3 (1.1 oz)	140	5	0	3	1	1	0	1	9
Miss Meringue										
Meringue Chocolate	1 pkg (1 oz)	100	0	0	0	0	0	0	1	23
New Morning										
Honey Grahams	2 (1.1 oz)	130	3	0	0	–	–	0	1	6
Newman's Own										
Fig Newmans Low Fat Organic	2 (1.1 oz)	110	2	0	1	0	1	0	tr	12
Newtons										
Fig Fat Free	2 (1 oz)	90	0	0	0	0	0	0	1	12
Fruit Thins Cranberry Citrus Oat	3 (1 oz)	140	5	0	1	3	1	0	1	7
Fruit Thins Fig And Honey	3 (1.1 oz)	140	5	0	1	3	1	0	2	7
Strawberry	2 (1 oz)	100	2	0	0	1	0	0	0	13
Nilla Wafers										
Cookies	8 (1 oz)	140	6	50	2	3	1	0	0	11
Nonni's										
Biscotti Bites Almond Dark Chocolate	3 (1 oz)	120	4	25	3	–	–	0	1	8
Biscotti Bites Classic Almond	4 (1 oz)	130	4	25	2	–	–	0	1	8
Biscotti Decadence	1 (0.8 oz)	100	4	20	2	–	–	0	1	9
Biscotti Originali	1 (0.7 oz)	90	3	20	1	–	–	0	0	7
Biscotti Salted Caramel	1 (0.8 oz)	100	4	20	2	–	–	0	0	11
Biscotti Triple Milk Chocolate	1 (0.8 oz)	110	5	20	3	–	–	0	1	10
Thinaddictives Cinnamon Raisin	1 pkg (0.7 oz)	100	3	20	0	–	–	0	1	7
Thinaddictives Pistachio Almond	1 pkg (0.7 oz)	100	4	30	1	–	–	0	1	5
Pepperidge Farm										
Bordeaux	4	130	5	10	4	–	–	0	tr	12
Brussels	3	150	7	5	4	–	–	0	1	11
Butter Chessmen	3	120	5	20	3	–	–	0	tr	5
Chesapeake Dark Chocolate Pecan	1 (0.9 oz)	130	6	<5	4	–	–	0	0	10
Geneva	3	160	9	0	4	–	–	0	1	8
Homestyle Gingerman	4	130	4	10	2	–	–	0	tr	13

FOOD	PORTION	CALS	TOTAL FAT	CHOL	SAT FAT	POLY FAT	MONO FAT	TRANS FAT	FIBER	SUGAR
Homestyle Sugar	3	150	7	10	3	–	–	0	tr	11
Lemon	4 (1.1 oz)	160	8	5	3	–	–	0	0	8
Lexington Crispy Milk Chocolate Toffee Almond	1	130	7	10	3	–	–	0	1	10
Maui Crispy Milk Chocolate Coconut Almond	1	130	7	5	4	–	–	0	1	9
Milano	3	180	10	10	5	–	–	0	tr	11
Milano Melts Chocolate Creme	2	140	7	<5	2	–	–	0	1	11
Milano Melts Dark Classic Creme	2	140	7	<5	2	3	2	0	1	11
Pirouettes Chocolate Hazelnut	2	120	4	0	2	–	–	0	0	10
Sausalito Milk Chocolate Macadamia Nut	1	130	6	<5	4	–	–	0	0	10
Soft Baked Mystic Sugar	1 (1.1 oz)	140	5	10	2	–	–	0	1	9
Soft Baked Sanibel Snickerdoodle	1	140	5	10	2	–	–	0	tr	9
Soft Baked Santa Cruz Oatmeal Raisin	1	130	5	<5	2	–	–	0	2	13
Tahiti	2	170	10	5	6	–	–	0	2	8
Tim Tam Chocolate Creme	2	190	10	<5	5	–	–	0	tr	18
Verona Strawberry	3	140	5	15	3	–	–	0	tr	9
Simply Shari's										
Gluten Free Almond Shortbread	2 (1 oz)	120	6	15	4	–	–	0	0	7
Gluten Free Chocolate Chip	2 (1 oz)	120	6	10	3	–	–	0	1	9
Gluten Free Fudge Brownies	2 (1 oz)	130	7	10	4	–	–	0	1	10
Gluten Free Shortbread	2 (1 oz)	130	6	15	4	–	–	0	0	8
SnackWell's										
Creme Sandwich	2 (0.9 oz)	110	3	0	1	1	1	0	0	9
Special K										
Pastry Crisps Chocolatey Delight	1 (0.88 oz)	100	2	0	1	–	–	0	tr	7
Stella D'Oro										
Margherite Combination	2 (1 oz)	130	5	10	3	1	2	0	tr	7
Swiss Fudge	3 (1.2 oz)	170	9	<5	5	1	3	0	tr	12
Titan										
High Protein Chocolate Chip	1 (1.4 oz)	150	6	10	3	–	–	0	3	5
High Protein Oatmeal Raisin	1 (1.4 oz)	150	5	10	3	–	–	0	2	5
High Protein Peanut Butter	1 (1.4 oz)	150	5	5	3	–	–	0	2	5

FOOD	PORTION	CALS	TOTAL FAT	CHOL	SAT FAT	POLY FAT	MONO FAT	TRANS FAT	FIBER	SUGAR
Voortman										
Shortbread	1 (0.6 oz)	90	5	0	1	–	–	0	0	4
Sugar Free Oatmeal	1 (0.7 oz)	70	4	0	1	–	–	0	tr	0
Walkers										
Shortbread Rounds	1 (0.6 oz)	90	5	15	3	–	–	0	0	3
WOW										
Chocolate Brownie	1 (1.4 oz)	161	9	38	5	–	–	0	1	15
Chocolate Chip Gluten Free	1 (1.4 oz)	170	8	31	5	–	–	–	1	14
Lemon Burst Gluten Free	1 (1.4 oz)	180	8	35	5	–	–	–	tr	10
Peanut Butter	1 (1.4 oz)	170	10	25	3	–	–	–	1	12
REFRIGERATED										
chocolate chip	1 (0.42 oz)	59	3	3	1	tr	1	–	–	–
chocolate chip dough	1 oz	126	6	7	2	1	3	–	–	–
oatmeal	1 (0.4 oz)	56	3	3	1	tr	1	–	–	–
oatmeal raisin	1 (0.4 oz)	56	3	3	1	tr	1	–	–	–
peanut butter	1 (0.4 oz)	60	3	4	1	1	2	–	–	–
peanut butter dough	1 oz	130	7	8	2	1	4	–	–	–
sugar	1 (0.42 oz)	58	3	4	1	tr	2	–	–	–
sugar dough	1 oz	124	6	8	2	1	3	–	–	–
TAKE-OUT										
biscotti w/ nuts chocolate dipped	1 (1.3 oz)	117	6	18	3	–	–	–	1	11
black & white	1 lg (3 oz)	302	9	58	5	–	–	–	1	31
finikia	1 (1.2 oz)	171	5	27	5	–	–	–	1	5
koulourakia butter cookie twist	1 (0.9 oz)	113	6	32	3	–	–	–	tr	5
linzer tart	1 (2.4 oz)	280	14	40	4	–	–	–	0	12
CORIANDER										
leaf dried	1 tsp	2	tr	0	tr	tr	tr	0	tr	tr
leaf fresh	¼ cup	1	tr	0	–	–	–	–	–	–
seed	1 tsp	5	tr	0	tr	tr	tr	0	1	–
CORN										
CANNED										
cream style	½ cup	93	1	0	tr	tr	tr	–	–	–
w/ red & green peppers	½ cup	86	1	0	tr	tr	tr	–	–	–
white	½ cup	66	1	0	tr	tr	tr	–	–	–
yellow	½ cup	66	1	0	tr	tr	tr	–	1	–
Butter Kernel										
Gold & White	½ cup (4.4 oz)	60	1	0	0	–	–	0	2	3

FOOD	PORTION	CALS	TOTAL FAT	CHOL	SAT FAT	POLY FAT	MONO FAT	TRANS FAT	FIBER	SUGAR
Whole Kernel No Salt Added	½ cup (4.4 oz)	70	1	0	0	–	–	0	2	3
Del Monte										
Cream Style No Salt Added	½ cup (4.4 oz)	60	1	0	0	0	0	0	2	7
Whole Kernel	½ cup (4.4 oz)	90	1	0	0	0	0	0	3	6
Whole Kernel No Salt Added	½ cup (4.4 oz)	90	1	0	0	0	0	0	3	6
Green Giant										
Cream Style Sweet	½ cup (4.5 oz)	90	1	0	0	–	–	0	1	7
Mexicorn	½ cup (3.3 oz)	90	1	0	–	–	–	0	1	6
Super Sweet Yellow & White	⅓ cup (2.6 oz)	60	1	0	0	–	–	0	1	3
Whole Kernel	½ cup (4.3 oz)	90	1	0	0	–	–	0	1	6
Jake & Amos										
Pickled Dill Baby Corn	2 tbsp	5	0	0	0	0	0	0	0	0
DRIED										
Crunchies										
Freeze Dried Corn Snack	⅓ cup (1 oz)	130	7	0	1	–	–	0	4	0
Freeze Dried Sweet Buttered	½ cup (1 oz)	100	2	0	0	–	–	0	3	5
Sunrich Naturals										
Toasted Corn Cool Ranch	1 pkg (1 oz)	100	2	1	tr	–	–	0	1	1
FRESH										
white cooked	½ cup	89	1	0	tr	tr	tr	–	–	–
white raw	½ cup	66	1	0	tr	tr	tr	–	–	–
yellow cooked	½ cup	89	1	0	tr	tr	tr	–	–	–
yellow cooked	1 ear (2.7 oz)	83	1	0	tr	tr	tr	–	–	–
yellow raw	1 ear (3 oz)	77	1	0	tr	tr	1	–	–	–
yellow raw	½ cup	66	1	0	tr	tr	tr	–	–	–
FROZEN										
cooked	½ cup	67	tr	0	tr	tr	tr	–	–	–
on the cob cooked	1 ear (2.2 oz)	59	tr	0	tr	tr	tr	–	–	–
TAKE-OUT										
fritters	1 (1 oz)	62	2	12	tr	1	1	–	1	–
on the cob w/ butter cooked	1 ear	155	3	6	2	tr	1	–	–	–
scalloped	1 cup	257	11	152	3	3	4	0	3	11

CORN CHIPS (see CHIPS)

CORNISH HEN (see CHICKEN)

CORNMEAL

FOOD	PORTION	CALS	TOTAL FAT	CHOL	SAT FAT	POLY FAT	MONO FAT	TRANS FAT	FIBER	SUGAR
cornmeal mush as prep w/ water	1 cup	223	1	0	tr	tr	tr	0	5	tr

FOOD	PORTION	CALS	TOTAL FAT	CHOL	SAT FAT	POLY FAT	MONO FAT	TRANS FAT	FIBER	SUGAR
cornmeal yellow	½ cup (2.2 oz)	236	1	0	tr	tr	tr	0	1	tr
whole grain blue	½ cup (1.9 oz)	201	3	0	–	–	–	0	5	0
yellow self-rising	½ cup (3 oz)	296	2	0	tr	1	1	0	5	–
Quaker										
Instant Original not prep	1 pkg (1 oz)	100	0	0	0	0	0	0	1	0
TAKE-OUT										
corn pone	1 piece (2.1 oz)	128	3	0	1	1	1	0	2	tr
fritter puerto rican style	1 (1.4 oz)	106	7	8	2	2	2	–	tr	tr
harina de maiz	1 cup (4 oz)	167	2	8	1	tr	1	–	1	20
harina de maiz con coco	½ cup (4.6 oz)	383	27	0	24	tr	1	–	3	21
hush puppies	1 (0.8 oz)	74	3	10	tr	2	1	0	1	tr
johnnycake	1 piece (1.7 oz)	134	4	35	1	1	1	0	2	4

CORNSTARCH

cornstarch	1 tbsp (0.3 oz)	34	0	0	0	0	0	0	tr	0
cornstarch	¼ cup (1.1 oz)	122	tr	0	tr	tr	tr	0	tr	0

COTTAGE CHEESE

creamed large curd	½ cup (4 oz)	110	5	19	2	tr	1	–	0	3
creamed small curd	½ cup (3.7 oz)	103	5	18	2	tr	1	–	0	3
dry curd	½ cup (2.5 oz)	52	tr	5	tr	tr	tr	–	0	1
lowfat 1%	½ cup (4 oz)	81	1	5	1	tr	tr	–	0	3
lowfat 1% lactose reduced	½ cup (4 oz)	84	1	5	1	tr	tr	–	1	3
Breakstone's										
2% Lowfat 30% Less Sodium	½ cup (4.4 oz)	90	3	15	2	–	–	0	0	4
4% Fat Small Curd	½ cup (4.4 oz)	120	5	25	3	–	–	0	0	5
Lactaid										
Lowfat	½ cup (4 oz)	80	1	10	1	–	–	0	0	3

COTTONSEED

kernels roasted	1 tbsp	51	4	0	1	2	1	–	–	–

COUSCOUS

cooked	1 cup (5.5 oz)	176	tr	0	tr	tr	tr	–	2	–
dry	1 cup (6.1 oz)	650	1	0	tr	tr	tr	–	9	–
Bob's Red Mill										
Pearl not prep	⅓ cup (2 oz)	210	1	0	0	–	–	0	0	0
Pearl Tricolor not prep	⅓ cup (2 oz)	210	1	0	0	–	–	0	0	0
Pearl Whole Wheat not prep	⅓ cup (2 oz)	190	1	0	0	–	–	0	5	0

FOOD	PORTION	CALS	TOTAL FAT	CHOL	SAT FAT	POLY FAT	MONO FAT	TRANS FAT	FIBER	SUGAR
Lundberg										
Brown Rice Roasted Garlic & Olive Oil not prep	¼ pkg (1.6 oz)	150	2	0	0	–	–	0	2	1
Brown Rice Roasted Plain Original not prep	⅙ pkg (1.6 oz)	150	2	0	0	–	–	0	3	1
Near East										
Roasted Garlic & Olive Oil as prep	1 cup	220	5	0	1	–	–	0	2	1
CRAB										
CANNED										
blue	½ cup	67	1	60	tr	tr	tr	–	0	0
blue drained	1 can (6.5 oz)	124	2	111	tr	1	tr	–	0	0
Chicken Of The Sea										
Fancy	⅓ can (2 oz)	40	0	50	0	0	0	0	0	0
Jumbo Lump	⅓ can (2 oz)	35	1	50	0	–	–	0	0	1
FRESH										
alaska king meat only steamed	3 oz	82	1	45	tr	tr	tr	–	0	0
blue cooked flaked	1 cup (4 oz)	120	2	118	tr	1	tr	–	0	0
dungeness steamed	3 oz	94	1	65	tr	tr	tr	–	0	–
queen steamed	3 oz	98	1	60	tr	tr	tr	–	0	0
TAKE-OUT										
alaska king leg steamed	1 leg (4.7 oz)	130	2	71	tr	1	tr	–	0	0
baked	1 (3.8 oz)	160	2	184	tr	1	1	–	–	–
cakes	2 (4.2 oz)	186	9	180	2	3	3	–	0	–
crab imperial	1 crab (6.8 oz)	289	15	242	3	4	6	–	0	3
crab salad	1 serv (5.5 oz)	285	21	109	3	11	5	–	1	1
crab thermidor	1 serv (6.4 oz)	456	37	313	22	2	11	–	tr	tr
deviled	1 serv (4.5 oz)	254	13	126	3	4	5	–	1	6
dungeness steamed	1 crab (4.5 oz)	140	2	97	tr	1	tr	–	0	–
empanada de jueyes	1 (4.4 oz)	341	16	45	4	2	9	–	2	7
fried crab puffs	4 (3.2 oz)	323	18	85	10	1	6	–	1	tr
salmorejo de jueyes (in tomato sauce)	1 serv (4.5 oz)	215	14	99	2	2	9	–	tr	1
soft-shell breaded & fried	1 med (2.3 oz)	216	13	79	3	4	5	–	1	1
taco de jueyes	1 (4.2 oz)	266	14	79	5	2	7	–	2	1
CRACKER CRUMBS										
cracker meal	1 cup	440	2	0	tr	1	tr	0	3	tr
graham cracker crumbs	1 cup	355	8	0	1	3	3	0	2	26

FOOD	PORTION	CALS	TOTAL FAT	CHOL	SAT FAT	POLY FAT	MONO FAT	TRANS FAT	FIBER	SUGAR
Mary's Gone Crackers										
Just The Crumbs Gluten Free	½ cup (1.4 oz)	160	3	0	0	2	1	0	3	0
CRACKERS										
melba toast round	1	12	tr	0	tr	tr	tr	0	tr	tr
oyster cracker	¼ cup	48	1	0	tr	tr	1	0	tr	tr
saltines	1	13	tr	0	tr	tr	tr	0	tr	tr
Annie's Homegrown										
Cheddar Bunnies Original	50 (1 oz)	140	6	0	1	–	–	0	0	1
Cheez-It										
Baby Swiss	25 (1 oz)	150	7	0	2	4	2	0	tr	0
Cheddar Jack	25 (1 oz)	140	7	0	2	3	2	0	tr	0
Colby	25 (1 oz)	150	8	0	2	4	2	0	tr	0
Crunchmaster										
Ancient Grains Cracked Pepper & Herb	14 (1 oz)	130	3	0	0	–	–	0	1	0
Crisps Cheezy Gluten Free	60 (1 oz)	120	3	0	0	–	–	0	2	2
Crisps Grammy Gluten Free	30 (1 oz)	130	2	0	0	–	–	0	1	5
Multi-Grain Sea Salt Gluten Free	16 (1 oz)	120	3	0	0	–	–	0	3	2
Multi-Seed Original Gluten Free	15 (1 oz)	140	5	0	1	–	–	0	2	0
Kim's Magic Pop										
Onion	1 (5 g)	15	0	0	0	0	0	0	0	0
Manischewitz										
Tam Tams Original	10 (1 oz)	110	4	0	1	–	–	0	0	1
Mary's Gone Crackers										
Herb Wheat & Gluten Free Organic	13 (1 oz)	140	5	0	1	3	2	0	3	0
Original Wheat & Gluten Free Organic	13 (1 oz)	140	5	0	1	3	2	0	3	0
Mediterranean Crackers										
Feta & Oregano	3 (0.6 oz)	91	5	0	3	–	–	0	0	1
Mediterranean Snacks										
Hummuz Crispz Olive Tapenade	14 (1 oz)	120	3	0	1	–	–	0	1	2
Hummuz Crispz Roasted Garlic	14 (1 oz)	120	3	0	1	–	–	0	1	2
Hummuz Crispz Roasted Red Pepper	14 (1 oz)	120	3	0	1	–	–	0	1	2

FOOD	PORTION	CALS	TOTAL FAT	CHOL	SAT FAT	POLY FAT	MONO FAT	TRANS FAT	FIBER	SUGAR
Lentil Cracked Pepper Gluten Free	22 (1 oz)	120	3	0	0	–	–	0	3	tr
Lentil Sea Salt Gluten Free	18 (1 oz)	110	3	0	0	–	–	0	1	2
Pepperidge Farm										
Baked Naturals Cheese Crisps Four Cheese Medley	20	140	5	<5	1	2	3	0	1	3
Baked Naturals Cracker Chips Simply Cheddar Multigrain	27	130	4	0	1	2	1	0	2	4
Baked Naturals Cracker Chips Simply Potato	26	140	5	0	1	–	–	0	2	3
Baked Naturals Wheat Crisps Toasted Wheat	17	140	5	0	1	–	–	0	2	5
Golden Butter	2	35	1	0	0	0	1	0	0	tr
Goldfish Cheddar	55	140	5	<5	1	2	3	0	tr	tr
Goldfish Colors	55	140	5	<5	1	1	3	0	1	tr
Goldfish Grahams Chocolate	37 (1.1 oz)	130	4	0	1	1	2	0	2	11
Goldfish Original	55	150	6	0	1	2	3	0	tr	tr
Goldfish Pretzel	43	130	3	0	1	1	1	0	tr	tr
Harvest Wheat	2	50	2	0	0	1	2	0	tr	2
Jingos Fiesta Cheddar	23	140	4	0	4	1	3	0	1	2
Jingos Lime & Sweet Chili	23	140	4	0	0	1	3	0	1	2
Snack Sticks Toasted Sesame	12	140	5	0	1	–	–	0	2	1
Premium										
Saltines Unsalted Tops	5 (0.5 oz)	70	2	0	0	1	0	0	0	0
Saltines w/ Whole Grain	6 (0.5 oz)	60	2	0	0	1	0	0	tr	0
Ritz										
Roasted Vegetable	5 (0.5 oz)	80	4	0	1	2	1	0	0	1
Special K										
Cracker Chips Cheddar	27 (1 oz)	110	3	0	1	1	1	0	3	1
Cracker Chips Sea Salt	30 (1 oz)	110	3	0	0	1	1	0	3	0
Cracker Chips Southwest Ranch	27 (1 oz)	110	3	0	1	2	1	0	3	1
Triscuit										
Fire Roasted Tomato	1 oz	120	4	0	1	–	–	0	3	0
Garden Herb	1 oz	120	4	0	1	–	–	0	3	0
Hint Of Salt	1 oz	130	5	0	1	–	1	0	3	0
Original	1 oz	120	5	0	1	–	–	0	3	0
Reduced Fat	1 oz	120	3	0	1	–	–	0	3	0
Rosemary & Olive Oil	1 oz	120	4	0	1	–	–	0	3	0

FOOD	PORTION	CALS	TOTAL FAT	CHOL	SAT FAT	POLY FAT	MONO FAT	TRANS FAT	FIBER	SUGAR
Thin Crisps Original	1 oz	130	5	0	1	–	–	0	3	0
Thin Crisps Quattro Formaggio	1.1 oz	140	5	0	1	–	1	0	3	1
Wellaby's										
Cheese Ups Classic Cheese Gluten Free	1 cup (1 oz)	122	5	15	3	–	–	0	tr	0
Cheese Ups Parmesan	1 cup (1 oz)	122	5	15	3	–	–	0	tr	0
Feta Oregano & Olive Oil Gluten Free	8 (1.1 oz)	130	59	15	3	–	–	0	1	1
Original Cheese Mini Gluten Free	8 (1.1 oz)	130	5	15	3	–	–	0	1	1
CRANBERRIES										
cranberry orange relish	¼ cup	118	tr	0	tr	tr	tr	0	2	28
dried	½ cup	85	tr	0	tr	tr	tr	0	2	18
fresh chopped	1 cup	13	tr	0	tr	tr	tr	0	1	1
fresh whole	1 cup	11	tr	0	tr	tr	tr	0	1	1
sauce	1 slice (2 oz)	86	tr	0	tr	tr	tr	0	1	22
sauce	¼ cup	109	tr	0	tr	tr	tr	0	1	26
Dole										
Fresh Whole	1 cup (3.3 oz)	45	0	0	0	0	0	0	4	4
Ocean Spray										
Jellied Sauce	¼ cup (2.5 oz)	110	0	0	0	0	0	0	tr	21
CRANBERRY BEANS										
canned	½ cup	108	tr	0	tr	tr	tr	–	8	–
dried cooked w/o salt	½ cup	120	tr	0	tr	tr	tr	–	9	–
CRANBERRY JUICE										
cranberry juice cocktail low calorie w/ vitamin C	8 oz	46	tr	0	0	0	0	0	0	11
cranberry juice cocktail w/ vitamin C	8 oz	137	tr	0	tr	tr	tr	0	0	30
unsweetened	8 oz	116	tr	0	tr	tr	tr	0	tr	31
Apple & Eve										
100% Juice	8 oz	130	0	0	0	0	0	0	–	30
Ocean Spray										
Cran•Energy	8 oz	35	0	0	0	0	0	0	–	8
Old Orchard										
Cranberry Naturals Classic Cranberry	8 oz	80	0	0	0	0	0	0	–	18

FOOD	PORTION	CALS	TOTAL FAT	CHOL	SAT FAT	POLY FAT	MONO FAT	TRANS FAT	FIBER	SUGAR
CRAYFISH										
cooked	3 oz	97	1	151	tr	tr	tr	–	0	0
raw	3 oz	76	1	118	tr	tr	tr	–	0	0
raw	8	24	tr	37	tr	tr	tr	–	0	0
CREAM (see also WHIPPED TOPPINGS)										
clotted cream	2 tbsp (1 oz)	164	18	48	–	–	–	–	0	–
creme fraiche	2 tbsp (1 oz)	100	11	40	–	–	–	–	0	–
half & half	1 pkg (0.5 oz)	20	2	6	1	tr	tr	–	0	tr
half & half	1 tbsp (0.5 oz)	20	2	6	1	tr	tr	–	0	tr
half & half	¼ cup (2.1 oz)	79	7	22	4	tr	2	–	0	tr
half & half fat free	4 oz	67	2	6	1	tr	tr	–	0	6
heavy whipping	½ cup (4.2 oz)	411	44	163	27	2	13	–	0	tr
heavy whipping	1 tbsp (0.5 oz)	52	6	21	3	tr	2	–	0	tr
heavy whipping whipped	½ cup (2.1 oz)	207	22	82	14	1	6	–	0	tr
light coffee	1 pkg (0.4 oz)	22	2	7	1	tr	1	–	0	tr
light coffee	½ cup (4.2 oz)	234	23	79	14	1	7	–	0	tr
light coffee	1 tbsp (0.5 oz)	29	3	10	2	tr	1	–	0	tr
whipped pressurized can	4 tbsp (0.4 oz)	31	3	9	2	tr	1	–	0	1
whipped pressurized can	½ cup (1 oz)	77	7	23	4	tr	2	–	0	2
Lactaid										
Half & Half	2 tbsp (1 oz)	40	3	15	2	–	–	0	0	1
Straus										
Organic Half And Half	2 tbsp (1 oz)	35	3	15	2	–	–	0	0	1
CREAM CHEESE										
cream cheese	1 pkg (3 oz)	297	30	93	19	1	8	–	–	–
cream cheese	1 oz	99	10	31	6	tr	3	–	–	–
Kelly's Kitchen										
Cranberry Almond Spread	2 tbsp (1 oz)	90	7	20	4	–	–	0	0	6
Philadelphia										
⅓ Less Fat	2 tbs (1.1 oz)	70	6	20	4	–	–	0	0	2
Fat Free	1 oz	30	0	5	0	0	0	0	0	1
Original	1 oz	100	9	35	6	–	–	0	0	1
Whipped Chive	2 tbsp (0.8 oz)	50	5	15	3	–	–	0	0	1
CREAM CHEESE SUBSTITUTES										
Follow Your Heart										
Vegan	1 oz	90	9	0	3	–	–	0	2	1
Go Veggie!										
Cream Cheese Dairy Free	2 tbsp (1 oz)	90	9	0	5	2	3	0	0	0

FOOD	PORTION	CALS	TOTAL FAT	CHOL	SAT FAT	POLY FAT	MONO FAT	TRANS FAT	FIBER	SUGAR
Tofutti										
Better Than Cream Cheese All Flavors	2 tbsp (1 oz)	60	5	0	2	–	–	0	0	0
CREAM OF TARTAR										
cream of tartar	1 tsp	8	0	0	0	0	0	0	0	0
CREPES										
basic crepe unfilled	1 (7 in)	112	6	78	2	1	2	0	tr	2
Ekizian										
Chickpea Crepe	1 (7 in) (1.5 oz)	212	13	2	2	2	8	0	3	3
Tandoor Chef										
Masala Dosa	1 (3 oz)	162	6	0	2	–	–	0	2	1
CROAKER										
atlantic breaded & fried	3 oz	188	11	71	3	2	5	–	–	–
atlantic raw	3 oz	89	3	52	1	tr	1	–	0	0
CROISSANT										
apple	1 (2 oz)	145	5	18	3	tr	1	–	1	–
butter	1 lg (2.4 oz)	272	14	45	8	1	4	–	2	8
butter mini	1 (1 oz)	114	6	19	3	tr	2	–	1	3
cheese	1 (1.5 oz)	174	9	24	4	1	3	–	1	5
chocolate	1 (2 oz)	237	14	34	8	1	4	–	2	6
TAKE-OUT										
w/ egg & cheese	1 (4.5 oz)	368	25	216	14	1	8	–	–	–
w/ egg & sausage	1 (5 oz)	497	34	237	15	3	13	–	2	8
w/ egg cheese & bacon	1 (4.1 oz)	385	24	253	12	2	8	–	1	8
w/ egg cheese & ham	1 (5.1 oz)	402	24	264	12	2	7	–	1	8
w/ egg cheese & sausage	1 (5.6 oz)	539	39	280	17	3	15	–	1	8
w/ ham & cheese	1 (4 oz)	338	20	64	12	1	6	–	1	4
CROUTONS										
plain	1 cup (1 oz)	122	2	0	tr	tr	1	–	2	–
Chatham Village										
Cheese & Garlic	2 tbsp (7 g)	40	3	0	0	–	–	0	0	0
Mrs. Cubbison's										
Asiago Cheese Ciabatta	2 tbsp (0.2 oz)	30	2	0	0	–	–	0	0	0
Seasoned Texas Toast	2 tbsp (0.2 oz)	30	2	0	0	–	–	0	0	1
Pepperidge Farm										
Seasoned	6	30	1	0	0	0	1	0	tr	tr
Zesty Italian	6	30	1	0	0	0	1	0	tr	tr

FOOD	PORTION	CALS	TOTAL FAT	CHOL	SAT FAT	POLY FAT	MONO FAT	TRANS FAT	FIBER	SUGAR
CUCUMBER										
fresh peeled	1 sm (5.5 oz)	19	tr	0	tr	tr	tr	0	1	2
fresh peeled	1 slice (7 g)	1	tr	0	tr	0	0	0	0	tr
fresh peeled	1 med (7.2 oz)	24	tr	0	tr	tr	tr	0	1	3
fresh peeled sliced	1 cup (4.2 oz)	14	tr	0	tr	tr	tr	0	1	2
fresh w/ peel sliced	½ cup (1.8 oz)	34	tr	0	tr	tr	tr	0	tr	1
fresh whole w/ peel	1 lg (10.6 oz)	45	tr	0	tr	tr	tr	0	2	5
TAKE-OUT										
cucumber raita	1 serv (3.3 oz)	40	3	6	2	tr	1	–	1	3
cucumber salad w/ onions + oil & vinegar	1 cup (5.6 oz)	183	15	0	2	7	6	0	1	8
cucumber salad w/ sour cream dressing	1 cup (4.7 oz)	63	5	13	3	tr	1	–	1	2
kimchee	½ cup (1.8 oz)	36	2	0	tr	–	–	–	tr	3
tzatziki	½ cup (3.4 oz)	72	6	5	1	–	–	–	1	3
CUMIN										
seed	1 tbsp (6 g)	22	1	0	tr	tr	1	0	1	tr
seed	1 tsp (2 g)	8	tr	0	tr	tr	tr	0	tr	tr
CURRANTS										
black fresh	½ cup	36	tr	0	tr	tr	tr	–	–	–
zante dried	½ cup	204	tr	0	tr	tr	tr	–	–	–
CURRY										
curry powder	1 tsp	7	tr	0	tr	tr	tr	–	1	tr
curry sauce mix as prep	1 cup	120	6	0	1	2	3	–	–	–
curry sauce mix as prep w/ milk	1 cup	270	15	35	6	3	5	–	–	–
paste	1 tube (6 oz)	465	36	16	12	10	13	tr	12	13
Tandoor Chef										
Chicken Curry	1 pkg (9 oz)	315	12	40	2	–	–	0	1	2
Kofta Curry	1 pkg (9.9 oz)	400	19	0	3	–	–	0	9	8
Thai Kitchen										
Red Curry Paste	1 tbsp (0.5 oz)	15	0	0	0	0	0	0	0	1
TAKE-OUT										
beef curry	1 cup	432	31	68	7	8	14	–	3	6
beef kurma	1 serv (10 oz)	611	47	114	26	4	15	–	6	3
chicken curry ½ breast	1 serv	160	9	45	2	2	4	–	1	3
chicken curry boneless	1 serv (6.2 oz)	219	12	62	2	3	1	–	2	4
chicken curry leg & thigh	1 serv	180	10	51	2	3	4	–	1	3
chickpea curry	1 serv (8.3 oz)	305	15	12	8	2	5	–	15	1

FOOD	PORTION	CALS	TOTAL FAT	CHOL	SAT FAT	POLY FAT	MONO FAT	TRANS FAT	FIBER	SUGAR
eggplant curry	1 serv (8 oz)	241	19	0	9	3	7	–	5	–
lamb curry	1 cup	257	14	90	4	3	5	–	1	1
potato curry	1 serv (5.5 oz)	791	60	12	14	16	27	–	14	5
sambhar dhal curry	1 serv (10 oz)	177	7	0	4	1	2	–	8	–
shrimp curry	1 cup (8.3 oz)	276	14	250	4	4	6	–	1	8

CUSK
fillet baked	3 oz	106	1	50	–	–	–	–	0	0

CUSTARD
MIX
egg custard as prep w/ 2% milk	1 serv (3.5 oz)	112	3	49	1	tr	1	tr	0	5
egg custard as prep w/ whole milk	1 serv (3.5 oz)	122	4	51	2	tr	1	–	0	5
flan as prep w/ 2% milk	1 serv (3.5 oz)	103	2	7	1	tr	tr	–	0	–
flan as prep w/ whole milk	1 serv (3.5 oz)	113	3	12	2	tr	1	–	0	–

Jell-O
Flan as prep	¼ pkg	140	3	9	2	–	–	0	0	20

READY-TO-EAT
Kozy Shack
Flan Creme Caramel Gluten Free	1 pkg (4 oz)	140	3	35	2	–	–	0	0	27

TAKE-OUT
baked	½ cup (5 oz)	147	6	118	3	1	2	–	0	16
flan	½ cup (5.4 oz)	222	6	138	3	1	2	–	0	35
flan de calabaza	1 serv (3.5 oz)	225	10	112	2	2	4	0	tr	22
flan de coco	½ cup (4.3 oz)	345	13	145	8	1	3	–	tr	49
flan de pina	1 serv (4.2 oz)	186	5	222	2	1	2	–	tr	27
flan de pini	½ cup (4.6 oz)	202	6	240	2	1	2	–	tr	29
puerto rican corn custard	½ cup (4.9 oz)	553	34	0	30	1	2	–	5	51
tocino del cielo heaven's delight	1 cup	856	21	967	7	3	9	–	0	154
zabaione	½ cup (2 oz)	135	5	213	2	1	2	–	0	–

CUTTLEFISH
steamed	3 oz	134	1	190	tr	tr	tr	–	–	–

DANDELION GREENS
fresh cooked	½ cup	17	tr	0	–	–	–	–	–	–
raw chopped	½ cup	13	tr	0	–	–	–	–	–	–

FOOD	PORTION	CALS	TOTAL FAT	CHOL	SAT FAT	POLY FAT	MONO FAT	TRANS FAT	FIBER	SUGAR
DANISH PASTRY										
READY-TO-EAT										
Entenmann's										
Pecan Danish Ring	⅛ ring (1.9 oz)	240	14	15	4	–	–	0	1	11
TAKE-OUT										
cheese	1 (2.5 oz)	266	16	11	5	2	8	–	1	5
cinnamon	1 (5 oz)	572	32	30	8	4	18	–	2	28
fruit	1 (5 oz)	527	27	162	7	3	14	–	3	39
lemon	1 (2.5 oz)	263	13	28	2	1	4	–	1	–
raisin nut	1 (2.3 oz)	280	16	30	4	3	9	–	1	17
DATES										
deglet noor chopped	¼ cup (1.3 oz)	104	tr	0	tr	tr	tr	0	3	23
deglet noor dried	1 (7 g)	20	tr	0	tr	tr	tr	0	1	5
jujube fresh	1 oz	30	tr	0	–	–	–	–		
medjool	1 (0.8 oz)	66	tr	0	–			0	2	16
Dole										
California Chopped	¼ cup (1.4 oz)	120	0	0	0	0	0	0	3	26
DEER (see JERKY, VENISON)										
DELI MEATS/COLD CUTS (see also BEEF, CHICKEN, HAM, MEAT SUBSTITUTES, TURKEY)										
barbecue loaf pork & beef	1 slice (0.8 oz)	40	2	9	1	tr	1	–	0	–
beerwurst beef	2 oz	155	13	35	5	1	6	–	1	0
berliner pork & beef	1 slice (0.8 oz)	53	4	11	1	tr	2	–	0	1
blood sausage	1 slice (0.9 oz)	95	9	30	3	1	4	–	0	tr
bologna beef	1 slice (1 oz)	88	8	16	3	tr	3	–	0	0
bologna beef & pork	1 slice (1 oz)	87	7	17	3	tr	3	–	0	1
bologna beef & pork lowfat	1 slice (1 oz)	64	5	11	2	tr	3	–	0	0
bologna beef lowfat	1 slice (1 oz)	57	4	12	2	tr	2	–	0	0
bologna beef reduced sodium	1 slice (1 oz)	88	8	16	3	tr	4	–	0	0
braunschweiger pork	1 slice (1 oz)	92	8	50	3	1	4	–	0	0
corned beef brisket	2 oz	90	5	35	2	–	–	–	0	0
dutch brand loaf pork & beef	1 slice (1.3 oz)	104	9	23	3	1	4	–	tr	0
headcheese pork	1 slice (1.6 oz)	71	5	31	2	1	3	–	0	0
honey loaf pork & beef	1 slice (1 oz)	35	1	10	tr	tr	1	–	0	0
lebanon bologna beef	2 slices (1 oz)	105	6	31	2	tr	3	–	0	0
mortadella beef & pork	1 slice (0.5 oz)	47	4	8	1	tr	2	–	0	0
olive loaf pork	2 slices (2 oz)	134	9	22	3	1	4	–	0	0
pastrami beef	1 slice (1 oz)	41	2	19	1	tr	1	–	tr	tr

FOOD	PORTION	CALS	TOTAL FAT	CHOL	SAT FAT	POLY FAT	MONO FAT	TRANS FAT	FIBER	SUGAR
peppered loaf pork & beef	1 slice (1 oz)	41	2	13	1	tr	1	–	0	0
pepperoni pork & beef	15 slices (1 oz)	135	12	34	5	1	5	–	tr	tr
picnic loaf pork & beef	1 slice (1 oz)	65	5	11	2	1	2	–	0	–
salami cooked beef & pork	1 slice (0.8 oz)	58	5	15	2	tr	2	–	0	0
salami hard pork	3 slices (0.9 oz)	14	8	27	3	1	4	–	0	0
salami hard pork & beef less sodium	1 slice (1 oz)	113	9	26	3	1	4	–	tr	2
sandwich spread pork & beef	¼ cup	141	10	23	4	2	5	–	tr	0
summer sausage thuringer cervelat	2 oz	203	17	41	6	1	7	–	0	tr
Boar's Head										
Bologna Beef	2 oz	150	13	35	4	0	5	0	0	0
Braunschweiger Liverwurst Lite	2 oz	120	8	50	5	1	3	0	0	0
Capocollo Hot & Sweet	1 oz	80	7	25	3	1	3	0	0	0
Mortadella	2 oz	160	14	30	5	1	3	0	0	0
Olive Loaf	2 oz	130	12	20	5	1	6	0	0	tr
Prosciutto Di Parma	1 oz	60	4	25	1	–	–	–	0	0
Foster Farms										
Bologna Chicken	1 slice (1 oz)	60	5	25	–	–	–	0	0	0
Hebrew National										
Bologna Beef	2 slices (2 oz)	170	15	30	6	–	–	1	0	0
Bologna Lean Beef	4 slices (2 oz)	90	5	20	2	–	–	0	–	–
Salami Beef	2 slices (2 oz)	150	13	30	5	–	–	1	0	0
Salami Lean Beef	4 slices (2 oz)	90	5	25	2	–	–	0	–	–
DILL										
seed	1 tsp	6	tr	0	tr	tr	tr	0	tr	–
sprigs fresh	5 (0.3 oz)	0	tr	0	tr	tr	tr	0	–	–
weed dry	1 tbsp	8	tr	0	tr	–	–	0	tr	–

DINNER (*see also* ASIAN FOOD, CURRY, PASTA DINNERS, POT PIE, SPANISH FOOD)

FOOD	PORTION	CALS	TOTAL FAT	CHOL	SAT FAT	POLY FAT	MONO FAT	TRANS FAT	FIBER	SUGAR
Candle Cafe										
Ginger Miso Stir Fry	1 pkg (9 oz)	200	6	0	1	–	–	0	4	9
Seitan Piccata w/ Lemon Caper Sauce	1 pkg (9 oz)	210	4	0	1	–	–	0	4	6
Dinty Moore										
Big Bowl Scalloped Potatoes & Ham	½ can	280	16	40	7	–	–	–	2	1

FOOD	PORTION	CALS	TOTAL FAT	CHOL	SAT FAT	POLY FAT	MONO FAT	TRANS FAT	FIBER	SUGAR
Healthy Choice										
Bacon & Smokey Cheddar Chicken	1 pkg (8.6 oz)	240	6	45	3	2	2	0	3	2
Beef Tips Portabello	1 pkg (11.2 oz)	270	6	45	2	1	3	0	6	12
Country Breaded Chicken	1 pkg (10.6 oz)	340	9	30	2	4	3	0	6	15
Fire Roasted Tomato Chicken	1 pkg (11.6 oz)	310	5	35	2	2	2	0	6	18
Fresh Mixers Creamy Roasted Garlic Chicken	1 pkg (7.4 oz)	310	6	10	2	–	–	0	6	3
Fresh Mixers Steak Portobello	1 pkg (7.5 oz)	290	6	15	2	–	–	0	5	4
Fresh Mixers Sweet Hickory BBQ Chicken	1 pkg (7.9 oz)	370	3	35	1	–	–	0	5	16
Grilled Chicken Monterey	1 pkg (10.9 oz)	320	8	40	3	2	3	0	6	12
Lemon Pepper Fish	1 pkg (10.6 oz)	300	5	25	1	2	2	0	5	15
Lunch Steamers Garlic Herb Shrimp	1 pkg (8.5 oz)	260	7	30	2	2	4	0	5	8
Lunch Steamers Lemon Herb Chicken	1 pkg (8.7 oz)	210	4	25	1	1	2	0	4	2
Lunch Steamers Rosemary Chicken & Sweet Potatoes	1 pkg (8.9 oz)	170	3	30	1	1	1	0	5	10
Pineapple Chicken	1 pkg (9 oz)	380	7	10	1	4	2	0	4	29
Portabella Spinach Parmesan	1 pkg (9.3 oz)	270	7	10	3	1	4	0	5	3
Salisbury Steak	1 pkg (8 oz)	170	5	30	2	1	2	0	4	2
Spicy Caribbean Chicken	1 pkg (8.5 oz)	310	2	20	1	1	1	0	5	16
Turkey Breast & Cranberries	1 pkg (10.7 oz)	250	4	35	1	1	2	0	6	12
Lean Cuisine										
Cafe Cuisine Chicken & Vegetables	1 pkg (10.5 oz)	220	4	30	2	1	1	0	3	5
Cafe Cuisine Chicken Marsala	1 pkg (8.1 oz)	250	9	25	3	3	3	0	2	4
Cafe Cuisine Lemon Pepper Fish	1 pkg (9 oz)	290	8	25	2	3	2	0	2	4
Cafe Cuisine Orange Chicken	1 pkg (9 oz)	300	7	25	2	3	3	0	2	11
Cafe Cuisine Roasted Garlic Chicken	1 pkg (8.8 oz)	170	6	40	2	2	1	0	0	3
Cafe Cuisine Steak Tips Portabello	1 pkg (7.5 oz)	150	4	20	2	0	1	0	3	4
Casual Cuisine Flatbread Melts Steakhouse Ranch	1 pkg (6.25 oz)	350	9	30	4	2	3	0	4	7
Comfort Classics Baked Chicken	1 pkg (8.6 oz)	240	7	30	2	3	2	0	2	4

FOOD	PORTION	CALS	TOTAL FAT	CHOL	SAT FAT	POLY FAT	MONO FAT	TRANS FAT	FIBER	SUGAR
Comfort Cuisine Beef Pot Roast	1 pkg (9 oz)	210	6	25	2	1	2	0	3	3
Comfort Cuisine Meatloaf w/ Gravy & Whipped Potatoes	1 pkg (9.4 oz)	250	8	45	3	2	3	0	3	2
Comfort Cuisine Roasted Turkey Breast w/ Dressing	1 pkg (9.75 oz)	290	4	20	1	2	1	0	3	27
Comfort Cuisine Salisbury Steak w/ Mac & Cheese	1 pkg (9.5 oz)	260	8	40	4	1	3	0	3	3
Dinnertime Selects Balsamic Glazed Chicken	1 pkg (12 oz)	330	7	40	3	2	3	0	4	11
Dinnertime Selects Chicken Florentine	1 pkg (13.25 oz)	410	9	45	4	2	3	0	6	13
Dinnertime Selects Chicken Portabello	1 pkg (12 oz)	390	8	55	1	4	3	0	2	2
Dinnertime Selects Salisbury Steak	1 pkg (12.5 oz)	270	9	45	4	2	3	0	5	10
Market Creations Chicken Poblano	1 pkg (10.5 oz)	300	5	40	2	1	1	0	5	7
Market Creations Shrimp Scampi	1 pkg (10.5 oz)	250	7	58	4	1	2	0	4	4
Market Creations Sweet & Spicy Ginger Chicken	1 pkg (10.5 oz)	280	3	30	1	1	0	0	4	12
Simple Favorites Quesadilla BBQ Chicken	1 pkg (5 oz)	280	6	20	3	1	2	0	2	7
Simple Favorites Stuffed Cabbage	1 pkg (9.5 oz)	210	6	15	2	2	2	0	3	6
Simple Favorites Swedish Meatballs	1 pkg (9.1 oz)	290	8	35	3	2	3	0	3	4
Spa Cuisine Chicken Mediterranean	1 pkg (10.5 oz)	240	4	25	1	2	1	0	5	7
Spa Cuisine Chicken In Peanut Sauce	1 pkg (9 oz)	280	6	25	1	2	3	0	5	5
Spa Cuisine Chicken Pecan	1 pkg (9 oz)	310	7	35	1	3	2	0	5	13
Spa Cuisine Lemon Chicken	1 pkg (9 oz)	290	9	25	2	4	2	0	5	8
Spa Cuisine Lemongrass Chicken	1 pkg (9.4 oz)	250	5	25	1	2	1	0	5	7
Spa Cuisine Rosemary Chicken	1 pkg (8.25 oz)	210	4	30	2	1	1	0	5	5
Spa Cuisine Salmon w/ Basil	1 pkg (9.5 oz)	210	5	20	2	2	1	0	5	2

FOOD	PORTION	CALS	TOTAL FAT	CHOL	SAT FAT	POLY FAT	MONO FAT	TRANS FAT	FIBER	SUGAR
Meal Mart										
Stuffed Cabbage Beef Hungarian Style	¼ pkg (2.5 oz)	210	5	30	1	–	–	0	2	12
Saffron Road										
Chicken Biryani	1 pkg (11 oz)	400	12	55	2	–	–	0	3	4
Chicken Tikka Masala w/ Basmati Rice	1 pkg (11 oz)	290	8	40	2	–	–	0	4	2
Lamb Saag w/ Basmati Rice	1 pkg (11 oz)	300	9	45	3	–	–	0	4	1
Lamb Vindaloo w/ Basmati Rice	1 pkg (11 oz)	340	7	40	2	–	–	0	5	2
Moroccan Lamb Stew	1 pkg (11 oz)	230	12	40	3	–	–	0	2	6
Simply Sensible										
Beef Pot Roast & Gravy w/ Mashed Potatoes	½ pkg (8.5 oz)	220	5	40	2	–	–	0	1	1
Beef Tips & Gravy w/ Brown Rice	1 cup (7 oz)	200	4	30	1	–	–	0	1	0
Zing Chicken & Brown Rice	1 cup (7 oz)	230	2	35	0	–	–	0	3	10
The Fillo Factory										
Fillo Pie Spinach & Cheese	⅕ pie (4.8 oz)	270	14	30	7	–	–	0	2	1
Weight Watchers										
Smart Ones Chicken w/ Broccoli & Cheese	1 pkg (11.8 oz)	340	8	65	4	1	2	0	3	6
Zatarain's										
Blackened Chicken w/ Yellow Rice	1 pkg (10.5 oz)	470	13	25	2	–	–		3	3
Jambalaya w/ Sausage	1 pkg (12 oz)	500	14	25	4	–	–		3	3
Red Beans & Rice w/ Sausage	1 pkg (12 oz)	510	20	30	7	–	–		5	5
Rice Bowl Big Easy	1 pkg (10 oz)	430	12	45	5	–	–		5	3
Sausage & Chicken Gumbo w/ Rice	1 pkg (12 oz)	300	14	30	4	–	–		2	3
DIP										
shrimp cream cheese	¼ cup (2 oz)	152	14	74	6	2	3	–	tr	1
spinach sour cream	¼ cup	155	15	13	4	7	4	–	1	1
Cedar's										
Tzatziki Cucumber Garlic	2 tbsp (1 oz)	35	3	5	1	–	–	0	0	1
Cheez Whiz										
Original	1 serv (1.2 oz)	90	7	5	2	–	–	0	0	2
Fritos										
Bean	2 tbsp (1.2 oz)	35	1	0	0	–	–	0	2	0
Chili Cheese	2 tbsp (1.2 oz)	45	3	1	1	–	–	1	tr	1

FOOD	PORTION	CALS	TOTAL FAT	CHOL	SAT FAT	POLY FAT	MONO FAT	TRANS FAT	FIBER	SUGAR
Lay's										
Country Ranch Mix as prep w/ sour cream	2 tbsp (1.1 oz)	70	6	10	4	–	–	0	0	0
French Onion	2 tbsp (1.2 oz)	60	5	<5	0	–	–	0	0	0
Mrs. Dash										
French Onion Mix Salt Free not prep	¾ tsp (2 g)	5	0	0	0	0	0	0	–	–
Salpica										
Chipotle Hummus Bean	2 tbsp (1 oz)	40	1	0	0	0	0	0	1	0
Cowgirl White Bean	2 tbsp (1 oz)	25	0	0	0	0	0	0	1	0
Salsa Con Queso	2 tbsp (1 oz)	20	1	0	0	0	0	0	0	4
Tostitos										
Creamy Spinach	2 tbsp (1.1 oz)	50	4	<5	0	–	–	0	tr	tr
Dip Creations Mix Freshly Made Guacamole as prep w/ avocados	2 tbsp (1.1 oz)	50	4	0	1	–	–	0	2	0
Zesty Bean & Cheese Medium	2 tbsp (1.2 oz)	45	2	0	1	–	–	0	2	tr
Victoria										
Artichoke	1 tbsp (1 oz)	30	2	0	1	–	–	0	1	2
Want'ems										
Sweet Chili Fusion	2 tbsp (1.1 oz)	50	0	0	0	0	0	0	0	11
Thai Mango Fusion	2 tbsp (1.1 oz)	40	0	0	0	0	0	0	0	8
DOCK										
fresh cooked	3 ½ oz	20	1	0	–	–	–	–	–	–
raw chopped	½ cup	15	tr	0	–	–	–	–	–	–
DOUGHNUTS										
chocolate glazed	1 med (1.5 oz)	175	8	24	2	1	5	–	1	13
chocolate w/ chocolate icing	1 med (2 oz)	218	12	4	4	1	6	–	1	13
creme filled	1 (3 oz)	307	21	20	5	3	10	–	1	12
custard filled	1 (2.3 oz)	235	16	16	4	2	8	–	1	9
french cruller glazed	1 med (1.4 oz)	169	8	5	2	1	4	–	1	14
jelly filled	1 (3 oz)	289	16	22	4	2	9	–	1	18
old fashioned plain	1 med (2 oz)	226	13	5	4	1	7	4	1	9
plain chocolate frosted	1 med (1.5 oz)	194	11	8	6	1	4	4	1	11
plain glazed	1 med (1.6 oz)	192	10	14	3	1	6	–	1	–
whole wheat sugared	1 med (1.6 oz)	162	9	9	1	3	4	–	1	10
Entenmann's										
Crumb	1 (1.9 oz)	230	10	10	4	–	–	0	tr	20

FOOD	PORTION	CALS	TOTAL FAT	CHOL	SAT FAT	POLY FAT	MONO FAT	TRANS FAT	FIBER	SUGAR
Glazed	1 (2 oz)	250	13	10	6	–	–	0	tr	20
Mini Rich Frosted Chocolate	1 (1.1 oz)	170	12	5	7	–	–	0	0	8
Old Fashion Plain	1 (1.7 oz)	230	14	15	6	–	–	0	tr	10
Pop'Ems Cinnamon	4 (2 oz)	250	13	0	6	–	–	0	tr	16
Pop'Ems Glazed Crullers	2 (1.6 oz)	210	12	10	5	–	–	0	0	17
Pop'Ems Holes Rich Frosted	4 (2.1 oz)	320	23	10	14	–	–	0	tr	17
Rich Frosted	1 (1.9 oz)	240	19	10	11	–	–	0	tr	16
TAKE-OUT										
andagi okinawan doughnut	1 (0.7 oz)	84	5	7	1	2	2	–	0	–
malasada portuguese ball	1 (1.1 oz)	118	5	22	1	2	2	–	0	–
DRINK MIXERS										
whiskey sour mix not prep	1 pkg (0.6 oz)	64	0	0	0	0	0	0	–	–
whiskey sour mix	2 oz	55	0	0	0	0	0	0	0	–
Arizona										
Pina Colada Virgin Cocktail	8 oz	90	1	0	0	–	–	0	0	20
Go Cocktails!										
On-The-Go Sugar Free Appletini	1 pkg (1.9 g)	5	0	0	0	0	0	0	0	0
On-The-Go Sugar Free Cosmo	1 pkg (2.2 g)	5	0	0	0	0	0	0	0	0
On-The-Go Sugar Free Lemon Drop	1 pkg (2.5 g)	5	0	0	0	0	0	0	0	0
On-The-Go Sugar Free Margarita	1 pkg (2.78 g)	5	0	0	0	0	0	0	0	0
Margaritaville										
Margarita Mix Mango	4 oz	120	0	0	0	0	0	0	–	26
Margarita Mix Original Lime	4 oz	110	0	0	0	0	0	0	–	26
Modmix										
Mojito	2 oz	50	0	0	0	0	0	0	0	13
Organic Citrus Margarita	2 oz	70	0	0	0	0	0	0	0	18
Organic French Martini	2 oz	50	0	0	0	0	0	0	0	12
Organic Lavender Lemon Drop	2 oz	55	0	0	0	0	0	0	0	13
Organic Pomegranate Cosmopolitan	2 oz	55	0	0	0	0	0	0	0	13
Organic Wasabi Bloody Mary	2 oz	20	0	0	0	0	0	0	0	3
Old Orchard										
Daiquiri Mixer Strawberry frzn as prep	8 oz	120	0	0	0	0	0	0	–	30

FOOD	PORTION	CALS	TOTAL FAT	CHOL	SAT FAT	POLY FAT	MONO FAT	TRANS FAT	FIBER	SU
Margarita Mixer frzn as prep	8 oz	120	0	0	0	0	0	0	–	30
Pina Colada Mixer frzn as prep	8 oz	120	0	0	0	0	0	0	–	30
Prometheus Springs										
Capsaicin Spiced Elixir Citrus Cayenne	8 oz	70	0	0	0	0	0	0	–	17
Capsaicin Spiced Elixir Lychee Wasabi	8 oz	80	0	0	0	0	0	0	–	20
Capsaicin Spiced Elixir Mango Chili	8 oz	70	0	0	0	0	0	0	–	16
Capsaicin Spiced Elixir Spicy Pear	8 oz	70	0	0	0	0	0	0	–	16
DRUM										
freshwater fillet baked	5.4 oz	236	10	126	2	4	2	–	0	0
freshwater baked	3 oz	130	5	70	1	1	2	–	0	0
DUCK										
boneless roasted	½ duck (7.8 oz)	444	25	197	9	3	8	–	0	0
boneless w/o skin roasted	3.5 oz	201	11	89	4	1	4	–	0	0
boneless w/o skin roasted diced	1 cup (4.9 oz)	281	16	125	6	2	5	–	0	0
chinese pressed	3 oz	162	8	28	3	1	4	–	1	9
chinese pressed diced	1 cup (4.9 oz)	267	14	46	4	2	6	–	1	14
pekin breast boneless w/ skin roasted	1 (4.2 oz)	242	13	163	4	2	7	–	0	0
pekin breast w/o skin broiled	3 oz	133	2	136	1	tr	1	–	0	0
pekin leg w/ skin w/o bone roasted	1 (3.2 oz)	200	10	105	3	2	5	–	0	0
pekin leg w/o skin & bone roasted	1 (2.6 oz)	134	5	79	1	1	2	–	0	0
w/ skin & bone roasted	½ duck (13 oz)	1287	108	321	37	14	49	–	0	0
w/ skin & bone roasted	1 serv (6 oz)	583	49	145	17	6	22	–	0	0
wing roasted bone removed	1 (1.1 oz)	101	8	25	3	1	4	–	0	0
TAKE-OUT										
breast battered & fried bone removed	½ (3.2 oz)	199	10	94	3	2	3	–	tr	tr
leg battered & fried bone removed	1 (2.5 oz)	155	8	73	3	1	2	–	tr	tr

FOOD	PORTION	CALS	TOTAL FAT	CHOL	SAT FAT	POLY FAT	MONO FAT	TRANS FAT	FIBER	SUGAR
DUMPLING										
Crazy Cuizine										
Potstickers Chicken w/ Sauce	8 (5 oz)	220	6	25	2	–	–	0	1	2
Potstickers Pork w/o Sauce	8 (5 oz)	240	8	20	3	–	–	0	1	1
Fujisan										
Chicken Shumai Dumplings	3 (3 oz)	130	2	20	0	–	–	0	0	2
Healthy Choice										
Sweet Asian Potstickers Entree	1 pkg (9.9 oz)	340	5	0	1	2	2	0	5	14
Lean Cuisine										
Market Creations Pot Stickers Chicken	1 pkg (10 oz)	270	6	14	1	2	1	0	5	16
Simple Favorites Asian Pot Stickers	1 pkg (9 oz)	260	4	10	1	1	1	0	2	9
Panni										
Spaetzle Authentic German not prep	2 oz	200	2	55	1	–	–	0	2	0
Pepperidge Farm										
Apple	1	230	11	0	6	–	–	0	1	13
Peach	1	250	11	0	6	–	–	0	1	18
Saffron Road										
Manchurian Dumplings w/ Rice	1 pkg (11 oz)	340	11	0	1	–	–	0	2	5
TAKE-OUT										
apple	1 (6.7 oz)	661	34	0	7	11	15	–	3	30
cherry	1 (2.7 oz)	238	12	0	2	5	5	–	1	13
cornmeal	1 (2.8 oz)	134	4	62	1	1	1	0	2	1
fried pork	1 (3.5 oz)	338	21	27	5	6	9	–	1	1
fried puerto rican style	1 med (1.1 oz)	117	7	0	1	2	3	–	tr	1
gyoza potstickers vegetable	8 (4.9 oz)	210	4	0	1	–	–	–	5	7
peach	1 (2.7 oz)	253	12	0	2	4	5	–	1	12
piroshki meat filled	1 (3.4 oz)	348	22	23	6	5	9	–	1	tr
steamed meat	1 (1.3 oz)	41	1	18	tr	tr	tr	–	tr	tr
DURIAN										
fresh	3.5 oz	141	2	0	–	–	–	–	–	–
EDAMAME (see SOYBEANS)										
EEL										
fresh cooked	3 oz	200	13	137	3	1	8	–	0	0

FOOD	PORTION	CALS	TOTAL FAT	CHOL	SAT FAT	POLY FAT	MONO FAT	TRANS FAT	FIBER	SUGA
fresh cooked	1 fillet (5.6 oz)	375	24	257	5	2	15	–	0	0
raw	3 oz	156	10	107	2	1	6	–	0	0

EGG (see also EGG DISHES)
CHICKEN

FOOD	PORTION	CALS	TOTAL FAT	CHOL	SAT FAT	POLY FAT	MONO FAT	TRANS FAT	FIBER	SUGA
fresh large	1 (1.8 oz)	72	5	186	2	1	2	tr	0	tr
fresh medium	1 (1.5 oz)	63	4	164	1	1	2	tr	0	tr
fresh small	1 (1.3 oz)	54	4	141	1	1	1	tr	0	tr
hard or soft cooked	1	77	5	186	2	1	2	–	0	1
pickled	1	72	5	198	2	1	2	–	0	1
poached	1	73	5	184	2	1	2	–	0	tr
scrambled plain	1 (2 oz)	61	7	169	2	1	3	tr	0	1
sunny side up	2	155	12	365	3	2	5	–	0	1
white raw	1 (1.1 oz)	17	tr	0	0	0	0	–	0	tr
yolk raw	1 (0.5 oz)	55	4	184	2	1	2	–	0	tr

Jake & Amos

FOOD	PORTION	CALS	TOTAL FAT	CHOL	SAT FAT	POLY FAT	MONO FAT	TRANS FAT	FIBER	SUGA
Pickled Red Beet Eggs	2 (5.3 oz)	200	8	345	3	–	–	0	0	21

Land O Lakes

FOOD	PORTION	CALS	TOTAL FAT	CHOL	SAT FAT	POLY FAT	MONO FAT	TRANS FAT	FIBER	SUGA
All Natural Brown Large ALA Omega-3	1 (1.8 oz)	70	5	185	2	–	–	0	0	0

Nature's Design

FOOD	PORTION	CALS	TOTAL FAT	CHOL	SAT FAT	POLY FAT	MONO FAT	TRANS FAT	FIBER	SUGA
Whole Peeled Egg	1 (1.5 oz)	70	4	190	2	–	–	0	–	–

Pete & Gerry's

FOOD	PORTION	CALS	TOTAL FAT	CHOL	SAT FAT	POLY FAT	MONO FAT	TRANS FAT	FIBER	SUGA
Heirloom	1 (1.8 oz)	70	5	215	2	–	–	0	–	–

Safest Choice

FOOD	PORTION	CALS	TOTAL FAT	CHOL	SAT FAT	POLY FAT	MONO FAT	TRANS FAT	FIBER	SUGA
Pasteurized Fresh	1 lg (1.8 oz)	70	5	186	2	1	2	0	0	0

OTHER POULTRY

FOOD	PORTION	CALS	TOTAL FAT	CHOL	SAT FAT	POLY FAT	MONO FAT	TRANS FAT	FIBER	SUGA
duck 100 year old	1 (1 oz)	49	3	173	–	–	–	–	–	–
duck cooked	1 (2.5 oz)	129	10	616	3	1	5	–	0	1
duck preserved hard core	1 (1.8 oz)	80	6	220	2	–	–	–	0	0
duck preserved soft core	1 (1.8 oz)	80	6	220	2	–	–	–	0	0
duck salted	1 (1 oz)	54	4	184	–	–	–	–	–	–
goose cooked	1 (5 oz)	265	19	1223	5	2	8	–	0	1
quail canned	1 (0.3 oz)	14	1	75	tr	tr	tr	–	0	tr
quail cooked	1 (0.5 oz)	24	2	42	1	tr	0	–	0	0
turkey raw	1 (2.8 oz)	135	9	737	3	1	4	–	0	–

EGG DISHES
Aunt Jemima

FOOD	PORTION	CALS	TOTAL FAT	CHOL	SAT FAT	POLY FAT	MONO FAT	TRANS FAT	FIBER	SUGA
Eggs & Sausage	1 pkg (6.2 oz)	320	21	310	5	–	–	–	2	3
Omelet Ham & Cheese	1 pkg (5.2 oz)	240	14	195	6	–	–	0	2	2
Scramble Ham & Egg	1 pkg (6.8 oz)	260	13	195	4	–	–	–	2	4

FOOD	PORTION	CALS	TOTAL FAT	CHOL	SAT FAT	POLY FAT	MONO FAT	TRANS FAT	FIBER	SUGAR
IHOP At Home										
Omelet Crisper Bacon & Cheese	1 (3.7 oz)	240	14	100	5	–	–	0	tr	2
Omelet Crisper Egg & Cheese	1 (3.7 oz)	210	12	125	4	–	–	0	tr	2
Omelet Crisper Sausage & Cheese	1 (3.7 oz)	230	13	95	5	–	–	0	tr	2
Weight Watchers										
Smart Ones Smart Morning Wrap Egg Sausage & Cheese	2 (4 oz)	240	8	30	3	2	3	0	7	2
TAKE-OUT										
deviled	1 half	62	5	121	1	2	2	–	0	tr
eggs benedict	2	825	64	784	30	7	22	–	2	3
omelet cheese	3 eggs	387	29	588	11	4	10	–	0	6
omelet mushroom	3 eggs	251	17	511	5	3	7	–	1	4
omelet mushroom & onion	3 eggs	294	20	600	6	4	8	–	1	5
omelet plain	3 eggs	338	25	736	7	4	10	–	0	4
omelet spanish	3 eggs	496	38	626	9	9	16	–	3	11
omelet spinach	3 eggs	279	19	568	6	3	8	–	1	4
omelet western	3 eggs	355	23	537	7	4	10	–	tr	4
salad	½ cup	353	34	344	6	15	10	–	0	1
tortilla de amarillo omelet w/ plantain	3 eggs	536	35	467	7	14	12	–	3	21
EGG ROLLS										
egg roll wrapper fresh	1 (1.1 oz)	93	tr	3	tr	tr	tr	0	1	–
Lean Cuisine										
Casual Cuisine Spring Rolls Fajita Chicken	½ pkg	200	7	30	2	4	2	0	2	3
Casual Cuisine Spring Rolls Garlic Chicken	½ pkg	200	8	20	2	4	3	0	2	4
Simple Favorites Eggroll Vegetable	1 pkg (9 oz)	320	4	0	1	2	1	0	2	12
TAKE-OUT										
chicken	1 (3 oz)	140	4	15	2	–	–	–	4	5
lobster	1 (4.8 oz)	270	7	0	2	–	–	–	6	4
lumpia vegetable & shrimp	2 (3 oz)	120	0	10	0	–	–	–	2	1
meat & shrimp	1 (4.8 oz)	320	12	10	3	–	–	–	4	3
pork & shrimp	1 (5 oz)	300	10	15	4	–	–	–	7	6
shrimp	1 (2.2 oz)	156	7	11	2	2	4	–	2	4
spicy pork	1 (3 oz)	200	9	5	2	–	–	–	3	3

FOOD	PORTION	CALS	TOTAL FAT	CHOL	SAT FAT	POLY FAT	MONO FAT	TRANS FAT	FIBER	SUG
spring roll deep fried	1 (0.8 oz)	70	4	3	2	1	2	–	1	–
vegetable	1 (3 oz)	170	4	0	1	–	–	–	4	4

EGGNOG

eggnog	1 qt	1368	76	596	45	3	23	–	–	–
eggnog	1 cup	342	19	149	11	1	6	–	–	–
eggnog flavor mix as prep w/ milk	9 oz	260	8	33	5	tr	2	–	–	–
Lactaid										
Eggnog	½ cup (4 oz)	170	9	60	5	–	–	0	0	19
Straus										
Organic	4 oz	160	10	70	5	–	–	0	0	13
Turkey Hill										
EggNog	½ cup (4.2 oz)	190	9	65	5	–	–	0	0	23
Light Vanilla	½ cup (4.2 oz)	150	5	45	3	–	–	0	0	22
TAKE-OUT										
eggnog	1 cup	306	22	63	14	–	–	–	0	–

EGGPLANT

cubed cooked w/ oil	1 cup	133	8	0	1	2	4	–	5	6
pickled	½ cup	33	tr	0	tr	tr	tr	–	2	3
slices grilled	1 (2 oz)	36	2	0	tr	1	1	–	1	2
Victoria										
In Vinegar	¼ cup (1 oz)	5	0	0	0	0	0	0	1	1
TAKE-OUT										
baba ghannouj	¼ cup	55	4	0	–	–	–	–	–	–
caponata	2 tbsp (1 oz)	30	2	0	–	–	–	–	–	2
iman bayildi eggplant w/ onion & tomato	1 serv (15.6 oz)	345	28	0	4	–	–	–	2	6
indian eggplant runi	1 serv	180	14	0	4	–	–	–	1	1
moussaka	1 serv (9 oz)	372	24	54	6	8	9	–	5	6
papoutsaki little shoes	1 serv (15.5 oz)	245	16	40	7	–	–	–	1	1
tempura	1 serv (1.5 oz)	118	10	0	5	1	4	–	1	0

ELDERBERRIES

fresh	1 cup (5 oz)	106	1	0	tr	tr	tr	0	10	–

ELDERBERRY JUICE

elderberry	7 oz	76	0	0	0	0	0	0	–	–

FOOD	PORTION	CALS	TOTAL FAT	CHOL	SAT FAT	POLY FAT	MONO FAT	TRANS FAT	FIBER	SUGAR
ELK										
eye of round roasted	3.5 oz	151	3	63	1	tr	1	tr	0	0
ground cooked	3.5 oz	143	3	70	1	tr	1	tr	0	0

ENERGY BARS (see also CEREAL BARS, FRUIT AND NUT BARS, NUTRITION SUPPLEMENTS)

FOOD	PORTION	CALS	TOTAL FAT	CHOL	SAT FAT	POLY FAT	MONO FAT	TRANS FAT	FIBER	SUGAR
Halo										
Honey Graham	1 (1.3 oz)	150	5	0	1	–	–	0	2	8
Nutty Marshmallow	1 (1.3 oz)	150	6	0	1	–	–	0	2	9
Rocky Road	1 (1.3 oz)	160	8	0	2	–	–	0	2	9
S'Mores	1 (1.3 oz)	150	5	0	1	–	–	0	2	13
Journey										
Coconut Curry	1 (1.75 oz)	220	11	0	4	–	–	0	5	10
Hickory Barbecue	1 (1.75 oz)	170	6	0	1	–	–	0	4	6
Pizza Marinara	1 (1.75 oz)	170	6	0	1	–	–	0	4	5
LaraBar										
Pineapple Upside Down Cake	1 (1.6 oz)	180	7	0	1	2	5	0	4	10
Luna										
Blueberry Bliss	1 (1.7 oz)	180	5	0	2	–	–	0	3	13
Chocolate Raspberry	1 (1.7 oz)	170	5	0	2	–	–	0	5	13
Fiber Chocolate Raspberry	1 (1.4 oz)	110	4	0	1	–	–	0	7	11
Fiber Vanilla Blueberry	1 (1.4 oz)	110	3	0	0	–	–	0	7	11
Mini LemonZest	1 (0.7 oz)	80	2	0	1	–	–	0	1	6
Mini White Chocolate Macadamia	1 (0.7 oz)	80	3	0	1	–	–	0	1	5
Nutz Over Chocolate	1 (1.7 oz)	180	6	0	3	–	–	0	3	10
Protein Chocolate Peanut Butter	1 (1.6 oz)	190	8	0	4	–	–	0	3	12
Protein Cookie Dough	1 (1.6 oz)	170	6	0	4	–	–	0	1	14
Protein Mint Chocolate Chip	1 (1.6 oz)	170	5	0	4	–	–	0	3	13
Vanilla Almond	1 (1.7 oz)	190	6	0	2	–	–	0	3	11
Marathon										
Snickers Chewy Chocolatey Peanut	1 (1.9 oz)	210	8	5	3	–	–	0	5	15
Snickers Crunchy Dark Chocolate	1 (1.6 oz)	150	5	5	3	–	–	0	7	9
Snickers Crunchy Multi-Grain	1 (1.9 oz)	220	7	5	3	–	–	0	3	17
Nogii										
No Gluten High Protein Peanut Butter & Chocolate	1 (2 oz)	230	8	0	3	–	–	0	2	10

FOOD	PORTION	CALS	TOTAL FAT	CHOL	SAT FAT	POLY FAT	MONO FAT	TRANS FAT	FIBER	SUGAR
Premier										
Protein Bar Double Chocolate Crunch	1 (2.5 oz)	270	6	20	4	–	–	0	2	9
Protein Bar Yogurt Peanut Crunch	1 (2.5 oz)	290	8	10	5	–	–	0	1	10
Quest										
Cravings Protein Peanut Butter Cups	2 (1.8 oz)	240	17	<5	8	–	–	0	3	1
Natural Protein Chocolate Peanut Butter	1 (2.1 oz)	160	5	5	1	–	–	0	17	1
Natural Protein Cinnamon Roll	1 (2.1 oz)	170	6	5	0	–	–	0	17	1
Natural Protein Peanut Butter & Jelly	1 (2.1 oz)	210	10	<5	2	–	–	0	17	2
Natural Protein Vanilla Almond Crunch	1 (2.1 oz)	200	9	<5	1	–	–	0	18	1
Rise Bar										
Energy + Cherry Almond	1 (1.6 oz)	200	11	0	2	–	–	0	3	11
Protein + Almond Honey	1 (2.1 oz)	280	16	0	2	–	–	0	4	13
Protein + Crunchy Carob Chip	1 (2.1 oz)	260	15	5	1	–	–	0	5	13
Think5										
Red Berry	1 (2.5 oz)	240	4	0	1	–	–	0	3	7
Titan										
High Protein Chocolate Peanut Butter Crunch	1 (2.8 oz)	320	13	10	7	–	–	0	1	5
High Protein Cookies And Cream	1 (2.8 oz)	330	9	5	7	–	–	0	tr	5

ENERGY DRINKS

FOOD	PORTION	CALS	TOTAL FAT	CHOL	SAT FAT	POLY FAT	MONO FAT	TRANS FAT	FIBER	SUGAR
Arizona										
Energy Low Carb	1 can (8 oz)	10	0	0	0	0	0	0	–	3
Rx Energy Fast Shot Natural Green Tea	1 bottle (2 oz)	10	0	0	0	0	0	0	–	3
Sports Orange	8 oz	50	0	0	0	0	0	0	0	13
Bing										
Energy Drink	1 can (12 oz)	40	0	0	0	0	0	0	–	10
EX										
Aqua Vitamins Lemon Lime	1 bottle (16.9 oz)	110	0	0	0	0	0	0	–	26
Chillout	1 can (8.4 oz)	80	0	0	0	0	0	0	–	20

FOOD	PORTION	CALS	TOTAL FAT	CHOL	SAT FAT	POLY FAT	MONO FAT	TRANS FAT	FIBER	SUGAR
Pure Energy	1 can (8.4 oz)	70	0	0	0	0	0	0	–	15
Slim Energy	1 can (8.4 oz)	20	0	0	0	0	0	0	–	2
Facedrink										
The Social Drink	1 bottle (2.5 oz)	3	0	0	0	0	0	0	–	0
Fever										
Stimulation Beverage All Flavors	8 oz	130	0	0	0	0	0	0	–	31
Gatorade										
G Series Fit 02 Perform	8 oz	10	0	0	0	0	0	0	–	2
G2 Natural Perform	8 oz	20	0	0	0	0	0	0	–	5
Hero										
Energy Shot	1 bottle (2 oz)	0	0	0	0	0	0	0	0	0
Honeydrop										
Alive Blood Orange & Honey	8 oz	40	0	0	0	0	0	0	–	10
Mamma Chia										
All Flavors	8 oz	120	4	0	–	–	–	0	6	14
Nawgan										
Berry Caffeine Free	1 can (11.5 oz)	40	0	0	0	0	0	0	–	10
Torocco Orange	1 can (11.5 oz)	45	0	0	0	0	0	0	–	11
Ocean Spray										
Cranergy Cranberry	8 oz	35	0	0	0	0	0	0	–	8
Palo										
Mamajuana	7 oz	50	0	0	0	0	0	0	–	13
Premier										
Nitro Shot	1 (1.8 oz)	75	0	0	0	0	0	0	0	15
Rocket Shot Berry Blast	1 (1.8 oz)	30	0	0	0	0	0	0	–	7
Pyure										
O.E.O. Shot All Flavors	1 bottle (2 oz)	0	0	0	0	0	0	0	0	0
Recharge										
Lemon as prep	8 oz	10	0	0	0	0	0	0	–	tr
Tropical as prep	8 oz	10	0	0	0	0	0	0	–	tr
Scheckter's										
Organic Energy	1 can (8.4 oz)	112	0	0	0	0	0	0	–	26
Organic Energy Lite	1 can (8.4 oz)	78	0	0	0	0	0	0	–	17
SoCal										
Just Chill	1 can (8.4 oz)	50	0	0	0	0	0	0	–	12
Solixir										
Blackberry	1 can	50	0	0	0	0	0	0	–	11
Orange	1 can	55	0	0	0	0	0	0	–	12
Pomegranate	1 can	60	0	0	0	0	0	0	–	13

FOOD	PORTION	CALS	TOTAL FAT	CHOL	SAT FAT	POLY FAT	MONO FAT	TRANS FAT	FIBER	SUGAR
Steaz										
Berry Organic	8 oz	90	0	0	0	0	0	0	–	23
ENGLISH MUFFIN										
READY-TO-EAT										
crumpets	1 (1.5 oz)	80	0	0	0	0	0	0	tr	1
plain	1 (2 oz)	129	1	0	tr	tr	tr	0	2	2
whole wheat	1 (2.3 oz)	134	1	0	tr	1	tr	–	4	5
Matthew's										
Golden White	1 (2.1 oz)	140	2	0	0	0	0	0	0	2
Nature's Own										
100 Calorie Multi Grain	1 (2 oz)	100	1	0	0	–	–	0	7	3
Original	1 (2 oz)	130	1	0	0	1	0	0	tr	1
Pepperidge Farm										
100% Whole Wheat	1	140	2	0	1	1	0	0	3	4
Original	1	130	2	0	1	1	0	0	1	1
Thomas'										
10 Grain	1 (2.1 oz)	130	1	0	0	0	0	0	6	2
100% Whole Wheat	1 (2 oz)	120	1	0	0	0	0	0	3	2
Corn	1 (2.1 oz)	150	1	0	0	0	0	0	1	3
Honey Wheat	1 (2 oz)	130	1	0	0	0	0	0	1	2
Light Multi-Grain	1 (2 oz)	100	1	0	0	0	0	0	8	tr
Multi-Grain	1 (2 oz)	150	3	0	0	2	1	0	2	3
Original	1 (2 oz)	120	1	0	0	0	0	0	1	1
TAKE-OUT										
w/ butter	1 (2.2 oz)	189	6	13	2	1	2	–	–	–
w/ cheese & sausage	1 (4 oz)	365	22	46	9	3	9	–	1	2
w/ egg cheese & canadian bacon	1 (4.9 oz)	307	13	234	5	2	4	–	1	3
w/ egg cheese & sausage	1 (5.8 oz)	472	30	269	11	5	11	–	tr	2
EPAZOTE										
fresh	1 tbsp (1 g)	<1	0	0	–	–	–	0	tr	–
fresh sprig	1 (2 g)	1	tr	0	–	–	–	–	tr	–
EPPAW										
raw	½ cup	75	1	0	–	–	–	–	–	–
FALAFEL										
Falafel Republic										
Traditional	3 (3 oz)	210	7	0	0	–	–	0	6	1

FOOD	PORTION	CALS	TOTAL FAT	CHOL	SAT FAT	POLY FAT	MONO FAT	TRANS FAT	FIBER	SUGAR
TAKE-OUT										
falafel	1 (1.2 oz)	57	3	0	tr	1	tr	–	–	–

FAT (*see also* BUTTER, BUTTER SUBSTITUTES, MARGARINE, OIL)

FOOD	PORTION	CALS	TOTAL FAT	CHOL	SAT FAT	POLY FAT	MONO FAT	TRANS FAT	FIBER	SUGAR
bacon grease	1 tbsp	116	13	12	5	1	6	–	0	0
beef shortening	1 tbsp	115	13	13	6	1	5	–	0	0
beef suet	1 oz	242	27	19	15	1	9	–	0	0
chicken	1 tbsp (0.4 oz)	115	13	11	4	3	6	–	0	0
duck	1 tbsp (0.4 oz)	113	13	13	4	2	6	–	0	0
goose	1 tbsp	115	13	13	4	1	7	–	0	0
lamb new zealand	1 oz	182	19	25	10	1	7	–	0	0
lard	1 tbsp (0.5 oz)	115	13	12	5	1	6	–	0	0
lard	1 cup (7.2 oz)	1849	205	195	80	23	93	–	0	0
meat pan drippings	½ tbsp	124	14	14	6	1	6	–	0	0
pork raw	1 oz	230	25	16	9	3	12	0	0	0
salt pork	1 cube (1 oz)	215	23	26	8	3	11	0	0	0
shortening	1 tbsp	113	13	0	3	5	5	–	0	0
shortening	1 cup	1812	205	0	41	78	75	–	0	0
turkey	1 tbsp	116	13	13	4	3	6	0	0	0
whale blubber	1 oz	248	28	0	–	–	–	–	0	0
More Than Gourmet										
Duck Rendered	1 tbsp (0.5 oz)	130	14	15	4	–	–	0	0	0
Spectrum										
Organic Shortening	1 tbsp (0.5 oz)	110	13	0	6	2	5	0	0	0
Shortening Butter Flavor Organic	1 tbsp (0.4 oz)	110	12	0	6	1	5	0	0	0

FAVA BEANS

FOOD	PORTION	CALS	TOTAL FAT	CHOL	SAT FAT	POLY FAT	MONO FAT	TRANS FAT	FIBER	SUGAR
canned	½ cup	91	tr	0	tr	tr	tr	–	–	–
fava fresh cooked	½ cup	94	tr	0	tr	tr	tr	–	5	2

FEIJOA

FOOD	PORTION	CALS	TOTAL FAT	CHOL	SAT FAT	POLY FAT	MONO FAT	TRANS FAT	FIBER	SUGAR
fresh	1 (1.75 oz)	25	tr	0	–	–	–	–	–	–
puree	1 cup	119	2	0	–	–	–	–	–	–

FENNEL

FOOD	PORTION	CALS	TOTAL FAT	CHOL	SAT FAT	POLY FAT	MONO FAT	TRANS FAT	FIBER	SUGAR
fresh bulb	1 (8.2 oz)	73	tr	0	–	–	–	0	7	–
fresh sliced	1 cup	27	tr	0	–	–	–	0	3	–
seed	1 tsp	7	tr	0	tr	tr	tr	0	1	–
stir fried	1 cup	85	6	0	1	2	3	–	3	5

FOOD	PORTION	CALS	TOTAL FAT	CHOL	SAT FAT	POLY FAT	MONO FAT	TRANS FAT	FIBER	SUGAR
FENUGREEK										
seed	1 tsp	12	tr	0	tr	–	–	0	1	–
FIBER										
apple fiber	0.5 oz	40	1	0	–	–	–	0	7	0
FIDDLEHEAD FERNS										
fresh	3.5 oz	34	tr	0	–	–	–	–	–	–
FIG JUICE										
Smart Juice										
Organic 100% Juice	8 oz	131	0	0	0	0	0	0	1	29
FIGS										
calimyrna	3 (5.4 oz)	120	0	0	0	0	0	0	4	11
canned in heavy syrup	½ cup	114	tr	0	tr	tr	tr	0	3	27
canned in light syrup	½ cup	87	tr	0	tr	tr	tr	0	2	20
canned water pack	½ cup	66	tr	0	tr	tr	tr	0	3	15
dried california	½ cup (3.5 oz)	200	1	0	–	–	–	0	17	–
dried cooked	½ cup	139	1	0	tr	tr	tr	0	5	30
dried small	1 (1.4 oz)	30	tr	0	tr	tr	tr	0	1	7
fresh large	1 (2.2 oz)	47	tr	0	tr	tr	tr	0	2	10
Fruit Bliss										
Soft Dried	2-3 (1.5 oz)	110	0	0	0	0	0	0	5	20
Jenny										
Kalamata Crown Natural Sundried	4 (1.5 oz)	120	0	0	0	0	0	0	5	21
FIREWEED										
leaves chopped	¼ cup (0.2 oz)	6	tr	0	–	–	–	0	1	–
plant	1 (0.8 oz)	23	1	0	–	–	–	0	2	–
FISH (*see also individual names,* FISH SUBSTITUTES, SUSHI)										
FROZEN										
breaded fillet	1 (2 oz)	155	7	64	2	2	3	–	–	–
sticks	1 stick (1 oz)	76	3	31	1	1	1	–	–	–
Dr. Praeger's										
Fish Sticks Potato Crusted	3 (2.3 oz)	120	6	25	1	–	–	0	tr	0
Gorton's										
Grilled Fillets Lemon Pepper	1 (3.8 oz)	90	3	60	1	1	1	0	0	0
TAKE-OUT										
amuk bok kum korean stir fried fish cake	1 cup (7.6 oz)	267	7	65	1	3	3	–	3	–

FOOD	PORTION	CALS	TOTAL FAT	CHOL	SAT FAT	POLY FAT	MONO FAT	TRANS FAT	FIBER	SUGAR
jamaican brown fish stew	1 serv	426	22	84	5	–	–	–	2	–
taramasalata	2 tbsp	124	14	10	–	–	–	–	–	–

FISH OIL

FOOD	PORTION	CALS	TOTAL FAT	CHOL	SAT FAT	POLY FAT	MONO FAT	TRANS FAT	FIBER	SUGAR
cod liver	1 tbsp	123	14	78	3	3	6	0	0	0
herring	1 tbsp	123	14	104	3	2	8	0	0	0
menhaden	1 tbsp	123	14	71	4	5	4	0	0	0
salmon	1 tbsp	123	14	66	3	5	4	0	0	0
sardine	1 tbsp	123	14	97	4	4	5	0	0	0

Nordic Naturals

FOOD	PORTION	CALS	TOTAL FAT	CHOL	SAT FAT	POLY FAT	MONO FAT	TRANS FAT	FIBER	SUGAR
Nordic Omega-3 Gummies Tangerine Treats	2 pieces	20	0	0	0	0	0	0	–	3

Spectrum

FOOD	PORTION	CALS	TOTAL FAT	CHOL	SAT FAT	POLY FAT	MONO FAT	TRANS FAT	FIBER	SUGAR
Cod Liver Oil w/ Lemon	1 tsp (4.5 g)	40	5	25	1	2	2	0	–	–

FISH SUBSTITUTES
Vegetarian Plus

FOOD	PORTION	CALS	TOTAL FAT	CHOL	SAT FAT	POLY FAT	MONO FAT	TRANS FAT	FIBER	SUGAR
Vegetarian Fish Fillets	1 (2 oz)	220	19	0	3	–	–	0	2	0

FLAXSEED
Spectrum

FOOD	PORTION	CALS	TOTAL FAT	CHOL	SAT FAT	POLY FAT	MONO FAT	TRANS FAT	FIBER	SUGAR
Ground Organic	2 tbsp (0.5 oz)	80	5	0	1	4	1	0	4	tr

FLOUNDER

FOOD	PORTION	CALS	TOTAL FAT	CHOL	SAT FAT	POLY FAT	MONO FAT	TRANS FAT	FIBER	SUGAR
fresh cooked	1 fillet (4.5 oz)	148	2	86	tr	1	tr	–	0	0
fresh cooked	3 oz	99	1	58	tr	tr	tr	–	0	0

Beacon Light

FOOD	PORTION	CALS	TOTAL FAT	CHOL	SAT FAT	POLY FAT	MONO FAT	TRANS FAT	FIBER	SUGAR
Fillets Wild Caught baked	3 oz	100	1	50	0	–	–	0	0	0

TAKE-OUT

FOOD	PORTION	CALS	TOTAL FAT	CHOL	SAT FAT	POLY FAT	MONO FAT	TRANS FAT	FIBER	SUGAR
breaded & fried	3.2 oz	211	11	31	3	6	2	–	–	–
stuffed w/ crab	1 piece (7.6 oz)	332	11	160	2	3	4	–	1	2

FLOUR

FOOD	PORTION	CALS	TOTAL FAT	CHOL	SAT FAT	POLY FAT	MONO FAT	TRANS FAT	FIBER	SUGAR
all-purpose enriched bleached	½ cup (2.2 oz)	228	1	0	tr	tr	tr	0	2	tr
all-purpose self-rising	½ cup (2.2 oz)	221	1	0	tr	tr	tr	0	2	tr
all-purpose unbleached	½ cup (2.2 oz)	228	1	0	tr	tr	tr	0	2	tr
arrowroot	½ cup (2.2 oz)	228	tr	0	tr	tr	tr	0	2	–
bread flour	½ cup (2.4 oz)	247	1	0	tr	tr	tr	0	2	tr
buckwheat whole groat	½ cup (2.1 oz)	201	2	0	tr	1	1	0	6	2
cake	½ cup (2.4 oz)	248	1	0	tr	tr	tr	0	1	tr

FOOD	PORTION	CALS	TOTAL FAT	CHOL	SAT FAT	POLY FAT	MONO FAT	TRANS FAT	FIBER	SUGAR
carob	1 tbsp (0.2 oz)	13	tr	0	tr	tr	tr	0	2	3
carob	½ cup (1.8 oz)	114	tr	0	tr	tr	tr	0	21	25
chickpea besan	½ cup (1.6 oz)	178	3	0	tr	1	1	0	5	5
peanut lowfat	½ cup (1.1 oz)	128	7	0	1	2	3	0	5	–
potato	½ cup (2.8 oz)	286	tr	0	tr	tr	tr	0	5	3
rice brown	½ cup (2.8 oz)	287	2	0	tr	1	1	0	4	1
rice white	½ cup (2.8 oz)	289	1	0	tr	tr	tr	0	2	tr
rye dark	½ cup (2.2 oz)	207	2	0	tr	1	tr	0	15	1
rye light	½ cup (1.8 oz)	187	1	0	tr	tr	tr	0	7	1
soy lowfat	½ cup (1.5 oz)	165	4	0	1	2	1	0	7	5
triticale whole grain	½ cup (2.3 oz)	220	1	0	tr	1	tr	0	10	–
whole wheat	½ cup (2.1 oz)	203	1	0	tr	tr	tr	0	7	tr
JK Gourmet										
Almond	¼ cup (1 oz)	170	14	0	1	–	–	0	3	1
Jovial										
Organic Einkorn	⅓ cup (1 oz)	100	1	0	0	–	–	0	2	0
King Arthur										
Whole Wheat Unbleached	¼ cup (1.1 oz)	110	1	0	0	–	–	0	4	0
Lundberg										
Brown Rice	¼ cup (1.1 oz)	110	2	0	0	–	–	0	2	1
Manischewitz										
Potato Starch	1 tbsp (0.4 oz)	30	0	0	0	0	0	0	0	0
Pillsbury										
All Purpose	¼ cup (1.1 oz)	110	0	0	0	0	0	0	tr	tr
Bread Flour	¼ cup (1.1 oz)	110	0	0	0	0	0	0	tr	0
Self Rising	¼ cup (1.1. oz)	100	0	0	0	0	0	0	tr	0
Whole Wheat	¼ cup (1.1 oz)	110	1	0	0	–	–	0	3	tr
Simpli										
Whole Oat Gluten Free	¼ cup (1.1 oz)	110	3	0	0	–	–	0	3	0

FOOD COLORS

FOOD	PORTION	CALS	TOTAL FAT	CHOL	SAT FAT	POLY FAT	MONO FAT	TRANS FAT	FIBER	SUGAR
blue	1 tsp	0	0	0	0	0	0	0	0	0
orange	1 tsp	0	0	0	0	0	0	0	0	0
red	1 tsp	<1	0	0	0	0	0	0	0	0
yellow	1 tsp	tr	0	0	0	0	0	0	0	0

FRENCH BEANS

FOOD	PORTION	CALS	TOTAL FAT	CHOL	SAT FAT	POLY FAT	MONO FAT	TRANS FAT	FIBER	SUGAR
dried cooked	1 cup	228	1	0	tr	1	tr	–	17	–

FRENCH FRIES (see POTATO)

FRENCH TOAST

FOOD	PORTION	CALS	TOTAL FAT	CHOL	SAT FAT	POLY FAT	MONO FAT	TRANS FAT	FIBER	SUGAR
french toast frzn	1 slice (2 oz)	126	4	48	1	1	1	–	1	–

FOOD	PORTION	CALS	TOTAL FAT	CHOL	SAT FAT	POLY FAT	MONO FAT	TRANS FAT	FIBER	SUGAR
Aunt Jemima										
Cinnamon Sticks	4 (3.1 oz)	270	10	0	3	–	–	0	1	11
Homestyle	2 slices (4.1 oz)	220	5	75	1	–	–	0	1	7
Whole Grain	2 slices (4 oz)	210	5	75	2	–	–	0	3	8
Farm Rich										
Toast Sticks	4 (3.7 oz)	270	11	0	2	–	–	0	1	7
Toast Sticks Cinnamon Sprinkle	4 (3.7 oz)	290	10	0	2	–	–	0	2	15
IHOP At Home										
Breakfast Sandwich Canadian Bacon	1 (4.3 oz)	200	8	105	3	–	–	0	tr	5
Breakfast Sandwich Maple Sausage	1 (4.8 oz)	290	16	125	6	–	–	0	tr	5
Stuffed Pastries Apple Cinnamon	1 (2.1 oz)	180	6	5	1	–	–	0	tr	10
Stuffed Pastries Blueberry	1 (2.1 oz)	200	9	5	2	–	–	0	1	6
Stuffed Pastries Cream Cheese	1 (2.1 oz)	210	9	15	4	–	–	0	tr	10
Van's										
Cinnamon Wheat Free	2 slices (2.8 oz)	190	4	0	0	–	–	0	1	12
Sticks	2 (2.8 oz)	190	5	0	0	–	–	0	1	9
Weight Watchers										
Smart Ones French Toast w/ Turkey Sausage	1 pkg (4.4 oz)	280	8	120	3	2	1	0	2	18
TAKE-OUT										
home prepared w/ 2% milk	1 slice (2.3 oz)	149	7	75	2	2	3	–	–	–
w/ butter & syrup	2 slices (8.1 oz)	520	14	58	6	2	5	–	–	–

FROG LEGS
TAKE-OUT

FOOD	PORTION	CALS	TOTAL FAT	CHOL	SAT FAT	POLY FAT	MONO FAT	TRANS FAT	FIBER	SUGAR
as prep w/ seasoned flour & fried	1 (0.8 oz)	70	5	12	–	–	–	–	–	–

FRUCTOSE

FOOD	PORTION	CALS	TOTAL FAT	CHOL	SAT FAT	POLY FAT	MONO FAT	TRANS FAT	FIBER	SUGAR
liquid	1 oz	84	0	0	0	0	0	0	0	23
powder	¼ cup (1.7 oz)	180	0	0	0	0	0	0	0	45
powder	1 tsp (4.2 g)	15	0	0	0	0	0	0	0	4

FOOD	PORTION	CALS	TOTAL FAT	CHOL	SAT FAT	POLY FAT	MONO FAT	TRANS FAT	FIBER	SUGAR
FRUIT AND NUT BARS *(see also* CEREAL BARS, ENERGY BARS*)*										
Cavewoman Bars										
Baklava	1 (2 oz)	190	9	0	1	–	–	0	5	26
PB&J	1 (2 oz)	210	7	0	1	–	–	0	4	27
Pineapple Upside Down Cake Raw	1 (2 oz)	190	6	0	0	–	–	0	4	31
Goodnessknows										
Nutty Apple	1 (1.2 oz)	150	7	0	2	3	1	0	2	12
Very Cranberry	1 (1.2 oz)	150	7	0	2	3	1	0	2	11
Kind										
Apple Cinnamon Nut	1 (1.4 oz)	180	10	0	1	–	–	0	5	12
Blueberry Vanilla & Cashew	1 (1.4 oz)	180	9	0	2	–	–	0	2	11
Orchard Bar										
Blueberry Pomegranate & Almond	1 (1.6 oz)	180	6	0	0	–	–	0	2	19
Pineapple Coconut & Macadamia	1 (1.6 oz)	190	7	0	2	–	–	0	2	18
Strawberry Raspberry & Walnut	1 (1.6 oz)	190	7	0	1	–	–	0	2	18
Pure										
Organic Apple Cinnamon	1 (1.7 oz)	190	8	0	1	–	–	0	3	20
Organic Chocolate Almond	1 (1.7 oz)	190	8	0	1	–	–	0	5	17
Organic Cranberry Orange	1 (1.7 oz)	190	8	0	1	–	–	0	3	19
Organic Peanut Raisin Crunch	1 (1.5 oz)	200	12	0	2	–	–	0	5	9
Organic Superfruit Nutty Crunch	1 (1.5 oz)	190	11	0	2	–	–	0	5	12
Organic Wild Blueberry	1 (1.7 oz)	190	8	0	1	–	–	0	3	19
FRUIT AND VEGETABLE DRINKS										
It Tastes RAAW										
Passion Fruit Wheatgrass	8 oz	100	0	0	0	0	0	0	1	21
Pineapple Cucumber	8 oz	105	0	0	0	0	0	0	1	24
Strawberry Purple Carrot	8 oz	100	0	0	0	0	0	0	6	23
Naked										
Berry Veggie	8 oz	130	1	0	0	–	–	0	5	18
Green Machine	8 oz	140	0	0	0	0	0	0	0	28
Orange Carrot	8 oz	120	0	0	0	0	0	0	1	26

FOOD	PORTION	CALS	TOTAL FAT	CHOL	SAT FAT	POLY FAT	MONO FAT	TRANS FAT	FIBER	SUGAR
Smart Juice										
Organic 100% Juice Pomegranate Purple Carrot	8 oz	137	0	0	0	0	0	0	0	33
Tropicana										
Farmstand 100% Juice Peach Mango	8 oz	120	0	0	0	0	0	0	–	28

FRUIT DRINKS (see also individual names, SMOOTHIES, VEGETABLE JUICE, YOGURT DRINKS)
FROZEN

FOOD	PORTION	CALS	TOTAL FAT	CHOL	SAT FAT	POLY FAT	MONO FAT	TRANS FAT	FIBER	SUGAR
Dole										
Orange Peach Mango not prep	¼ cup	120	0	0	0	0	0	0	0	23

MIX

FOOD	PORTION	CALS	TOTAL FAT	CHOL	SAT FAT	POLY FAT	MONO FAT	TRANS FAT	FIBER	SUGAR
Crystal Light										
Fusion Fruit Punch as prep	8 oz	5	0	0	0	0	0	0	0	0
Immunity Cherry Pomegranate as prep	8 oz	5	0	0	0	0	0	0	–	0
Strawberry Orange Banana as prep	8 oz	5	0	0	0	0	0	0	0	0

READY-TO-DRINK

FOOD	PORTION	CALS	TOTAL FAT	CHOL	SAT FAT	POLY FAT	MONO FAT	TRANS FAT	FIBER	SUGAR
fruit punch	6 oz	87	tr	0	0	0	0	–	–	–
Apple & Eve										
Mango Passion 100% Juice	8 oz	120	0	0	0	0	0	0	–	26
Capri Sun										
Super V All Flavors	1 pkg (6 oz)	70	0	0	0	0	0	0	3	14
Dole										
Orange Peach Mango	8 oz	120	0	0	0	0	0	0	–	27
Paradise Blend	8 oz	120	0	0	0	0	0	0	0	24
Pina Colada	8 oz	120	0	0	0	0	0	0	0	24
Strawberry Kiwi	8 oz	120	0	0	0	0	0	0	0	26
Fave										
Orange Tangerine Pineapple	8 oz	60	1	0	0	–	–	0	0	12
Strawberry Banana Kiwi	8 oz	60	0	0	0	–	0	0	0	12
Fizzy Lizzy										
Raspberry Lemon	1 bottle (12 oz)	120	0	0	0	0	0	0	–	28
Genesis Today										
Boost Pomegranate Berry 100% Juice	8 oz	130	0	0	0	0	0	0	1	27
Honest Ade										
Superfruit Punch	8 oz	48	0	0	0	0	0	0	–	12

FOOD	PORTION	CALS	TOTAL FAT	CHOL	SAT FAT	POLY FAT	MONO FAT	TRANS FAT	FIBER	SUGAR
Minute Maid										
Citrus Punch	8 oz	90	0	0	0	0	0	0	–	25
Enhanced Mango Tropical	1 bottle	120	0	0	0	0	0	0	4	25
Fruit Punch	8 oz	90	0	0	0	0	0	0	–	25
Pomegranate Blueberry 100% Juice	8 oz	120	1	0	–	–	–	0	–	29
Tropical Punch	8 oz	90	0	0	0	0	0	0	–	25
Naked										
Peach Guava Reduced Calorie 100% Juice	8 oz	100	0	0	0	0	0	0	0	20
Pomegranate Acai	8 oz	160	1	0	0	–	–	0	0	31
Power-C Machine	8 oz	120	0	0	0	0	0	0	0	23
Protein Zone	8 oz	220	2	30	1	–	–	0	0	28
Protein Zone Double Berry	8 oz	220	2	10	1	–	–	0	0	29
Red Machine 100% Juice	8 oz	170	5	0	1	3	1	0	3	25
Ocean Spray										
Blueberry Pomegranate	8 oz	120	0	0	0	0	0	0	–	30
Ruby Tangerine	8 oz	110	0	0	0	0	0	0	–	28
White Cran-Peach	8 oz	110	0	0	0	0	0	0	–	27
Old Orchard										
100% Juice Acai Pomegranate	8 oz	130	0	0	0	0	0	0	–	29
100% Juice Berry Blend	8 oz	130	0	0	0	0	0	0	–	29
100% Juice Cherry Pomegranate	8 oz	130	0	0	0	0	0	0	–	29
Cranberry Grape Cocktail	8 oz	31	0	0	0	0	0	0	–	6
Healthy Balance Apple Kiwi Strawberry Cocktail	8 oz	31	0	0	0	0	0	0	–	6
Pomegranate Blueberry Acai Cocktail	8 oz	31	0	0	0	0	0	0	–	6
Very Cherre 100% Juice Tart Cherry Cranberry	8 oz	130	0	0	0	0	0	0	–	21
R.W. Knudsen										
Razzleberry 100% Juice	8 oz	120	0	0	0	0	0	0	0	27
Sensible Sippers Organic Fruit Punch	1 box (4.23 oz)	30	0	0	0	0	0	0	–	7
TreeTop										
Apple Berry	8 oz	120	0	0	0	0	0	0	–	28
Apple Cranberry 100% Juice	8 oz	120	0	0	0	0	0	0	–	23

FOOD	PORTION	CALS	TOTAL FAT	CHOL	SAT FAT	POLY FAT	MONO FAT	TRANS FAT	FIBER	SUGAR
Apple Fruit Punch 100% Juice	8 oz	120	0	0	0	0	0	0	–	25
Apple Grape 100% Juice	8 oz	130	0	0	0	0	0	0	–	26
Apple Pear 100% Juice	1 box (3.5 oz)	100	0	0	0	0	0	0	–	21
Kiwi Strawberry 100% Juice	1 bottle (10 oz)	130	0	0	0	0	0	0	–	30
Ochango 100% Juice	1 bottle (10 oz)	170	0	0	0	0	0	0	–	33
Orange Passionfruit 100% Juice	8 oz	110	0	0	0	0	0	0	–	24
Pineapple Orange 100% Juice	8 oz	120	0	0	0	0	0	0	–	23
V8										
V-Fusion Black Cherry Pomegranate	1 can (8.4 oz)	60	0	0	0	0	0	0	0	12
V-Fusion Tangerine Raspberry	1 can (8.4 oz)	60	0	0	0	0	0	0	0	13
Welch's										
Sparkling Mango Passion Fruit	8 oz	130	0	0	0	0	0	0	–	31

FRUIT MIXED (see also individual names, FRUIT AND NUT BARS)
CANNED

FOOD	PORTION	CALS	TOTAL FAT	CHOL	SAT FAT	POLY FAT	MONO FAT	TRANS FAT	FIBER	SUGAR
fruit cocktail in heavy syrup	½ cup	93	tr	0	tr	tr	tr	–	–	–
fruit cocktail juice pack	½ cup	56	tr	0	tr	tr	tr	–	–	–
fruit cocktail water pack	½ cup	40	tr	0	tr	tr	tr	–	–	–
fruit salad in heavy syrup	½ cup	94	tr	0	tr	tr	tr	–	–	–
fruit salad in light syrup	½ cup	73	tr	0	tr	tr	tr	–	–	–
fruit salad juice pack	½ cup	62	tr	0	tr	tr	tr	–	–	–
fruit salad water pack	½ cup	37	tr	0	tr	tr	tr	–	–	–
mixed fruit in heavy syrup	½ cup	92	tr	0	tr	tr	tr	–	–	–
tropical fruit salad in heavy syrup	½ cup	110	tr	0	–	–	–	–	–	–
Del Monte										
Citrus Salad	½ cup (4.4 oz)	50	0	0	0	0	0	0	1	8
Fruit Cocktail Lite	½ cup (4.4 oz)	60	0	0	0	0	0	0	1	14
Mixed Fruit Chunks In Mango Passion Fruit Juice	1 pkg (6 oz)	120	0	0	0	0	0	0	3	20
Snack Cups Cherry Mixed Fruit	1 pkg (4 oz)	70	0	0	0	0	0	0	–	15
Superfruit Peach Chunks Pomegranate & Orange Juice	1 pkg (6 oz)	100	0	0	0	0	0	0	3	12

FOOD	PORTION	CALS	TOTAL FAT	CHOL	SAT FAT	POLY FAT	MONO FAT	TRANS FAT	FIBER	SUGAR
Superfruit Pear Chunks In Acai & Blackberry Juice	1 pkg (6 oz)	120	0	0	0	0	0	0	3	24
Tropical Fruit	1 pkg (4 oz)	70	0	0	0	0	0	0	–	16
Tropical Fruit Salad In 100% Juice	½ cup (4.4 oz)	80	0	0	0	0	0	0	1	20
Dole										
Cherry Mixed Fruit In Fruit Juice	1 pkg (4 oz)	70	0	0	0	0	0	0	1	16
Tropical Fruit In Fruit Juice	1 pkg (4 oz)	60	0	0	0	0	0	0	1	14
DRIED										
mixed	11 oz pkg	712	1	0	tr	tr	1	–	–	–
Crunchies										
Freeze Dried Mixed Fruit	¼ cup (7 g)	25	0	0	0	0	0	0	1	4
Fruit Bliss										
Soft Dried Medley	¼ pkg (1.5 oz)	90	0	0	0	0	0	0	3	14
FROZEN										
mixed fruit sweetened	1 cup	245	tr	0	tr	tr	tr	–	–	–
REFRIGERATED										
Del Monte										
Fruit Naturals Mixed Berries	1 pkg (6 oz)	100	1	0	0	0	0	0	3	20

FRUIT SNACKS

FOOD	PORTION	CALS	TOTAL FAT	CHOL	SAT FAT	POLY FAT	MONO FAT	TRANS FAT	FIBER	SUGAR
fruit leather	1 bar (0.8 oz)	81	1	0	1	tr	tr	–	–	–
fruit leather pieces	1 pkg (0.9 oz)	92	2	0	tr	1	1	–	–	–
fruit leather pieces	1 oz	97	2	0	tr	1	1	–	–	–
fruit leather rolls	1 lg (0.7 oz)	73	1	0	tr	tr	tr	–	–	–
fruit leather rolls	1 sm (0.5 oz)	49	tr	0	tr	tr	tr	–	–	–
Annie's Homegrown										
Orchard Fruit Bites Grape	1 pkg (0.6 oz)	60	0	0	0	0	0	0	1	12
Orchard Fruit Bites Strawberry	1 pkg (0.6 oz)	60	0	0	0	0	0	0	1	12
Organic Bunny Fruit Snacks Lemonade	1 pkg (0.6 oz)	70	0	0	0	0	0	0	–	10
Organic Bunny Fruit Tropical Treat	1 pkg (0.8 oz)	70	0	0	0	0	0	0	–	10
Dole										
Real Fruit Bites Apple	1 pkg (0.7 oz)	80	2	0	2	–	–	0	0	11
Froose										
All Flavors	1 pkg (0.9 oz)	70	0	0	0	0	0	0	3	9

FOOD	PORTION	CALS	TOTAL FAT	CHOL	SAT FAT	POLY FAT	MONO FAT	TRANS FAT	FIBER	SUGAR
Funky Monkey										
Applemon	1 pkg (0.42 oz)	40	0	0	0	0	0	0	1	9
Bananamon	1 pkg (0.42 oz)	45	0	0	0	0	0	0	1	9
Carnaval Mix	1 pkg (0.42 oz)	45	0	0	0	0	0	0	1	9
Jivealime	1 pkg (0.42 oz)	45	0	0	0	0	0	0	1	8
MangoOJ	1 pkg (0.42 oz)	35	0	0	0	0	0	0	1	8
Pink Pineapple	1 pkg (0.42 oz)	45	0	0	0	0	0	0	1	9
Purple Funk	1 pkg (0.42 oz)	50	0	0	0	0	0	0	1	8
Juicefuls										
Berry Mania	1 pkg (0.9 oz)	80	0	0	0	0	0	0	–	11
Kaia Foods										
Fruit Leather Lime Ginger	1 (1 oz)	50	0	0	0	0	0	0	2	7
Fruit Leather Vanilla Pear	1 (1 oz)	60	0	0	0	0	0	0	3	9
Kettle Valley										
100% Fruit Bar All Flavors	1 (0.7 oz)	70	0	0	0	0	0	0	1	12
Fruit Twists All Flavors	1 (0.6 oz)	60	0	0	0	0	0	0	1	12
Mott's										
Medleys Assorted Fruit	1 pkg (0.8 oz)	80	0	0	0	0	0	0	–	12
Revolution Foods										
Organic Mashups Strawberry Banana	1 pkg (3.2 oz)	60	0	0	0	0	0	0	1	9
Sun-Rype										
Fruit Bar Mango Strawberry	1 (1.3 oz)	120	0	0	0	0	0	0	3	27
Fruit Bar Strawberry	1 (1.3 oz)	130	0	0	0	0	0	0	2	29
Tasty										
All Flavors	1 pkg (0.8 oz)	130	0	0	0	0	0	0	0	17
That's It										
Bar 1 Apple + 1 Pear	1 (1.2 oz)	100	0	0	0	0	0	0	3	24
Bar 1 Apple + 10 Cherries	1 (1.2 oz)	100	0	0	0	0	0	0	3	22
Bar 1 Apple + 3 Apricots	1 (1.2 oz)	100	0	0	0	0	0	0	3	23
The Good Bean										
The Fruit & No-Nut Bar Apricot Coconut	1 (1.4 oz)	130	5	0	2	–	–	0	5	12
The Fruit & No-Nut Bar Chocolate Berry	1 (1.4 oz)	140	5	0	1	–	–	0	5	11
The Fruit & No-Nut Bar Fruit & Seeds Trail Mix	1 (1.4 oz)	130	5	0	1	–	–	0	5	11
TreeTop										
Fruit Snacks All Natural	1 pkg (0.9 oz)	80	0	0	0	0	0	0	–	15

FOOD	PORTION	CALS	TOTAL FAT	CHOL	SAT FAT	POLY FAT	MONO FAT	TRANS FAT	FIBER	SUGAR
Welch's										
Mixed Fruit	1 pkg (0.9 oz)	80	0	0	0	0	0	0	0	11
Mixed Fruit Reduced Sugar	1 pkg (0.9 oz)	70	0	0	0	0	0	0	–	8
GARLIC										
clove	1	4	tr	0	tr	tr	0	–	tr	tr
fresh chopped	1 tbsp	18	tr	0	tr	tr	tr	–	tr	tr
powder	1 tsp	9	tr	0	tr	tr	tr	–	tr	1
Garlic It!										
Caramelized	1 tbsp (0.5 oz)	80	8	0	1	–	–	0	0	0
Dijon	1 tbsp (0.5 oz)	80	8	0	1	–	–	0	0	0
Savory Basil	1 tbsp (0.5 oz)	80	8	0	1	–	–	0	0	0
Thai Peanut	1 tbsp (0.5 oz)	90	9	0	1	–	–	0	0	0
Tomato Curry	1 tbsp (0.5 oz)	50	3	0	tr	–	–	0	tr	6
Jake & Amos										
Sweet Pickled Garlic	1 oz	36	0	0	0	0	0	0	0	7
Rinaldo's Organic										
Gold Nuggets	1 tsp	10	1	0	0	–	–	0	0	0
Victoria										
Chopped In Water	1 tsp (5 g)	0	0	0	0	0	0	0	0	0
GEFILTE FISH										
sweet	1 piece (1.5 oz)	35	1	12	tr	tr	tr	–	–	–
Manischewitz										
In Jelly	1 (2.2 oz)	70	2	25	0	–	–	0	0	0
Jellied Reduced Sodium	1 (2.2 oz)	70	2	25	0	–	–	0	0	0
Pieces In Liquid	7 (2 oz)	45	2	15	0	–	–	0	0	0
GELATIN										
MIX										
Jell-O										
Apricot as prep	1 serv	80	0	0	0	0	0	0	–	19
Cherry as prep	1 serv	80	0	0	0	0	0	0	–	19
Lime as prep	1 serv	80	0	0	0	0	0	0	–	19
Margarita as prep	1 serv	80	0	0	0	0	0	0	–	19
Orange as prep	1 serv	80	0	0	0	0	0	0	–	19
Orange Sugar Free as prep	1 serv	10	0	0	0	0	0	0	0	0
Peach Sugar Free as prep	1 serv	10	0	0	0	0	0	0	0	0
Watermelon as prep	1 serv	80	0	0	0	0	0	0	0	19

FOOD	PORTION	CALS	TOTAL FAT	CHOL	SAT FAT	POLY FAT	MONO FAT	TRANS FAT	FIBER	SUGAR
READY-TO-EAT										
Del Monte										
Mixed Fruit In Cherry Gel	1 pkg (4.5 oz)	90	0	0	0	0	0	0	0	20
Dole										
Mixed Fruit In Cherry Gel Sugar Free	1 pkg (4.3 oz)	60	0	0	0	0	0	0	1	5
Mixed Fruit In Peach Gel	1 pkg (4.3 oz)	100	0	0	0	0	0	0	1	22
Pineapple In Lime Gel	1 pkg (4.3 oz)	90	0	0	0	0	0	0	1	22
Jell-O										
Cherry & Black Cherry	1 pkg (3.2 oz)	10	0	0	0	0	0	0	0	0
Raspberry & Orange Sugar Free	1 pkg (3.2 oz)	10	0	0	0	0	0	0	0	0
Strawberry	1 pkg (3.5 oz)	70	0	0	0	0	0	0	–	17
Strawberry Sugar Free	1 pkg (3.2 oz)	10	0	0	0	0	0	0	0	0
Snack Pack										
Gels Cherry No Sugar Added	1 pkg (3.5 oz)	10	0	0	0	0	0	0	tr	0
Gels Strawberry	1 pkg (3.5 oz)	100	0	0	0	0	0	0	0	22
GIBLETS										
capon simmered	1 cup (5 oz)	238	8	629	3	2	2	–	0	0
chicken fried	1 cup (5 oz)	402	20	647	6	5	6	–	0	–
chicken simmered	1 cup (5 oz)	289	17	419	6	2	7	0	0	0
turkey simmered	1 (3.3 oz)	164	6	495	2	1	1	tr	0	0
GINGER										
ground	1 tsp	6	tr	0	tr	tr	tr	–	tr	tr
pickled	1 tbsp (0.3 oz)	9	0	0	0	0	0	0	0	–
preserved	1.5 oz	34	0	0	0	0	0	–	1	7
root fresh	5 slices	9	tr	0	tr	tr	tr	–	tr	tr
root fresh sliced	¼ cup	19	tr	0	tr	tr	tr	–	1	tr
GINKGO NUTS										
canned	1 oz	32	tr	0	tr	tr	tr	–	–	–
dried	1 oz	99	tr	0	tr	tr	tr	–	–	–
raw	1 oz	52	tr	0	tr	tr	tr	–	–	–
GIZZARDS										
chicken simmered	1 cup (5 oz)	212	4	536	1	1	1	tr	0	0
turkey simmered	1 (3 oz)	103	3	171	1	tr	1	0	0	0
Foster Farms										
Chicken Gizzards & Hearts fresh	4 oz	150	8	150	–	–	–	0	0	0

FOOD	PORTION	CALS	TOTAL FAT	CHOL	SAT FAT	POLY FAT	MONO FAT	TRANS FAT	FIBER	SUGAR
GNOCCHI										
spinach	12 (4 oz)	220	1	0	0	–	–	0	5	2
Racconto										
Potato Whole Wheat as prep w/o salt	1 cup (5.8 oz)	248	0	0	0	0	0	0	8	tr
Solterra										
Original Potato	¼ pkg (3 oz)	100	0	0	0	0	0	0	2	1
Spinach	¼ pkg (3 oz)	100	0	0	0	0	0	0	2	1
GOAT										
diced boiled	1 cup (4.7 oz)	190	4	100	1	tr	2	–	0	0
fried boneless	3 oz	130	4	62	1	1	1	–	0	0
ribs cooked	3 (4.8 oz)	196	4	104	1	tr	2	–	0	0
roasted boneless	3 oz	122	3	64	1	tr	1	–	0	0
TAKE-OUT										
stew puerto rican style	1 cup (6.2 oz)	460	31	112	6	3	20	–	1	2
GOJI BERRIES										
dried	1 oz	106	3	0	–	–	–	0	2	–
GOOSE										
boneless roasted	2.7 oz	231	17	69	5	2	8	–	0	0
meat only raw	6.5 oz	298	13	155	5	2	3	–	0	0
w/ skin & bone roasted	1 serv (6.6 oz)	573	41	171	13	5	19	–	0	0
wild boneless roasted diced	1 cup (4.9 oz)	426	31	127	10	4	14	–	0	0
GOOSEBERRIES										
canned in light syrup	1 cup	184	1	0	tr	tr	tr	0	6	–
fresh	1 cup (5.3 oz)	66	1	0	tr	tr	tr	0	6	–
GRAINS										
Village Harvest										
Wheatberry & Barley	½ cup	260	3	0	1	–	–	0	10	1
Whole Grain Creations w/ Cranberries & Almonds	¾ cup (4.3 oz)	220	4	0	1	–	–	0	6	6
Whole Grain Medley Farro & Red Rice	1 cup (5 oz)	290	3	0	0	–	–	0	4	0
GRAPE JUICE										
bottled unsweetened	1 cup	154	tr	0	tr	tr	tr	0	tr	38
Fizzy Lizzy										
Yakima Grape	1 bottle (12 oz)	120	0	0	0	0	0	0	–	30

FOOD	PORTION	CALS	TOTAL FAT	CHOL	SAT FAT	POLY FAT	MONO FAT	TRANS FAT	FIBER	SUGAR
Kedem										
Organic	8 oz	140	0	0	0	0	0	0	–	33
Manischewitz										
Concord Purple	8 oz	160	0	0	0	0	0	0	–	39
Minute Maid										
100% Juice Grape Blend	8 oz	150	0	0	0	0	0	0	–	34
Old Orchard										
100% Juice	8 oz	130	0	0	0	0	0	0	–	29
100% Juice White	8 oz	130	0	0	0	0	0	0	–	29
R.W. Knudsen										
100% Juice	8 oz	130	0	0	0	0	0	0	tr	31
TreeTop										
Vineyard Grape 100% Juice	1 bottle (10 oz)	160	0	0	0	0	0	0	–	33
Welch's										
100% White	8 oz	160	0	0	0	0	0	0	–	38
Concord Grape Light	8 oz	45	0	0	0	0	0	0	–	11
Fruit Fizz Concord Grape Blast	1 can (8.4 oz)	70	0	0	0	0	0	0	–	18
Healthy Start 100% Juice	8 oz	140	0	0	0	0	0	0	–	36
White Light Juice Beverage	8 oz	45	0	0	0	0	0	0	–	11
GRAPE LEAVES										
canned	1 (4 g)	3	tr	0	tr	tr	tr	0	–	–
fresh raw	1 (3 g)	3	tr	0	tr	tr	tr	0	tr	tr
Galil										
Stuffed	5 (4.2 oz)	200	11	0	1	–	–	0	3	2
TAKE-OUT										
dolmas w/ beef & rice	1 (0.7 oz)	50	4	5	1	tr	2	0	1	1
dolmas w/ lamb & rice	1 (0.7 oz)	56	4	5	1	1	3	0	1	1
dolmas w/ rice	1 (2 oz)	92	6	0	1	1	5	0	2	2
GRAPEFRUIT										
CANNED										
sections juice pack	½ cup (4.4 oz)	46	tr	0	tr	tr	tr	0	1	11
sections light syrup	½ cup (4.5 oz)	76	tr	0	tr	tr	tr	0	1	19
sections water pack	½ cup (4.3 oz)	44	tr	0	tr	tr	tr	0	1	11
Del Monte										
Red In Light Syrup	½ cup (4.4 oz)	90	0	0	0	0	0	0	1	17
FRESH										
pink or red	½ (4.6 oz)	52	tr	0	tr	tr	tr	0	2	8
sections pink or red	1 cup (8.1 oz)	97	tr	0	tr	tr	tr	0	4	16

FOOD	PORTION	CALS	TOTAL FAT	CHOL	SAT FAT	POLY FAT	MONO FAT	TRANS FAT	FIBER	S
sections white	1 cup (8.1 oz)	76	tr	0	tr	tr	tr	0	3	1
white	½ (4.1 oz)	39	tr	0	tr	tr	tr	0	1	9
Ocean Spray										
Sweet Ruby	½ med (5.4 oz)	60	0	0	0	0	0	0	6	1C
Sunkist										
Fresh	½ med (5.4 oz)	60	0	0	0	0	0	0	2	11
GRAPEFRUIT JUICE										
canned sweetened	1 cup (8.8 oz)	115	tr	0	tr	tr	tr	0	tr	28
canned unsweetened	1 cup (8.7 oz)	94	tr	0	tr	tr	tr	0	tr	22
pink fresh	1 cup (8.7 oz)	96	tr	0	tr	tr	tr	0	–	–
white fresh	1 cup (8.7 oz)	96	tr	0	tr	tr	tr	0	tr	22
Apple & Eve										
Ruby Red	8 oz	130	0	0	0	0	0	0	–	32
Fizzy Lizzy										
Grapefruit	1 bottle (12 oz)	100	0	0	0	0	0	0	–	25
Minute Maid										
100% Juice + Calcium frzn not prep	2 oz	100	0	0	0	0	0	0	–	2C
Ruby Red	8 oz	130	0	0	0	0	0	0	–	32
Ocean Spray										
100% Juice White	8 oz	90	0	0	0	0	0	0	–	17
Old Orchard										
Ruby Red Cocktail	8 oz	31	0	0	0	0	0	0	–	6
GRAPES										
muscadine	10–12 (3.5 oz)	76	0	0	0	0	0	0	3	–
scuppernongs	10–12 (3.5 oz)	68	0	0	0	0	0	0	3	–
seedless red or green	1 cup	110	tr	0	tr	tr	tr	0	1	24
seedless red or green	20	69	tr	0	tr	tr	tr	0	1	15
thompson seedless in heavy syrup	½ cup	93	tr	0	tr	tr	tr	0	1	24
thompson seedless water pack	½ cup	49	tr	0	tr	tr	tr	0	1	12
with seeds red or green	1 cup	106	tr	0	tr	tr	tr	0	1	24
with seeds red or green	20	80	tr	0	tr	tr	tr	0	1	18
Crunch Pak										
Sweet Seedless	⅓ pkg	40	0	0	0	0	0	0	tr	9
Dole										
Fresh	26 (4.4 oz)	90	0	0	0	0	0	0	1	20

FOOD	PORTION	CALS	TOTAL FAT	CHOL	SAT FAT	POLY FAT	MONO FAT	TRANS FAT	FIBER	SUGAR
Sunkist										
Fresh	1 cup (5.3 oz)	110	0	0	0	0	0	0	1	23
GRAVY										
CANNED										
beef	1 can (10 oz)	155	7	9	3	tr	3	–	–	–
beef	1 cup	124	6	7	3	tr	2	–	–	–
chicken	1 cup	189	14	5	3	4	6	–	–	–
mushroom	1 cup	120	6	0	1	2	3	–	–	–
turkey	1 cup	122	5	5	1	1	2	–	–	–
Campbell's										
Beef	¼ cup (2 oz)	25	1	<5	1	–	–	0	0	tr
Mushroom	¼ cup (2.1 oz)	20	1	<5	–	–	–	0	0	1
Heinz										
HomeStyle Classic Chicken	¼ cup (2 oz)	15	0	0	0	0	0	0	0	0
HomeStyle Rich Mushroom	¼ cup (2.1 oz)	20	1	0	0	–	–	0	0	0
HomeStyle Savory Beef	¼ cup (2 oz)	25	1	0	1	–	–	0	0	0
Roasted Turkey Fat Free	¼ cup (2.1 oz)	20	0	0	0	0	0	0	0	0
Manischewitz										
Beef Savory	¼ cup (2.1 oz)	20	1	0	0	–	–	0	0	0
Chicken Reduced Sodium	¼ cup (2.1 oz)	20	1	0	0	–	–	0	0	0
Chicken Classic	¼ cup (2.1 oz)	20	1	0	0	–	–	0	0	0
Roasted Turkey	¼ cup (2.1 oz)	25	1	0	0	–	–	0	0	0
MIX										
au jus as prep w/ water	1 cup	32	1	1	1	tr	1	–	–	–
brown as prep w/ water	1 cup	75	2	2	1	tr	1	–	–	–
chicken as prep	1 cup	83	2	3	1	tr	1	–	–	–
mushroom as prep	1 cup	70	1	1	1	tr	tr	–	–	–
onion as prep w/ water	1 cup	77	1	tr	tr	tr	tr	–	–	–
pork as prep	1 cup	76	2	3	1	tr	1	–	–	–
turkey as prep	1 cup	87	2	3	1	tr	1	–	–	–
Loney's										
Brown as prep	¼ cup (2.1 oz)	15	0	0	0	0	0	0	0	0
Turkey as prep	¼ cup (2.1 oz)	20	0	0	0	0	0	0	0	0
TAKE-OUT										
au jus	1 cup	62	6	6	2	1	3	–	tr	tr
giblet gravy	¼ cup	45	3	23	1	1	1	0	tr	tr
GREAT NORTHERN BEANS										
canned	1 cup	299	1	0	tr	tr	tr	–	13	–
dried cooked	1 cup	209	1	0	tr	tr	tr	–	12	–

FOOD	PORTION	CALS	TOTAL FAT	CHOL	SAT FAT	POLY FAT	MONO FAT	TRANS FAT	FIBER	SUG
GREEN BEANS										
CANNED										
drained	1 cup	27	tr	0	tr	tr	tr	–	3	1
Butter Kernel										
Cut	½ cup (4.2 oz)	20	0	0	0	0	0	0	2	2
Cut No Salt Added	½ cup (4.2 oz)	20	0	0	0	0	0	0	2	2
Del Monte										
Cut	½ cup (4.2 oz)	20	0	0	0	0	0	0	2	1
Cut No Salt Added	½ cup (4.2 oz)	20	0	0	0	0	0	0	2	2
FRESH										
cooked w/o salt	1 cup	44	tr	0	tr	tr	tr	–	4	2
raw	1 cup	34	tr	0	tr	tr	tr	0	4	2
raw whole beans	10	17	tr	0	tr	tr	tr	–	2	1
Ready Pac										
Fast 'N Fresh as prep	1 cup (3 oz)	30	0	0	0	0	0	0	3	1
FROZEN										
cooked	1 cup	38	tr	0	tr	tr	tr	0	4	2
Lisa's Organics										
Whole In Garlic Oil Sauce	½ pkg (4 oz)	60	2	0	0	–	–	0	3	4
TAKE-OUT										
casserole w/ mushroom sauce	1 cup	108	6	2	2	3	1	–	3	3
pickled	½ cup	19	tr	0	tr	tr	tr	–	2	1
GROUNDCHERRIES										
fresh	½ cup	37	tr	0	–	–	–	–	–	–
GROUPER										
cooked	1 fillet (7.1 oz)	238	3	95	1	1	1	–	0	0
cooked	3 oz	100	1	40	tr	tr	tr	–	0	0
raw	3 oz	78	1	31	tr	tr	tr	–	0	0
GUAVA										
fresh	1 (1.9 oz)	37	1	0	tr	tr	tr	–	3	5
fresh cut up	1 cup (5.8 oz)	112	2	0	tr	1	tr	–	9	15
fresh strawberry	1 (6 g)	4	tr	0	tr	tr	tr	–	tr	–
fresh strawberry cut up	1 cup (8.6 oz)	168	1	0	tr	1	tr	–	13	–
guava paste	1 piece (1.1 oz)	90	tr	0	tr	tr	tr	–	tr	23
GUINEA HEN										
boneless w/o skin raw	½ hen (9.3 oz)	290	7	166	2	2	2	–	0	0
w/ skin raw	½ hen (12 oz)	545	22	255	6	5	8	–	0	0

FOOD	PORTION	CALS	TOTAL FAT	CHOL	SAT FAT	POLY FAT	MONO FAT	TRANS FAT	FIBER	SUGAR
HADDOCK										
fresh broiled	4 oz	127	1	84	tr	tr	tr	0	0	0
roe raw	1 oz	37	tr	103	–	–	–	–	–	–
smoked	1 oz	33	tr	22	tr	tr	tr	0	0	0
TAKE-OUT										
breaded & fried	4 oz	229	10	88	2	3	4	0	1	1
HAGGIS										
scottish haggis	1 serv (6.4 oz)	473	32	77	15	3	12	0	5	3
HALIBUT										
atlantic & pacific cooked	½ fillet (5.6 oz)	223	5	65	1	1	2	–	0	0
atlantic & pacific cooked	3 oz	119	2	35	tr	1	1	–	0	0
atlantic & pacific raw	3 oz	93	2	27	tr	1	1	–	0	0
greenland baked	5.6 oz	380	28	94	5	3	17	–	0	0
greenland baked	3 oz	203	15	50	2	1	9	–	0	0
HAM										
boneless extra lean roasted	3 oz	123	5	45	2	tr	2	0	0	0
boneless steak pan broiled	1 (4.8 oz)	170	7	62	2	1	3	tr	0	6
canned extra lean roasted	3 oz	116	4	26	1	tr	2	0	0	–
canned lean roasted	3 oz	142	7	35	2	1	3	0	0	–
center slice lean & fat roasted	3 oz	173	11	46	4	1	5	0	0	–
deviled	¼ cup	188	17	35	6	2	8	0	0	0
ham salad spread	2 tbsp	65	5	11	2	1	2	0	0	0
patty grilled	1 patty (2 oz)	205	19	43	7	2	9	0	0	0
prosciutto	4 slices (1.3 oz)	72	3	26	1	tr	1	0	0	0
sliced	3 slices (2.9 oz)	137	7	48	2	1	4	0	1	0
sliced extra lean	3 slices (2.2 oz)	69	2	30	1	tr	1	0	0	0
whole roasted	3 oz	207	14	53	5	2	7	0	0	0
Boar's Head										
Rosemary & Sundried Tomato	2 oz	70	3	10	1	0	2	0	0	0
Jones										
Steak Extra Lean	3 oz	100	4	50	1	–	–	0	–	–
TAKE-OUT										
croquette	1 (2.2 oz)	149	9	18	2	2	4	0	tr	2
salad	½ cup	287	23	237	5	1	6	–	tr	–

FOOD	PORTION	CALS	TOTAL FAT	CHOL	SAT FAT	POLY FAT	MONO FAT	TRANS FAT	FIBER
spam musubi	1 serv (6 oz)	253	6	14	2	1	3	–	1
thick slice fried	1 (2.2 oz)	140	9	33	3	2	4	0	0

HAMBURGER
Al Fresco
FOOD	PORTION	CALS	TOTAL FAT	CHOL	SAT FAT	POLY FAT	MONO FAT	TRANS FAT	FIBER
Chicken Burger Buffalo Style	1 (3.4 oz)	130	7	75	2	–	–	0	0
Chicken Burger Sweet Italian	1 (3.4 oz)	140	8	75	2	–	–	0	0

Farm Rich
FOOD	PORTION	CALS	TOTAL FAT	CHOL	SAT FAT	POLY FAT	MONO FAT	TRANS FAT	FIBER
Cheeseburgers Mini Bacon	2 (2.2 oz)	150	7	15	4	–	–	0	1

Foster Farms
FOOD	PORTION	CALS	TOTAL FAT	CHOL	SAT FAT	POLY FAT	MONO FAT	TRANS FAT	FIBER
Cheeseburgers Mini Chicken w/ BBQ Sauce	1 (1.3 oz)	90	4	18	2	–	–	0	0

TAKE-OUT
FOOD	PORTION	CALS	TOTAL FAT	CHOL	SAT FAT	POLY FAT	MONO FAT	TRANS FAT	FIBER
cheeseburger + condiments	1 reg (4.5 oz)	347	17	46	7	3	6	0	1
double hamburger + condiments	1 reg (5.8 oz)	384	19	66	7	1	8	0	2
single patty + condiments	1 reg (4 oz)	299	11	33	4	1	4	0	2

HAMBURGER SUBSTITUTES (see also MEAT SUBSTITUTES)
Asherah's Gourmet
FOOD	PORTION	CALS	TOTAL FAT	CHOL	SAT FAT	POLY FAT	MONO FAT	TRANS FAT	FIBER
Organic Vegan Burger Chipotle	1 (4 oz)	180	5	0	3	–	–	0	5
Organic Vegan Burgers Original	1 (4 oz)	180	5	0	3	–	–	0	5

Boca
FOOD	PORTION	CALS	TOTAL FAT	CHOL	SAT FAT	POLY FAT	MONO FAT	TRANS FAT	FIBER
All American Flame Grilled	1 (2.5 oz)	120	5	<5	2	2	1	0	4

Harmony Valley
FOOD	PORTION	CALS	TOTAL FAT	CHOL	SAT FAT	POLY FAT	MONO FAT	TRANS FAT	FIBER
Vegetarian Hamburger Mix as prep	1 (3 oz)	120	5	0	3	–	–	0	4

Quorn
FOOD	PORTION	CALS	TOTAL FAT	CHOL	SAT FAT	POLY FAT	MONO FAT	TRANS FAT	FIBER
Classic Burger	1 (2.1 oz)	90	3	5	1	1	2	0	3
Vegan Burger	1 (2.1 oz)	100	4	0	1	–	–	0	2

Tandoor Chef
FOOD	PORTION	CALS	TOTAL FAT	CHOL	SAT FAT	POLY FAT	MONO FAT	TRANS FAT	FIBER
Vegetable Masala Burger	1 (2.5 oz)	120	8	0	1	–	–	0	1

HAZELNUTS
FOOD	PORTION	CALS	TOTAL FAT	CHOL	SAT FAT	POLY FAT	MONO FAT	TRANS FAT	FIBER
chocolate hazelnut spread	2 tbsp (1.3 oz)	200	11	0	11	0	0	–	2	2
chopped	¼ cup (1 oz)	181	17	0	1	2	13	0	3
ground	¼ cup (0.7 oz)	118	11	0	1	1	9	0	1
whole	¼ cup (1.2 oz)	212	21	0	2	3	15	0	3
whole nuts	21 (1 oz)	178	17	0	1	2	13	0	3

FOOD	PORTION	CALS	TOTAL FAT	CHOL	SAT FAT	POLY FAT	MONO FAT	TRANS FAT	FIBER	SUGAR
Kettle Brand										
Butter Unsalted	2 tbsp (1 oz)	180	17	0	1	2	14	0	3	1
HEART										
beef simmered	3 oz	140	4	180	1	1	1	0	0	0
chicken cooked	1 (3 g)	5	tr	6	tr	tr	tr	0	0	0
chicken diced simmered	½ cup	134	6	175	2	2	1	0	0	–
lamb braised	3 oz	157	7	212	3	1	2	0	0	–
pork braised	1 (4.5 oz)	191	7	285	2	2	2	0	0	–
turkey simmered	½ cup	94	3	133	1	1	1	0	0	0
veal braised	3 oz	158	6	150	2	2	1	0	0	–
HEARTS OF PALM										
canned	1 (1.2 oz)	9	tr	0	tr	tr	tr	0	1	–
canned	½ cup	20	tr	0	tr	tr	tr	0	2	–
HERBAL TEA (see TEA/HERBAL TEA)										
HERBS/SPICES (see also individual names)										
garam masala	1 tsp	8	tr	0	–	–	–	–	–	–
poultry seasoning	1 tsp	5	tr	0	tr	tr	tr	0	tr	tr
pumpkin pie spice	1 tsp (1.7 g)	6	tr	0	tr	tr	tr	0	tr	tr
Emeril's										
Original Essence	½ tsp (2 g)	0	0	0	0	0	0	0	–	–
McCormick										
Grill Mates Rub Applewood	2 tsp	15	0	0	0	0	0	0	0	1
Meat Tenderizer Seasoned	¼ tsp (1 g)	0	0	0	0	0	0	0	0	0
Modern Day Masala										
Organic Garam Masala	1 tsp (3 g)	10	0	0	0	0	0	0	1	–
Mrs. Dash										
Seasoning Mix Salt Free Beef Stew	1½ tsp (4 g)	15	0	0	0	0	0	0	–	–
Seasoning Mix Salt Free Chili	1¼ tsp (4.5 g)	15	0	0	0	0	0	0	–	–
Seasoning Mix Salt Free Fajita	1½ tsp (4.5 oz)	15	0	0	0	0	0	0	–	–
Seasoning Mix Salt Free Meatloaf	1 tsp (3 g)	10	0	0	0	0	0	0	–	–
Seasoning Mix Salt Free Pot Roast	1 tsp (4.5 oz)	10	0	0	0	0	0	0	–	1
Seasoning Mix Salt Free Sloppy Joe	1½ tsp (4.5 g)	15	0	0	0	0	0	0	0	2
Seasoning Mix Salt Free Taco	1 tbsp (6 g)	20	0	0	0	0	0	0	–	–

FOOD	PORTION	CALS	TOTAL FAT	CHOL	SAT FAT	POLY FAT	MONO FAT	TRANS FAT	FIBER	SUGAR
Old Bay										
Seasoning	¼ tsp (0.6 g)	0	0	0	0	0	0	0	0	0
Seasoning 30% Less Sodium	¼ tsp (0.6 g)	0	0	0	0	0	0	0	0	0
Simply Asia										
Five Spice Spicy Szechwan	¼ tsp	0	0	0	0	0	0	0	0	0
Sweet & Spicy Saigon Seasoning	¼ tsp	0	0	0	0	0	0	0	0	0
HERRING										
atlantic baked	4 oz	230	13	87	3	3	5	0	0	0
dried salted	1 fillet (1.4 oz)	161	9	61	2	2	4	0	0	0
pickled	1 oz	74	5	4	1	tr	3	0	0	–
pickled in cream sauce	1 oz	72	5	5	1	tr	3	0	0	tr
roe	1 tbsp	39	2	105	tr	1	tr	0	0	0
smoked kippered	1 oz	62	4	23	1	1	1	0	0	0
TAKE-OUT										
breaded fried	1 serv (4 oz)	225	14	67	3	4	6	0	1	1
HIBISCUS										
flowers dried sweetened	⅓ cup	100	0	0	0	0	0	0	2	21
HICKORY NUTS										
dried	1 oz	187	18	0	2	6	9	–	–	–
HOMINY										
white canned	1 cup	119	1	0	tr	1	tr	0	4	3
yellow canned	½ cup	115	1	0	tr	1	tr	0	4	–
Bush's										
Golden	½ cup (4.6 oz)	60	0	0	0	0	0	0	3	0
HONEY										
honey	¼ cup (3 oz)	258	0	0	0	0	0	0	tr	70
honey	1 tbsp (0.7 oz)	64	0	0	0	0	0	0	–	17
orange blossom	1 tbsp	60	0	0	0	0	0	0	0	16
wild honey	1 tbsp	60	0	0	0	0	0	0	–	16
Dutch Gold										
Organic Wildflower	1 tbsp (0.7 oz)	60	0	0	0	0	0	0	0	16
Maple Grove Farms										
Honey Maple Spread	2 tbsp (1.5 oz)	160	0	0	0	0	0	0	–	37
HONEYDEW										
balls frzn	1 cup (8 oz)	83	tr	0	tr	tr	tr	0	2	19
fresh cut up	1 cup	61	tr	0	tr	tr	tr	0	1	14

FOOD	PORTION	CALS	TOTAL FAT	CHOL	SAT FAT	POLY FAT	MONO FAT	TRANS FAT	FIBER	SUGAR
fresh wedge	⅛ melon (4.5 oz)	45	tr	0	tr	tr	tr	0	1	10
whole fresh	1 (35 oz)	360	1	0	tr	tr	1	0	8	81
Dole										
Fresh	⅒ med (4.7 oz)	50	0	0	0	0	0	0	1	11

HORSE
roasted	3 oz	149	5	58	2	1	2	–	0	0

HORSERADISH
sauce	1 tbsp	7	tr	0	tr	tr	tr	–	1	1
wasabi root raw	1 (5.9 oz)	184	1	0	–	–	–	0	13	–
wasabi root raw sliced	½ cup (2.3 oz)	71	tr	0	–	–	–	0	5	–
Manischewitz										
Sauce Original	1 tsp (5 g)	15	2	5	0	–	–	0	0	1
Zatarain's										
Prepared	1 tbsp (0.5 oz)	15	0	0	0	0	0	0	0	0

HOT CHOCOLATE
mix not prep	1 pkg (1 oz)	111	1	0	1	tr	tr	–	1	18
mix w/ no calorie sweetener as prep w/ water	8 oz	72	1	0	tr	tr	tr	–	2	7
mix w/ sugar as prep w/ nonfat milk	8 oz	209	1	5	1	tr	tr	–	1	29
mix w/ sugar as prep w/ water	8 oz	138	1	0	1	tr	tr	–	1	23
Nestle										
Hot Cocoa Mix Fat Free as prep	1 pkg	20	0	0	0	0	0	0	tr	4
TAKE-OUT										
chocolate caliente w/ lowfat milk	1 serv (8.4 oz)	221	9	12	6	tr	3	–	1	25
chocolate caliente w/ whole milk	1 serv (8.4 oz)	276	17	38	10	1	5	–	1	23
hot chocolate	1 cup (8.7 oz)	192	6	20	4	tr	2	tr	3	24
mexican hot chocolate	1 cup	173	6	18	4	–	–	–	1	–

HOT DOG (see also HOT DOG SUBSTITUTES)
beef	1 (1.5 oz)	149	13	24	5	1	6	–	0	2
beef & pork	1 (1.5 oz)	137	12	23	5	1	6	–	1	0
beef lowfat	1 (2 oz)	133	11	23	5	tr	6	–	0	0

FOOD	PORTION	CALS	TOTAL FAT	CHOL	SAT FAT	POLY FAT	MONO FAT	TRANS FAT	FIBER	SUGAR
chicken	1 (1.5 oz)	116	9	45	2	2	4	–	0	0
fat free	1 (2 oz)	62	1	23	tr	tr	tr	–	0	0
low sodium	1 (2 oz)	180	16	35	7	1	8	–	0	0
lowfat	1 (2 oz)	88	6	25	2	1	3	–	0	0
pork and beef cheese smokie	1 (1.5 oz)	141	12	29	5	1	6	–	0	1
turkey	1 (1.5 oz)	102	8	48	3	2	3	–	0	0
Abeles & Heymann										
Beef Uncured Reduced Fat & Sodium	1 (1.7 oz)	120	9	30	4	–	–	–	0	0
Al Fresco										
Chicken Uncured	1 (1.5 oz)	60	3	30	1	–	–	0	0	0
Applegate Farms										
The Great Uncured Beef	1 (2 oz)	110	8	30	3	–	–	0	0	0
The Great Uncured Chicken	1 (1.7 oz)	70	4	35	1	–	–	0	0	0
The Great Uncured Turkey	1 (1.7 oz)	60	4	25	1	–	–	0	0	0
Uncured Beef	1 (1.5 oz)	70	6	20	2	–	–	0	0	0
Uncured Big Apple	1 (2 oz)	110	9	30	4	–	–	0	0	0
Foster Farms										
Chicken	1 (2 oz)	140	12	30	–	–	–	0	0	tr
Corn Dog Chili Cheese	1 (2.6 oz)	190	9	25	3	–	–	0	1	4
Corn Dog Extreme Cheese	1 (2.6 oz)	200	10	20	4	–	–	0	0	4
Corn Dogs Honey Crunchy	1 (2.6 oz)	180	9	25	3	–	–	0	0	6
Corn Dogs Mini	4 (2.7 oz)	210	12	45	–	–	–	0	1	0
Turkey	1 (2 oz)	140	12	25	–	–	–	0	0	tr
Hebrew National										
Beef	1 (1.7 oz)	150	14	25	6	–	–	1	0	0
Beef 97% Fat Free	1 (1.6 oz)	40	1	10	0	–	–	0	0	0
Beef Franks In A Blanket	5 (2.8 oz)	300	24	10	8	–	–	3	1	tr
Beef Jumbo	1 (3 oz)	270	25	45	10	–	–	1	0	0
Oscar Mayer										
Turkey Uncured	1 (2 oz)	120	9	35	3	–	–	0	–	1
State Fair										
Classic Corn Dog	1 (2.7 oz)	210	10	25	3	–	–	0	0	7
Corn Dog Beef	1 (2.7 oz)	220	10	20	4	–	–	0	0	8
Corn Dog Mini	6 (3 oz)	230	12	35	4	–	–	0	1	6
TAKE-OUT										
corndog	1	460	19	79	5	3	9	–	–	–
w/ bun chili	1	297	13	51	5	1	7	–	–	–
w/ bun plain	1	242	15	44	5	2	7	–	–	–

FOOD	PORTION	CALS	TOTAL FAT	CHOL	SAT FAT	POLY FAT	MONO FAT	TRANS FAT	FIBER	SUGAR
HOT DOG SUBSTITUTES										
Morningstar Farms										
Veggie Dogs	1 (1.4 oz)	50	1	0	0	0	0	0	tr	2
HUMMUS										
Athenos										
Artichoke & Garlic	2 tbsp (0.9 oz)	50	3	0	0	0	0	0	1	1
Cucumber Dill	2 tbsp (0.9 oz)	50	3	0	0	–	–	0	1	1
Greek Style	2 tbsp (0.9 oz)	50	3	0	0	–	–	0	1	1
Original	2 tbsp (0.9 oz)	50	3	0	0	–	–	0	1	1
Roasted Red Pepper	2 tbsp (0.9 oz)	50	3	0	0	–	–	0	1	1
Cedar's										
Artichoke Spinach	2 tbsp (1 oz)	70	4	0	0	–	–	0	1	1
Fountain Of Health										
Traditional	1 oz	70	5	0	1	–	–	0	1	1
Margaritaville										
Cilantro Jalapeno	1 oz	70	5	0	1	–	–	0	1	1
Island Lemon	1 oz	70	6	0	1	–	–	0	1	1
Nasoya										
Super Classic Original	2 tbsp (1 oz)	50	3	0	0	2	1	0	1	1
Sabra										
Classic Singles	1 (2 oz)	150	11	0	2	–	–	0	3	1
Greek Olive	2 tbsp (1 oz)	70	6	0	1	–	–	0	1	0
Roasted Pine Nut	2 tbsp (1 oz)	80	7	0	1	–	–	0	1	0
Spinach & Artichoke	2 tbsp (1 oz)	70	6	0	1	–	–	0	1	0
TAKE-OUT										
hummus	¼ cup (2.2 oz)	109	5	0	1	1	3	–	3	tr
HYACINTH BEANS										
dried cooked	1 cup	228	1	0	–	–	–	–	–	–

ICE CREAM AND FROZEN DESSERTS (*see also* ICES AND ICE POPS, SHERBET, YOGURT FROZEN)

FOOD	PORTION	CALS	TOTAL FAT	CHOL	SAT FAT	POLY FAT	MONO FAT	TRANS FAT	FIBER	SUGAR
chocolate	½ cup (4 fl oz)	143	7	22	4	tr	2	–	–	13
dixie cup chocolate	1 (3.5 fl oz)	125	6	20	4	tr	2	–	–	11
dixie cup strawberry	1 (3.5 fl oz)	112	5	17	–	–	–	–	–	9
dixie cup vanilla	1 (3.5 fl oz)	116	6	25	4	tr	2	–	–	9
freeze dried ice cream chocolate strawberry & vanilla	1 pkg (0.75 oz)	158	5	1	2	–	–	–	1	10
strawberry	½ cup (4 fl oz)	127	6	19	–	–	–	–	–	10

FOOD	PORTION	CALS	TOTAL FAT	CHOL	SAT FAT	POLY FAT	MONO FAT	TRANS FAT	FIBER	SUGAR
vanilla	½ cup (4 fl oz)	132	7	29	4	tr	2	–	–	10
vanilla soft serve	½ cup	111	2	10	1	tr	1	–	–	–
Arctic Zero										
Chocolate	½ cup (2.6 oz)	37	0	0	0	0	0	0	2	6
Chocolate Coated Bars All Flavors	1 (2 oz)	85	5	5	4	–	–	0	1	5
Coffee	½ cup (2.6 oz)	37	0	0	0	0	0	0	2	5
Mint Chocolate Cookie	½ cup (2.6 oz)	37	0	0	0	0	0	0	2	5
Pumpkin Spice	½ cup (2.6 oz)	45	0	10	0	0	0	0	2	7
Vanilla Maple	½ cup (2.6 oz)	37	0	0	0	0	0	0	2	7
Carvel										
Cake Original Ice Cream	⅙ cake (3.2 oz)	250	13	30	10	–	–	0	1	21
Clemmy's										
Bar Sugar Free Cherry Vanilla	1 (1.9 oz)	70	3	15	2	–	–	0	5	0
Bar Sugar Free Chocolate Fudge	1 (2.2 oz)	70	3	10	2	–	–	0	5	0
Bar Sugar Free Orange Creme	1 (2 oz)	70	3	15	2	–	–	0	5	0
Butter Pecan Sugar Free	½ cup (2.6 oz)	180	14	60	7	–	–	0	5	0
Chocolate Sugar Free	½ cup (2.6 oz)	160	11	65	7	–	–	0	5	0
Ice Cream Os Sugar Free	1 (1.75 oz)	100	7	10	5	–	–	0	2	0
Peanut Butter Chocolate Chip Sugar Free	½ cup (2.6 oz)	200	15	55	8	–	–	0	5	0
Toasted Almond Sugar Free	½ cup (2.7 oz)	180	13	65	7	–	–	0	5	0
Vanilla Bean Sugar Free	½ cup (2.5 oz)	150	11	65	7	–	–	0	5	0
Dove										
Miniatures Dark Chocolate Variety Pack	5 (3.1 oz)	320	21	30	13	–	–	0	3	24
Miniatures Milk Chocolate Variety Pack	5 (3.1 oz)	340	22	30	14	–	–	0	1	29
Mint Chocolate Chunk	½ cup (2.4 oz)	180	11	30	7	–	–	0	1	14
Unconditional Chocolate	½ cup (2.5 oz)	200	12	25	8	–	–	0	2	17
Vanilla Chocolate Chunk	½ cup (2.3 oz)	180	11	30	7	–	–	0	0	15
Good Karma										
Organic Rice Divine Bar Chocolate Chocolate	1 (2.4 oz)	200	13	0	7	–	–	0	1	12
Organic Rice Divine Chocolate Chip	½ cup (2.6 oz)	170	9	0	3	–	–	0	2	13

FOOD	PORTION	CALS	TOTAL FAT	CHOL	SAT FAT	POLY FAT	MONO FAT	TRANS FAT	FIBER	SUGAR
Organic Rice Divine Coconut Mango	½ cup (2.6 oz)	150	6	0	1	–	–	0	1	14
Organic Rice Divine Key Lime Pie	½ cup (2.6 oz)	140	6	0	0	–	–	0	1	13
Halo Top Creamery										
Light Chocolate	½ cup (3 oz)	80	4	43	2	–	–	0	5	4
Light Lemon Cake	½ cup (2.5 oz)	70	3	43	2	–	–	0	4	4
Light Strawberry	½ cup (2.6 oz)	70	3	43	2	–	–	0	4	4
Light Vanilla Bean	½ cup (2.5 oz)	70	3	43	2	–	–	0	4	4
Healthy Choice										
Bar Fudge	1 (2.2 oz)	80	2	5	1	1	0	0	4	4
Bar Low Fat Sorbet & Cream	1 (2.2 oz)	80	1	<5	0	0	0	0	tr	12
Sandwich Vanilla	1 (2.4 oz)	150	2	<5	1	–	–	0	0	14
Lactaid										
Butter Pecan	½ cup (4 oz)	170	11	30	5	–	–	0	0	11
Chocolate	½ cup (2.5 oz)	160	8	30	5	–	–	0	0	13
Vanilla	½ cup (4 oz)	150	8	35	5	–	–	0	0	12
Lifeway										
Frozen Kefir Tart And Tangy Original	½ cup (2.5 oz)	90	1	5	1	–	–	0	0	16
Frozen Kefir Tart And Tangy Pomegranate	½ cup (2.5 oz)	90	1	5	0	–	–	0	0	16
Frozen Kefir Tart And Tangy Strawberry	½ cup (2.5 oz)	90	1	5	0	–	–	0	0	16
Greek Style Fro-Yo Honey Swirl	½ cup (2.5 oz)	110	1	10	0	–	–	0	0	17
Magnum										
Classic	1 bar (2.7 oz)	240	16	25	10	–	–	0	tr	21
Dark	1 bar (2.7 oz)	240	17	25	11	–	–	0	2	18
Double Caramel	1 bar (3.2 oz)	320	20	25	14	–	–	0	1	29
White	1 bar (2.7 oz)	250	16	25	14	–	–	0	0	23
McConnell's										
Dutchman's Chocolate	½ cup (3.7 oz)	230	17	75	10	–	–	0	1	19
Golden State Vanilla	½ cup (3.7 oz)	250	18	80	11	–	–	0	0	20
Mint Chip	½ cup (3.7 oz)	250	17	75	10	–	–	0	0	24
Salted Caramel Chip	½ cup (3.7 oz)	270	18	75	11	–	–	0	0	24
Turkish Coffee	½ cup (3.7 oz)	250	18	80	10	–	–	0	1	19
Straus										
I'm Organic Coffee	4 oz	240	15	70	10	–	–	0	0	19
I'm Organic Raspberry	½ cup (4 oz)	230	14	65	9	–	–	0	1	19

FOOD	PORTION	CALS	TOTAL FAT	CHOL	SAT FAT	POLY FAT	MONO FAT	TRANS FAT	FIBER	SUGAR
I'm Organic Vanilla Bean	4 oz	240	15	70	10	–	–	0	0	19
Organic Brown Sugar Banana	½ cup (3.2 oz)	250	11	55	7	–	–	0	0	31
Tofutti										
Cuties Chocolate	1 (1.3 oz)	130	1	0	0	–	–	0	0	9
Cuties Vanilla	1 (1.3 oz)	130	6	0	1	–	–	0	0	9
Flowers Chocolate Covered	1 (1.4 oz)	180	8	0	2	–	–	0	2	19
Marry Me Dessert Bars	1 bar (2.5 oz)	168	8	0	3	–	–	0	tr	18
Yours Truly Cones	1 (2.6 oz)	220	13	0	3	–	–	0	2	21
Weight Watchers										
Smart Ones Sundae Chocolate Fudge Brownie	1 (2.3 oz)	140	3	5	2	0	1	0	tr	14
Smart Ones Sundae Turtle	1 (2.2 oz)	130	3	5	1	1	2	0	0	10
TAKE-OUT										
cone vanilla light soft serve	1 (4.6 oz)	164	6	28	4	tr	2	–	–	–
gelato chocolate hazelnut	½ cup (5.3 oz)	370	29	92	4	2	16	–	2	21
gelato vanilla	½ cup (3 oz)	211	15	151	8	1	4	–	0	18
ice cream pie no crust	1 slice (3.4 oz)	218	14	56	9	1	4	–	1	18
mud pie	⅛ pie (8 oz)	698	32	53	15	4	11	–	3	64
sundae caramel	1 (5.4 oz)	303	9	25	5	1	3	–	–	–
sundae hot fudge	1 (5.4 oz)	284	9	21	5	tr	2	–	–	–
sundae strawberry	1 (5.4 oz)	269	8	21	4	1	3	–	–	–

ICE CREAM CONES AND CUPS

brown sugar cone	1 (10 g)	40	tr	0	tr	tr	tr	–	tr	3
wafer cone	1	17	tr	0	tr	tr	tr	0	tr	tr
waffle cone	1 lg	121	2	0	tr	1	1	0	1	2

ICE CREAM TOPPINGS

marshmallow cream	1 oz	88	tr	0	–	–	–	–	–	–
marshmallow cream	1 jar (7 oz)	615	tr	0	–	–	–	–	–	–
nuts in syrup	2 tbsp	184	9	0	1	6	2	0	1	15
pineapple	2 tbsp (1.5 oz)	106	tr	0	tr	tr	tr	0	tr	9
strawberry	1 cup (11.5 oz)	863	1	0	–	–	–	–	–	–
strawberry	2 tbsp (1.5 oz)	107	tr	0	–	–	–	–	–	–
Smucker's										
Plate Scrapers Chocolate Fudge	2 tbsp (1.4 oz)	120	3	0	1	–	–	0	tr	14

ICED TEA

MIX

Crystal Light

FOOD	PORTION	CALS	TOTAL FAT	CHOL	SAT FAT	POLY FAT	MONO FAT	TRANS FAT	FIBER	SUGAR
Antioxidant Sugar Free Green Tea Raspberry as prep	8 oz	5	0	0	0	0	0	0	–	0
On The Go White Peach Tea as prep	8 oz	5	0	0	0	0	0	0	0	0
Pure Sugar Free Mixed Berry as prep	8 oz	15	0	0	0	0	0	0	0	3

READY-TO-DRINK

Arizona

FOOD	PORTION	CALS	TOTAL FAT	CHOL	SAT FAT	POLY FAT	MONO FAT	TRANS FAT	FIBER	SUGAR
Black & White	8 oz	50	0	0	0	0	0	0	0	14
Diet Black Tea Peach	8 oz	0	0	0	0	0	0	0	0	tr
Green Tea Lemonade	8 oz	50	0	0	0	0	0	0	0	13
Organic Green Tea	8 oz	50	0	0	0	0	0	0	0	13

Honest Tea

FOOD	PORTION	CALS	TOTAL FAT	CHOL	SAT FAT	POLY FAT	MONO FAT	TRANS FAT	FIBER	SUGAR
Assam Black	8 oz	17	0	0	0	0	0	0	–	5
Green Dragon	8 oz	30	0	0	0	0	0	0	–	8
Green Tea Zero Calorie Passion Fruit	8 oz	0	0	0	0	0	0	0	0	0
Half & Half	8 oz	48	0	0	0	0	0	0	–	12
Heavenly Lemon Tulsi	8 oz	30	0	0	0	0	0	0	–	8
Jasmine Green Energy	8 oz	17	0	0	0	0	0	0	–	5
Just Green	8 oz	0	0	0	0	0	0	0	0	0
Pearfect White	8 oz	35	0	0	0	0	0	0	–	9
White Mango Acai	8 oz	35	0	0	0	0	0	0	–	9

Lipton

FOOD	PORTION	CALS	TOTAL FAT	CHOL	SAT FAT	POLY FAT	MONO FAT	TRANS FAT	FIBER	SUGAR
Diet Green Tea w/ Citrus	8 oz	0	0	0	0	0	0	0	0	0
Diet Green Tea w/ Watermelon	8 oz	0	0	0	0	0	0	0	–	0
Green Tea 100% Natural Citrus	8 oz	70	0	0	0	0	0	0	–	18
Green Tea 100% Natural Passionfruit Mango	8 oz	50	0	0	0	0	0	0	–	13

Old Orchard

FOOD	PORTION	CALS	TOTAL FAT	CHOL	SAT FAT	POLY FAT	MONO FAT	TRANS FAT	FIBER	SUGAR
Green Tea w/ Lemon & Honey	8 oz	45	0	0	0	0	0	0	0	12
Red Tea w/ Currant	8 oz	45	0	0	0	0	0	0	–	12

FOOD	PORTION	CALS	TOTAL FAT	CHOL	SAT FAT	POLY FAT	MONO FAT	TRANS FAT	FIBER	SUGAR
POM										
Green Tea Pomegranate Lychee	8 oz	70	0	0	0	0	0	0	–	17
Pomegranate Blackberry	8 oz	80	0	0	0	0	0	0	–	18
Rooibee Red Tea										
Unsweetened	1 bottle (12.5 oz)	0	0	0	0	0	0	0	0	0
Vanilla Chai	1 bottle (12.5 oz)	90	0	0	0	0	0	0	–	20
Watermelon Mint Organic	1 bottle (12.5 oz)	80	0	0	0	0	0	0	–	20
Spindrift										
Sparkling Half & Half	8 oz	80	0	0	0	0	0	0	0	20
Steaz										
Iced Green Tea Blueberry Pomegranate	8 oz	40	0	0	0	0	0	0	–	10
Iced Green Tea Super Fruit Organic	8 oz	40	0	0	0	0	0	0	–	9
Iced Green Tea Unsweetened Lemon Organic	8 oz	0	0	0	0	0	0	0	0	0
Iced Green Tea w/ Coconut Water Organic	8 oz	40	0	0	0	0	0	0	–	9
Sparkling Green Tea Blueberry Pomegranate	8 oz	0	0	0	0	0	0	0	0	0
Tea Of A Kind										
All Flavors	8 oz	10	0	0	0	0	0	0	–	3

ICES AND ICE POPS
Del Monte

FOOD	PORTION	CALS	TOTAL FAT	CHOL	SAT FAT	POLY FAT	MONO FAT	TRANS FAT	FIBER	SUGAR
Fruit Chillers Arctic Strawberry Cup	1 (4.5 oz)	170	0	0	0	0	0	0	2	26
Fruit Chillers Frosty Peach Cup	1 (4.5 oz)	170	0	0	0	0	0	0	2	26
Fruit Chillers Grape Berry Blast Tube	1	55	0	0	0	0	0	0	1	11
Fruit Chillers Strawberry Snow Storm Tube	1	55	0	0	0	0	0	0	1	11
Dole										
Fruit Bars Strawberry	1 (2.75 oz)	90	0	0	0	0	0	0	0	22

FOOD	PORTION	CALS	TOTAL FAT	CHOL	SAT FAT	POLY FAT	MONO FAT	TRANS FAT	FIBER	SUGAR
Super Fruit Bars Acai Blueberry	1 (2.75 oz)	90	0	0	0	0	0	0	0	21
Dreyer's										
Outshine Bar Coconut Waters w/ Banana	1 (3 oz)	60	0	0	0	0	0	0	0	13
Outshine Bar Coconut Waters w/ Pineapple	1 (3 oz)	60	0	0	0	0	0	0	0	14
Outshine Bar Seasonal Picks Peach	1 (3 oz)	90	0	0	0	0	0	0	0	21
Outshine Bar Seasonal Picks Raspberry	1 (3 oz)	80	0	0	0	0	0	0	0	18
Minute Maid										
Soft Frozen Lemonade Lemon	1 pkg	70	0	0	0	0	0	0	–	13
Soft Frozen Limeade Cherry	1 pkg	70	0	0	0	0	0	0	–	13

INDIAN FOOD (see ASIAN FOOD)

JACKFRUIT

FOOD	PORTION	CALS	TOTAL FAT	CHOL	SAT FAT	POLY FAT	MONO FAT	TRANS FAT	FIBER	SUGAR
canned in syrup	½ cup (3.1 oz)	82	tr	0	–	–	–	–	1	–
fresh sliced	1 cup (5.8 oz)	157	1	0	tr	tr	tr	0	3	31

JALAPENO (see PEPPERS)

JAM/JELLY/PRESERVES

FOOD	PORTION	CALS	TOTAL FAT	CHOL	SAT FAT	POLY FAT	MONO FAT	TRANS FAT	FIBER	SUGAR
apple butter	1 tbsp (0.6 oz)	31	tr	0	tr	tr	tr	0	tr	6
jam all flavors	1 tbsp (0.7 oz)	56	tr	0	tr	0	tr	0	tr	10
jam all flavors	1 pkg (0.5 oz)	39	tr	0	tr	0	tr	0	tr	7
jam apricot	1 tbsp (0.7 oz)	48	tr	0	tr	0	0	0	tr	9
jam diet all flavors	1 tbsp (0.5 oz)	18	tr	0	tr	tr	tr	0	tr	5
jelly all flavors	1 tbsp (0.7 oz)	51	0	0	0	0	0	0	tr	10
jelly reduced sugar all flavors	1 tbsp (0.7 oz)	34	tr	0	tr	tr	0	0	tr	9
jelly diet all flavors	1 tbsp (0.7 oz)	25	tr	0	tr	tr	tr	0	1	7
orange marmalade	1 tbsp (0.7 oz)	49	0	0	0	0	0	0	tr	12
preserves all flavors	1 tbsp (0.7 oz)	56	tr	0	tr	0	tr	0	tr	10
Bonne Maman										
Jelly Muscat Grape	1 tbsp (0.7 oz)	50	0	0	0	0	0	0	–	13
Orange Marmalade	1 tbsp (0.7 oz)	50	0	0	0	0	0	0	–	13
Preserves Apricot	1 tbsp (0.7 oz)	50	0	0	0	0	0	0	–	13
Preserves Cherry	1 tbsp (0.7 oz)	50	0	0	0	0	0	0	–	13
Preserves Golden Plum Mirabelle	1 tbsp (0.7 oz)	50	0	0	0	0	0	0	–	12

FOOD	PORTION	CALS	TOTAL FAT	CHOL	SAT FAT	POLY FAT	MONO FAT	TRANS FAT	FIBER	SUGAR
Jake & Amos										
Jam Fig	1 tbsp (0.5 oz)	35	0	0	0	0	0	0	0	8
Jam Hot Pepper	1 tbsp	43	0	0	0	0	0	0	–	8
Jam Rhubarb	1 tbsp (0.7 oz)	40	0	0	0	0	0	0	0	11
Jenkins Jellies										
Fiery Figs Pepper Jelly	1 tbsp (0.7 oz)	50	0	0	0	0	0	0	–	11
Guava Brava	1 tbsp (0.7 oz)	50	0	0	0	0	0	0	–	11
Hell Fire Pepper Jelly	1 tbsp (0.7 oz)	40	0	0	0	0	0	0	1	10
Passion Fire Pepper Jelly	1 tbsp (0.7 oz)	45	0	0	0	0	0	0	–	12
Smucker's										
Jam Blackberry	1 tbsp (0.7 oz)	50	0	0	0	0	0	0	–	12
Jam Concord Grape	1 tbsp (0.7 oz)	50	0	0	0	0	0	0	–	12
Jam Red Plum	1 tbsp (0.7 oz)	50	0	0	0	0	0	0	–	12
Jam Seedless Red Raspberry	1 tbsp (0.7 oz)	50	0	0	0	0	0	0	–	12
Jelly Apple	2 tbsp (0.7 oz)	50	0	0	0	0	0	0	–	12
Jelly Concord Grape	1 tbsp (0.7 oz)	50	0	0	0	0	0	0	–	12
Jelly Strawberry	1 tbsp (0.7 oz)	50	0	0	0	0	0	0	–	12
Orange Marmalade Low Sugar	2 tbsp (0.7 oz)	25	0	0	0	0	0	0	–	5
Preserves Apricot Low Sugar	1 tbsp (0.6 oz)	25	0	0	0	0	0	0	–	5
Simply Fruit Black Cherry	1 tbsp (0.7 oz)	40	0	0	0	0	0	0	–	8
Simply Fruit Peach	1 tbsp (0.7 oz)	40	0	0	0	0	0	0	–	8
Simply Fruit Strawberry	1 tbsp (0.7 oz)	40	0	0	0	0	0	0	–	8
Trappist										
Jelly Hot Pepper	1 tbsp (0.7 oz)	50	0	0	0	0	0	0	–	13
Welch's										
Grape Jelly	1 tbsp (0.7 oz)	50	0	0	0	0	0	0	–	13
Natural Spread Concord Grape	1 tbsp (0.6 oz)	30	0	0	0	0	0	0	–	8
Natural Spread Strawberry	1 tbsp (0.6 oz)	30	0	0	0	0	0	0	–	8

JAPANESE FOOD (see ASIAN FOOD, SUSHI)

JELLY (see JAM/JELLY/PRESERVES)

JELLYFISH

pickled	½ cup (1 oz)	10	tr	1	tr	tr	tr	0	0	0

JERKY

beef	1 oz	122	8	14	3	tr	3	–	1	3
pork	1 oz	122	8	14	3	tr	3	–	1	3
venison	1 oz	119	7	39	3	1	2	–	0	4

FOOD	PORTION	CALS	TOTAL FAT	CHOL	SAT FAT	POLY FAT	MONO FAT	TRANS FAT	FIBER	SUGAR
Jerky For Life										
Beef Steak Black Pepper & Garlic	¼ pkg (1 oz)	50	2	5	1	–	–	0	0	0
Beef Steak Jalapeno	¼ pkg (1 oz)	50	2	5	1	–	–	0	–	0
King Kalibur										
Black Angus Beef Sticks	1 (1.2 oz)	93	5	14	3	–	–	0	0	4
Krave										
Beef Chili Lime	1 oz	50	2	10	0	–	–	0	0	2
Beef Pineapple Orange	1 oz	80	2	20	1	–	–	0	0	6
Beef Sweet Chipotle	1 oz	80	2	20	1	–	–	0	0	7
Pork Smoky Grilled Teriyaki	1 oz	70	2	15	0	–	–	0	0	8
Turkey Basil Citrus	1 oz	100	0	25	0	–	–	0	0	16
Matador										
Beef Original	1 pkg (1.4 oz)	110	2	40	1	–	–	0	0	7
Snack Stick Original	1 (1 oz)	150	13	30	5	–	–	0	0	0
Oh Boy! Oberto										
Beef Hickory	1 oz	80	1	10	0	–	–	0	0	6
Beef Original	1 oz	80	1	10	1	–	–	0	0	5
Beef Peppered	1 oz	80	1	10	0	–	–	0	0	5
Original Thin	1 pkg (1.2 oz)	90	2	15	1	–	–	0	0	1
Pepperoni Bite Size Sticks	6 (1.1 oz)	160	13	35	5	–	–	0	0	1
Smok-A-Roni	2 (1 oz)	140	12	35	5	–	–	0	0	1
Sticks Original	1 pkg (1 oz)	130	10	35	4	–	–	0	0	0
Tender Style	1 pkg (0.4 oz)	45	3	10	2	–	–	0	0	1
Perky Jerky										
Beef	1 pkg (1 oz)	90	2	25	1	–	–	0	0	5
Turkey	1 pkg (1 oz)	50	0	0	0	0	0	0	0	2
Simply Snackin										
Dried Beef Sirloin w/ Apples & Cherries	1 pkg (1 oz)	60	1	10	0	1	0	0	0	3
Dried Chicken Breast w/ Black Bean Salsa	1 pkg (1 oz)	60	0	20	0	0	0	0	0	tr
Teriyaki Dried Beef Sirloin w/ Pineapples	1 pkg (1 oz)	60	1	10	0	–	–	0	0	2
Teriyaki Dried Chicken Breast w/ Mangoes & Papayas	1 pkg (1 oz)	60	0	20	0	0	0	0	0	2
Sunrich Naturals										
Fruit Bar Sour Apple	1 (0.7 oz)	70	0	0	0	0	0	0	1	12
Fruit Bar Strawberry Kiwi	1 (0.7 oz)	70	0	0	0	0	0	0	1	12

FOOD	PORTION	CALS	TOTAL FAT	CHOL	SAT FAT	POLY FAT	MONO FAT	TRANS FAT	FIBER	SUGAR
Umpqua Indian Foods										
Brew Pub Steak Jerky Beef Flavored	¼ pkg (1 oz)	90	3	15	1	–	–	0	–	5
Steak Jerky Original	¼ pkg (1 oz)	60	2	15	1	–	–	0	0	0
JICAMA										
fresh	1 sm (12.8 oz)	139	tr	0	tr	tr	tr	–	18	7
raw sliced	1 cup	46	tr	0	tr	tr	tr	0	6	2
JUJUBE										
dried	1 oz	82	tr	0	–	–	–	0	–	–
JUTE										
cooked	1 cup	32	tr	0	tr	tr	tr	–	2	1
KALE										
chopped cooked w/o salt	1 cup	36	1	0	tr	tr	tr	0	3	2
fresh cooked w/ fat	1 cup	69	4	0	1	1	2	–	2	2
scotch chopped cooked w/o salt	1 cup	36	1	0	tr	tr	tr	0	2	–
KANGAROO										
kangaroo	3 oz	120	2	56	–	–	–	–	–	–
KEFIR										
kefir	8 oz	98	2	10	1	tr	1	0	0	12
Green Valley										
Organic Lactose Free Blueberry Pom Acai	1 pkg (6 oz)	150	3	10	2	–	–	0	0	19
Organic Lactose Free Plain	8 oz	90	3	10	2	–	–	0	0	4
Helios										
Organic Nonfat Plain	8 oz	100	0	0	0	0	0	0	2	12
Organic Nonfat Raspberry	8 oz	160	0	5	0	0	0	0	2	27
Organic Nonfat Vanilla	8 oz	160	0	5	0	0	0	0	2	27
Lifeway										
BioKefir For Digestion All Flavors	1 bottle (3.5 oz)	60	0	0	0	0	0	0	2	9
Greek Style	8 oz	210	14	55	9	–	–	0	–	12
Lowfat Coconut Chia	8 oz	140	2	10	2	–	–	0	1	20
Lowfat Mango	8 oz	140	2	10	2	–	–	0	–	20
Lowfat Strawberry	8 oz	140	2	10	2	–	–	0	–	20
Nonfat Plain	8 oz	90	0	5	0	0	0	0	–	12
Nonfat Raspberry	8 oz	150	0	5	0	0	0	0	–	27

FOOD	PORTION	CALS	TOTAL FAT	CHOL	SAT FAT	POLY FAT	MONO FAT	TRANS FAT	FIBER	SUGAR
Organic Whole Milk Plain	8 oz	160	8	30	5	–	–	0	–	12
Original	8 oz	150	8	30	5	–	–	0	0	12
Probugs All Flavors	1 pkg (4 oz)	100	4	15	2	–	–	0	–	10
Slim6 Plain	8 oz	110	2	10	2	–	–	0	2	6
The Greek Gods										
Honey & Strawberry	8 oz	230	3	10	2	–	–	0	0	37
Plain	8 oz	140	3	10	2	–	–	0	0	17
Vanilla Honey	8 oz	220	3	10	2	–	–	0	0	38
KETCHUP										
banana	1 tsp	10	0	0	0	0	0	0	0	2
ketchup	1 pkg (0.3 oz)	10	tr	0	tr	tr	tr	0	0	2
ketchup	¼ cup (2.1 oz)	67	tr	0	tr	tr	tr	0	tr	13
ketchup	1 tbsp (0.6 oz)	19	tr	0	tr	tr	tr	0	tr	4
low sodium	1 tbsp	15	tr	0	tr	tr	tr	0	0	3
Annie's Homegrown										
Organic	1 tbsp (0.6 oz)	15	0	0	0	0	0	0	–	4
Del Monte										
Tomato	1 tbsp (0.6 oz)	15	0	0	0	0	0	0	0	4
Fischer & Wieser										
Chipotle Chili	1 tbsp (0.7 oz)	15	0	0	0	0	0	0	–	2
Heinz										
No Salt Added	1 tbsp (0.6 oz)	20	0	0	0	0	0	0	0	4
Reduced Sugar	1 tbsp (0.6 oz)	5	0	0	0	0	0	0	0	1
Hunt's										
Ketchup	1 tbsp (0.6 oz)	20	0	0	0	0	0	0	0	4
Ketchup No Salt Added	1 tbsp (0.6 oz)	25	0	0	0	0	0	0	0	4
OrganicVille										
No Added Sugar	1 tbsp (0.6 oz)	20	0	0	0	0	0	0	0	3
KIDNEY										
beef simmered	3 oz	134	4	609	1	1	1	tr	0	0
lamb braised	3 oz	116	3	480	1	1	1	0	0	–
pork braised	3 oz	128	4	408	1	tr	1	0	0	0
veal braised	3 oz	139	5	672	1	1	1	0	0	0
KIDNEY BEANS										
canned	½ cup	108	1	0	tr	tr	tr	0	6	2
dried cooked w/o salt	½ cup	112	tr	0	tr	tr	tr	0	6	tr
Vitarroz										
Light Red	½ cup (4.2 oz)	100	0	0	0	0	0	0	5	1

FOOD	PORTION	CALS	TOTAL FAT	CHOL	SAT FAT	POLY FAT	MONO FAT	TRANS FAT	FIBER	SUGAR
KIWI										
fresh	1 med (2.6 oz)	46	tr	0	tr	tr	tr	0	2	7
fresh	1 lg (3.2 oz)	56	tr	0	tr	tr	tr	0	3	8
KNISH										
Gabila's										
Potato	1 (4.5 oz)	180	3	0	0	–	–	0	2	tr
TAKE-OUT										
cheese	1 (2.1 oz)	205	12	56	3	3	5	–	1	tr
meat	1 sm (1.8 oz)	174	11	48	3	2	5	–	1	tr
meat	1 lg (5.6 oz)	524	32	144	8	7	15	–	2	1
potato	1 sm (2.1 oz)	213	12	52	3	4	6	–	1	tr
potato	1 lg (6.3 oz)	616	35	149	8	10	16	–	2	2
KOHLRABI										
raw sliced	1 cup	36	tr	0	tr	tr	tr	0	4	4
sliced cooked w/o salt	1 cup	48	tr	0	tr	tr	tr	0	2	5
TAKE-OUT										
creamed	1 cup	150	9	6	2	2	4	–	1	6
KUMQUATS										
canned in syrup	1	13	tr	0	tr	tr	tr	0	1	3
fresh	1	13	tr	0	tr	tr	tr	0	1	2
LAMB										
australian ground 85% lean not prep	4 oz	288	23	82	11	1	9	2	0	0
cubed lean & fat braised	4 oz	253	10	122	4	1	4	0	0	0
cubed lean broiled	4 oz	211	8	102	3	1	3	0	0	0
ground broiled	4 oz	321	22	110	9	2	9	0	0	0
leg roasted	4 oz	213	15	74	6	1	6	0	0	0
loin chop lean & fat broiled	1 chop (4 oz)	222	16	72	7	1	7	0	0	0
rib chop lean & fat broiled	1 chop (1.6 oz)	165	14	46	6	1	6	0	0	0
rib roast baked	4 oz	386	31	109	13	2	13	0	0	0
shank lean & fat braised	4 oz	360	20	157	8	1	8	0	0	0
shoulder chop lean & fat cooked	1 chop (5.5 oz)	274	20	91	8	2	8	0	0	0
shoulder w/ bone braised	4 oz	231	17	77	7	1	7	0	0	0
LAMB DISHES										
Tandoor Chef										
Lamb Vindaloo frzn	1 pkg (9.4 oz)	360	15	80	5	–	–	0	3	5
Samosa Lamb frzn	2 (2 oz)	150	8	15	3	–	–	0	1	1

FOOD	PORTION	CALS	TOTAL FAT	CHOL	SAT FAT	POLY FAT	MONO FAT	TRANS FAT	FIBER	SUGAR
TAKE-OUT										
keema w/ coconut milk	1 serv (8 oz)	380	28	88	18	1	7	–	6	9
moroccan pilaf w/ bulgur	1 serv	327	13	54	2	–	–	–	–	–
moussaka	4 in sq (16 oz)	659	43	96	11	13	16	–	8	10
shepherd's pie	1 (21.3 oz)	742	31	103	8	7	14	–	9	9
stew w/ potatoes & vegetables	1 cup	260	6	58	2	1	2	–	4	3
LAMBSQUARTERS										
chopped cooked w/ salt	1 cup	58	1	0	tr	tr	tr	0	4	–
LECITHIN										
lecithin	1 tbsp	104	14	0	2	6	2	–	0	0
LEEKS										
chopped cooked w/o salt	¼ cup	8	tr	0	tr	tr	tr	0	tr	–
cooked	1 (4.4 oz)	38	tr	0	tr	tr	tr	0	1	–
freeze dried	1 tbsp	1	0	0	0	0	0	0	0	–
LEMON										
fresh	1 med (4 oz)	22	tr	0	tr	tr	tr	0	5	–
peel	1 tsp	1	0	0	0	0	0	0	tr	tr
peel	1 tbsp	3	tr	0	tr	tr	tr	0	1	tr
wedge	1 (7 g)	2	tr	0	tr	tr	tr	0	tr	tr
Sunkist										
Fresh	1 med (2 oz)	15	0	0	0	0	0	0	2	2
LEMON EXTRACT										
lemon extract	½ tsp	12	tr	0	–	–	–	–	0	0
LEMON JUICE										
bottled	1 oz	6	tr	0	tr	tr	tr	0	tr	1
bottled	1 tbsp	3	tr	0	tr	tr	tr	0	tr	tr
fresh	1 oz	8	0	0	0	0	0	0	tr	1
from 1 lemon	1.6 oz	12	0	0	0	0	0	0	tr	1
from wedge	6 g	1	0	0	0	0	0	0	0	tr
Italian Volcano										
Organic	2 tbsp (1 oz)	9	0	0	0	0	0	0	0	1
Izze										
Esque Sparkling Limon	1 bottle (12 oz)	50	0	0	0	0	0	0	–	11
KeVita										
Sparkling Probiotic Drink Lemon Ginger Organic	8 oz	45	0	0	0	-0	0	0	–	9

FOOD	PORTION	CALS	TOTAL FAT	CHOL	SAT FAT	POLY FAT	MONO FAT	TRANS FAT	FIBER	SUGAR
Volcano										
Organic Lemon Burst	2 tbsp (1 oz)	0	0	0	0	0	0	0	0	0
LEMONADE										
MIX										
Crystal Light										
Sugar Free as prep	8 oz	5	0	0	0	0	0	0	0	0
READY-TO-DRINK										
Honest Ade										
Classic Zero Calorie	8 oz	0	0	0	0	0	0	0	0	0
Minute Maid										
Just 15 Calories	8 oz	15	0	0	0	0	0	0	–	2
Lemonade	8 oz	110	0	0	0	0	0	0	–	28
Pink Light	8 oz	15	0	0	0	0	0	0	–	3
Santa Cruz										
Organic Peach	8 oz	100	0	0	0	0	0	0	0	25
Organic Strawberry	8 oz	90	0	0	0	0	0	0	–	22
Simply										
Lemonade	8 oz	120	0	0	0	0	0	0	–	28
Spindrift										
Sparkling	8 oz	80	0	0	0	0	0	0	0	19
Sunkist										
Sparkling	8 oz	110	0	0	0	0	0	0	–	29
Tropicana										
Trop50 Raspberry	8 oz	50	0	0	0	0	0	0	–	12
V8										
V-Fusion Strawberry	1 can (8.4 oz)	60	0	0	0	0	0	0	0	11
Welch's										
Sparkling	8 oz	140	0	0	0	0	0	0	–	35
LEMONGRASS										
fresh	1 tbsp	5	tr	0	tr	tr	tr	0	–	–
LENTILS										
dried cooked	1 cup	230	1	0	tr	tr	tr	0	16	4
TAKE-OUT										
lentil loaf	1 slice (1.6 oz)	83	4	0	tr	2	1	–	3	1
middle eastern lentil salad	1 serv (4.5 oz)	158	3	0	tr	–	–	–	–	–
yemiser selatta ethiopian lentil salad	1 serv (3 oz)	115	7	0	1	–	–	–	2	1

FOOD	PORTION	CALS	TOTAL FAT	CHOL	SAT FAT	POLY FAT	MONO FAT	TRANS FAT	FIBER	SUGAR
LETTUCE (see also SALAD)										
arugula	6 leaves (0.4 oz)	3	tr	0	tr	tr	tr	0	tr	tr
arugula shredded	1 cup	5	tr	0	tr	tr	tr	0	tr	tr
boston	1 head (5.7 oz)	21	tr	0	tr	tr	tr	0	2	2
boston chopped	6 leaves	7	tr	0	tr	tr	tr	0	1	1
cornsalad field salad	1 cup (1.9 oz)	7	tr	0	–	–	–	–	1	–
iceberg	1 lg head (26.5 oz)	106	1	0	tr	1	tr	0	9	15
iceberg	6 med leaves	7	tr	0	tr	tr	tr	0	1	1
iceberg shredded	1 cup	10	tr	0	tr	tr	tr	0	1	1
looseleaf outer leaves	6 (5 oz)	22	tr	0	tr	tr	tr	0	2	1
looseleaf shredded	1 cup	5	tr	0	tr	tr	tr	0	1	tr
red leaf	6 leaves (3.6 oz)	16	tr	0	tr	tr	tr	0	1	tr
red leaf shredded	1 cup	4	tr	0	tr	tr	tr	0	tr	tr
romaine	3 leaves (3 oz)	14	tr	0	tr	tr	tr	0	2	1
romaine heart	6 leaves (1.3 oz)	6	tr	0	tr	tr	tr	0	1	tr
romaine shredded	1 cup	8	tr	0	tr	tr	tr	0	1	1
Dole										
Just Lettuce	1½ cups (3 oz)	15	0	0	0	0	0	0	1	1
Romaine Chopped	1½ cups (3 oz)	15	0	0	0	0	0	0	1	2
Mann's										
Green Leaf Singles	6 leaves (3 oz)	15	0	0	0	0	0	0	2	2
Ready Pac										
Baby Arugula	4 cups (3 oz)	20	0	0	0	0	0	0	1	2
Shredded Iceberg	1 cup (3 oz)	10	0	0	0	0	0	0	1	1
Simply Lettuce	2½ cups (3 oz)	15	0	0	0	0	0	0	1	1
River Ranch										
Iceberg Shreds	2 cups (3 oz)	10	0	0	0	0	0	0	1	2
LIMA BEANS										
CANNED										
lima beans	½ cup	95	tr	0	tr	tr	tr	0	6	–
Del Monte										
Green	½ cup (4.4 oz)	80	0	0	0	0	0	0	4	0
DRIED										
cooked	½ cup	150	tr	0	tr	tr	tr	0	5	1
LIME										
fresh	1 (2.4 oz)	20	tr	0	tr	tr	tr	0	1	1
wedge	1 (8 g)	2	tr	0	tr	tr	tr	0	tr	tr

FOOD	PORTION	CALS	TOTAL FAT	CHOL	SAT FAT	POLY FAT	MONO FAT	TRANS FAT	FIBER	SUGAR
Sunkist										
Fresh	1 med (2.4 oz)	20	0	0	0	0	0	0	2	0
LIME JUICE										
bottled	1 oz	6	tr	0	tr	tr	tr	0	tr	tr
fresh	1 oz	8	tr	0	tr	tr	tr	0	tr	1
from 1 lime	1.1 oz	11	tr	0	tr	tr	tr	0	tr	1
Honest Ade										
Limeade	8 oz	48	0	0	0	0	0	0	–	12
Minute Maid										
Limonada Limeade	8 oz	120	0	0	0	0	0	0	–	31
Sunkist										
Cherry Limeade	8 oz	120	0	0	0	0	0	0	–	29
Volcano										
Organic Lime Burst	2 tbsp (1 oz)	0	0	0	0	0	0	0	0	0
Welch's										
Sparkling Limeade Raspberry	8 oz	140	0	0	0	0	0	0	–	33
LINGCOD										
baked	3 oz	93	1	57	tr	tr	tr	–	0	0
fillet baked	5.3 oz	164	2	101	tr	1	1	–	0	0
LIQUOR (see ALCOHOL DRINKS, BEER AND ALE, CHAMPAGNE, MALT, WINE)										
LIVER (see also PATE)										
beef braised	1 slice (2.4 oz)	130	4	269	1	tr	tr	0	0	0
beef pan-fried	1 slice (2.8 oz)	142	4	309	1	1	tr	0	0	0
chicken fried	3 oz	146	5	479	2	1	1	0	0	0
chicken simmered	3 oz	142	6	479	2	1	1	0	0	0
duck raw	1 (1.5 oz)	60	2	227	1	tr	tr	–	0	–
goose raw	1 (3.3 oz)	125	4	484	1	tr	1	–	0	–
lamb braised	3 oz	187	7	426	3	1	2	0	0	–
lamb fried	3 oz	202	11	419	4	2	2	–	0	–
moose braised	3 oz	132	4	331	–	1	1	0	–	–
pork braised	3 oz	140	4	302	1	1	1	0	0	–
turkey simmered	1 liver (2.9 oz)	227	17	322	6	2	8	0	0	0
veal braised	1 slice (2.8 oz)	154	5	409	2	1	1	0	0	0
veal pan fried	1 slice (2.4 oz)	129	4	325	1	1	1	0	0	0
TAKE-OUT										
calves liver w/ onions	1 serv (5 oz)	177	4	335	1	1	1	0	1	2

FOOD	PORTION	CALS	TOTAL FAT	CHOL	SAT FAT	POLY FAT	MONO FAT	TRANS FAT	FIBER	SUGAR
LLAMA										
llama	3 oz	120	3	60	–	–	–	–	–	–
LOBSTER										
northern cooked	1 cup	142	1	104	tr	tr	tr	–	–	–
northern cooked	3 oz	83	1	61	tr	tr	tr	–	–	–
northern raw	1 lobster (5.3 oz)	136	1	143	–	–	–	–	–	–
northern raw	3 oz	77	1	81	–	–	–	–	–	–
spiny steamed	1 (5.7 oz)	233	3	146	tr	1	1	–	–	–
spiny steamed	3 oz	122	2	76	tr	1	tr	–	–	–
TAKE-OUT										
newburg	1 cup	485	27	455	–	–	–	–	–	–
LOGANBERRIES										
fresh	½ cup (2.5 oz)	40	tr	0	tr	tr	tr	0	4	6
frzn thawed	½ cup (2.6 oz)	40	tr	0	tr	tr	tr	0	4	6
LONGANS										
fresh	1	2	0	0	0	0	0	0	–	–
LOQUATS										
fresh	1 lg (0.7 oz)	9	tr	0	tr	tr	tr	0	tr	–
fresh	1 sm (0.5 oz)	6	tr	0	tr	tr	tr	0	tr	–
fresh cubed	½ cup (2.6 oz)	35	tr	0	tr	tr	tr	0	1	–
LOTUS										
root raw sliced	10 slices	45	tr	0	tr	tr	tr	–	–	–
root sliced cooked	10 slices	59	tr	0	tr	tr	tr	–	–	–
seeds dried	1 oz	94	1	0	tr	tr	tr	–	–	–
LOX (see SALMON)										
LUPINES										
dried cooked	1 cup	197	5	0	1	1	2	–	–	–
LYCHEES										
canned in syrup	1 (0.7 oz)	19	tr	0	tr	tr	tr	0	tr	5
canned in syrup	½ cup (4.4 oz)	114	tr	0	tr	tr	tr	0	1	28
dried	1 (2.5 g)	7	tr	0	tr	tr	tr	0	tr	2
fresh	1 (0.3 oz)	6	tr	0	tr	tr	tr	0	tr	1
fresh cut up	½ cup (3.3 oz)	63	tr	0	tr	tr	tr	0	1	14

FOOD	PORTION	CALS	TOTAL FAT	CHOL	SAT FAT	POLY FAT	MONO FAT	TRANS FAT	FIBER	SUGAR
MACADAMIA NUTS										
dry roasted w/ salt	11 nuts (1 oz)	200	22	0	4	1	17	–	1	2
oil roasted	1 oz	204	22	0	3	tr	17	–	–	–
MACE										
ground	1 tsp	8	1	0	tr	tr	tr	0	tr	–
MACKEREL										
CANNED										
jack	1 cup	296	12	150	4	3	4	–	0	0
jack	1 can (12.7 oz)	563	23	285	7	6	8	–	0	0
Chicken Of The Sea										
Jack In Water	⅓ cup	90	4	55	2	–	–	–	0	0
FRESH										
atlantic cooked	3 oz	223	15	64	4	4	6	–	0	0
atlantic raw	3 oz	174	12	60	3	4	3	–	0	0
jack baked	3 oz	171	9	51	2	2	3	–	0	0
jack fillet baked	6.2 oz	354	18	106	5	4	6	–	0	0
king baked	3 oz	114	2	58	tr	1	1	–	0	0
king fillet baked	5.4 oz	207	4	105	1	1	2	–	0	0
pacific baked	3 oz	171	9	51	2	2	3	–	0	0
pacific fillet baked	6.2 oz	354	18	106	5	4	6	–	0	0
spanish cooked	3 oz	134	5	62	2	2	2	–	0	0
spanish fillet cooked	1 (5.1 oz)	230	9	107	3	3	3	–	0	0
spanish raw	3 oz	118	5	65	2	1	1	–	0	0
SMOKED										
atlantic	3.5 oz	296	24	93	5	5	12	–	0	0
MAHI MAHI										
fresh baked	4 oz	192	13	49	4	2	4	0	0	tr
MALANGA										
dasheen mashed	1 cup	226	tr	0	tr	tr	tr	–	8	1
dasheen pieces boiled	1 cup	212	tr	0	tr	tr	tr	–	8	1
pieces fried	1 cup	304	11	0	2	3	5	–	8	1
root raw	1 (10.7 oz)	299	1	0	tr	–	–	–	5	–
MALT										
malt liquor	1 bottle (12 oz)	148	0	0	0	0	0	0	tr	tr

FOOD	PORTION	CALS	TOTAL FAT	CHOL	SAT FAT	POLY FAT	MONO FAT	TRANS FAT	FIBER	SUGAR
nonalcoholic	1 bottle (12 oz)	133	tr	0	tr	tr	tr	–	0	29

MALTED MILK

chocolate as prep w/ milk	1 cup	179	5	16	3	tr	1	–	1	15
chocolate flavor powder	3 heaping tsp (0.7 oz)	79	1	0	tr	tr	tr	–	1	5
natural flavor as prep w/ milk	1 cup	186	6	21	3	tr	2	–	tr	22
natural flavor powder	3 heaping tsp (0.7 oz)	87	2	7	1	tr	tr	–	tr	12

MAMMY APPLE

fresh	1	431	4	0	–	–	–	–	–	–

MANGO

dried	½ cup (1.8 oz)	74	tr	0	tr	tr	tr	0	3	38
dried	1 slice (5 g)	16	tr	0	tr	tr	tr	0	tr	4
fresh	1 (7.3 oz)	135	1	0	tr	tr	tr	0	4	31
fresh sliced	½ cup (3 oz)	54	tr	0	tr	tr	tr	0	2	12
pickled	1 slice (1 oz)	38	tr	0	tr	tr	tr	0	tr	9
Crunchies										
Freeze Dried	¼ cup (6 g)	20	0	0	0	0	0	0	1	3
Crunchy N'Yummy										
Organic Freeze Dried	1 pkg (1 oz)	100	0	0	0	0	0	0	tr	0
Del Monte										
Diced In Light Syrup	1 pkg (4 oz)	70	0	0	0	0	0	0	1	17
Dole										
Chunks frzn	¾ cup (4.9 oz)	90	0	0	0	0	0	0	2	21
Fresh	½ (3.6 oz)	70	0	0	0	0	0	0	2	15

MANGO JUICE

nectar canned	1 cup (8.8 oz)	128	tr	0	tr	tr	tr	0	1	31
It Tastes RAAW										
Mango Guarana	8 oz	90	0	0	0	0	0	0	0	25
Naked										
Mighty Mango	8 oz	150	0	0	0	0	0	0	0	30
Old Orchard										
Nectar Cocktail	8 oz	75	0	0	0	0	0	0	–	17
TreeTop										
100% Juice	8 oz	190	0	0	0	0	0	0	3	34
Ultra Lo-Gly										
Mango Mojito	1 bottle (10 oz)	35	0	0	0	0	0	0	0	7

FOOD	PORTION	CALS	TOTAL FAT	CHOL	SAT FAT	POLY FAT	MONO FAT	TRANS FAT	FIBER	SUGAR
Welch's										
Mango Twist Cocktail	8 oz	150	0	0	0	0	0	0	–	37
MANGOSTEEN										
canned in syrup	½ cup (3.4 oz)	72	1	0	–	–	–	0	2	–
Nature's Guru										
Instant Mangosteen Fruit Powder	1 pkg (0.9 oz)	70	0	0	0	0	0	0	0	3
Xango										
Single Supplement	1 pkg (1 oz)	13	0	0	0	0	0	0	–	3
MARGARINE										
margarine butter blend	1 tbsp (0.5 oz)	101	11	2	2	3	4	2	0	0
squeeze	1 pkg (0.2 oz)	36	4	0	1	2	1	–	0	0
squeeze liquid	1 tbsp (0.5 oz)	102	11	0	2	5	4	–	0	0
stick	1 stick (4 oz)	810	91	0	17	27	44	17	0	0
stick	1 tbsp (0.5 oz)	100	11	0	2	3	5	2	0	0
tub diet	1 tbsp (0.5 oz)	26	3	0	tr	1	1	–	0	0
tub fat free	1 tbsp (0.5 oz)	27	tr	0	tr	tr	tr	tr	0	0
tub light	1 tbsp (0.5 oz)	59	7	0	1	3	2	1	0	–
tub salted	1 tbsp (0.5 oz)	101	11	0	2	4	5	1	0	0
whipped salted	1 tbsp (0.3 oz)	67	8	0	1	3	3	–	0	0
Blue Bonnet										
Light Stick	1 tbsp (0.5 oz)	50	5	0	1	2	2	1	0	0
Soft Spread	1 tbsp (0.5 oz)	60	6	0	1	3	2	0	0	0
Soft Spread Light	1 tbsp (0.5 oz)	40	5	0	1	2	1	0	0	0
Sticks	1 tbsp (0.5 oz)	70	8	0	2	3	2	2	0	0
Brummel & Brown										
Spread w/ Natural Yogurt	1 tbsp (0.5 oz)	45	5	0	2	3	1	0	0	0
I Can't Believe It's Not Butter										
Original	1 tbsp (0.5 oz)	70	8	0	2	4	2	–	0	0
Original Soft	1 tbsp (0.5 oz)	70	8	0	2	4	2	0	0	0
Spray	2 sprays (1 g)	0	0	0	0	0	0	0	0	0
Olivio										
Original Olive Oil	1 tbsp (0.5 oz)	80	8	0	2	2	5	0	0	0
Parkay										
Original Spread	1 tbsp (0.4 oz)	70	7	0	2	4	2	0	0	0
Spray	5 sprays (1 g)	0	0	0	0	0	0	0	0	0
Squeeze	1 tbsp (0.5 oz)	70	8	0	2	5	2	0	0	0
Stick	1 tbsp (0.5 oz)	80	9	0	2	3	3	2	0	0

FOOD	PORTION	CALS	TOTAL FAT	CHOL	SAT FAT	POLY FAT	MONO FAT	TRANS FAT	FIBER	SUGAR
Smart Balance										
Buttery Sticks Omega-3	1 tbsp (0.5 g)	100	11	15	5	2	3	0	0	0
MARINADE (see SAUCE)										
MARIONBERRY JUICE										
TreeTop										
Grower's Best 100% Juice	8 oz	130	0	0	0	0	0	0	–	30
MARJORAM										
dried	1 tsp	2	tr	0	tr	tr	tr	0	tr	tr
MARSHMALLOW										
chocolate coated	1 (0.4 oz)	41	1	0	1	tr	tr	–	tr	6
coconut coated	1 (0.4 oz)	33	1	0	tr	tr	tr	–	tr	5
marshmallow regular	1 (0.3 oz)	23	tr	0	tr	tr	tr	0	0	4
miniatures	10 (0.3 oz)	22	tr	0	tr	tr	tr	0	0	4
miniatures	1 cup (1.8 oz)	159	tr	0	tr	tr	tr	0	tr	29
MATZO										
brie	1 piece (0.5 oz)	54	3	21	1	1	1	0	tr	3
egg	1 (1 oz)	109	1	23	tr	tr	tr	0	1	–
matzo ball	1 med (1.2 oz)	48	2	36	tr	tr	1	0	tr	tr
plain	1 (1 oz)	111	tr	0	tr	tr	tr	0	1	–
whole wheat	1 (1 oz)	98	tr	0	tr	tr	tr	0	3	–
Manischewitz										
Egg	1 (1.2 oz)	100	0	0	0	0	0	0	0	0
Everything	1 (1 oz)	80	0	0	0	0	0	0	0	1
Farfel	¼ cup (0.6 oz)	70	0	0	0	0	0	0	0	1
Matzo	1 (1 oz)	110	0	0	0	0	0	0	0	0
Matzo Meal	¼ cup (1 oz)	110	0	0	0	0	0	0	1	1
Matzo Meal Whole Grain	¼ cup (1 oz)	120	1	0	0	–	–	0	4	1
Whole Wheat	1 (1 oz)	110	1	0	0	–	–	0	3	0
MAYONNAISE										
imitation	1 tbsp	35	3	4	tr	2	1	0	0	1
light	1 tbsp (0.5 oz)	36	3	2	1	2	1	tr	0	1
mayonnaise	2 tbsp (1 oz)	188	21	12	3	12	5	tr	0	1
Cains										
All Natural	1 tbsp (0.5 oz)	100	11	5	2	–	–	0	0	0
Fat Free	1 tbsp (0.5 oz)	10	0	0	0	0	0	0	0	1
Light	1 tbsp (0.5 oz)	50	5	5	0	–	–	0	0	1
Sandwich Spread	1 tbsp (0.5 oz)	70	7	5	1	–	–	0	0	2

FOOD	PORTION	CALS	TOTAL FAT	CHOL	SAT FAT	POLY FAT	MONO FAT	TRANS FAT	FIBER	SUGAR
w/ Olive Oil	1 tbsp (0.5 oz)	50	5	5	1	3	2	0	0	tr
Nasoya										
Nayonaise Original	1 tbsp (0.5 oz)`	35	4	1	0	–	–	0	0	0
Spectrum										
Canola Squeeze	1 tbsp (0.5 oz)	100	11	5	1	4	7	0	0	0
Canola Squeeze Light Eggless Vegan	1 tbsp (0.5 oz)	35	4	0	0	1	3	0	0	0

MEAT SUBSTITUTES (see also BACON SUBSTITUTES, CHICKEN SUBSTITUTES, HAMBURGER SUBSTITUTES, MEATBALL SUBSTITUTES, SAUSAGE SUBSTITUTES, TURKEY SUBSTITUTES)

FOOD	PORTION	CALS	TOTAL FAT	CHOL	SAT FAT	POLY FAT	MONO FAT	TRANS FAT	FIBER	SUGAR
Quorn										
Beef-Style Grounds	⅔ cup (3 oz)	90	2	0	1	1	1	0	5	1
Viana										
Veggie Doner Kebab	½ cup (3 oz)	210	14	0	3	–	–	1	2	2

MEATBALL SUBSTITUTES

FOOD	PORTION	CALS	TOTAL FAT	CHOL	SAT FAT	POLY FAT	MONO FAT	TRANS FAT	FIBER	SUGAR
meatless	2 (1.3 oz)	71	3	0	1	2	1	–	2	tr
Franklin Farms										
Portabella Veggiballs Gluten Free	3 (3 oz)	140	1	0	0	–	–	0	4	3
Morningstar Farms										
Meal Starters Veggie Meatballs	5 (2.8 oz)	130	5	0	1	3	1	0	3	tr
Nate's										
Classic	3 (1.5 oz)	90	5	0	0	–	–	0	2	tr
Savory Mushroom	3 (1.5 oz)	100	5	0	0	–	–	0	2	tr
Zesty Italian	3 (1.5 oz)	90	5	0	0	–	–	0	2	tr
Quorn										
Meatless Meatballs	3-4 (2.4 oz)	90	2	5	1	1	1	0	1	1
Tandoor Chef										
Malai Kofta	½ pkg (5 oz)	260	17	60	7	–	–	0	0	9

MEATBALLS

FOOD	PORTION	CALS	TOTAL FAT	CHOL	SAT FAT	POLY FAT	MONO FAT	TRANS FAT	FIBER	SUGAR
beef cocktail	1 (0.2 oz)	18	1	6	tr	tr	1	–	0	0
beef lg	1 (1.5 oz)	111	7	37	3	tr	3	–	0	0
beef med	1 (1 oz)	74	5	25	2	tr	2	–	0	0
chicken cocktail	1 (0.2 oz)	12	tr	6	tr	tr	tr	–	0	tr
chicken lg	1 (1.5 oz)	71	3	36	1	1	1	–	tr	1
chicken med	1 (1 oz)	47	2	24	tr	tr	1	–	tr	1
turkey med	1 (1 oz)	47	2	24	tr	tr	1	–	tr	1
venison	1 (1.5 oz)	69	3	37	1	1	tr	–	tr	1

FOOD	PORTION	CALS	TOTAL FAT	CHOL	SAT FAT	POLY FAT	MONO FAT	TRANS FAT	FIBER	SUGAR
Al Fresco										
Chicken Teriyaki Ginger	4 (3 oz)	200	8	75	3	–	–	0	0	8
Chicken Tomato & Basil	4 (3 oz)	160	9	65	3	–	–	0	0	2
Coleman										
Chicken Buffalo Style	4	160	12	60	4	–	–	0	0	0
Chicken Chipotle Cheddar	4 (2.6 oz)	180	14	55	4	–	–	0	0	0
Chicken Italian w/ Parmesan	7 (2.6 oz)	150	10	60	3	–	–	0	1	0
Chicken Pesto Parmesan	4 (2.6 oz)	170	12	60	4	–	–	0	0	0
Chicken Spinach Fontina Cheese & Roasted Garlic	4 (2.6 oz)	130	9	55	3	–	–	0	0	0
Chicken Sun-Dried Tomato Basil & Provolone	4 (2.6 oz)	150	9	65	3	–	–	0	0	0
Dinty Moore										
Meatball Stew	½ can	250	15	40	6	–	–	–	1	3
Farm Rich										
Original	6 (3 oz)	240	20	45	8	–	–	0	2	1
Turkey	5 (3.1 oz)	150	9	55	4	–	–	–	2	1
Foster Farms										
Turkey	3 (2.9 oz)	150	7	40	–	–	–	0	0	tr
Hans All Natural										
Chicken Buffalo Style	4	160	12	60	4	–	–	0	0	0
Chicken Sweet Basil Parmesan	4	170	12	60	4	–	–	0	0	0
Mom Made										
Bite-Size Turkey	9 (3 oz)	140	4	65	2	–	–	0	0	1
Saffron Road										
Lamb Koftis w/ Rice	1 pkg (11 oz)	340	11	30	3	–	–	0	4	8
Shady Brook										
Turkey Meatballs Appetizer Size + Sweet & Sour Sauce	6 + 2 tbsp sauce	235	10	65	3	–	–	0	tr	11
TAKE-OUT										
albondigas w/ sauce	3 + sauce (5.3 oz)	372	27	102	8	6	10	–	1	3
porcupine w/ tomato sauce	3 + sauce	160	7	34	3	tr	3	–	1	3
swedish w/ cream sauce	3 + sauce (4.7 oz)	215	12	86	5	1	5	–	tr	2
sweet & sour	3 + sauce (4.5 oz)	188	11	67	3	tr	5	–	1	1

MEXICAN FOOD (see SALSA, SPANISH FOOD, TORTILLA)

FOOD	PORTION	CALS	TOTAL FAT	CHOL	SAT FAT	POLY FAT	MONO FAT	TRANS FAT	FIBER	SUGAR
MILK										
CANNED										
condensed sweetened	1 cup (10.7 oz)	982	27	104	17	1	7	–	0	166
condensed sweetened	1 tbsp (0.7 oz)	61	2	6	1	tr	tr	–	0	10
evaporated nonfat	1 tbsp (0.5 oz)	12	tr	1	tr	tr	tr	–	1	2
evaporated nonfat	1 cup (9 oz)	200	1	10	tr	tr	tr	–	0	29
Borden										
Sweetened Condensed	2 tbsp (1.4 oz)	130	3	10	2	–	–	0	0	22
Meyenberg										
Goat Evaporated	4 oz	145	8	27	5	2	tr	–	–	10
DRIED										
buttermilk	1 tbsp (0.2 oz)	25	tr	4	tr	tr	tr	–	0	3
buttermilk	¼ cup (1 oz)	111	2	20	1	tr	tr	–	0	14
nonfat instant	1 tbsp (0.6 oz)	61	tr	3	tr	tr	tr	–	0	9
nonfat instant	1 pkg (3.2 oz)	326	1	16	tr	tr	tr	–	0	47
whole milk	¼ cup (1.1 oz)	159	9	31	5	tr	3	–	0	12
Meyenberg										
Goat Powdered	1 scoop (1 oz)	90	0	10	0	–	–	0	0	11
REFRIGERATED										
1%	1 cup (8.6 oz)	102	3	12	2	tr	1	–	0	13
2%	1 cup (8.6 oz)	122	5	20	3	tr	1	–	0	12
buttermilk lowfat	1 cup (8.6 oz)	98	2	10	1	tr	1	–	0	12
fat free	1 cup (8.6 oz)	83	tr	5	tr	tr	tr	–	0	12
goat	1 cup (8.6 oz)	168	10	27	7	tr	3	–	0	11
human	1 cup (8.6 oz)	172	11	34	5	1	4	–	0	7
indian buffalo	1 cup (8.6 oz)	237	17	46	11	tr	4	–	0	–
sheep	1 cup (8.6 oz)	265	17	66	11	1	4	–	0	–
whole	1 cup (8.6 oz)	149	8	24	5	tr	2	–	0	12
Lactaid										
Fit & Creamy Lowfat	8 oz	120	3	15	2	–	–	0	0	12
Whole	8 oz	160	8	35	5	–	–	0	0	12
Meyenberg										
Goat Low Fat	8 oz	89	2	8	2	1	tr	–	–	9
Goat Whole	8 oz	142	7	25	4	2	tr	–	–	11
Over The Moon										
Fat Free	8 oz	120	0	5	0	0	0	0	0	16
Straus										
Organic Cream Top Whole	8 oz	150	8	35	5	–	–	0	0	11
Organic Fat Free	8 oz	90	0	5	0	0	0	0	0	12
Organic Whole Milk	8 oz	170	7	35	5	–	–	0	0	7

FOOD	PORTION	CALS	TOTAL FAT	CHOL	SAT FAT	POLY FAT	MONO FAT	TRANS FAT	FIBER	SUGAR
MILK DRINKS										
chocolate milk	1 cup (8.8 oz)	208	8	30	5	tr	2	–	2	24
chocolate milk lowfat	1 cup (8.8 oz)	158	3	8	2	tr	1	–	1	25
DrSears										
Cool Fuel Chocolate	1 pkg (8 oz)	190	6	0	1	–	–	0	4	9
Cool Fuel Chocolate Banana	1 pkg (8 oz)	190	6	0	1	–	–	0	4	9
Cool Fuel Vanilla	1 pkg (8 oz)	190	6	0	1	–	–	0	4	9
Lactaid										
Chocolate Milk 1% Fat	8 oz	150	3	15	2	–	–	0	tr	23
MojoMilk										
Chocolate Mix not prep	1 pkg (4.5 g)	20	1	0	0	–	–	0	0	2
Probiotic Chocolate Milk not prep	1 pkg (4.5 g)	20	1	0	0	–	–	0	0	2
Rockin' Recovery										
Intense Recovery Protein Fortified Lowfat Milk Chocolate	1 bottle (12 oz)	300	5	30	3	–	–	0	1	44
Intense Recovery Protein Fortified Lowfat Milk Vanilla	1 bottle (12 oz)	280	4	30	3	–	–	0	0	42
Muscle Builder Protein Fortified Milk Chocolate	1 bottle (12 oz)	190	5	30	3	–	–	0	3	6
Muscle Recovery Protein Fortified Lowfat Milk Chocolate No Sugar Added	1 bottle (12 oz)	240	4	20	3	–	–	0	1	23
Refuel Protein Fortified Lowfat Milk Strawberry	1 bottle (12 oz)	280	4	30	3	–	–	0	0	42
TruMoo										
Chocolate Milk Fat Free	8 oz	130	0	5	0	0	0	0	0	22
Chocolate Milk Lowfat	8 oz	150	3	10	2	–	–	0	0	22
Strawberry Milk Fat Free	8 oz	130	0	5	0	–	–	0	0	22
MILK SUBSTITUTES										
soy milk	1 cup	79	5	0	1	2	1	–	–	–
Good Karma										
Flax Milk Original	8 oz	60	3	0	0	2	0	0	0	11
Flax Milk Unsweetened	8 oz	25	3	0	0	2	0	0	0	0
Flax Milk Vanilla	8 oz	60	3	0	0	2	0	0	0	11
Whole Grain Rice Original Organic	8 oz	100	3	0	0	1	2	0	3	9

FOOD	PORTION	CALS	TOTAL FAT	CHOL	SAT FAT	POLY FAT	MONO FAT	TRANS FAT	FIBER	SUGAR
Whole Grain Rice Vanilla Organic	8 oz	120	3	0	0	1	2	0	3	13
Pacific Foods										
7 Grain Original Organic	1 cup (8 oz)	140	2	0	0	–	–	0	1	16
Almond Original Unsweetened Organic	8 oz	35	3	0	0	–	–	0	0	0
Hazelnut Original	8 oz	110	4	0	0	–	–	0	1	14
Hemp Original	8 oz	140	5	0	1	4	1	0	1	14
Oat Original Organic	1 cup (8 oz)	130	3	0	0	–	–	0	2	19
Rice All Natural Plain	1 cup (8 oz)	130	2	0	0	–	–	0	0	14
Soy Original Unsweetened Organic	1 cup (8 oz)	90	5	0	1	–	–	0	2	2
Soy Ultra Plain	1 cup (8 oz)	120	4	0	1	–	–	0	1	8
Simpli										
Naked Oat Vanilla	8 oz	100	3	0	0	–	–	0	2	10
Sol										
Sunflower Original	8 oz	70	4	0	1	–	–	0	1	7
Sunflower Unsweetened	8 oz	45	4	0	1	–	–	0	1	0
Sunflower Vanilla	8 oz	90	4	0	1	–	–	0	1	12
Sunrich Naturals										
Soymilk Original Plain	8 oz	110	5	0	1	3	1	0	1	9
Soymilk Vanilla	8 oz	130	5	0	1	3	1	0	1	11
Vitasoy										
Organic Lite Plus Original	8 oz	60	2	0	tr	1	tr	0	0	5
Organic Lite Plus Vanilla	8 oz	80	2	0	tr	1	tr	0	0	11
Organic Mint Chocolate	8 oz	160	4	0	1	3	1	0	1	24
Organic Original	8 oz	90	4	0	1	2	1	0	1	7
Organic Vanilla	8 oz	110	4	0	1	2	1	0	1	12

MILKFISH (AWA)

FOOD	PORTION	CALS	TOTAL FAT	CHOL	SAT FAT	POLY FAT	MONO FAT	TRANS FAT	FIBER	SUGAR
baked	4 oz	215	10	76	–	–	–	–	0	0

MILKSHAKE

FOOD	PORTION	CALS	TOTAL FAT	CHOL	SAT FAT	POLY FAT	MONO FAT	TRANS FAT	FIBER	SUGAR
chocolate	1 serv (10.6 oz)	357	8	33	5	tr	2	–	1	63
malted milk shake	1 serv (10 oz)	402	14	51	8	1	4	–	1	58
vanilla	1 (11 oz)	351	9	38	6	tr	3	–	0	56
Special K										
Protein Shake Dark Chocolate	1 bottle (10 oz)	190	5	0	1	–	–	0	5	18

FOOD	PORTION	CALS	TOTAL FAT	CHOL	SAT FAT	POLY FAT	MONO FAT	TRANS FAT	FIBER	SUGAR
MILLET										
cooked	1 cup (6.1 oz)	207	2	0	tr	1	tr	–	2	–
MINERAL WATER (see WATER)										
MISO										
miso	½ cup	284	8	0	1	5	2	–	7	–
MOLASSES										
blackstrap	1 tbsp (0.7 oz)	47	0	0	0	0	0	0	–	–
molasses	¼ cup (3 oz)	244	tr	0	tr	tr	tr	–	0	47
molasses	1 tbsp (0.7 oz)	58	tr	0	tr	tr	tr	0	0	11
MONKFISH										
baked	3 oz	82	2	27	–	–	–	–	0	0
MOOSE										
roasted	4 oz	142	1	83	tr	tr	tr	0	0	0
MOTH BEANS										
dried cooked	1 cup	207	1	0	tr	tr	tr	–	–	–
MOUSSE										
TAKE-OUT										
chocolate	½ cup	454	32	283	18	2	10	–	1	30
fish timbale	1 cup	329	25	210	15	1	7	–	0	1
MUFFIN										
FROZEN										
Garden Lites										
Veggie Muffins Zucchini Chocolate	1 (2 oz)	120	4	20	2	–	–	0	5	11
MIX										
Jiffy										
Banana as prep	1	170	6	42	2	–	–	0	tr	10
Bran w/ Dates as prep	1	160	6	42	2	–	–	0	2	9
Corn as prep	1	170	6	39	2	–	–	0	tr	7
Oatmeal as prep	1	170	6	45	3	–	–	0	tr	8
TAKE-OUT										
blueberry	1 (5 oz)	546	27	56	5	13	7	0	2	38
corn	1 lg (5 oz)	424	12	36	2	4	3	–	5	10
oat bran	1 lg (5 oz)	375	10	0	2	6	2	–	6	11
pumpkin w/ raisins & nuts	1 med (4 oz)	351	8	81	1	3	3	–	2	43

FOOD	PORTION	CALS	TOTAL FAT	CHOL	SAT FAT	POLY FAT	MONO FAT	TRANS FAT	FIBER	SUGAR
MULBERRIES										
fresh	20 (1 oz)	13	tr	0	tr	tr	tr	0	1	2
fresh	½ cup (2.5 oz)	30	tr	0	tr	tr	tr	0	1	6
MULLET										
striped cooked	3 oz	127	4	54	1	1	1	–	0	0
striped raw	3 oz	99	3	42	1	1	1	–	0	0
MUNG BEANS										
dried cooked	1 cup	213	1	0	tr	tr	tr	–	–	–
MUNGO BEANS										
dried cooked	1 cup	190	1	1	tr	1	tr	–	–	–
MUSHROOMS										
CANNED										
caps	8 (1.6 oz)	12	tr	0	tr	tr	tr	0	1	1
caps pickled	6 (0.8 oz)	5	tr	0	tr	tr	0	0	tr	tr
chanterelle	3.5 oz	12	1	0	–	–	–	–	6	–
pickled	1 cup	33	tr	0	tr	tr	0	0	1	2
pieces	½ cup	20	tr	0	tr	tr	tr	0	1	1
straw	1 cup	58	1	0	tr	tr	tr	0	5	–
Jake & Amos										
Pickled Dill Mushrooms	1 serv (1 oz)	5	0	0	0	0	0	0	tr	0
Victoria										
Marinated	¼ cup (1 oz)	20	2	0	0	–	–	0	0	0
DRIED										
chanterelle	1 oz	25	tr	0	–	–	–	–	17	–
shiitake	1 (3.6 g)	11	tr	0	tr	tr	tr	0	tr	tr
tree ear	½ cup (0.4 oz)	36	tr	0	–	–	–	–	–	–
FRESH										
brown italian or crimini sliced	1 cup	19	tr	0	tr	tr	tr	0	tr	1
brown italian or crimini whole	1 (0.7 oz)	5	tr	0	tr	tr	0	0	tr	tr
chanterelle	3.5 oz	11	tr	0	–	–	–	–	6	–
enoki raw	1 lg (5 g)	2	tr	0	tr	tr	0	0	tr	tr
enoki sliced	1 cup	29	tr	0	tr	tr	tr	0	2	tr
enoki whole	1 cup	28	tr	0	tr	tr	tr	0	2	tr
maitake diced	1 cup	26	tr	0	tr	tr	tr	0	2	1
maitake whole	1 (6.6 g)	2	tr	0	tr	tr	tr	0	tr	tr
morel	3.5 oz	9	tr	0	–	–	–	–	7	–

FOOD	PORTION	CALS	TOTAL FAT	CHOL	SAT FAT	POLY FAT	MONO FAT	TRANS FAT	FIBER	SUGAR
oyster	1 sm (0.5 oz)	5	tr	0	tr	tr	tr	0	tr	tr
oyster sliced	1 cup	30	tr	0	tr	tr	tr	0	2	1
portabella raw	1 cap (3 oz)	22	tr	0	tr	tr	tr	0	1	2
portabella sliced grilled	1 cup (4.2 oz)	42	1	0	tr	tr	0	0	3	0
shiitake cooked	4 (2.5 oz)	40	tr	0	tr	tr	tr	0	2	3
shiitake pieces cooked	1 cup	81	tr	0	tr	tr	tr	0	3	5
white	1 (0.6 oz)	4	tr	0	tr	tr	tr	0	tr	tr
white sliced cooked	1 cup	28	tr	0	tr	tr	tr	0	2	0
white sliced raw	½ cup	8	tr	0	tr	tr	tr	0	tr	1
Dole										
Raw	½ cup (1.2 oz)	9	0	0	0	0	0	0	0	0
FROZEN										
Alexia										
Mushroom Bites w/ Roasted Garlic & Olive Oil	¼ pkg (2 oz)	110	5	0	1	3	1	0	2	tr
Farm Rich										
Breaded	5 (3 oz)	120	2	0	0	–	–	0	1	0
TAKE-OUT										
battered fried	1 lg (0.6 oz)	39	3	1	tr	1	1	–	tr	1
creamed	1 cup	171	11	7	3	3	4	–	3	7
stuffed	1 (0.8 oz)	67	4	3	1	1	1	–	1	1
MUSSELS										
blue raw	3 oz	73	2	24	tr	1	tr	–	–	–
blue raw	1 cup	129	3	42	1	1	1	–	–	–
fresh blue cooked	3 oz	147	4	48	1	1	1	–	–	–
MUSTARD										
dry mustard	1 tsp	15	1	0	tr	tr	1	–	–	–
hot chinese	1 tsp	3	tr	0	tr	tr	tr	0	tr	tr
organic yellow	1 tsp	5	0	0	0	0	0	0	0	0
seed	1 tsp	15	1	0	tr	tr	1	0	1	tr
yellow prepared	1 tbsp	3	tr	0	tr	tr	tr	0	tr	tr
Annie's Homegrown										
Organic Dijon	1 tsp (5 g)	5	0	0	0	0	0	0	–	–
Beaver										
Hickory Bacon	1 tsp (5 g)	10	0	0	0	0	0	0	0	0
Gold's										
New York Deli	1 tsp (5 g)	0	0	0	0	0	0	0	0	0
Inglehoffer										
Organic Honey	1 tsp (5 g)	10	0	0	0	0	0	0	–	2
Organic Stone Ground	1 tsp (5)	10	0	0	0	0	0	0	–	–

FOOD	PORTION	CALS	TOTAL FAT	CHOL	SAT FAT	POLY FAT	MONO FAT	TRANS FAT	FIBER	SUGAR
Jack & Amos										
Sweet Dipping	1 tbsp (0.5 oz)	30	1	10	0	–	–	0	0	4
OrganicVille										
Stone Ground No Sugar Added	1 tbsp (5 g)	5	0	0	0	0	0	0	0	0
Zatarain's										
Creole	1 tsp (7 g)	10	1	0	–	–	–	–	0	0
MUSTARD GREENS										
canned	1 cup	23	tr	0	tr	tr	tr	0	3	tr
fresh as prep w/ fat	1 cup	50	3	0	1	1	1	–	3	tr
fresh chopped boiled w/o salt	1 cup	21	tr	0	tr	tr	tr	0	3	tr
fresh raw chopped	1 cup	15	tr	0	tr	tr	tr	0	2	1
frozen chopped boiled w/o salt	1 cup	28	tr	0	tr	tr	tr	0	4	tr
NAVY BEANS										
canned	1 cup	296	1	0	tr	tr	tr	–	–	–
dried cooked	1 cup	259	1	0	tr	tr	tr	–	–	–
NECTARINE										
fresh	1 sm (4.5 oz)	57	tr	0	tr	tr	tr	0	2	10
fresh	1 lg (5.5 oz)	69	1	0	tr	tr	tr	0	3	12
fresh sliced	1 cup (5 oz)	63	tr	0	tr	tr	tr	0	2	11
Dole										
Fresh	1 med (5 oz)	60	0	0	0	0	0	0	2	11
NEUFCHATEL										
neufchatel	1 pkg (3 oz)	215	19	63	11	1	5	–	0	3
neufchatel	1 oz	72	6	21	4	tr	2	–	0	1
Philadelphia										
⅓ Less Fat	1 oz	70	6	20	4	–	–	0	0	1
NOODLES										
cellophane	1 cup	492	tr	0	tr	tr	tr	–	–	–
chow mein	1 cup (1.6 oz)	237	14	0	2	7	3	–	2	–
egg	1 cup (38 g)	145	2	36	tr	tr	tr	–	–	–
egg cooked	1 cup (5.6 oz)	213	2	53	tr	1	1	–	2	–
japanese soba cooked	1 cup (4 oz)	113	tr	0	tr	tr	tr	–	–	–
japanese somen cooked	1 cup (6.2 oz)	231	tr	0	tr	tr	tr	–	–	–
rice cooked	1 cup (6.2 oz)	192	tr	0	tr	tr	tr	–	2	–
spinach/egg cooked	1 cup (5.6 oz)	211	3	53	1	1	1	–	4	–

FOOD	PORTION	CALS	TOTAL FAT	CHOL	SAT FAT	POLY FAT	MONO FAT	TRANS FAT	FIBER	SUGAR
Light 'N Fluffy										
Egg Extra Wide not prep	⅙ pkg (2 oz)	210	3	70	1	–	–	0	2	2
Manischewitz										
Egg Fine not prep	1½ cups (2 oz)	210	3	60	1	–	–	0	2	2
Whole Grain Yolk Free Extra Wide not prep	1¼ cups (2 oz)	180	1	0	0	–	–	0	6	2
Yolk Free Medium	1¾ cups (2 oz)	210	1	0	0	–	–	–	2	2
Pennsylvania Dutch										
Fine Egg not prep	1 cup (2 oz)	220	3	65	1	–	–	0	2	2
Thai Kitchen										
Red Rice	¼ pkg (2 oz)	200	1	0	0	–	–	0	1	1

NUT BUTTERS (see also individual nut names, PEANUT BUTTER)

FOOD	PORTION	CALS	TOTAL FAT	CHOL	SAT FAT	POLY FAT	MONO FAT	TRANS FAT	FIBER	SUGAR
NuttZo										
Omega-3 Organic Seven Nut & Seed Butter	2 tbsp (1.1 oz)	180	16	0	2	–	–	0	3	1
Omega-3 Organic Seven Nut & Seed Butter Dark Chocolate	2 tbsp (1.1 oz)	180	13	0	2	–	–	0	3	1
Omega-3 Organic Seven Nut & Seed Butter No Peanuts	2 tbsp (1.1 oz)	110	15	0	3	–	–	0	3	1

NUTMEG

FOOD	PORTION	CALS	TOTAL FAT	CHOL	SAT FAT	POLY FAT	MONO FAT	TRANS FAT	FIBER	SUGAR
ground	1 tsp	12	1	0	1	tr	tr	0	1	1
nutmeg butter	1 tbsp	120	14	0	12	0	1	–	0	0

NUTRITION SUPPLEMENTS (see also CEREAL BARS, ENERGY BARS, ENERGY DRINKS)

FOOD	PORTION	CALS	TOTAL FAT	CHOL	SAT FAT	POLY FAT	MONO FAT	TRANS FAT	FIBER	SUGAR
BANa										
Hydration Drink	1 bottle (16.9 oz)	0	0	0	0	0	0	0	–	–
Be Happy										
Health Guard	1 bottle (2 oz)	40	0	0	0	0	0	0	0	9
Fiber One										
Protein Bar Caramel Nut	1 (1.17 oz)	130	6	0	3	–	–	0	5	7
Protein Bar Coconut Almond	1 (1.17 oz)	140	6	0	4	–	–	0	5	7
Joint Juice										
Cranberry Pomegranate	1 bottle (8 oz)	20	0	0	0	0	0	0	–	2
Easy Shot Glucosamine Chondroitin	2.5 tbsp (1.25 oz)	15	0	0	0	0	0	0	–	2
Easy Shot Hyal-Joint	2.5 tbsp (1.25 oz)	15	0	0	0	0	0	0	–	2
On The Go Blueberry Acai	1 pkg (6 g)	20	0	0	0	0	0	0	–	–

FOOD	PORTION	CALS	TOTAL FAT	CHOL	SAT FAT	POLY FAT	MONO FAT	TRANS FAT	FIBER	SUG
Orgain										
Organic Meal Replacement All Flavors	1 pkg (11 oz)	255	7	20	0	–	–	0	2	12
Premier										
Protein Shake Chocolate	1 (11 oz)	160	3	25	1	–	–	0	3	1
Protein Shake Strawberry	1 (11 oz)	160	3	25	1	–	–	0	2	1
Protein Shake Vanilla	1 (11 oz)	160	3	25	1	–	–	0	2	1
Special K										
Protein Meal Bar Chocolate Caramel	1 (1.59 oz)	170	5	0	4	–	–	0	5	15
NUTS MIXED (see also individual names)										
dry roasted w/ peanuts salted	¼ cup	203	18	0	2	4	11	0	3	–
dry roasted w/ peanuts w/o salt	¼ cup	203	18	0	2	4	11	0	3	–
mixed nuts chocolate covered	¼ cup (1.5 oz)	240	17	5	7	–	–	–	2	17
oil roasted w/ peanuts salted	1 oz	172	15	0	2	4	8	tr	2	1
oil roasted w/o peanuts salted	1 oz	172	14	0	2	4	8	0	2	1
oil roasted w/o peanuts w/o salt	¼ cup	221	20	0	3	4	12	0	2	–
Frito Lay										
Deluxe Mixed	¼ cup	170	16	0	3	–	–	0	2	1
Planters										
Bar Big Triple Nut	1 (1.6 oz)	220	12	0	2	–	–	0	3	12
Lightly Salted	1 oz	170	15	0	2	–	8	0	2	1
Mixed	1 oz	170	15	0	2	–	8	0	2	1
Nut-rition Men's Health	28 (1 oz)	170	15	0	2	4	8	0	3	1
Unsalted	1 oz	170	15	0	2	–	–	0	2	1
Simple Squares										
Nut & Honey Bar Rosemary	1 (1.6 oz)	230	17	0	5	–	–	0	3	10
Nut & Honey Bar Sage	1 (1.6 oz)	230	17	0	5	–	–	0	3	10
Whole Food Bar Cinnamon Clove	1 (1.6 oz)	230	17	0	5	–	–	0	3	9
OCTOPUS										
dried boiled	3 oz	144	2	84	tr	tr	tr	–	0	0
fresh steamed	3 oz	139	2	81	tr	tr	tr	–	0	0

FOOD	PORTION	CALS	TOTAL FAT	CHOL	SAT FAT	POLY FAT	MONO FAT	TRANS FAT	FIBER	SUGAR
smoked	1 oz	40	1	23	tr	tr	tr	–	0	0
Matiz										
Pulpo In Olive Oil	½ pkg (2 oz)	107	5	36	1	–	–	0	0	0
TAKE-OUT										
ensalada de pulpo	1 cup	299	21	52	3	2	14	–	2	4

OHELOBERRIES

FOOD	PORTION	CALS	TOTAL FAT	CHOL	SAT FAT	POLY FAT	MONO FAT	TRANS FAT	FIBER	SUGAR
fresh	1 cup	39	tr	0	–	–	–	–	–	–

OIL

FOOD	PORTION	CALS	TOTAL FAT	CHOL	SAT FAT	POLY FAT	MONO FAT	TRANS FAT	FIBER	SUGAR
almond	1 tbsp	120	14	0	1	2	10	–	0	0
almond	1 cup	1927	218	0	1	2	10	–	0	0
apricot kernel	1 cup	1927	218	0	14	64	131	–	0	0
apricot kernel	1 tbsp	120	14	0	1	4	8	–	0	0
avocado	1 tbsp	124	14	0	2	2	10	–	0	0
avocado	1 cup	1927	218	0	25	29	154	–	0	0
babassu palm	1 tbsp	120	14	0	11	tr	2	–	0	0
butter oil	1 cup	1795	204	524	127	8	59	–	0	0
butter oil	1 tbsp	112	13	33	8	1	4	–	0	0
canola	1 tbsp	124	14	0	2	3	8	–	0	0
canola	1 cup	1927	218	0	15	65	128	–	0	0
coconut	1 tbsp	117	14	0	12	tr	1	0	0	0
corn	1 cup (7.6 oz)	1962	218	0	28	119	60	–	0	0
corn	1 tbsp (0.5 oz)	122	14	0	2	7	4	–	0	0
cottonseed	1 cup	1927	218	0	56	113	39	–	0	0
cottonseed	1 tbsp	120	14	0	4	7	2	–	0	0
cupu assu	1 tbsp	120	14	0	7	1	5	–	0	0
grapeseed	1 tbsp	120	14	0	1	10	2	0	0	0
hazelnut	1 cup	1927	218	0	1	1	11	–	0	0
hazelnut	1 tbsp	120	14	0	1	1	11	–	0	0
mustard	1 cup	1927	218	0	25	46	129	–	0	0
mustard	1 tbsp	124	14	0	2	3	8	–	0	0
oat	1 tbsp	120	14	0	3	6	5	–	0	0
olive	1 tbsp	119	14	0	2	1	10	–	0	0
olive	1 cup	1909	216	0	26	18	159	–	0	0
palm	1 tbsp	120	14	0	7	1	5	–	0	0
palm	1 cup	1927	218	0	107	20	81	–	0	0
palm kernel	1 cup	1879	218	0	178	3	25	–	0	0
palm kernel	1 tbsp	117	14	0	11	tr	2	–	0	0
peanut	1 tbsp	119	14	0	2	4	6	–	0	0
peanut	1 cup	1909	216	0	36	69	100	–	0	0

FOOD	PORTION	CALS	TOTAL FAT	CHOL	SAT FAT	POLY FAT	MONO FAT	TRANS FAT	FIBER	S
peppermint	1 tsp	42	4	0	–	–	–	–	0	0
poppyseed	1 tbsp	120	14	0	2	9	3	–	0	0
rice bran	1 tbsp	120	14	0	3	5	5	–	0	0
safflower	1 cup	1927	218	0	20	162	26	–	0	0
safflower	1 tbsp	120	14	0	1	10	2	–	0	0
sesame	1 tbsp	120	14	0	2	6	5	–	0	0
sheanut	1 tbsp	120	14	0	6	1	6	–	0	0
soybean	1 cup	1927	218	0	31	126	51	–	0	0
soybean	1 tbsp	120	14	0	2	8	3	–	0	0
sunflower	1 cup	1927	218	0	23	143	43	–	0	0
sunflower	1 tbsp	120	14	0	1	9	3	–	0	0
teaseed	1 tbsp	120	14	0	3	3	7	–	0	0
tomatoseed	1 tbsp	120	14	0	3	7	3	–	0	0
vegetable	1 cup	1927	218	0	2	7	4	–	0	0
vegetable	1 tbsp	120	14	0	2	7	4	–	0	0
walnut	1 tbsp	120	14	0	1	9	3	–	0	0
walnut	1 cup	1927	218	0	20	138	50	–	0	0
wheat germ	1 tbsp	120	14	0	3	8	2	–	0	0
Bella Sun Luci										
Olive Extra Virgin Cold Pressed	1 tbsp (0.5 oz)	120	14	0	2	–	–	0	0	0
Carotino										
Palm Fruit Oil	1 tbsp (0.5 oz)	121	14	0	6	2	7	0	0	0
Red Palm & Canola	1 tbsp	120	14	0	2	3	8	0	0	0
Pam										
All Varieties	¼ sec spray	0	0	0	0	0	0	0	0	0
Penny's PopSurprise										
Organic Extra Virgin Olive Spicy	1 tbsp (0.5 oz)	130	14	0	2	3	9	0	0	0
Pillsbury										
Baking Spray w/ Flour	⅙ sec spray	0	0	0	0	0	0	0	0	0
Planters										
100% Pure Peanut	1 tbsp (0.5 oz)	120	14	0	3	–	6	0	0	0
Pompeian										
Olive	1 tbsp	130	14	0	–	–	–	–	–	–
Sadaf										
Avocado Cold Pressed	1 tbsp (0.5 oz)	130	14	0	2	3	9	0	0	0
Grapeseed	1 tbsp (0.5 oz)	120	14	0	2	10	3	0	0	0
Light Olive	1 tbsp (0.5 oz)	120	14	0	2	1	11	0	0	0

FOOD	PORTION	CALS	TOTAL FAT	CHOL	SAT FAT	POLY FAT	MONO FAT	TRANS FAT	FIBER	SUGAR
Sonoma Gourmet										
Dip-N-Toss Olive Oil Basil Parmesan	1 tbsp (0.5 oz)	120	13	0	0	2	–	0	0	0
Spectrum										
Almond	1 tbsp (0.5 oz)	120	14	0	1	4	9	0	0	0
Apricot Kernel	1 tbsp (0.5 oz)	120	14	0	1	4	9	0	0	0
Avocado	1 tbsp (0.5 oz)	120	14	0	2	2	10	0	0	0
Coconut Organic	1 tbsp (0.5 oz)	120	14	0	12	1	1	0	0	0
Flaxseed w/ Lemon	1 tbsp (0.5 oz)	120	14	0	2	10	3	0	–	–
Grapeseed	1 tbsp (0.5 oz)	120	14	1	1	10	3	0	0	0
Olive Organic	1 tbsp (0.5 oz)	120	14	0	2	2	11	0	0	0
Sesame	1 tbsp (0.5 oz)	120	14	0	2	6	6	0	0	0
Walnut	1 tbsp (0.5 oz)	120	14	0	2	9	3	0	0	0
OKRA										
CANNED										
pickled	6 pods (2.3 oz)	18	tr	0	tr	tr	tr	0	2	1
FRESH										
cooked w/ salt	8 pods	19	tr	0	tr	tr	tr	0	2	2
luffa chinese okra cooked	1 cup	39	tr	0	tr	tr	tr	0	4	4
sliced cooked w/ salt	½ cup	18	tr	0	tr	tr	tr	0	2	2
TAKE-OUT										
batter dipped fried	10 pieces (2.6 oz)	142	10	2	1	5	3	–	2	3
OLIVES										
black	2 med (0.3 oz)	8	1	0	tr	1	tr	0	tr	0
greek	1 (0.5 oz)	16	1	0	tr	1	tr	0	tr	0
green	2 lg (0.3 oz)	11	1	0	tr	tr	1	0	tr	tr
green	1 sm (0.2 oz)	8	1	0	tr	tr	1	0	tr	tr
green	2 med (0.2 oz)	10	1	0	tr	tr	1	0	tr	tr
green	2 extra lg (0.5 oz)	19	2	0	tr	tr	1	0	tr	tr
green chopped	¼ cup (1.2 oz)	48	5	0	1	tr	4	0	1	tr
green olive tapenade	1 tbsp	25	3	0	0	–	–	–	0	1
green stuffed	2 lg (0.3 oz)	12	1	0	tr	1	tr	0	tr	tr
green stuffed	2 med (0.3 oz)	10	1	0	tr	1	tr	0	tr	tr
green stuffed	¼ cup (1.3 oz)	47	5	0	1	tr	4	0	1	tr
green stuffed	2 sm (0.2 oz)	9	1	0	tr	tr	1	0	tr	tr
ripe	2 sm (0.2 oz)	7	1	0	tr	tr	0	0	tr	0

FOOD	PORTION	CALS	TOTAL FAT	CHOL	SAT FAT	POLY FAT	MONO FAT	TRANS FAT	FIBER	SUG
ripe	2 extra lg (0.4 oz)	12	1	0	tr	tr	tr	0	tr	0
ripe	2 lg (0.3 oz)	10	1	0	tr	tr	tr	0	tr	0
ripe sliced	¼ cup (1.2 oz)	35	3	0	tr	tr	2	0	1	0
spanish stuffed	5 (0.5 oz)	15	1	0	0	–	–	–	0	0
Kelly's Kitchen										
Blue Cheese Stuffed	2 (0.8 oz)	30	3	5	1	–	–	0	0	0
Matiz										
Olivada Spread Sweet	2 tbsp	87	6	0	1	–	–	0	1	9
Olivada Spread Traditional & Hot	2 tbsp	114	12	0	3	–	–	0	2	tr
Priorat Natur										
Natural Olives	10	30	3	0	0	–	–	0	1	tr
Progresso										
Tapenade	1 tbsp (0.5 oz)	20	2	0	0	–	–	0	0	0
Victoria										
Almond Stuffed	2 (0.5 oz)	25	3	0	–	0	2	0	0	0
Calamata	2 (0.5 oz)	30	3	0	1	0	–	0	2	0
Gaeta	3 (0.5 oz)	45	3	0	1	0	–	0	0	0
Jalapeno Stuffed	2 (0.5 oz)	20	2	0	–	0	1	0	0	0
Manzanilla Stuffed	5 (0.5 oz)	25	3	0	–	0	1	0	0	0
Queen Stuffed	2 (0.5 oz)	20	2	0	–	0	1	0	0	0
Zatarain's										
Cocktail	7 (0.5 oz)	25	3	0	1	–	–	–	0	0
Stuffed	6 (0.5 oz)	25	3	0	1	–	–	–	0	0
ONION										
CANNED										
cocktail	½ cup	41	tr	0	tr	tr	tr	–	2	4
DRIED										
flakes	1 tbsp	17	tr	0	tr	tr	tr	–	1	2
powder	1 tsp	7	tr	0	tr	tr	tr	–	tr	1
shallots	1 tbsp	3	0	0	0	0	0	0	–	–
FRESH										
cooked w/o salt	1 med (3.3 oz)	41	tr	0	tr	tr	tr	–	1	4
cooked w/o salt	1 sm (2 oz)	26	tr	0	tr	tr	tr	–	1	3
cooked w/o salt	1 lg (4.5 oz)	56	tr	0	tr	tr	tr	–	2	6
cooked w/o salt chopped	1 tbsp	7	tr	0	tr	tr	tr	–	tr	1
raw chopped	½ cup	32	tr	0	tr	tr	tr	–	1	3
raw chopped	1 tbsp	4	tr	0	tr	tr	tr	–	tr	tr

FOOD	PORTION	CALS	TOTAL FAT	CHOL	SAT FAT	POLY FAT	MONO FAT	TRANS FAT	FIBER	SUGAR
raw slice	1 (0.5 oz)	6	tr	0	tr	tr	tr	–	tr	1
raw sliced	½ cup	23	tr	0	0	tr	tr	–	1	2
scallions raw	1 med (0.5 oz)	5	tr	0	tr	tr	tr	–	tr	tr
scallions raw chopped	¼ cup	8	tr	0	tr	tr	tr	–	1	1
shallots raw chopped	¼ cup	29	tr	0	tr	tr	tr	–	–	–
sweet whole raw	1 (11.6 oz)	106	tr	0	tr	tr	tr	–	3	17
whole raw	1 med (4 oz)	44	tr	0	tr	tr	tr	–	2	5
whole raw	1 lg (5.3 oz)	60	tr	0	tr	tr	tr	–	3	6
whole raw	1 sm (2.5 oz)	28	tr	0	tr	tr	tr	–	1	3
Bland Farms										
Vidalia Sweet	1 (5 oz)	60	0	0	0	0	0	0	3	5
RealSweet										
Vidalia	1 (5.2 oz)	45	0	0	0	0	0	0	3	9
FROZEN										
Alexia										
Crispy Onion w/ Panko Breading & Sea Salt	6 (3 oz)	240	13	0	2	8	3	0	2	2
Onion Rings Multigrain w/ Sea Salt	6 (3 oz)	110	12	0	2	7	3	0	2	2
TAKE-OUT										
creamed	1 cup	187	9	7	2	3	4	–	2	10
fried	½ cup	57	5	0	–	–	–	–	1	tr
rings breaded & fried	8 to 9 (3 oz)	276	16	14	7	1	7	–	–	–

ORANGE
CANNED
Del Monte

FOOD	PORTION	CALS	TOTAL FAT	CHOL	SAT FAT	POLY FAT	MONO FAT	TRANS FAT	FIBER	SUGAR
Mandarin In Light Syrup	1 pkg (4 oz)	70	0	0	0	0	0	0	–	17
Mandarin No Sugar Added	½ cup (4.3 oz)	45	0	0	0	0	0	0	1	6
Dole										
Mandarin In Fruit Juice	1 pkg (4 oz)	80	0	0	0	0	0	0	1	18
FRESH										
california valencia	1 (4.2 oz)	59	tr	0	tr	tr	tr	0	3	–
california valencia sections	½ cup (3.2 oz)	44	tr	0	tr	tr	tr	0	2	–
cara cara navel	1 (5.4 oz)	80	0	0	0	0	0	0	3	14
florida	1 (5.3 oz)	69	tr	0	tr	tr	tr	0	4	14
florida sections	½ cup (3.2 oz)	43	tr	0	tr	tr	tr	0	2	8
fresh	1 med (4.6 oz)	62	tr	0	tr	tr	tr	0	3	12
fresh	1 sm (3.4 oz)	45	tr	0	tr	tr	tr	0	2	9
fresh	1 lg (6.5 oz)	86	tr	0	tr	tr	tr	0	4	17

FOOD	PORTION	CALS	TOTAL FAT	CHOL	SAT FAT	POLY FAT	MONO FAT	TRANS FAT	FIBER	SUG
navel	1 (4.9 oz)	69	tr	0	tr	tr	tr	0	3	12
navel sections	1 cup (5.8 oz)	81	tr	0	tr	tr	tr	0	4	14
peel	1 tbsp (0.2 oz)	3	tr	0	tr	tr	tr	0	1	tr
Dole										
Orange	1 med (4.2 oz)	60	0	0	0	0	0	0	3	13
Sunkist										
Cara Cara	1 med (5.4 oz)	80	0	0	0	0	0	0	3	14
Mandarin	1 (2.2 oz)	40	0	0	0	0	0	0	tr	8
Minneola Tangelo	1 (3.8 oz)	70	1	0	0	–	–	0	2	9
Moro	1 (5.4 oz)	70	1	0	0	–	–	0	3	14
Navel	1 med (5.4 oz)	80	0	0	0	0	0	0	3	14
Satsuma Mandarin	1 (3.8 oz)	50	0	0	0	0	0	0	2	10

ORANGE JUICE

FOOD	PORTION	CALS	TOTAL FAT	CHOL	SAT FAT	POLY FAT	MONO FAT	TRANS FAT	FIBER	SUG
chilled bottled	1 cup (8.7 oz)	112	1	0	tr	tr	tr	0	1	21
fresh	1 cup (8.7 oz)	112	1	0	tr	tr	tr	0	1	21
Dole										
100% Juice w/ Calcium	8 oz	120	0	0	0	0	0	0.	0	–
Genesis Today										
Omega Orange 100% Juice	8 oz	90	0	0	0	0	0	0	3	13
Italian Volcano										
Organic Blood Orange	8 oz	101	0	0	0	0	0	0	–	23
Izze										
Esque Sparkling Mandarin	1 bottle (12 oz)	50	0	0	0	0	0	0	–	11
Minute Maid										
100% Juice Heart Wise	8 oz	110	0	0	0	0	0	0	–	24
100% Juice No Pulp	8 oz	110	0	0	0	0	0	0	–	22
100% Juice w/ Calcium & Vitamin D	8 oz	110	0	0	0	0	0	0	–	24
Orangeade	8 oz	110	0	0	0	0	0	0	–	30
Old Orchard										
100% Juice	8 oz	130	0	0	0	0	0	0	–	29
Tropicana										
100% Juice	8 oz	110	0	0	0	0	0	0	–	22
TAKE-OUT										
orange julius	1 cup (9.2 oz)	212	tr	0	tr	tr	tr	–	tr	35

OREGANO

FOOD	PORTION	CALS	TOTAL FAT	CHOL	SAT FAT	POLY FAT	MONO FAT	TRANS FAT	FIBER	SUG
crumbled	1 tsp	3	tr	0	tr	tr	tr	0	tr	tr
ground	1 tsp	6	tr	0	tr	tr	tr	0	1	tr

FOOD	PORTION	CALS	TOTAL FAT	CHOL	SAT FAT	POLY FAT	MONO FAT	TRANS FAT	FIBER	SUGAR
ORGAN MEATS (see BRAINS, GIBLETS, GIZZARDS, HEART, KIDNEY, LIVER, SWEETBREAD)										
OROBLANCO										
Sunkist										
Fresh	½ (5.4 oz)	100	1	0	0	–	–	0	4	11
OSTRICH										
cooked	4 oz	195	8	92	2	1	2	–	0	0
cooked diced	1 cup (4.7 oz)	215	9	111	2	1	3	–	0	0
OYSTERS										
canned eastern	1 cup	112	4	89	1	1	tr	0	0	0
eastern baked	6 med	47	1	22	tr	tr	tr	0	0	–
eastern raw	6 med	50	1	21	tr	tr	tr	0	0	–
eastern sauteed	6 med	76	5	36	1	2	2	0	0	0
smoked	6	33	1	26	tr	tr	tr	0	0	0
Chicken Of The Sea										
Smoked In Oil	1 can (3.75 oz)	170	8	45	2	–	–	–	0	0
Whole	¼ can (2 oz)	80	3	35	1	–	–	–	0	0
TAKE-OUT										
breaded & fried	6	368	18	108	5	5	7	0	–	–
fritter	1 (1.4 oz)	121	6	36	1	2	3	0	tr	tr
oysters rockefeller	1 cup	302	17	90	8	2	5	0	4	2
stew	1 cup	208	13	78	8	1	3	0	0	9
PANCAKE/WAFFLE SYRUP										
light	¼ cup	98	0	0	0	0	0	0	0	20
pancake syrup	¼ cup	209	tr	0	tr	tr	tr	–	0	50
pancake syrup	1 pkg (2 oz)	156	tr	0	tr	tr	tr	–	0	38
Ali's All Natural										
All Flavors	¼ cup (2 oz)	5	0	0	0	0	0	0	tr	0
IHOP At Home										
Blueberry	¼ cup (2.1 oz)	200	0	0	0	0	0	0	–	21
Lite	¼ cup (2.1 oz)	110	0	0	0	0	0	0	–	26
Original	¼ cup (2.1 oz)	220	0	0	0	0	0	0	–	28
Strawberry	¼ cup (2.1 oz)	200	0	0	0	0	0	0	–	23
Sugar Free	¼ cup (2.1 oz)	20	0	0	0	0	0	0	–	0
Log Cabin										
Lite	¼ cup (2 oz)	100	0	0	0	0	0	0	–	22
Smucker's										
Breakfast Syrup Sugar Free	¼ cup (2.1 oz)	20	0	0	0	0	0	0	–	0

FOOD	PORTION	CALS	TOTAL FAT	CHOL	SAT FAT	POLY FAT	MONO FAT	TRANS FAT	FIBER	SUGAR
PANCAKES										
FROZEN										
Aunt Jemima										
Blueberry	3 (3.7 oz)	260	6	25	1	–	–	0	1	13
Buttermilk	3 (3.7 oz)	250	6	30	1	–	–	0	1	9
Buttermilk Lowfat	3 (3.6 oz)	200	2	25	0	–	–	0	1	8
Oatmeal	3 (3.7 oz)	230	4	25	2	–	–	0	4	11
Whole Grain	3 (3.6 oz)	240	6	20	1	–	–	0	3	9
Dr. Praeger's										
Sweet Potato Bites	1 (2 oz)	80	2	0	0	–	–	0	3	6
MIX										
Maple Grove Farms										
Buttermilk & Honey as prep	1	220	7	69	1	–	–	0	tr	36
Mix Gluten Free as prep	1	200	8	60	2	–	–	0	2	4
TAKE-OUT										
bu chu jun korean w/ vegetables	1 (4 oz)	83	4	21	1	1	1	–	1	–
buckwheat	1 (7 in)	142	5	45	1	1	2	0	2	4
norwegian lefse	1 (9 in) (2.7 oz)	163	5	8	2	1	1	–	2	2
pindaettok korean mung bean	1 (3.9 oz)	204	11	3	2	4	5	–	6	–
plain	1 (7 in)	183	3	7	1	1	1	0	1	10
potato	1 (1.3 oz)	70	4	26	1	1	2	0	1	tr
whole wheat	1 (7 in)	183	8	47	2	3	3	0	3	5
PANCREAS (see SWEETBREAD)										
PANINI (see SANDWICHES)										
PAPAYA										
canned in syrup	½ cup (2.3 oz)	50	tr	0	tr	tr	tr	0	1	11
dried	1 strip (0.8 oz)	59	tr	0	tr	tr	tr	0	3	9
fresh	1 sm (5.3 oz)	59	tr	0	tr	tr	tr	0	3	9
fresh	1 lg (13.3 oz)	148	1	0	tr	tr	tr	0	7	22
fresh cubed	1 cup (4.9 oz)	55	tr	0	tr	tr	tr	0	3	8
green cooked	½ cup (2.3 oz)	18	tr	0	tr	tr	tr	0	1	3
Crunchy N'Yummy										
Organic Papaya	1 pkg (1 oz)	55	0	0	0	0	0	0	2	0
Dole										
Fresh	½ (4.9 oz)	60	0	0	0	0	0	0	3	9

FOOD	PORTION	CALS	TOTAL FAT	CHOL	SAT FAT	POLY FAT	MONO FAT	TRANS FAT	FIBER	SUGAR
PAPAYA JUICE										
nectar	1 cup (8.8 oz)	142	tr	0	tr	tr	tr	0	2	35
Old Orchard										
Nectar Cocktail	8 oz	75	0	0	0	0	0	0	–	17
PAPRIKA										
dried	1 tsp	1	tr	0	tr	tr	tr	0	tr	tr
PARSLEY										
dried	1 tbsp	4	tr	0	tr	tr	tr	0	1	tr
freeze dried	1 tbsp	1	tr	0	–	–	–	0	tr	–
fresh chopped	¼ cup	5	tr	0	tr	tr	tr	0	1	tr
fresh chopped	1 tbsp	1	tr	0	tr	tr	tr	0	tr	tr
fresh sprigs	5 (1.8 oz)	18	tr	0	tr	tr	tr	0	2	tr
PARSNIPS										
fresh sliced cooked w/o salt	½ cup (2.7 oz)	55	tr	0	tr	tr	tr	0	3	4
whole cooked	1 (5.6 oz)	114	tr	0	tr	tr	tr	0	6	8
TAKE-OUT										
creamed	1 cup (8 oz)	237	11	7	3	3	5	–	5	10
PASSION FRUIT										
fresh	1 (0.6 oz)	17	tr	0	tr	tr	tr	0	2	2
fresh cut up	½ cup (4.1 oz)	114	1	0	tr	tr	tr	0	12	13
PASSION FRUIT JUICE										
nectar	1 cup (8.8 oz)	168	tr	0	tr	tr	tr	0	tr	43
yellow lilikoi	1 cup (8.7 oz)	138	tr	0	tr	tr	tr	0	1	34
Welch's										
Passion Fruit Cocktail	8 oz	150	0	0	0	0	0	0	–	37
PASTA (see also NOODLES, PASTA DINNERS, PASTA SALAD)										
DRY										
corn cooked	1 cup (4.9 oz)	176	1	0	tr	tr	tr	–	7	–
elbows not prep	1 cup	389	2	0	tr	tr	tr	–	–	–
elbows cooked	1 cup (4.9 oz)	197	1	0	tr	tr	tr	–	2	–
shells small cooked	1 cup (4 oz)	162	1	0	tr	tr	tr	–	2	–
spaghetti cooked	1 cup (4.9 oz)	197	1	0	tr	tr	tr	–	2	–
spinach spaghetti cooked	1 cup (4.9 oz)	182	1	0	tr	tr	tr	–	–	–
spirals cooked	1 cup (4.7 oz)	189	tr	0	tr	tr	tr	–	2	–
vegetable cooked	1 cup (4.7 oz)	172	tr	0	tr	tr	tr	–	6	–
whole wheat all shapes cooked	1 cup	174	tr	0	tr	tr	tr	–	4	–

FOOD	PORTION	CALS	TOTAL FAT	CHOL	SAT FAT	POLY FAT	MONO FAT	TRANS FAT	FIBER	SUGAR
Barilla										
Lasagne not prep	2 pieces (1.8 oz)	180	0	0	0	–	–	0	2	1
Piccolini Mini Penne not prep	2 oz	210	1	0	0	–	–	0	6	2
Plus Spaghetti not prep	2 oz	210	2	0	0	1	1	0	4	2
Rotini Tri-Color	2 oz	200	1	0	0	–	–	0	2	2
Spaghetti Whole Grain not prep	1/7 box (2 oz)	200	2	0	0	–	–	0	6	2
Tortellini Three Cheese not prep	2/3 cup (2 oz)	230	8	35	3	–	–	0	3	2
Heartland										
Gluten Free not prep	2 oz	200	1	0	0	–	–	0	1	0
Naturals Penne not prep	3/4 cup (2 oz)	210	1	0	0	–	–	0	2	2
Perfect Balance Elbow Macaroni not prep	1/2 cup (2 oz)	200	1	0	0	–	–	0	3	2
Whole Wheat Rotini not prep	3/4 cup (2 oz)	210	2	0	0	–	–	0	5	2
Lundberg										
Organic Spaghetti Brown Rice not prep	2 oz	190	3	0	1	–	–	0	4	1
Mara's Pasta										
100% Whole Wheat not prep	2 oz	190	1	0	0	–	–	0	7	0
Mueller's										
100% Whole Grain Spaghetti not prep	1/7 pkg (2 oz)	200	2	0	0	1	0	0	5	2
Racconto										
Essentials Heart Health Rigatoni not prep	1/6 pkg (2 oz)	190	1	0	0	–	–	0	7	0
Rienzi										
Catanisella Lunga	2 oz	200	1	0	0	–	–	0	1	2
Ronzoni										
Alphabets not prep	1/3 cup (2 oz)	210	1	0	0	–	–	0	2	2
Garden Delight Rotini not prep	2 oz	200	1	0	0	–	–	0	2	3
Quick Cook Penne Rigate not prep	3/4 cup (2 oz)	210	1	0	0	–	–	0	2	2
Smart Taste Angel Hair not prep	1/7 pkg (2 oz)	170	1	0	0	–	–	0	5	1
Wacky Mac										
Veggie Bows not prep	1/6 pkg (2 oz)	200	1	0	0	–	–	0	1	0

FOOD	PORTION	CALS	TOTAL FAT	CHOL	SAT FAT	POLY FAT	MONO FAT	TRANS FAT	FIBER	SUGAR
FRESH										
cooked	2 oz	75	1	33	tr	tr	tr	–	–	–
spinach cooked	2 oz	74	1	19	tr	tr	tr	–	–	–
Buitoni										
Angel Hair	⅓ pkg (2.8 oz)	230	2	40	0	–	–	0	2	1
Ravioli Four Cheese	1 serv (3.7 oz)	340	12	55	4	–	–	0	3	2
Reserva Quattro Formaggi Agnolotti	1 serv (4.4 oz)	360	17	90	9	–	–	0	2	2
Tortellini Spinach Cheese	1 serv (3.7 oz)	320	7	55	4	–	–	0	3	4
Tortellini Whole Wheat Cheese	1 serv (3.7 oz)	330	10	60	3	–	–	0	6	3
Nasoya										
Pasta Zero Plus Shirataki Fettuccine or Spaghetti	⅔ cup (4 oz)	20	0	0	0	0	0	0	3	0
Pasta Prima										
Ravioli Butternut Squash	½ pkg (4 oz)	250	6	45	4	–	–	0	2	2
Ravioli Gluten Free Butternut Squash	1 cup (3.5 oz)	180	4	30	3	–	–	0	2	2
Ravioli Gluten Free Five Cheese	1 cup (3.5 oz)	230	10	55	6	–	–	0	2	1
Ravioli Italian Sausage	½ pkg (4 oz)	290	13	60	6	–	–	0	2	1
Ravioli Lobster	½ pkg (4 oz)	250	7	55	4	–	–	0	2	2
Ravioli Spinach & Cheese	1 cup (3.5 oz)	210	7	35	3	–	–	0	2	1
FROZEN										
Pasta Prima										
Ravioli Spinach & Mozzarella	1 cup (4 oz)	200	5	27	2	–	–	0	4	0
Solterra										
Fettuccine Gluten Free	⅓ pkg (4 oz)	330	6	150	2	–	–	0	3	1
Tofutti										
Ravioli Dairy Free	4 (3.2 oz)	210	10	0	3	–	–	0	1	1
PASTA DINNERS (see also PASTA SALAD)										
CANNED										
Annie's Homegrown										
Organic Cheesy Ravioli	1 cup (8.5 oz)	180	4	5	2	–	–	–	3	9
Organic P'sghetti Loops	1 cup (8.4 oz)	190	4	0	1	–	–	–	2	9
Chef Boyardee										
Beef Ravioli	1 cup (8.6 oz)	230	8	15	3	–	–	0	3	5
Beefaroni	1 cup (8.7 oz)	240	10	15	4	–	–	0	3	5
Spaghetti & Meat Balls	1 cup (9 oz)	260	11	15	4	–	–	0	4	7

FOOD	PORTION	CALS	TOTAL FAT	CHOL	SAT FAT	POLY FAT	MONO FAT	TRANS FAT	FIBER	SUGAR
SpaghettiOs										
Sliced Franks	1 cup (8.8 oz)	220	6	20	2	1	3	0	4	9
FROZEN										
Buitoni										
Braised Beef & Sausage Ravioli w/ Creamy Marinara Sauce	½ pkg (11.9 oz)	590	19	120	9	–	–	1	5	9
Chicken & Mushroom Ravioli w/ Marsala Wine Sauce	½ pkg (10.9 oz)	530	20	110	11	–	–	1	5	7
Four Cheese & Spinach Ravioli w/ Tomato Basil Sauce	½ pkg (12.9 oz)	550	21	100	12	–	–	1	7	12
Grilled Chicken w/Spinach Cannelloni w/Alfredo Sauce	½ pkg (10.9 oz)	560	26	145	15	–	–	1	3	7
Candle Cafe										
Macaroni & Vegan Cheese	1 pkg (9 oz)	300	12	0	5	–	–	0	5	tr
Tofu Spinach Ravioli	1 pkg (9 oz)	320	10	0	3	–	–	0	4	4
Healthy Choice										
Chicken Fettuccini Alfredo	1 pkg (11.4 oz)	300	7	45	3	2	3	0	7	16
Hearty Beef Stroganoff	1 pkg (10.9 oz)	280	7	40	3	1	3	0	6	17
Lobster Cheese Ravioli	1 pkg (8.9 oz)	270	6	15	3	1	2	0	4	9
Roasted Red Pepper Marinara	1 pkg (8.5 oz)	270	6	5	2	1	3	0	5	6
Tortellini Primavera Parmesan	1 pkg (8.9 oz)	240	5	20	2	1	2	0	6	7
Lean Cuisine										
Cafe Cuisine Three Cheese Stuffed Rigatoni	1 pkg (9 oz)	230	6	20	4	1	2	0	4	6
Dinnertime Selects Chicken Fettuccini	1 pkg (12 oz)	330	6	40	3	1	1	0	4	3
Market Creations Tortelloni Mushroom	1 pkg (10 oz)	280	7	30	3	1	1	0	5	7
Simple Favorites Alfredo Pasta w/ Chicken & Broccoli	1 pkg (10 oz)	300	6	30	3	1	1	0	3	5
Simple Favorites Angel Hair Pomodoro	1 pkg (10 oz)	250	5	5	2	1	1	0	4	10
Simple Favorites Cheese Ravioli	1 pkg (8.5 oz)	220	5	35	3	1	1	0	3	8

FOOD	PORTION	CALS	TOTAL FAT	CHOL	SAT FAT	POLY FAT	MONO FAT	TRANS FAT	FIBER	SUGAR
Simple Favorites Chicken Fettuccini	1 pkg (9.25 oz)	270	6	40	3	1	2	0	0	6
Simple Favorites Fettuccini Alfredo	1 pkg (9.25 oz)	330	7	15	3	2	1	0	3	6
Simple Favorites Lasagna Chicken Florentine	1 pkg (10 oz)	280	6	30	2	2	2	0	3	6
Simple Favorites Lasagna Classic Five Cheese	1 pkg (11.5 oz)	350	7	20	3	1	2	0	4	11
Simple Favorites Lasagna w/ Meat Sauce	1 pkg (10.5 oz)	320	8	30	4	0	2	0	4	8
Simple Favorites Macaroni & Cheese	1 pkg (10 oz)	290	7	20	4	1	2	0	1	7
Simple Favorites Spaghetti w/Meat Sauce	1 pkg (11.5 oz)	300	4	15	1	1	1	0	4	9
Simple Favorites Spaghetti w/Meatballs	1 pkg (9.5 oz)	270	6	25	2	1	2	0	3	6
Spa Cuisine Ravioli Butternut Squash	1 pkg (9.9 oz)	260	7	20	2	3	1	0	5	11
Mom Made										
Cheesy Mac	1 pkg (7 oz)	200	3	10	2	–	–	0	4	4
Spaghetti w/Turkey Meatballs & Sauce	1 pkg (7 oz)	180	4	35	1	–	–	–	3	3
Tabatchnick										
Macaroni & Cheese	1 serv (7.5 oz)	250	8	20	4	–	–	0	tr	4
Weight Watchers										
Chicken & Broccoli Alfredo	1 pkg (11.8 oz)	300	4	50	2	1	1	0	4	3
Smart Ones Sesame Chicken	1 pkg (11.8 oz)	360	7	30	1	3	2	0	6	10
Smart Ones Ziti w/Meatballs & Cheese	1 pkg (11.7 oz)	390	9	50	4	2	3	0	6	8
MIX										
Annie's Homegrown										
Gluten Free Rice Pasta & Cheddar as prep	1 cup	280	4	10	3	–	–	0	1	4
Mac & Cheese Lower Sodium as prep	1 cup	280	4	10	3	–	–	0	2	5
Organic 5-Grain Elbows & White Cheddar as prep	1 cup	270	4	10	2	–	–	0	3	5

FOOD	PORTION	CALS	TOTAL FAT	CHOL	SAT FAT	POLY FAT	MONO FAT	TRANS FAT	FIBER	SUGA
Organic Classic Mac & Cheese as prep	1 cup	280	4	10	2	–	–	0	2	5
Organic Peace Pasta & Parmesan as prep	1 cup	270	4	10	2	–	–	0	2	4
Organic Shells & Real Aged Wisconsin Cheddar as prep	1 cup	270	4	10	3	–	–	0	2	5
Organic Skillet Meals Beef Stroganoff as prep	1 cup	360	18	60	8	–	–	0	1	3
Organic Skillet Meals Cheesy Lasagna as prep	1 cup	440	18	81	9	–	–	0	1	6
Organic Skillet Meals Tuna Spirals as prep	1 cup	320	8	36	5	–	–	0	2	4
Shells & White Cheddar as prep	1 cup	270	5	10	2	–	–	0	2	5
Kraft										
Macaroni & Cheese White Cheddar as prep	⅓ pkg	380	15	10	4	–	–	0	0	7
Simply Shari's										
Mac & Cheese Gluten Free as prep	¼ pkg (4 oz)	280	6	15	3	–	–	0	2	1
REFRIGERATED										
Simply Sensible										
Lasagna w/ Meat Sauce	½ pkg (8 oz)	200	5	20	2	0	2	0	2	8
Mediterranean Style Chicken	1½ cups (7.2 oz)	250	6	20	1	–	–	0	2	3
SHELF-STABLE										
Barilla										
Mezze Penne w/ Tomato & Basil Sauce	1 pkg (9 oz)	320	5	0	1	–	–	0	6	8
Healthy Choice										
Balsamic Vegetable Medley	1 pkg (6.9 oz)	290	3	0	1	–	–	0	7	6
Fresh Mixers Rotini & Zesty Marinara Sauce	1 pkg (9.9 oz)	300	4	0	1	–	–	0	7	11
Fresh Mixers Ziti & Meat Sauce	1 pkg (6.9 oz)	340	6	20	2	–	–	0	8	10
Pasta Margherita	1 pkg (6.9 oz)	270	4	0	1	–	–	0	4	7
TAKE-OUT										
lasagna meatless	1 piece (9 oz)	356	11	38	7	1	3	0	3	8
lasagna w/ meat	1 piece (8 oz)	362	14	56	7	1	4	0	3	6
lasagna w/ vegetables	1 serv (9 oz)	315	10	33	6	1	3	–	4	8

FOOD	PORTION	CALS	TOTAL FAT	CHOL	SAT FAT	POLY FAT	MONO FAT	TRANS FAT	FIBER	SUGAR
macaroni & cheese w/ ham	1 cup	542	33	61	13	4	13	0	3	7
manicotti cheese w/ marinara sauce	1 (5 oz)	229	10	83	6	1	3	0	1	3
manicotti cheese w/ meat sauce	1 (5 oz)	239	11	86	6	1	4	0	3	1
pasta w/ pesto sauce	1 cup	370	25	10	4	6	13	0	2	1
ravioli cheese & spinach w/ cream sauce	1 cup	362	17	160	6	3	6	0	2	5
ravioli cheese w/tomato sauce	1 cup	335	14	158	6	2	5	–	2	4
ravioli meat w/ marinara sauce	1 cup	372	16	168	5	2	7	0	3	5
rigatoni w/ sausage sauce	¾ cup	260	12	59	4	0	5	–	3	–
spaghetti w/ red clam sauce	1 cup	285	8	17	1	1	5	0	3	3
spaghetti w/ sauce & meatballs	2 cups	670	26	114	8	5	10	0	12	15
spaghetti w/ white clam sauce	1 cup	456	20	50	3	3	13	–	3	1
tortellini cheese w/ tomato sauce	1 cup	332	14	158	6	2	5	–	2	4
tortellini meat w/ marinara sauce	1 cup	281	10	90	3	2	4	0	2	3
tortellini spinach w/ marinara sauce	1 cup	238	8	72	2	2	3	0	2	3

PASTA SALAD
TAKE-OUT

FOOD	PORTION	CALS	TOTAL FAT	CHOL	SAT FAT	POLY FAT	MONO FAT	TRANS FAT	FIBER	SUGAR
pasta salad w/ crab vegetables mayonnaise	1 cup	317	16	32	2	9	4	–	2	2
pasta salad w/ shrimp vegetables & mayonnaise	1 cup (6.2 oz)	335	17	65	3	9	4	–	2	6
tortellini salad cheese filled w/ vinaigrette dressing	1 cup	333	18	144	7	5	6	0	1	1

PATE

FOOD	PORTION	CALS	TOTAL FAT	CHOL	SAT FAT	POLY FAT	MONO FAT	TRANS FAT	FIBER	SUGAR
chicken liver canned	1 tbsp	26	2	51	1	tr	1	0	0	0
liver w/ truffle	1 serv (2 oz)	183	16	59	6	2	8	0	–	–
mushroom anchovy pate	1 (2.25 oz)	130	11	5	2	–	–	–	1	1
pate de foie gras smoked canned	1 tbsp	60	6	20	2	tr	3	0	0	–
pork pate	1 oz	107	10	51	4	1	5	–	0	1

FOOD	PORTION	CALS	TOTAL FAT	CHOL	SAT FAT	POLY FAT	MONO FAT	TRANS FAT	FIBER	SUGAR
pork pate en croute	1 oz	91	7	32	3	1	3	–	tr	tr
rabbit pate	1 oz	66	5	21	3	1	1	–	–	–
shrimp pate	1 can (2.25 oz)	140	10	25	2	–	–	–	0	1
PEACH										
CANNED										
halves in heavy syrup	½ cup (2.6 oz)	85	tr	0	tr	tr	tr	0	2	20
halves in light syrup	1 half (3.4 oz)	53	tr	0	tr	tr	tr	0	1	13
halves juice pack	1 half (3.4 oz)	43	tr	0	tr	tr	tr	0	1	10
peach sauce	½ cup	120	0	0	0	0	0	0	1	31
pickled	½ cup (4.2 oz)	143	tr	0	tr	tr	tr	0	1	34
pickled whole	1 (3.1 oz)	104	tr	0	tr	tr	tr	0	1	25
slices juice pack	½ cup (4.4 oz)	55	tr	0	tr	tr	tr	0	2	13
slices light syrup	½ cup (4.4 oz)	68	tr	0	tr	tr	tr	0	2	17
slices water pack	½ cup (4.3 oz)	29	tr	0	tr	tr	tr	0	2	6
spiced in heavy syrup	½ cup (4.2 oz)	91	tr	0	tr	tr	tr	0	2	23
Del Monte										
Diced In Light Syrup	1 pkg (4 oz)	70	0	0	0	0	0	0	–	16
Freestone Slices Lite	½ cup (4.4 oz)	60	0	0	0	0	0	0	1	13
Peaches In Strawberry Banana Gel	1 pkg (4.5 oz)	60	0	0	0	0	0	0	–	12
Sliced 100% Juice	½ cup (4.4 oz)	60	0	0	0	0	0	0	1	14
Sliced In Heavy Syrup	½ cup (4.5 oz)	100	0	0	0	0	0	0	1	23
DRIED										
halves	½ cup (2.8 oz)	191	1	0	tr	tr	tr	0	7	33
halves	1 (0.5 oz)	31	tr	0	tr	tr	tr	0	1	5
halves cooked w/o sugar	½ cup (4.5 oz)	99	tr	0	tr	tr	tr	0	4	22
FRESH										
peach	1 lg (6.1 oz)	68	tr	0	tr	tr	tr	0	3	15
peach	1 med (5.3 oz)	58	tr	0	tr	tr	tr	0	2	13
sliced	½ cup (2.7 oz)	30	tr	0	tr	tr	tr	0	1	6
Dole										
Peach	1 lg (5.2 oz)	60	0	0	0	0	0	0	2	12
FROZEN										
Dole										
Sliced	¾ cup (4.9 oz)	50	0	0	0	0	0	0	1	10
REFRIGERATED										
Dole										
Fruit Crisp Peach	1 pkg (4 oz)	150	4	0	0	–	–	0	2	20
Parfait Peaches & Creme	1 pkg (4.3 oz)	120	2	0	2	–	–	0	1	21

FOOD	PORTION	CALS	TOTAL FAT	CHOL.	SAT FAT	POLY FAT	MONO FAT	TRANS FAT	FIBER	SUGAR
PEACH JUICE										
nectar	1 cup (8.7 oz)	134	tr	0	tr	tr	tr	0	2	33
Froose										
Playful Peach	1 box (4.2 oz)	80	0	0	0	0	0	0	3	7
Minute Maid										
Fruit Drink	8 oz	120	0	0	0	0	0	0	–	30
PEANUT BUTTER (see also individual nut names, NUT BUTTER)										
chunky	2 tbsp (1.1 oz)	188	16	0	3	5	8	–	3	3
no sugar added	2 tbsp (1.1 oz)	208	18	0	3	5	9	–	3	1
reduced sodium	2 tbsp (1.1 oz)	202	16	0	2	5	8	–	2	3
smooth	2 tbsp (1.1 oz)	188	16	0	3	5	8	–	2	3
Jake & Amos										
Schmier	1 tbsp (0.6 oz)	60	3	0	1	–	–	0	0	8
Kettle Brand										
Organic Unsalted	2 tbsp (1 oz)	160	14	0	3	4	7	0	2	3
Peanut Butter & Co.										
Cinnamon Raisin Swirl	2 tbsp (1.1 oz)	160	11	0	2	–	–	0	2	9
Dark Chocolate Dreams	2 tbsp (1.1 oz)	170	13	0	3	–	–	0	2	7
Old Fashioned Crunchy	2 tbsp (1.1 oz)	190	16	0	2	–	–	0	2	1
The Bee's Knees	2 tbsp (1.1 oz)	180	14	0	3	–	–	0	1	8
Planters										
Creamy or Crunchy	2 tbsp (1.1 oz)	180	15	0	3	–	7	0	2	3
Natural Creamy	2 tbsp (1.1 oz)	190	17	0	4	–	8	0	3	3
Smart Balance										
Creamy or Chunky Omega-3	2 tbsp (1.1 oz)	190	16	0	3	2	12	0	2	3
Smucker's										
Chunky	2 tbsp (1.1 oz)	200	16	0	3	5	8	0	2	1
Creamy Honey	2 tbsp (1.2 oz)	200	16	0	3	–	–	0	2	4
Creamy No Salt Added	2 tbsp (1.1 oz)	210	16	0	3	–	–	0	2	1
Creamy Reduced Fat	2 tbsp (1.2 oz)	190	12	0	2	4	6	0	2	2
Goober Grape	3 tbsp (1.9 oz)	240	13	0	3	–	–	0	2	21
Goober Peanut Butter & Chocolate Spread	3 tbsp (2 oz)	230	11	0	2	–	–	0	2	23
Wild Squirrel										
Chocolate Coconut	2 tbsp (1.1 oz)	200	17	0	3	–	–	0	3	2
Cinnamon Raisin	2 tbsp (1.1 oz)	180	15	0	2	–	–	0	3	3
Honey Pretzel	2 tbsp (1.1 oz)	190	16	0	2	–	–	0	2	2
PEANUTS										
chocolate coated	¼ cup	193	12	3	5	2	5	0	2	14

FOOD	PORTION	CALS	TOTAL FAT	CHOL	SAT FAT	POLY FAT	MONO FAT	TRANS FAT	FIBER	SUGAR
chocolate coated	1	21	1	0	1	tr	1	0	tr	2
cooked w/ salt	½ cup	286	20	0	3	6	10	0	8	2
dry roasted w/ salt	28 (1 oz)	164	14	0	2	4	7	0	1	2
dry roasted w/o salt	28 (1 oz)	164	14	0	2	4	7	0	2	1
dry roasted w/o salt	¼ cup	214	18	0	3	6	9	0	3	2
honey roasted	¼ cup	191	16	0	3	5	8	0	3	5
sugar coated	¼ cup	203	13	0	2	4	6	0	2	16
yogurt coated	¼ cup	230	16	0	7	3	5	0	2	15
Frito Lay										
Salted In Shells	1 oz	160	14	0	2	–	–	0	2	1
Planters										
Bar Big Double	1 (1.6 oz)	220	13	0	3	–	–	0	3	12
Dry Roasted	1 oz	160	14	0	2	–	7	0	2	2
Dry Roasted Lightly Salted	1 oz	160	14	0	2	–	7	0	2	1
Dry Roasted Unsalted	1 oz	170	14	0	2	–	7	0	2	1
Honey & Dry Roasted	1 oz	160	13	0	2	–	6	0	2	4
Roasted In Milk Chocolate	¼ cup (1.4 oz)	210	15	5	5	–	–	0	2	15
Virginia Cocktail Peanuts										
Jalapeno	⅕ can (1 oz)	170	13	0	2	–	–	0	5	tr
Milk Chocolate	⅓ pkg (1.5 oz)	230	14	0	9	–	–	0	4	14
Sea Salt	⅕ can (1 oz)	170	13	0	2	–	–	0	5	tr
Toffee	⅕ can (1 oz)	210	7	0	1	–	–	0	2	14
Unsalted	⅕ can (1 oz)	170	13	0	2	–	–	0	5	tr
PEAR										
CANNED										
halves in heavy syrup	1 (1.7 oz)	36	tr	0	tr	tr	tr	0	1	8
halves in heavy syrup	½ cup (3.5 oz)	74	tr	0	tr	tr	tr	0	3	17
halves in light syrup	1 (2.7 oz)	43	tr	0	tr	tr	tr	0	1	9
halves juice pack	1 (2.7 oz)	38	tr	0	tr	tr	tr	0	1	7
halves juice pack	½ cup (4.4 oz)	62	tr	0	tr	tr	tr	0	2	12
halves light syrup	½ cup (4.4 oz)	72	tr	0	tr	tr	tr	0	2	15
halves water pack	1 (2.7 oz)	22	tr	0	tr	tr	tr	0	1	5
Del Monte										
Halves Lite	½ cup (4.4 oz)	60	0	0	0	0	0	0	1	14
Dole										
Diced In Fruit Juice	1 pkg (4 oz)	90	0	0	0	0	0	0	2	18
DRIED										
halves	½ cup (3.2 oz)	236	1	0	tr	tr	tr	0	7	56
halves	1 (0.6 oz)	47	tr	0	tr	tr	tr	0	1	11

FOOD	PORTION	CALS	TOTAL FAT	CHOL	SAT FAT	POLY FAT	MONO FAT	TRANS FAT	FIBER	SUGAR
halves	5 (3 oz)	229	1	0	tr	tr	tr	0	7	54
halves cooked w/o sugar	½ cup (4.5 oz)	162	tr	0	tr	tr	tr	0	8	35
Crunchies										
Freeze Dried	¼ cup (6 g)	20	0	0	0	0	0	0	1	3
FRESH										
asian	1 lg (9.6 oz)	116	1	0	tr	tr	tr	0	10	19
asian	1 med (4.3 oz)	51	tr	0	tr	tr	tr	0	4	9
pear	1 med (6.2 oz)	103	tr	0	tr	tr	tr	0	6	17
pear	1 lg (8.1 oz)	133	tr	0	tr	tr	tr	0	7	23
pear	1 sm (5.2 oz)	86	tr	0	tr	tr	tr	0	5	15
sliced w/ skin	1 cup (4.9 oz)	81	tr	0	tr	tr	tr	0	4	14
Dole										
Pear	1 med (5.8 oz)	100	0	0	0	0	0	0	5	16
PEAR JUICE										
nectar canned	1 cup (8.8 oz)	150	tr	0	tr	tr	tr	0	2	38
Smart Juice										
Organic 100% Juice	8 oz	110	0	0	0	0	0	0	2	25
PEAS										
CANNED										
green	½ cup (4.4 oz)	66	tr	0	tr	tr	tr	0	4	4
green low sodium	½ cup (4.4 oz)	66	tr	0	tr	tr	tr	0	4	4
Bush's										
Crowder Peas	½ cup (4.6 oz)	80	0	0	0	0	0	0	5	0
Field Peas w/ Snaps	½ cup (4.6 oz)	80	0	0	0	0	0	0	2	0
Purple Hull	½ cup (4.6 oz)	90	0	0	0	0	0	0	5	0
Butter Kernel										
Sweet	½ cup (4.4 oz)	60	0	0	0	0	0	0	4	6
Del Monte										
Sweet	½ cup (4.4 oz)	60	0	0	0	0	0	0	3	6
Sweet No Salt Added	½ cup (4.4 oz)	60	0	0	0	0	0	0	3	6
DRIED										
split cooked w/o salt	1 cup (6.9 oz)	231	1	0	tr	tr	tr	0	16	6
Crunchies										
Freeze Dried Organic	¼ cup (0.5 oz)	50	1	0	0	–	–	0	3	8
Goya										
Green Split Peas not prep	¼ cup (1.6 oz)	110	0	0	0	0	0	0	11	1
FRESH										
green cooked w/o salt	½ cup (2.8 oz)	67	tr	0	tr	tr	tr	0	4	5
green raw	½ cup (2.5 oz)	59	tr	0	tr	tr	tr	0	4	4

FOOD	PORTION	CALS	TOTAL FAT	CHOL	SAT FAT	POLY FAT	MONO FAT	TRANS FAT	FIBER	SUGAR
snap peas cooked w/o salt	1 cup (5.6 oz)	67	tr	0	tr	tr	tr	0	5	6
snap peas raw	10 (1.2 oz)	14	tr	0	tr	tr	tr	0	1	1
snap peas raw	1 cup (2.2 oz)	26	tr	0	tr	tr	tr	0	2	3
Dole										
Sugar Snap Peas	1 cup (3 oz)	35	0	0	0	0	0	0	2	3
Eat Smart										
Sugar Snap	1 serv (3 oz)	40	0	0	0	0	0	0	2	3
Mann's										
Snow Peas	1 serv (3 oz)	35	0	0	0	0	0	0	2	3
FROZEN										
creamed	1 cup (4.3 oz)	132	6	4	2	2	2	–	4	6
green cooked w/o salt	½ cup (2.8 oz)	62	tr	0	tr	tr	tr	0	4	4
Birds Eye										
Baby Sweet Peas	⅔ cup (3 oz)	70	0	0	0	0	0	0	4	4
Lisa's Organics										
Sweet Peas In Parmesan Herb Sauce	½ pkg (4 oz)	80	1	0	0	–	–	0	3	0
PECANS										
candied	1 oz	190	17	0	3	4	10	–	5	4
chopped dried w/o salt	¼ cup (0.9 oz)	188	20	0	2	6	11	–	3	1
halves dried w/o salt	¼ cup (0.9 oz)	171	18	0	2	6	12	–	2	1
halves dried w/o salt	19 (1 oz)	196	20	0	2	6	12	–	3	1
halves oil roasted w/ salt	15 (1 oz)	203	21	0	2	7	12	–	3	1
oil roasted w/ salt	¼ cup (1 oz)	197	21	0	2	6	11	–	3	1
Planters										
Halves	1 oz	200	20	0	2	–	–	0	3	1
Sante										
Cinnamon Pecan	¼ cup (1 oz)	190	17	0	2	5	10	0	2	5
PECTIN										
liquid	1 oz	3	0	0	0	0	0	0	1	0
powder	1 pkg (1.75 oz)	162	tr	0	tr	tr	tr	0	4	–
PEPEAO										
dried	¼ cup	18	tr	0	–	–	–	0	–	–
raw sliced	1 cup	25	tr	0	–	–	–	0	–	–
PEPPER										
black	1 tsp	5	tr	0	tr	tr	tr	0	1	tr
cayenne	1 tsp	6	tr	0	tr	tr	tr	0	1	tr
white	1 tsp	7	tr	0	tr	tr	tr	0	1	–

FOOD	PORTION	CALS	TOTAL FAT	CHOL	SAT FAT	POLY FAT	MONO FAT	TRANS FAT	FIBER	SUGAR
Badia										
Lemon Pepper	¼ tsp (0.9 g)	0	0	0	0	0	0	0	0	0
McCormick										
Lemon Pepper w/ Garlic & Onion California Style	¼ tsp (0.6 g)	0	0	0	0	0	0	0	0	0
PEPPERMINT										
fresh chopped	2 tbsp	2	tr	0	tr	tr	tr	0	tr	–
PEPPERS										
CANNED										
chili green hot	1 (2.6 oz)	15	tr	0	tr	tr	tr	–	1	2
chili green hot chopped	½ cup (2.4 oz)	14	tr	0	tr	tr	tr	–	1	2
green halves	1 cup (4.9 oz)	25	tr	0	tr	tr	tr	–	2	–
jalapeno	1 (0.8 oz)	6	tr	0	tr	tr	tr	–	1	tr
jalapeno chopped	1 cup (4.8 oz)	37	1	0	tr	1	tr	–	4	3
Gedney										
Hot Banana Pepper Rings	¼ cup (1 oz)	10	0	0	0	0	0	0	0	0
Jalapeno Sliced	¼ cup (1 oz)	10	0	0	0	0	0	0	0	2
Jake & Amos										
Mild Sweet Stuffed	2 tbsp	15	0	0	0	0	0	0	0	0
Kelly's Kitchen										
Peppadew Stuffed w/ Garlic & Herb Spread	2 (1 oz)	90	7	16	5	–	–	0	tr	4
Matiz										
Organic Piquillo Peppers	2	20	0	0	0	0	0	0	tr	3
Piparras	½ jar (1 oz)	5	0	0	0	0	0	0	0	0
Victoria										
Jalapeno Hot Roasted	1 oz	10	0	0	0	0	0	0	1	0
Red & Green Roasted	⅓ cup (4.6 oz)	24	0	0	0	0	0	0	1	2
DRIED										
ancho	1 tsp	3	tr	0	–	–	–	0	tr	–
ancho	1 (0.6 oz)	48	1	0	tr	1	tr	–	4	–
casabel	1 tsp	3	tr	0	–	–	–	0	tr	–
chili hot sun-dried	¼ cup (0.3 oz)	30	1	0	tr	tr	tr	–	3	4
chili hot sun-dried	1 (0.5 g)	2	tr	0	tr	tr	tr	–	tr	tr
chipotle smoked	1 tsp	3	tr	0	–	–	–	0	tr	–
green freeze dried	1 tbsp (0.4 g)	1	tr	0	tr	tr	tr	–	tr	1
guajillo	1 tsp	3	tr	0	–	–	–	0	tr	–
mulato	1 tsp	3	tr	0	–	–	–	0	tr	–
pasilla	1 tsp	3	tr	0	–	–	–	0	tr	–

FOOD	PORTION	CALS	TOTAL FAT	CHOL	SAT FAT	POLY FAT	MONO FAT	TRANS FAT	FIBER	SUGAR
pasilla	1 (7 g)	24	1	0	–	–	–	–	2	–
red sweet freeze-dried	1 tbsp (0.4 g)	1	tr	0	tr	tr	tr	–	tr	tr
FRESH										
banana	1 lg (2.6 oz)	20	tr	0	tr	tr	tr	–	3	1
banana	1 cup (4.4 oz)	33	1	0	tr	tr	tr	–	4	2
banana	1 (4 in) (1.2 oz)	9	tr	0	tr	tr	tr	–	1	1
chili green hot	1 (1.6 oz)	18	tr	0	tr	tr	tr	–	1	2
chili green hot chopped	½ cup (2.6 oz)	30	tr	0	tr	tr	tr	–	1	4
chili red hot	1 (1.6 oz)	18	tr	0	tr	tr	tr	–	1	2
chili red hot chopped	½ cup (2.6 oz)	30	tr	0	tr	tr	tr	–	1	4
green chopped	1 cup (5.2 oz)	30	tr	0	tr	tr	tr	–	3	4
green chopped fried	1 cup (4 oz)	146	14	0	2	7	3	–	2	3
green chopped or strips cooked w/o salt	1 cup (4.7 oz)	38	tr	0	tr	tr	tr	–	2	4
green sweet	1 med (4.2 oz)	24	tr	0	tr	tr	tr	–	2	3
habanero	1 tsp	9	tr	0	–	–	–	–	1	–
hungarian	1 (0.9 oz)	8	tr	0	tr	tr	tr	–	tr	1
jalapeno	1 (0.5 oz)	4	tr	0	tr	tr	0	–	tr	1
jalapeno sliced	1 cup (3.2 oz)	26	tr	0	tr	tr	tr	–	3	4
red	1 lg (5.6 oz)	51	tr	0	tr	tr	tr	–	3	7
red	1 med (4.2 oz)	37	tr	0	tr	tr	tr	–	3	5
red chopped	1 cup (5.2 oz)	46	tr	0	tr	tr	tr	–	3	6
red chopped cooked w/o salt	½ cup (2.4 oz)	19	tr	0	tr	tr	tr	–	1	3
red sweet	1 lg (5.8 oz)	33	tr	0	tr	tr	tr	–	3	4
red sweet ring	1 (0.4 oz)	2	tr	0	tr	tr	tr	–	tr	tr
serrano	1 (6 g)	2	tr	0	0	tr	0	–	tr	tr
serrano chopped	1 cup (3.7 oz)	34	tr	0	tr	tr	tr	–	4	4
yellow	1 lg (6.5 oz)	50	tr	0	–	–	–	–	2	–
yellow strips	10 (1.8 oz)	14	tr	0	–	–	–	–	1	–
FROZEN										
Farm Rich										
Stuffed Jalapeno	2 (1.7 oz)	120	8	10	3	–	–	0	0	1

PERCH
FRESH

FOOD	PORTION	CALS	TOTAL FAT	CHOL	SAT FAT	POLY FAT	MONO FAT	TRANS FAT	FIBER	SUGAR
cooked	3 oz	99	1	98	tr	tr	tr	–	0	0
cooked	1 fillet (1.6 oz)	54	1	53	tr	tr	tr	–	0	0
ocean perch atlantic cooked	1 fillet (1.8 oz)	60	1	27	tr	tr	tr	–	0	0
ocean perch atlantic cooked	3 oz	103	2	46	tr	tr	1	–	0	0

FOOD	PORTION	CALS	TOTAL FAT	CHOL	SAT FAT	POLY FAT	MONO FAT	TRANS FAT	FIBER	SUGAR
ocean perch atlantic raw	3 oz	80	1	36	tr	tr	1	–	0	0
raw	3 oz	77	1	76	tr	tr	tr	–	0	0

PERSIMMONS

dried japanese	1 (1.2 oz)	93	tr	0	–	–	–	0	5	–
fresh	1 (6 oz)	118	tr	0	tr	tr	tr	0	6	21

PHEASANT

breast boneless cooked	½ (4.4 oz)	312	15	113	4	2	7	0	0	0
cooked diced	1 cup	332	16	120	5	2	8	–	0	0
drumstick & thigh cooked	1 (2.6 oz)	184	9	67	3	1	4	0	0	0

PHYLLO

sheet	1 (0.7 oz)	57	1	0	tr	tr	1	–	tr	tr

Athens

Fillo Dough Sheets	5 (2 oz)	160	1	0	0	–	–	0	1	1
Kataifi Shredded Fillo Dough	⅛ pkg (2 oz)	120	2	0	0	–	–	0	tr	0
Mini Fillo Shells	2 (7 g)	25	1	0	0	–	–	0	0	0
Spanakopita Spinach & Cheese Appetizers	2 (2 oz)	160	8	20	2	–	–	0	1	1
Tyropita Three Cheese Appetizers	2 (2 oz)	180	11	25	5	–	–	0	0	1

Ekizian

Sheets	2 (4 oz)	433	9	62	4	3	2	0	3	2

PICANTE (see SALSA)

PICKLES

bread & butter	6 slices	39	tr	0	tr	tr	0	0	1	4
dill	1 lg (4.7 oz)	24	tr	0	tr	tr	tr	0	2	5
dill low sodium	1 med (2.3 oz)	12	tr	0	tr	tr	tr	0	1	–
dill sliced	6 slices	7	tr	0	tr	tr	tr	0	1	1
sweet gherkin	1 (1.2 oz)	41	tr	0	tr	tr	tr	0	tr	5
tsukemono japanese pickles sliced	¼ cup	10	tr	0	tr	tr	tr	0	1	1

B&G

Crunchy Kosher Dill Gherkins	1 (1 oz)	5	0	0	0	0	0	0	–	–

Claussen

Sandwich Slices Hearty Garlic	2 (1.2 oz)	5	0	0	0	0	0	0	–	tr

FOOD	PORTION	CALS	TOTAL FAT	CHOL	SAT FAT	POLY FAT	MONO FAT	TRANS FAT	FIBER	SUGAR
Gedney										
Dill	½ lg (1 oz)	5	0	0	0	0	0	0	0	0
Kosher Dill Babies	3 (1 oz)	5	0	0	0	0	0	0	0	0
State Fair Norwegian Dills	1 med (1 oz)	5	0	0	0	0	0	0	0	tr
Sweet Bread & Butter Chips	5 (1 oz)	30	0	0	0	0	0	0	0	7
Jake & Amos										
Bread & Butter Chips	2 tbsp	20	0	0	0	0	0	0	0	2
Mt. Olive										
Bread & Butter Spears	½ spear (1 oz)	20	0	0	0	0	0	0	–	4
Vlasic										
Farmer's Garden Deli Halves	½ (1 oz)	0	0	0	0	0	0	0	–	–
Kosher Dill Spears Reduced Sodium	⅔ spear (1 oz)	0	0	0	0	0	0	0	0	0
Stackers Kosher Dill	1 (1 oz)	0	0	0	0	0	0	0	–	0
Stackers Kosher Dill Reduced Sodium	1 (1 oz)	0	0	0	0	0	0	0	0	0

PIE (see also PIE CRUST, PIE FILLING)
FROZEN

FOOD	PORTION	CALS	TOTAL FAT	CHOL	SAT FAT	POLY FAT	MONO FAT	TRANS FAT	FIBER	SUGAR
Edwards										
Pie Slices Key Lime	1 slice (3.25 oz)	330	16	35	11	–	–	0	tr	33
Mom Made										
Munchie Apple	1 (2.5 oz)	220	10	0	5	–	–	0	1	8
MIX										
Jell-O										
No Bake Lemon Meringue as prep	⅛ pie	270	10	0	3	–	–	0	1	29
TAKE-OUT										
apple one crust	1 slice (5.3 oz)	363	14	0	3	4	6	–	2	36
apple tart	1 (4.2 oz)	370	19	0	5	5	7	–	1	20
apple two crust	1 slice (5.3 oz)	356	17	0	6	3	7	–	2	23
apricot tart	1 (4.2 oz)	356	17	0	4	5	7	–	2	20
apricot two crust	1 slice (5.3 oz)	417	19	0	5	5	8	–	3	28
banana cream	1 slice (5.1 oz)	387	20	73	5	5	8	–	1	17
blackberry one crust	1 slice (4.4 oz)	341	17	0	4	5	7	–	4	18
blackberry two crust	1 slice (5.3 oz)	394	19	0	4	5	8	–	5	24
blueberry one crust	1 slice (4.8 oz)	292	12	0	3	3	5	–	3	23
blueberry tart	1 (4.2 oz)	346	17	0	4	5	7	–	2	21
blueberry two crust	1 slice (5.3 oz)	348	15	0	3	5	6	–	2	15

FOOD	PORTION	CALS	TOTAL FAT	CHOL	SAT FAT	POLY FAT	MONO FAT	TRANS FAT	FIBER	SUGAR
cherry one crust	1 slice (4.8 oz)	312	12	0	3	3	5	–	2	30
cherry two crust	1 slice (5.3 oz)	390	17	0	4	3	9	–	1	21
chess	1 slice (3 oz)	365	18	128	8	3	6	–	1	37
chocolate cream	1 slice (5 oz)	380	18	73	7	3	7	–	2	29
coconut creme	1 slice (5 oz)	429	24	0	10	2	10	–	2	52
custard	1 slice (4.8 oz)	286	16	45	3	5	7	–	2	16
grasshopper	1 slice (3.5 oz)	341	19	96	8	3	7	–	1	23
key lime	1 slice (5 oz)	420	14	25	6	–	–	0	tr	28
lemon meringue	1 slice (4.8 oz)	367	12	62	2	3	5	–	2	33
lemon meringue tart	1 (4.1 oz)	298	14	68	3	4	5	–	1	22
mince two crust	1 slice (5.3 oz)	434	16	0	4	4	7	–	4	42
peach two crust	1 slice (5.3 oz)	334	15	0	2	6	6	–	1	9
pear two crust	1 slice (5.3 oz)	400	18	0	4	5	7	–	3	27
pecan	1 slice (4 oz)	456	21	36	4	4	12	–	4	32
pineapple two crust	1 slice (5.3 oz)	394	18	0	4	5	7	–	2	23
plum two crust	1 slice (5.3 oz)	441	21	0	5	6	8	–	2	29
prune one crust	1 slice (5.3 oz)	450	14	0	4	4	6	–	2	55
pumpkin	1 slice (5.4 oz)	323	15	31	3	5	6	–	4	21
raisin tart	1 (4.2 oz)	348	16	0	4	5	7	–	2	21
raisin two crust	1 slice (5.3 oz)	376	16	0	4	5	7	–	2	26
raspberry one crust	1 slice (4.8 oz)	330	13	5	3	4	5	–	6	29
raspberry two crust	1 slice (5.3 oz)	422	20	0	5	6	8	–	5	25
rhubarb two crust	1 slice (5.3 oz)	444	23	0	6	7	9	–	2	16
shoo-fly	1 slice (4 oz)	404	13	36	3	3	5	–	1	39
strawberry rhubarb two crust	1 slice (5.3 oz)	422	21	20	5	6	9	–	2	18
strawberry two crust	1 slice (6 oz)	386	16	0	4	5	6	–	3	29
sweet potato	1 piece (5.4 oz)	276	14	57	4	3	5	–	2	13

PIE CRUST

FOOD	PORTION	CALS	TOTAL FAT	CHOL	SAT FAT	POLY FAT	MONO FAT	TRANS FAT	FIBER	SUGAR
baked	⅙ crust (1 oz)	147	9	0	3	1	4	–	tr	1
chocolate wafer	⅛ crust (1.2 oz)	177	11	0	2	3	5	–	1	8
chocolate wafer tart shell	1 (0.8 oz)	111	7	0	1	2	3	–	tr	5
deep dish frzn	⅛ crust (1.8 oz)	266	16	0	5	2	8	–	1	–
graham cracker	⅙ crust (1.2 oz)	172	9	0	2	2	4	–	1	13
graham cracker tart shell	1 (0.8 oz)	109	5	0	1	2	3	–	tr	8

FOOD	PORTION	CALS	TOTAL FAT	CHOL	SAT FAT	POLY FAT	MONO FAT	TRANS FAT	FIBER	S\
puff pastry shell	1 (1.4 oz)	223	15	0	2	9	4	0	1	tr
tart shell	1 (1 oz)	149	10	0	3	1	5	–	tr	1
Jiffy										
Mix as prep	1/16 pkg	80	5	<5	2	–	–	0	0	0
Pepperidge Farm										
Puff Pastry Sheets frzn	1/6 sheet	160	10	0	5	–	–	0	1	1
Puff Pastry Shell frzn	1	180	11	0	6	–	–	0	2	1

PIE FILLING

FOOD	PORTION	CALS	TOTAL FAT	CHOL	SAT FAT	POLY FAT	MONO FAT	TRANS FAT	FIBER	S\
apple	1 cup	155	tr	0	tr	tr	0	0	2	34
blueberry	1 cup	474	1	0	tr	tr	tr	0	7	99
cherry	1 cup	317	2	0	tr	1	1	0	2	66
lemon	1 cup	923	18	348	4	4	8	–	1	166
pumpkin pie mix canned	1 cup (9.5 oz)	281	tr	0	tr	tr	tr	0	22	–
Comstock										
Apple No Sugar Added	1/3 cup (3 oz)	35	0	0	0	0	0	0	1	5
Apple Caramel	1/3 cup (3 oz)	90	0	0	0	0	0	0	1	21
Berry Medley	1/3 cup	90	0	0	0	0	0	0	1	16
Blackberry	1/3 cup (3 oz)	100	0	0	0	0	0	0	1	13
Blueberry More Fruit	1/3 cup (3 oz)	90	0	0	0	0	0	0	2	18
Cherry Dark Sweet	1/3 cup (3 oz)	70	0	0	0	0	0	0	0	14
Cherry More Fruit Lite	1/3 cup (3 oz)	90	0	0	0	0	0	0	0	16
Cherry No Sugar Added	1/3 cup (3 oz)	35	0	0	0	0	0	0	0	4
Key Lime Creme	1/3 cup (3.2 oz)	170	3	0	1	–	–	0	0	28
Lemon Creme	1/3 cup (3.2 oz)	130	2	0	1	–	–	0	0	20
Peach Country	1/3 cup (3 oz)	100	0	0	0	0	0	0	1	17
Strawberry	1/3 cup (3 oz)	100	0	0	0	0	0	0	0	10

PIEROGI

FOOD	PORTION	CALS	TOTAL FAT	CHOL	SAT FAT	POLY FAT	MONO FAT	TRANS FAT	FIBER	S\
potato	1 (1.3 oz)	70	2	22	1	tr	1	–	1	tr

PIGEON PEAS

FOOD	PORTION	CALS	TOTAL FAT	CHOL	SAT FAT	POLY FAT	MONO FAT	TRANS FAT	FIBER	S\
dried cooked	1 cup	204	1	0	tr	tr	tr	–	–	–
dried cooked w/ salt	1/2 cup (2.9 oz)	102	tr	0	tr	tr	tr	0	6	–

PIGNOLIA (see PINE NUTS)

PIG'S FEET

FOOD	PORTION	CALS	TOTAL FAT	CHOL	SAT FAT	POLY FAT	MONO FAT	TRANS FAT	FIBER	S\
cooked	1	201	14	93	4	1	7	0	0	0
pickled	1	177	14	70	5	1	7	0	0	tr

PIKE

FOOD	PORTION	CALS	TOTAL FAT	CHOL	SAT FAT	POLY FAT	MONO FAT	TRANS FAT	FIBER	S\
northern cooked	3 oz	96	1	43	tr	tr	tr	–	0	0

FOOD	PORTION	CALS	TOTAL FAT	CHOL	SAT FAT	POLY FAT	MONO FAT	TRANS FAT	FIBER	SUGAR
northern cooked	½ fillet (5.4 oz)	176	1	78	tr	tr	tr	–	0	0
northern raw	3 oz	75	1	33	tr	tr	tr	–	0	0
roe raw	1 oz	37	tr	103	–	–	–	–	–	–
walleye baked	3 oz	101	1	94	tr	tr	tr	–	0	0
walleye fillet baked	4.4 oz	147	2	137	tr	1	tr	–	0	0

PILLNUTS

canarytree dried	1 oz	204	23	0	9	2	11	–	–	–

PIMIENTOS

canned	1 tbsp	3	tr	0	tr	tr	tr	–	–	–
canned	1 slice	0	0	0	0	0	0	0	–	–

PINE NUTS

pine nuts dried	¼ cup (1.2 oz)	277	23	0	2	11	6	–	1	1
pinyon dried	20 (2 g)	13	1	0	tr	1	tr	–	tr	–
pinyon dried	1 oz	178	17	0	3	7	7	–	3	–

PINEAPPLE
CANNED

in heavy syrup crushed sliced or chunks	1 cup (8.9 oz)	198	tr	0	tr	tr	tr	0	2	50
in heavy syrup slice	1 (1.7 oz)	38	tr	0	tr	tr	tr	0	tr	8
in juice crushed sliced or chunks	1 cup (8.7 oz)	149	tr	0	tr	tr	tr	0	2	36
in light syrup crushed sliced or chunks	1 cup (8.8 oz)	131	tr	0	tr	tr	tr	0	2	32
in light syrup slice	1 (1.7 oz)	25	tr	0	tr	tr	tr	0	tr	6
in water crushed sliced or chunks	1 cup (8.6 oz)	79	tr	0	tr	tr	tr	0	2	18
juice pack slice	1 (1.6 oz)	28	tr	0	tr	tr	tr	0	tr	7
water pack slice	1 (1.6 oz)	15	tr	0	tr	tr	tr	0	tr	4

Del Monte

Crushed In 100% Juice	½ cup (4.3 oz)	70	0	0	0	0	0	0	1	15
Slices 100% Juice	2 (4 oz)	60	0	0	0	0	0	0	1	14

Dole

Crushed In Heavy Syrup	½ cups (4.3 oz)	90	0	0	0	0	0	0	1	22
Crushed Juice Pack	½ cup (4.3 oz)	70	0	0	0	0	0	0	1	16
Slices In Heavy Syrup	2 (4.1 oz)	90	0	0	0	0	0	0	1	22
Slices Juice Pack	2 (4 oz)	60	0	0	0	0	0	0	1	13

DRIED

dried	1 piece (1 oz)	71	tr	0	tr	tr	tr	0	2	14

FOOD	PORTION	CALS	TOTAL FAT	CHOL	SAT FAT	POLY FAT	MONO FAT	TRANS FAT	FIBER	SUGAR
Crunchies										
Freeze Dried	1 pkg (9 g)	35	0	0	0	0	0	0	tr	6
Crunchy N'Yummy										
Organic Freeze Dried	1 pkg (1 oz)	100	0	0	0	0	0	0	2	0
FRESH										
chunks	1 cup (5.8 oz)	82	tr	0	tr	tr	tr	0	2	16
slice	1 slice (3 oz)	42	tr	0	tr	tr	tr	0	1	8
whole	1 (2 lbs)	452	1	0	tr	tr	tr	0	13	89
Dole										
Pineapple	2 slices (3.9 oz)	60	0	0	0	0	0	0	2	12
FROZEN										
chunks sweetened	1 cup (8.6 oz)	211	tr	0	tr	tr	tr	0	3	52
Dole										
Chunks	¾ cup (4.9 oz)	70	0	0	0	0	0	0	2	3
Tropical Gold	1 pkg (3 oz)	45	0	0	0	0	0	0	1	8
PINEAPPLE JUICE										
canned unsweetened w/ vitamin C	1 cup (8.8 oz)	132	tr	0	tr	tr	tr	0	1	25
frzn unsweetened as prep w/ water	1 cup (8.8 oz)	130	tr	0	tr	tr	tr	0	1	31
Del Monte										
Juice	8 oz	110	0	0	0	0	0	0	0	23
Dole										
100% Juice	1 can (6 oz)	90	0	0	0	0	0	0	1	21
Fizzy Lizzy										
Pineapple	1 bottle (12 oz)	100	0	0	0	0	0	0	–	25
PINK BEANS										
dried cooked	1 cup	252	1	0	tr	tr	tr	–	–	–
PINTO BEANS										
dried cooked	1 cup	245	1	0	tr	tr	tr	0	15	1
TAKE-OUT										
stewed w/ viandas	1 cup	222	8	8	2	1	5	–	6	2
PISTACHIOS										
dry roasted w/ salt	49 nuts (1 oz)	161	13	0	2	4	7	0	3	2
dry roasted w/o salt	49 nuts (1 oz)	162	13	0	2	4	7	0	3	2
in shells	½ cup	165	13	0	2	4	7	0	3	2

FOOD	PORTION	CALS	TOTAL FAT	CHOL	SAT FAT	POLY FAT	MONO FAT	TRANS FAT	FIBER	SUGAR
Planters										
Dry Roasted In Shell	½ cup	160	13	0	2	4	7	0	3	2
Sante										
Candied	¼ cup (1 oz)	200	16	0	2	5	9	0	1	7
Wonderful										
Roasted & Salted In Shells	½ cup	160	14	0	2	4	7	0	3	2
PITANGA										
fresh	1	2	tr	0	–	–	–	–	–	–
fresh	1 cup	57	1	0	–	–	–	–	–	–
PIZZA (see also PIZZA CRUST)										
Bellatoria										
Fire Grilled Flatbread Buffalo Chicken	⅓ pie (5.8 oz)	340	17	45	7	–	–	0	5	4
Fire Grilled Flatbread Chicken Ranch w/ Uncured Bacon	¼ pie (4.5 oz)	270	13	45	5	–	–	0	3	3
Ultra Thin Crust Margherita	⅓ pie (4.9 oz)	280	16	30	6	–	–	0	1	2
Ultra Thin Crust Ultimate Pepperoni	¼ pie (4.3 oz)	300	18	45	8	–	–	0	1	3
Better 4 U!										
Four Cheese Gluten Free	¼ pie (4.6 oz)	200	7	15	3	–	–	0	1	3
Mediterranean Gluten Free	¼ pie (5.3 oz)	210	8	15	3	–	–	0	2	3
Roasted Vegetable Dairy Free Gluten Free	¼ pie (5 oz)	170	5	0	1	–	–	0	2	3
Thin Crust Four Cheese	⅓ pie (4.3 oz)	240	8	15	3	–	–	0	4	4
Thin Crust Uncured Pepperoni	⅓ pie (4.5 oz)	270	10	20	4	–	–	0	4	4
Bold Organics										
Deluxe	½ pie (6.7 oz)	460	24	10	5	–	–	0	5	12
Meat Lovers	½ pie (6 oz)	450	24	10	5	–	–	0	5	11
Vegan Cheese	½ pie (5.5 oz)	380	18	0	3	–	–	0	5	11
Veggie Lovers	½ pie (6.2 oz)	390	18	10	3	–	–	0	5	12
Farm Rich										
Pizza Slices Pepperoni	2 (3.5 oz)	280	14	30	7	–	–	0	1	6
Lean Cuisine										
Casual Cuisine Deep Dish Roasted Vegetable	1 pkg (6 oz)	320	5	5	2	1	1	0	3	6
Casual Cuisine Deep Dish Spinach & Mushroom	1 pkg (6 oz)	340	7	10	4	1	1	0	2	5

FOOD	PORTION	CALS	TOTAL FAT	CHOL	SAT FAT	POLY FAT	MONO FAT	TRANS FAT	FIBER	SUG
Casual Cuisine Deep Dish Three Meat	1 pkg (6.4 oz)	390	9	25	3	2	3	0	3	7
Casual Cuisine Flatbread Melts Chicken Philly	1 pkg (6.5 oz)	350	9	35	4	2	3	0	5	5
Casual Cuisine Traditional Deluxe	1 pkg (6 oz)	340	8	20	3	2	3	0	4	6
Casual Cuisine Traditional Four Cheese	1 pkg (6 oz)	350	6	10	2	2	2	0	3	6
Casual Cuisine Traditional Mushroom	1 pkg (6 oz)	300	5	5	2	2	1	0	4	5
Casual Cuisine Traditional Pepperoni	1 pkg (6 oz)	380	9	20	3	2	3	0	3	6
Casual Cuisine Wood Fire Bacon Alfredo	1 pkg (6 oz)	320	9	15	3	1	1	0	2	4
Casual Cuisine Wood Fire Margherita	1 pkg (6 oz)	310	7	15	3	2	2	0	3	7
Simple Favorites French Bread Cheese	1 pkg (6 oz)	340	7	15	3	1	2	0	5	7
Lunchables										
Extra Cheesy	1 pkg	280	9	25	5	–	–	0	3	6
Pizza w/ Pepperoni	1 pkg	310	13	30	6	–	–	0	3	6
Mom Made										
Munchie Cheese Pizza	1 (2.5 oz)	160	9	0	4	–	–	0	1	2
Pacific Foods										
BBQ Chicken	1/3 pie (4.5 oz)	270	9	25	5	–	–	0	1	3
Herb Garlic Chicken	1/3 pie (4.5 oz)	270	9	25	5	–	–	0	1	3
Supreme	1/3 pie (4.8 oz)	270	11	25	5	–	–	0	2	4
Simply Shari's										
Gluten Free Cheese	1/2 pie (5 oz)	290	11	65	5	–	–	0	2	3
Gluten Free Pepperoni	1/2 pie (5 oz)	320	13	75	6	–	–	0	2	3
Gluten Free Pesto Margherita	1/2 pie (5 oz)	340	15	60	5	–	–	0	3	3
Gluten Free Spinach Feta	1/4 pkg (5 oz)	280	10	65	5	–	–	0	2	4
Gluten Free Vegetable Margherita	1/4 pie (5 oz)	220	5	40	2	–	–	0	3	4
Solterra										
Cheese Margherita	1/2 pie (4.1 oz)	200	9	15	4	–	–	0	2	2
Vegan	1/2 pie (4.1 oz)	210	10	0	3	–	–	0	3	2
Tandoor Chef										
Naan Pizza Cilantro Pesto	1/2 pie (3.7 oz)	210	3	7	1	–	–	0	2	4
Naan Pizza Roasted Eggplant	1/2 pie (4.8 oz)	330	5	15	3	–	–	0	4	6

FOOD	PORTION	CALS	TOTAL FAT	CHOL	SAT FAT	POLY FAT	MONO FAT	TRANS FAT	FIBER	SUGAR
Tofutti										
Pan Crust Pizzaz Dairy Free	1 slice (2.7 oz)	180	7	0	2	–	–	0	1	6
Vitalicious										
VitaPizza Cheese & Tomato	1 (5.3 oz)	190	3	10	2	–	–	0	11	4
VitaPizza Meatless Pepperoni Supreme	1 (5.3 oz)	190	3	10	1	–	–	0	19	4
TAKE-OUT										
cheese	16 in pie	3384	144	294	61	25	40	–	23	44
cheese	⅛ of 16 in pie	423	18	37	8	3	5	–	3	5
cheese & vegetables	⅛ of 16 in pie	428	16	19	6	2	7	–	3	5
cheese deep dish individual	1 (5.5 oz)	460	24	20	9	–	–	–	2	4
ground beef	16 in pie	3753	172	299	68	18	75	–	20	25
ham & pineapple	⅛ of 16 in pie	439	16	29	6	2	7	–	3	7
no cheese	⅛ of 16 in pie	262	7	0	2	1	4	–	2	3
pepperoni	⅛ of 16 in pie	469	22	37	9	2	9	–	3	3
white pizza	⅛ of 16 in pie	484	17	38	9	1	6	–	2	1
PIZZA CRUST										
crust	1 slice (1.7 oz)	130	2	0	0	–	–	–	1	1
whole wheat	⅛ crust (2 oz)	120	2	0	0	–	–	0	4	0
Jiffy										
Crust Mix as prep	⅕ pie	140	3	0	1	–	–	0	tr	1
Stonefire										
Italian Thin w/ Sauce	1 serv (1.9 oz)	130	3	0	0	–	–	0	1	2
Stonebaked Original	⅙ (1.8 oz)	140	3	0	0	–	–	0	1	1
PLANTAINS										
cooked mashed	1 cup	232	tr	0	tr	tr	tr	–	5	28
sliced cooked	1 cup	179	tr	0	tr	tr	tr	–	4	22
Dole										
Fresh cooked	½ med (3.2 oz)	100	0	0	0	0	0	0	2	13
Isleno										
Chips	1 oz	150	9	0	1	–	–	0	2	0
TAKE-OUT										
mofongo	1 serv	320	3	7	1	tr	1	–	5	31
sweet baked w/ ice cream	1 serv	285	8	0	5	tr	2	–	3	35
PLUMS										
canned purple in heavy syrup	1 cup	163	tr	0	tr	tr	tr	0	3	39

FOOD	PORTION	CALS	TOTAL FAT	CHOL	SAT FAT	POLY FAT	MONO FAT	TRANS FAT	FIBER	SUC
canned purple juice pack	1 cup	146	tr	0	tr	tr	tr	0	2	35
canned purple water pack	1 cup	102	tr	0	tr	tr	tr	0	2	25
dried japanese	1	9	tr	0	tr	tr	tr	0	tr	1
fresh	1	30	tr	0	tr	tr	tr	0	1	7
pickled	1	34	tr	0	tr	tr	tr	0	tr	9
Dole										
Fresh	2 (5.3 oz)	70	0	0	0	0	0	0	2	15
Fruit Bliss										
Soft Dried	5 (1.5 oz)	100	0	0	0	0	0	0	3	17

POI

poi	1 cup	240	0	0	0	0	0	0	1	–

POKEBERRY SHOOTS

cooked	½ cup	16	tr	0	–	–	–	–	–	–
fresh	½ cup	18	tr	0	–	–	–	–	–	–

POLLACK

atlantic baked	3 oz	100	1	77	tr	1	tr	–	0	0
atlantic fillet baked	5.3 oz	178	2	137	tr	1	tr	–	0	0

POMEGRANATE

fresh	1 (5.4 oz)	105	tr	0	tr	tr	tr	0	1	26
POM										
Poms Fresh Arils	1 pkg (4.3 oz)	100	1	0	1	–	–	0	6	9

POMEGRANATE JUICE

KeVita

Sparkling Probiotic Drink Organic	8 oz	20	0	0	0	0	0	0	–	4

POM

100% Juice	8 oz	150	0	0	0	0	0	0	0	32
100% Juice Concentrate	3 tbsp (1.5 oz)	150	0	0	0	0	0	0	0	30
Lite Pomegranate Cocktail	8 oz	75	0	0	0	0	0	0	0	18
Lite Pomegranate Dragonfruit	8 oz	80	0	0	0	0	0	0	0	17
Pomegranate Blueberry	8 oz	150	0	0	0	0	0	0	0	31
Pomegranate Cherry	8 oz	150	0	0	0	0	0	0	0	29
Smart Juice										
Organic 100% Juice	8 oz	149	0	0	0	0	0	0	1	33
Ultra Lo-Gly										
Pomegranate	1 bottle (10 oz)	45	0	0	0	0	0	0	0	9

FOOD	PORTION	CALS	TOTAL FAT	CHOL	SAT FAT	POLY FAT	MONO FAT	TRANS FAT	FIBER	SUGAR
Pomegranate Mojita	1 bottle (10 oz)	40	0	0	0	0	0	0	0	7

POMPANO

FOOD	PORTION	CALS	TOTAL FAT	CHOL	SAT FAT	POLY FAT	MONO FAT	TRANS FAT	FIBER	SUGAR
smoked	2 oz	109	6	33	2	1	2	–	0	0
steamed or poached	4 oz	156	9	47	3	1	2	0	0	0

TAKE-OUT

FOOD	PORTION	CALS	TOTAL FAT	CHOL	SAT FAT	POLY FAT	MONO FAT	TRANS FAT	FIBER	SUGAR
battered & fried	4 oz	304	21	67	6	5	8	0	tr	tr
breaded & fried	4 oz	242	15	63	4	4	5	–	1	1

POPCORN (see also POPCORN CAKES)

FOOD	PORTION	CALS	TOTAL FAT	CHOL	SAT FAT	POLY FAT	MONO FAT	TRANS FAT	FIBER	SUGAR
air popped	1 cup (0.3 oz)	31	tr	0	tr	tr	tr	–	2	–
caramel coated w/ peanuts	⅔ cup (1 oz)	114	2	0	tr	1	1	–	1	11
cheese	1 cup (0.4 oz)	58	4	1	1	2	1	–	1	–
oil popped	1 cup (0.4 oz)	55	3	0	1	1	1	–	1	tr

Bachman

FOOD	PORTION	CALS	TOTAL FAT	CHOL	SAT FAT	POLY FAT	MONO FAT	TRANS FAT	FIBER	SUGAR
Regular	2¾ cups (1 oz)	160	10	0	1	–	–	0	6	0

Chip'ins

FOOD	PORTION	CALS	TOTAL FAT	CHOL	SAT FAT	POLY FAT	MONO FAT	TRANS FAT	FIBER	SUGAR
Chips Hot Buffalo Wing	18 (1 oz)	130	5	0	0	–	–	0	1	0
Chips Jalapeno Ranch	18 (1 oz)	130	4	0	0	–	–	0	1	0
Chips Sea Salt	18 (1 oz)	120	3	0	0	–	–	0	1	0
Chips White Cheddar	18 (1 oz)	130	4	0	0	–	–	0	1	1

Cracker Jack

FOOD	PORTION	CALS	TOTAL FAT	CHOL	SAT FAT	POLY FAT	MONO FAT	TRANS FAT	FIBER	SUGAR
The Original	½ cup (1 oz)	120	2	0	0	–	–	0	1	15

G.H.Cretors

FOOD	PORTION	CALS	TOTAL FAT	CHOL	SAT FAT	POLY FAT	MONO FAT	TRANS FAT	FIBER	SUGAR
Caramel Nut Crunch	½ cup (1 oz)	130	6	10	2	–	–	0	1	16
Chicago Mix	1¼ cups (1 oz)	140	8	10	2	–	–	0	1	10
Just The Caramel	¾ cup (1 oz)	120	5	10	2	–	–	0	1	17
Just The Cheese	2 cups (1 oz)	170	13	5	3	–	–	0	2	0
Kettle Corn	2 cups (1 oz)	130	7	0	1	–	–	0	2	6

Gaslamp Popcorn

FOOD	PORTION	CALS	TOTAL FAT	CHOL	SAT FAT	POLY FAT	MONO FAT	TRANS FAT	FIBER	SUGAR
Cinnamon Caramel	1 cup (1 oz)	140	6	10	4	0	2	0	1	15
Kettle Corn Sweet & Salty	2¼ cups (1 oz)	130	5	0	1	2	3	0	2	11
White Cheddar	2⅓ cups (1 oz)	140	7	5	5	0	2	0	2	2

LesserEvil

FOOD	PORTION	CALS	TOTAL FAT	CHOL	SAT FAT	POLY FAT	MONO FAT	TRANS FAT	FIBER	SUGAR
Fields Good Kettlecorn Black & White	1 cup (1 oz)	110	2	<5	1	–	–	0	1	15
Fields Good Kettlecorn Classic	1 cup (1.1 oz)	110	2	<5	1	–	–	0	1	14

Orville Redenbacher's

FOOD	PORTION	CALS	TOTAL FAT	CHOL	SAT FAT	POLY FAT	MONO FAT	TRANS FAT	FIBER	SUGAR
Microwave Smart Pop 94% Fat Free as prep	1 cup	15	0	0	0	0	0	0	1	–

FOOD	PORTION	CALS	TOTAL FAT	CHOL	SAT FAT	POLY FAT	MONO FAT	TRANS FAT	FIBER	SUGA
Popcorn Indiana										
Kettlecorn Cinnamon Sugar	2½ cups (1 oz)	130	5	0	0	–	–	0	2	7
Kettlecorn Sweet & Tangy BBQ	2½ cups (1 oz)	130	5	0	0	–	–	0	2	7
Original Movie Theater	2 cups (1 oz)	160	12	5	2	–	–	0	3	0
Smartfood										
Kettle Corn	1¼ cups (1 oz)	140	6	0	1	2	4	0	2	11
Reduced Fat White Cheddar	3 cups (1 oz)	130	6	0	1	–	–	0	3	0
White Cheddar	1¾ cups (1 oz)	160	10	<5	2	–	–	0	2	2
The Whole Earth										
Organic Kettle Corn Salty & Sweet	2 cups (1 oz)	120	5	0	0	–	–	0	2	9

POPCORN CAKES (see also RICE CAKES)

POPOVER

FOOD	PORTION	CALS	TOTAL FAT	CHOL	SAT FAT	POLY FAT	MONO FAT	TRANS FAT	FIBER	SUGA
home recipe as prep w/ 2% milk	1 (1.4 oz)	87	3	46	1	1	1	–	–	–
home recipe as prep w/ whole milk	1 (1.4 oz)	90	3	47	1	1	1	–	–	–

POPPY SEEDS

FOOD	PORTION	CALS	TOTAL FAT	CHOL	SAT FAT	POLY FAT	MONO FAT	TRANS FAT	FIBER	SUGA
poppy seeds	1 tbsp	47	4	0	tr	1	3	0	1	1

PORK (see also HAM, JERKY, PORK DISHES)
CANNED
Spam

FOOD	PORTION	CALS	TOTAL FAT	CHOL	SAT FAT	POLY FAT	MONO FAT	TRANS FAT	FIBER	SUGA
Classic	2 oz	180	16	40	6	–	–	–	0	0
Less Sodium	2 oz	180	16	40	6	–	–	0	0	0
Smoked	2 oz	180	16	40	6	–	–	–	0	0
Spread	2 oz	140	12	40	4	–	–	–	0	1
FRESH										
boston butt shoulder lean & fat braised	3 oz	227	15	83	6	2	7	tr	0	0
center cut boneless pork loin roast not prep	4 oz	188	9	73	2	1	2	tr	0	0
center loin chop bone in broiled	1 (3 oz)	178	9	71	3	–	–	tr	0	0
center rib chop lean & fat bone in broiled	1 (4 oz)	249	15	75	5	2	6	tr	0	0
country style ribs bone in lean & fat not prep	1 (4.5 oz)	242	15	95	3	1	4	tr	0	0

FOOD	PORTION	CALS	TOTAL FAT	CHOL	SAT FAT	POLY FAT	MONO FAT	TRANS FAT	FIBER	SUGAR
dehydrated oriental style	1 cup (0.8 oz)	135	14	15	5	2	6	0	0	0
fresh ham rump half lean & fat roasted	4 oz	278	16	106	6	2	7	0	0	0
fresh ham shank half lean & fat roasted	4 oz	319	22	102	8	2	10	0	0	0
fresh ham whole lean & fat roasted	4 oz	302	19	104	7	2	9	0	0	0
ground 96% lean grilled	1 patty (4 oz)	212	8	88	2	1	3	tr	0	0
ham hock cooked	1	167	12	56	4	1	5	0	0	0
shoulder chop bone in braised	1 (3 oz)	229	15	84	6	–	–	tr	0	0
spareribs lean & fat roasted	1 rack (3.4 lbs)	5534	473	1610	142	46	164	4	0	0
tail simmered	3 oz	336	30	110	11	3	14	–	0	0
tenderloin boneless lean only roasted	4 oz	162	4	83	1	1	2	tr	0	0
tenderloin roast boneless lean & fat roasted	4 oz	145	4	73	1	–	–	tr	0	0
top loin chop boneless lean only broiled	1 (5.1 oz)	251	9	104	3	1	4	tr	0	0
Hormel										
Always Tender Loin Filet Lemon Garlic	1 serv (4 oz)	130	5	45	2	–	–	0	0	0
Pork Chops Smoked Thin Cut Bone-In	3 oz	140	9	45	4	–	–	0	0	0
TAKE-OUT										
char siu chinese style	1 piece (0.4 oz)	28	2	7	1	0	1	–	0	–
chicharrones pork cracklings fried	1 cup	492	38	100	13	4	17	–	0	0
chop breaded & fried	1 lg (5 oz)	441	26	126	8	6	10	–	1	2
chop breaded & fried	1 med (3.4 oz)	304	18	87	5	4	7	–	1	1
chop stewed	1 lg (4.6 oz)	315	18	106	7	2	8	0	0	0

PORK DISHES
Lloyd's

FOOD	PORTION	CALS	TOTAL FAT	CHOL	SAT FAT	POLY FAT	MONO FAT	TRANS FAT	FIBER	SUGAR
Babyback Pork Ribs w/ Original BBQ Sauce	1 serv (5 oz)	340	21	110	9	–	–	–	0	12
TAKE-OUT										
kalua pork	1 cup (7 oz)	497	34	157	13	3	15	–	0	–
pork satay w/ peanut sauce	5 sticks (3.5 oz)	214	13	74	4	2	2	–	3	–

FOOD	PORTION	CALS	TOTAL FAT	CHOL	SAT FAT	POLY FAT	MONO FAT	TRANS FAT	FIBER	SUGAR
pulled pork w/ barbecue sauce	1 serv (5 oz)	240	14	55	5	–	–	1	1	12
spareribs barbecue w/ sauce	2 med (2.8 oz)	248	18	70	6	2	8	–	tr	1

PORK RINDS

pork skins	1 oz	154	9	27	3	1	4	–	0	0
pork skins barbecue	1 oz	152	9	33	3	1	4	–	–	–

Baken-ets

Pork Skins Hot 'N Spicy	9 (0.5 oz)	80	5	20	2	–	–	0	0	0
Pork Skins Traditional	9 (0.5 oz)	80	5	20	3	–	–	0	0	0

Lee's

Original	0.5 oz	80	5	20	2	1	3	0	0	0

Pepe's

Cracklin Strips Seasoned	0.5 oz	70	5	20	2	1	3	0	0	0

Southern Recipe

Bar-B-Q	0.5 oz	80	5	20	2	1	3	0	0	0
Dipper Cracklins Chile & Lime	0.5 oz	80	6	15	3	–	–	0	0	0
Hot & Spicy	⅕ pkg (0.5 oz)	80	5	20	2	1	3	0	0	0
Salt & Vinegar	0.5 oz	80	5	15	2	1	3	0	0	0

POT PIE

Pacific Foods

Organic Beef	1 cup (8 oz)	410	21	80	12	–	–	0	6	0
Organic Turkey	1 cup (8 oz)	400	19	70	11	–	–	0	7	1

TAKE-OUT

beef	1 (14.6 oz)	938	57	67	13	14	25	–	5	4
chicken	1 (14.6 oz)	897	52	113	16	12	21	–	6	5
ham	1 serv (11 oz)	752	45	38	10	13	20	–	4	3
oyster	1 serv (11.5 oz)	817	53	89	15	14	21	0	3	6
puerto rican pastelon de carne	1 piece (5 oz)	666	48	93	18	4	21	–	2	1
st. stephen's day pie	1 serv (16.7 oz)	549	29	198	16	–	–	–	6	5
tuna	1 (27 oz)	1715	102	92	30	26	40	–	10	10
vegetarian w/ meat substitute	1 (8 oz)	511	32	20	9	10	12	–	5	3

POTATO (see also CHIPS, KNISH, PANCAKES)
CANNED

potatoes	½ cup	54	tr	0	tr	tr	tr	–	–	–

FOOD	PORTION	CALS	TOTAL FAT	CHOL	SAT FAT	POLY FAT	MONO FAT	TRANS FAT	FIBER	SUGAR
Butter Kernel										
Whole	⅔ cup (5.4 oz)	60	0	0	0	0	0	0	2	0
Del Monte										
New Whole	2 med (5.5 oz)	70	0	0	0	0	0	0	1	1
FRESH										
baked skin only	1 skin (2 oz)	115	tr	0	tr	tr	tr	–	2	–
baked w/ skin	1 (6.5 oz)	220	tr	0	tr	tr	tr	–	–	–
baked w/o skin	½ cup	57	tr	0	tr	tr	tr	–	1	–
baked w/o skin	1 (5 oz)	145	tr	0	tr	tr	tr	–	2	–
boiled	½ cup	68	tr	0	tr	tr	tr	–	1	–
microwaved	1 (7 oz)	212	tr	0	tr	tr	tr	–	–	–
microwaved w/o skin	½ cup	78	tr	0	tr	tr	tr	–	–	–
raw w/o skin	1 (3.9 oz)	88	tr	0	tr	tr	tr	–	–	–
red new boiled	5 sm (5 oz)	120	0	0	0	0	0	0	2	3
Dole										
Idaho	1 (5.3 oz)	110	0	0	0	0	0	0	2	1
Green Giant										
Klondike Gourmet	5 sm (5.3 oz)	110	0	0	0	0	0	0	2	1
Masser's										
Roasted Russet Triple Washed	1 (5.3 oz)	110	0	0	0	0	0	0	2	1
FROZEN										
french fries	10 strips (2.3 oz)	99	4	0	2	tr	2	–	2	–
potato puffs	1	16	1	0	tr	tr	tr	–	–	–
potato puffs	½ cup	138	7	0	3	tr	3	–	–	–
Alexia										
Crispy Sweet Potato Puffs	⅔ cup (3 oz)	140	5	0	0	2	3	0	3	9
Hashed Browns Yukon Select w/ Onion Garlic & White Pepper	⅔ cup (3 oz)	60	0	0	0	0	0	0	2	tr
Oven Fries w/ Olive Oil Rosemary & Garlic	8 (3 oz)	110	3	0	0	0	2	0	3	tr
Oven Reds w/ Olive Oil Parmesan & Roasted Garlic	8 (3 oz)	120	4	0	1	0	2	0	2	0
Saute Reds w/ Portabella Mushrooms Green Beans & Onions	1 cup (6.4 oz)	200	12	0	2	1	10	0	4	2
Sweet Potato Fries w/ Sea Salt	12 (3 oz)	140	5	0	0	1	4	0	3	6

FOOD	PORTION	CALS	TOTAL FAT	CHOL	SAT FAT	POLY FAT	MONO FAT	TRANS FAT	FIBER	SUGAR
Waffle Cut Bruschetta Fries	1 cup (3 oz)	160	6	0	1	2	4	0	3	tr
Yukon Select Fries Organic	24 (3 oz)	110	4	0	0	1	2	0	3	0
Lean Cuisine										
Simple Favorites Cheddar Potato w/ Broccoli	1 pkg (10.25 oz)	210	4	15	2	0	1	0	4	6
Ore Ida										
Steak Fries	7 (3 oz)	110	3	0	1	–	–	0	2	tr
MIX										
au gratin as prep	½ cup	160	9	29	6	tr	3	–	–	–
instant mashed flakes as prep w/ whole milk & margarine	1 cup (7.4 oz)	237	12	8	3	3	5	–	5	–
instant mashed flakes not prep	½ cup	78	tr	0	tr	tr	tr	–	–	–
instant mashed granules as prep w/ whole milk & butter	½ cup	114	5	15	3	tr	1	–	–	–
instant mashed granules not prep	½ cup	372	1	0	tr	tr	tr	–	–	–
scalloped	½ cup	105	5	14	3	tr	1	–	–	–
Betty Crocker										
Mashed Creamy Butter as prep	⅔ cup	80	1	<5	1	–	–	0	3	1
Idahoan										
Mashed Buttery Homestyle as prep	½ cup	110	3	0	1	–	–	0	1	2
Mashed Roasted Garlic as prep	½ cup	110	3	0	1	–	–	0	1	2
TAKE-OUT										
au gratin w/ cheese	½ cup	178	10	18	4	1	4	–	–	–
baked topped w/ cheese sauce	1	475	29	19	11	6	11	–	–	–
baked topped w/ cheese sauce & bacon	1	451	26	30	10	5	10	–	–	–
baked topped w/ cheese sauce & broccoli	1 (12 oz)	403	21	20	9	4	8	–	–	–
baked topped w/ cheese sauce & chili	1	481	22	31	13	tr	7	–	–	–
baked topped w/ sour cream & chives	1	394	22	23	10	3	8	–	–	–

FOOD	PORTION	CALS	TOTAL FAT	CHOL	SAT FAT	POLY FAT	MONO FAT	TRANS FAT	FIBER	SUGAR
french fries	1 reg	235	12	0	4	2	6	–	–	–
hash browns	½ cup (2.5 oz)	151	9	9	4	tr	4	–	–	–
indian yogurt potatoes	1 serv	315	9	18	4	–	–	–	0	–
mashed	½ cup	111	4	2	1	1	2	–	–	–
o'brien	1 cup	157	3	7	2	tr	1	–	–	–
potato pancakes	1 (1.3 oz)	101	7	35	1	2	2	–	–	–
potato salad	½ cup	179	10	85	2	5	3	–	2	–
scalloped	½ cup	127	5	7	–	–	–	–	–	–
twice baked w/ cheese	1 half (10 oz)	392	18	54	10	–	–	–	4	–

POTATO STARCH

potato starch	1 oz	96	tr	0	–	–	–	–	–	–

POUT

ocean baked	3 oz	87	1	57	tr	tr	tr	–	0	0
ocean fillet baked	1 (4.8 oz)	140	2	92	1	tr	1	–	0	0

PRETZELS

chocolate covered	1 (0.4 oz)	47	1	1	tr	tr	1	0	tr	2
soft	1 lg (5 oz)	483	4	4	1	1	2	0	2	tr
twists salted	10 (2.1 oz)	229	2	0	tr	1	1	–	2	–
twists w/o salt	10 (2.1 oz)	229	2	0	tr	1	1	–	2	1
whole wheat	2 sm (1 oz)	103	1	0	tr	tr	tr	–	2	–
yogurt covered	1 (4 g)	19	1	0	1	tr	tr	0	tr	1
yogurt covered	1 cup (3 oz)	391	13	1	11	1	1	0	1	30
Annie's Homegrown										
Organic Bunnies	32 (1 oz)	100	1	0	0	–	–	0	1	1
Bachman										
Honey Wheat Splits	9 (1 oz)	110	1	0	0	–	–	0	1	3
Mini Low Sodium	17 (1 oz)	110	0	0	0	0	0	0	1	–
Original Twist	5 (1 oz)	100	1	0	0	–	–	0	1	1
Rolled Rods	2 (1 oz)	110	0	0	0	0	0	0	1	1
Thin N Rights	12 (1 oz)	120	1	0	0	–	–	0	1	1
Farm Rich										
Stuffed Bites frzn	3 (1.7 oz)	110	3	5	2	–	–	0	1	2
Mary's Gone Crackers										
Sticks & Twigs Sea Salt Organic	15 (1 oz)	150	5	0	1	3	2	0	4	0
Pepperidge Farm										
Baked Naturals Pretzel Thins Simply Pretzel	12	110	0	0	0	0	0	0	1	1

FOOD	PORTION	CALS	TOTAL FAT	CHOL	SAT FAT	POLY FAT	MONO FAT	TRANS FAT	FIBER	SUG
Rold Gold										
Braided Twists Honey Wheat	8 (1 oz)	110	1	0	0	–	–	0	1	3
Rods	3 (1 oz)	110	1	0	0	–	–	0	1	1
Sourdough	1 (0.8 oz)	90	1	0	0	–	–	0	2	tr
Sticks	53 (1 oz)	100	0	0	0	0	0	0	1	1
Tiny Twists Fat Free	18 (1 oz)	110	0	0	0	0	0	0	tr	tr
PRUNE JUICE										
jarred	1 cup	182	tr	0	tr	tr	tr	–	3	42
Del Monte										
100% Juice	8 oz	180	0	0	0	0	0	0	3	25
PRUNES										
cooked w/o sugar	½ cup	133	tr	0	tr	tr	tr	0	4	31
dried	1	20	tr	0	tr	tr	tr	0	1	3
Del Monte										
Dried	5 (1.4 oz)	100	0	0	0	0	0	0	3	15
PUDDING										
MIX										
Jell-O										
Banana Cream Instant as prep w/ 2% milk	½ cup	150	3	9	2	–	–	0	0	18
Butterscotch Cook & Serve as prep w/ 2% milk	½ cup	160	3	9	2	–	–	0	0	19
Chocolate Cook & Serve as prep w/ 2% milk	½ cup	150	3	9	2	–	–	0	0	15
Chocolate Cook & Serve Sugar Free Fat Free as prep w/ fat free milk	½ cup	70	0	0	0	0	0	0	0	0
Coconut Cream Instant as prep w/ 2% milk	½ cup	160	5	9	4	–	–	0	0	16
Rice Fat Free as prep w/ fat free milk	½ cup	140	0	0	0	0	0	0	0	13
Tapioca Fat Free Cook & Serve as prep w/ fat free milk	½ cup	130	0	0	0	0	0	0	0	15
Vanilla Instant as prep	1 serv	90	0	0	0	0	0	0	0	19
READY-TO-EAT										
Cocon										
Mixed Mini Pudding w/ Nata De Coco	2 (1 oz)	15	0	0	0	0	0	0	0	3

FOOD	PORTION	CALS	TOTAL FAT	CHOL	SAT FAT	POLY FAT	MONO FAT	TRANS FAT	FIBER	SUGAR
Jell-O										
Boston Cream Pie Sugar Free Reduced Calorie	1 pkg (3.7 oz)	60	1	0	1	–	–	0	0	0
Chocolate	1 pkg (4 oz)	120	2	0	2	–	–	0	1	19
Chocolate Fat Free	1 pkg (4 oz)	100	0	0	0	0	0	0	1	17
Chocolate Vanilla Swirl	1 pkg (4 oz)	110	2	0	2	–	–	0	1	19
Creme Brulee Sugar Free Reduced Calorie	1 pkg (3.7 oz)	70	2	10	1	–	–	0	0	0
Dulce De Leche Sugar Free Reduced Calorie	1 pkg (3.7 oz)	60	1	0	1	–	–	0	0	0
Orange Ice Cream Shop	1 pkg (3.9 oz)	120	3	10	2	–	–	0	0	18
Rice Sugar Free Reduced Calorie	1 pkg (3.7 oz)	70	2	10	1	–	–	0	0	0
Tapioca	1 pkg (4 oz)	110	2	0	2	–	–	0	0	19
Vanilla	1 serv (4 oz)	110	2	0	2	–	–	0	0	18
Vanilla Sugar Free Reduced Calorie	1 pkg (3.7 oz)	60	1	0	1	–	–	0	0	0
Kozy Shack										
Bread Pudding Apple Cinnamon	1 pkg (3.5 oz)	150	3	40	2	–	–	0	0	19
Butterscotch	1 pkg (4 oz)	120	2	10	1	–	–	0	0	19
Chocolate Lactose Free	1 pkg (4 oz)	130	4	15	2	–	–	0	1	17
Chocolate No Sugar Added	1 pkg (4 oz)	60	1	5	1	–	–	0	4	4
Rice Lactose Free	1 pkg (4 oz)	120	3	15	2	–	–	0	0	13
Rice No Sugar Added	1 pkg (4 oz)	70	1	10	0	–	–	0	3	5
Soda Shoppe Root Beer Float	1 pkg (3.7 oz)	100	1	10	0	–	–	0	0	17
Soda Shoppe Orange Cream Pop	1 pkg (3.7 oz)	110	1	10	0	–	–	0	0	17
Tapioca Lactose Free	1 pkg (4 oz)	120	3	15	2	–	–	0	0	15
Tapioca No Sugar Added	1 pkg (4 oz)	70	1	5	0	–	–	0	3	6
Snack Pack										
Banana Cream Pie	1 pkg (3.5 oz)	110	4	0	2	–	–	0	0	13
Butterscotch	1 pkg (3.5 oz)	110	3	0	2	–	–	0	0	16
Caramel Cream	1 pkg (3.5 oz)	120	3	0	2	–	–	1	0	17
Chocolate	1 pkg (3.5 oz)	130	3	0	2	–	–	0	tr	16
Chocolate Daredevil Triples	1 pkg (3.5 oz)	130	4	0	2	–	–	0	tr	18
Chocolate Fat Free	1 pkg (3.5 oz)	80	0	0	0	0	0	0	tr	15
Chocolate No Sugar Added	1 pkg (3.5 oz)	70	4	0	2	–	–	0	1	0
Lemon	1 pkg (3.5 oz)	130	3	0	2	–	–	0	0	20
Tapioca	1 pkg (3.5 oz)	120	4	0	2	–	–	0	0	15

FOOD	PORTION	CALS	TOTAL FAT	CHOL	SAT FAT	POLY FAT	MONO FAT	TRANS FAT	FIBER	SUGAR
Tapioca Fat Free	1 serv (3.5 oz)	80	0	0	0	0	0	0	0	13
Vanilla	1 pkg (3.5 oz)	120	4	0	2	–	–	0	1	14
SoYummi										
Dark Chocolate	1 pkg (3.5 oz)	110	3	0	0	–	–	0	4	11
Key Lime	1 pkg (3.5 oz)	115	4	0	0	1	1	0	2	11
Rice	1 pkg (3.5 oz)	110	2	0	1	1	0	0	2	6
TAKE-OUT										
bread w/ raisins	1 cup	306	9	124	3	2	3	0	2	29
coconut	1 cup	291	9	15	7	tr	1	0	2	38
corn	1 cup	328	13	185	6	1	4	–	4	17
guinataan coconut milk pudding	1 cup (9 oz)	331	11	0	9	0	0	–	3	–
indian pudding	½ cup	156	4	40	2	tr	1	0	1	16
noodle pudding kugel	1 cup	297	10	144	2	2	4	0	2	15
plum pudding	1 slice (1.5 oz)	125	5	22	3	tr	1	0	1	12
pumpkin	½ cup (4.6 oz)	139	4	4	1	tr	2	–	tr	19
rice pudding	1 cup	302	4	14	2	tr	1	0	1	37
sweet potato	½ cup	107	3	1	1	1	1	–	3	7
tapioca	1 cup	236	7	156	3	1	2	0	0	31
yorkshire	1 serv (3 oz)	177	8	57	–	–	–	–	tr	–
PUMMELO										
fresh white	1 (21.4 oz)	231	tr	0	–	–	–	0	6	–
sections white	1 cup (6.7 oz)	72	tr	0	–	–	–	–	2	–
Sunkist										
Fresh	¼ (5.3 oz)	90	1	0	0	–	–	0	4	11
PUMPKIN										
butter	1 tbsp	32	0	0	0	0	0	0	–	8
canned w/o salt	1 cup (8.6 oz)	83	1	0	tr	tr	tr	–	7	8
cooked mashed w/o salt	1 cup (8.6 oz)	49	tr	0	tr	tr	tr	–	3	3
flowers cooked w/o salt	1 cup (4.7 oz)	20	tr	0	tr	tr	tr	–	1	3
leaves cooked w/o salt	1 cup (2.5 oz)	15	tr	0	tr	tr	tr	–	2	tr
Farmer's Market										
Organic Puree	½ cup (4.3 oz)	50	0	0	0	0	0	0	4	4
Libby's										
Pumpkin	½ cup (4.3 oz)	40	1	0	0	–	–	0	5	4
TAKE-OUT										
indian sago	1 serv (2.3 oz)	75	5	0	2	1	2	–	3	3
pumpkin fritters	1 (1.2 oz)	84	3	3	1	tr	1	–	tr	8

FOOD	PORTION	CALS	TOTAL FAT	CHOL	SAT FAT	POLY FAT	MONO FAT	TRANS FAT	FIBER	SUGAR
PUMPKIN SEEDS										
kernels dried	¼ cup (1.1 oz)	180	16	0	3	7	5	tr	2	tr
kernels roasted w/o salt	¼ cup (1 oz)	169	14	0	3	6	5	tr	2	tr
whole roasted w/o salt	¼ cup (0.5 oz)	71	3	0	1	1	1	–	3	–
David										
Kernels	1 pkg (2.5 oz)	280	22	0	4	10	6	0	2	tr
Spitz										
Seasoned Hulled	¼ cup (1 oz)	180	15	0	3	8	4	0	4	0
Sunrich Naturals										
Pepitas Lightly Salted	1 pkg (1 oz)	160	14	0	3	–	–	0	2	0
PURSLANE										
cooked	1 cup	21	tr	0	–	–	–	–	–	–
fresh	1 cup	7	tr	0	–	–	–	–	–	–
QUAIL										
cooked bone removed	1 (2.7 oz)	177	11	65	3	3	4	0	0	0
QUICHE										
La Terra Fina										
Cheddar & Broccoli	⅕ pie (4.6 oz)	300	18	25	8	–	–	0	2	3
Lorraine	⅕ pie (4.6 oz)	320	19	30	8	–	–	0	1	2
Spinach & Artichoke	⅕ pie (4.6 oz)	290	17	20	7	–	–	0	2	2
TAKE-OUT										
cheese	⅛ (9 in) pie	566	44	240	21	5	15	–	1	1
lorraine	⅛ (9 in) pie	568	44	242	20	5	15	–	1	1
spinach	⅛ (9 in) pie	342	26	157	12	3	9	–	1	1
QUINCE										
fresh	1	53	tr	0	tr	tr	tr	–	–	–
Matiz										
Quince Paste	2 tbsp	83	0	0	0	0	0	0	1	13
QUINCE JUICE										
Smart Juice										
Organic 100% Juice	8 oz	110	0	0	0	0	0	0	0	21
QUINOA										
cooked	1 cup (6.5 oz)	222	4	0	–	–	–	0	5	–
quinoa not prep	¼ cup (1.5 oz)	156	3	0	tr	1	1	0	3	–
Simply Shari's										
Quinoa + Marinara Gluten Free as prep	¼ pkg (4 oz)	175	2	5	0	–	–	0	5	4

FOOD	PORTION	CALS	TOTAL FAT	CHOL	SAT FAT	POLY FAT	MONO FAT	TRANS FAT	FIBER	SUGAR
Village Harvest										
Whole Grain Medley Golden Quinoa	¾ cup (5 oz)	220	3	0	0	–	–	0	4	0
Whole Grain Medley Red Quinoa & Brown Rice	1 cup (5 oz)	300	4	0	1	–	–	0	3	0
RABBIT										
domestic w/o bone roasted	3 oz	167	7	70	2	1	2	–	0	0
wild w/o bone stewed	3 oz	147	3	104	1	1	1	–	0	0
RADICCHIO										
raw shredded	½ cup	5	tr	0	–	–	–	–	–	–
RADISHES										
chinese dried	½ cup	157	tr	0	tr	tr	tr	–	–	–
chinese raw	1 (12 oz)	62	tr	0	tr	tr	tr	–	–	–
chinese raw sliced	½ cup	8	tr	0	tr	tr	tr	–	–	–
chinese sliced cooked	½ cup	13	tr	0	tr	tr	tr	–	–	–
daikon dried	½ cup	157	tr	0	tr	tr	tr	–	–	–
daikon raw	1 (12 oz)	62	tr	0	tr	tr	tr	–	–	–
daikon raw sliced	½ cup	8	tr	0	tr	tr	tr	–	–	–
daikon sliced cooked	½ cup	13	tr	0	tr	tr	tr	–	–	–
red raw	10	7	tr	0	tr	tr	tr	–	–	–
red sliced	½ cup	10	tr	0	tr	tr	tr	–	–	–
white icicle raw	1 (0.5 oz)	2	tr	0	tr	tr	tr	–	–	–
white icicle raw sliced	½ cup	7	tr	0	tr	tr	tr	–	–	–
TAKE-OUT										
moo namul saengche korean salad	1 serv (3.7 oz)	34	tr	0	tr	–	–	–	2	6
RAISINS										
cinnamon coated	¼ cup	108	tr	0	tr	tr	tr	0	1	21
cooked	¼ cup	162	tr	0	tr	tr	tr	0	1	35
golden seedless	¼ cup	109	tr	0	tr	tr	tr	0	1	21
jumbo golden	¼ cup	130	0	0	0	0	0	0	2	29
milk chocolate coated	28 (1 oz)	109	4	1	2	tr	1	0	1	17
milk chocolate coated	¼ cup	176	7	1	4	tr	2	0	2	28
seedless	55 (1 oz)	86	tr	0	tr	tr	tr	0	1	17
Dole										
Golden Seedless	¼ cup (1.4 oz)	120	0	0	0	0	0	0	1	24
Sun-Maid										
Chocolate Covered	30 (1.4 oz)	160	6	5	4	–	–	0	2	24

FOOD	PORTION	CALS	TOTAL FAT	CHOL	SAT FAT	POLY FAT	MONO FAT	TRANS FAT	FIBER	SUGAR
RAMBUTAN										
canned in syrup	1 cup (4.3 oz)	123	tr	0	–	–	–	0	1	–
RASPBERRIES										
black fresh	1 cup	70	1	0	tr	tr	tr	0	9	6
canned in heavy syrup	½ cup	116	tr	0	tr	tr	tr	0	4	26
canned water pack	1 cup	43	1	0	tr	tr	tr	0	5	4
fresh	1 pt	162	2	0	tr	1	tr	0	20	14
fresh	1 cup	64	1	0	tr	tr	tr	0	8	5
frzn sweetened	1 cup	129	tr	0	tr	tr	tr	0	6	27
frzn unsweetened	1 cup	65	1	0	tr	tr	tr	0	8	6
Dole										
Fresh	1 cup (4.3 oz)	60	1	0	0	–	–	0	8	5
Raspberries frzn	1 cup (4.9 oz)	70	1	0	0	–	–	0	9	7
RASPBERRY JUICE										
Izze										
Esque Sparkling Black Raspberry	1 bottle (12 oz)	50	0	0	0	0	0	0	–	11
Old Orchard										
100% Juice	8 oz	130	0	0	0	0	0	0	–	29
RELISH										
hamburger	½ cup	158	1	0	tr	tr	tr	–	–	–
hamburger	1 tbsp	19	tr	0	tr	tr	tr	–	–	–
hot dog	1 tbsp	14	tr	0	tr	tr	tr	–	–	–
hot dog	½ cup	111	1	0	tr	tr	tr	–	–	–
sweet	½ cup	159	1	0	tr	tr	tr	–	–	–
sweet	1 tbsp	19	tr	0	tr	tr	tr	–	–	–
tomato	¼ cup (2.8 oz)	119	tr	0	tr	tr	tr	0	1	26
Gedney										
Sweet	1 tbsp (0.5 oz)	15	0	0	0	0	0	0	0	3
Jake & Amos										
Chow Chow Sweet & Sour	1 serv (4 oz)	140	0	0	0	0	0	0	5	19
Corn	2 tbsp	40	0	0	0	0	0	0	0	6
Green Tomato	1 serv (1 oz)	25	0	0	0	0	0	0	–	6
RHUBARB										
fresh	½ cup	13	tr	0	–	–	–	–	–	–
frozen	½ cup	60	tr	0	–	–	–	–	–	–
frzn as prep w/ sugar	½ cup	139	tr	0	–	–	–	–	–	–

FOOD	PORTION	CALS	TOTAL FAT	CHOL	SAT FAT	POLY FAT	MONO FAT	TRANS FAT	FIBER	SUGAR
RICE *(see also RICE CAKES, WILD RICE)*										
arborio	½ cup	100	0	0	–	–	–	0	–	–
brown long grain cooked	1 cup (6.8 oz)	216	2	0	tr	1	1	–	4	–
brown medium grain cooked	1 cup (6.8 oz)	218	2	0	tr	1	1	–	4	–
glutinous cooked	1 cup (6.1 oz)	169	tr	0	tr	tr	tr	–	2	–
starch	1 oz	98	0	0	0	0	0	0	–	–
white long grain cooked	1 cup (5.5 oz)	205	tr	0	tr	tr	tr	–	1	–
white long grain instant cooked	1 cup (5.8 oz)	162	tr	0	tr	tr	tr	–	1	–
white medium grain cooked	1 cup (6.5 oz)	242	tr	0	tr	tr	tr	–	1	–
white short grain cooked	1 cup (6.5 oz)	242	tr	0	tr	tr	tr	–	–	–
Birds Eye										
Steamfresh Whole Grain Brown Rice as prep	1 cup (4.8 oz)	150	1	0	0	–	–	0	2	0
Carolina										
White Medium Grain as prep	1 cup	160	0	0	0	0	0	0	1	0
Gourmet House										
Indian Basmati as prep	¾ cup	160	0	0	0	0	0	0	0	0
Italian Arborio as prep	¾ cup	160	0	0	0	0	0	0	tr	0
Organic Brown as prep	¾ pkg	150	1	0	0	–	–	0	1	0
Organic White as prep	¾ cup	150	0	0	0	0	0	0	0	0
Lundberg										
Organic Heat & Eat Short Grain	1 pkg (7.4 oz)	290	3	0	1	–	–	0	5	1
Organic Risotto Florentine not prep	¼ pkg (1.4 oz)	140	0	0	0	0	0	0	1	2
Organic Risotto Tuscan not prep	¼ pkg (1.4 oz)	140	0	0	0	0.	0	0	1	2
Risotto Butternut Squash not prep	¼ pkg (1.4 oz)	140	1	0	0	–	–	0	1	1
Mahatma										
Jasmine as prep	¾ cup	160	0	0	0	0	0	0	0	0
White as prep	¾ cup	150	0	0	0	0	0	0	0	0
Whole Grain Brown as prep	¾ cup	150	1	0	0	–	–	0	1	0
Minute										
Brown as prep	⅔ cup	150	2	0	0	–	–	0	2	0
Ready To Serve Brown & Wild Rice	1 pkg (4.4 oz)	230	5	0	1	–	–	0	5	0
Ready To Serve Pilaf	1 pkg (4.4 oz)	220	4	0	0	–	–	0	2	3
Ready To Serve Spanish Rice	1 pkg (4.4 oz)	230	5	0	1	–	–	0	2	1

FOOD	PORTION	CALS	TOTAL FAT	CHOL	SAT FAT	POLY FAT	MONO FAT	TRANS FAT	FIBER	SUGAR
Ready To Serve Whole Grain Brown	1 pkg (4.4 oz)	230	4	0	0	–	–	0	2	0
Steamers Broccoli & Cheese	1 cup (6.4 oz)	200	4	5	2	–	–	0	1	2
Steamers Fried Rice	1 cup (6.5 oz)	280	6	5	1	–	–	0	2	0
White as prep	1 cup	200	0	0	0	0	0	0	0	0
River Rice										
Brown as prep	¾ cup	150	0	0	0	0	0	0	1	0
Stahlbush Island Farms										
Organic Brown Rice & Black Beans frzn	1 cup (6.2 oz)	200	2	0	0	–	–	0	7	0
Success										
Boil-In-Bag Jasmine as prep	¾ cup	150	0	0	0	0	0	0	0	0
Boil-In-Bag White as prep	1 cup	190	0	0	0	0	0	0	0	0
Boil-In-Bag Whole Grain Brown as prep	1 cup	150	1	0	0	–	–	0	2	0
Uncle Ben's										
Whole Grain White Broccoli Cheddar as prep	1 cup	200	2	0	1	–	–	0	4	1
Whole Grain White Creamy Chicken as prep	1 cup	200	2	0	0	–	–	0	5	1
Whole Grain White Garden Vegetable as prep	1 cup	180	1	0	0	–	–	0	4	2
Whole Grain White Long Grain as prep	1 cup	170	1	0	0	–	–	0	4	1
Whole Grain White Sweet Tomato as prep	1 cup	210	2	0	1	–	–	0	5	4
Whole Grain White Taco as prep	1 cup	160	2	0	0	–	–	0	4	1
Village Harvest										
Whole Grain Creations w/ Corn & Black Beans frzn	¾ cup (4.3 oz)	140	2	0	0	–	–	0	4	4
Whole Grain Medley Brown Red & Wild Rice frzn	1 cup (5 oz)	250	3	0	1	–	–	0	3	0
Water Maid										
Medium Grain as prep	¾ cup	160	0	0	0	0	0	0	1	0
Zatarain's										
Black Eyed Peas & Rice as prep	1 cup	220	1	0	0	–	–	–	4	0
Caribbean Rice Mix as prep	1 cup	160	2	0	1	–	–	–	tr	0
Cheddar Broccoli as prep	1 cup	220	2	<5	1	–	–	–	tr	3
Yellow as prep	1 cup	190	0	0	0	0	0	–	tr	tr

FOOD	PORTION	CALS	TOTAL FAT	CHOL	SAT FAT	POLY FAT	MONO FAT	TRANS FAT	FIBER	SUGAR
TAKE-OUT										
dirty rice w/ chicken giblets	1 cup (6.9 oz)	291	10	107	5	1	3	–	1	tr
nasi goreng indonesian rice & vegetables	1 cup (4.9 oz)	130	0	0	0	0	0	–	1	1
pea palau rice & peas fried in ghee	1 serv	144	5	21	3	1	1	–	2	1
pilaf	½ cup	84	3	22	1	tr	1	–	3	–
spanish	¾ cup	363	27	35	10	4	12	–	–	–
RICE CAKES (see also POPCORN CAKES)										
Lundberg										
Eco-Farmed Apple Cinnamon	1 (0.7 oz)	80	1	0	0	–	–	0	1	2
Eco-Farmed Toasted Sesame	1 (0.7 oz)	70	0	0	0	0	0	0	1	0
Organic Caramel Corn	1 (0.7 oz)	80	1	0	0	–	–	0	1	2
Organic Flax w/ Tamari	1 (0.7 oz)	80	1	0	0	–	–	0	1	1
Organic Mochi Sweet	1 (0.7 oz)	60	1	0	0	–	–	0	1	0
Organic Popcorn Rice	1 (0.7 oz)	60	1	0	0	–	–	0	1	0
Organic Sesame Tamari	1 (0.7 oz)	60	1	0	0	–	–	0	1	0
Organic Wild Rice Lightly Salted	1 (0.6 oz)	70	0	0	0	0	0	0	1	0
Mother's										
Caramel	1 (0.5 oz)	45	0	0	0	0	0	0	–	3
Plain Salted	1 (0.3 oz)	35	0	0	0	0	0	0	–	–
Plain Unsalted	1 (0.3 oz)	35	0	0	0	0	0	0	–	–
Salted Butter	1 (0.3 oz)	35	0	0	0	0	0	0	–	–
Quaker										
Apple Cinnamon	1 (0.5 oz)	50	0	0	0	0	0	0	–	3
Butter Popped Corn	1 (0.3 oz)	35	0	0	0	0	0	0	–	0
Lightly Salted	1 (0.3 oz)	35	0	0	0	0	0	0	–	–
Quakes Chocolate	13 (1 oz)	120	2	0	0	–	–	0	1	7
Quakes Vanilla Creme Brulee	13 (1 oz)	120	1	0	0	–	–	0	1	8
ROCKFISH										
pacific cooked	3 oz	103	2	38	tr	1	tr	–	0	0
pacific cooked	1 fillet (5.2 oz)	180	3	66	1	1	1	–	0	0
pacific raw	3 oz	80	1	29	tr	1	tr	–	0	0
ROE (see also individual fish names)										
fresh baked	1 oz	58	2	136	1	1	1	0	0	–

ROLL

FROZEN

Alexia

FOOD	PORTION	CALS	TOTAL FAT	CHOL	SAT FAT	POLY FAT	MONO FAT	TRANS FAT	FIBER	SUGAR
Ancient Grain Artisan	1 (1.5 oz)	110	1	0	0	1	0	0	1	tr
Ciabatta Artisan	1 (1.5 oz)	120	2	0	0	1	1	0	2	1
Focaccia Artisan	1 (1.5 oz)	130	2	5	1	1	1	0	2	1
Sweet Potato Artisan	1 (1.5 oz)	120	3	10	1	1	1	0	2	4
Whole Grain Artisan	1 (1.5 oz)	110*	1	0	0	1	0	0	3	2
READY-TO-EAT										
bialy	1 (2.2 oz)	138	0	0	0	0	0	0	1	–
brioche sweet roll	1 (3.5 oz)	410	23	190	14	1	6	–	3	5
cheese	1 (2.3 oz)	238	12	50	4	1	6	–	1	–
cinnamon raisin	1 (2.1 oz)	223	10	40	2	4	3	–	1	19
dinner	1 (1 oz)	78	1	0	tr	1	tr	–	1	2
egg	1 (1.2 oz)	107	2	16	1	tr	1	–	1	2
french	1 (1.3 oz)	105	2	0	tr	tr	1	–	1	tr
garlic	1 (1.5 oz)	133	3	2	1	1	1	0	1	2
hamburger or hot dog	1 (1.5 oz)	120	2	0	tr	1	tr	–	1	3
hamburger or hot dog multi grain	1 (1.5 oz)	113	3	0	1	tr	1	–	2	3
hamburger or hot dog reduced calorie	1 (1.5 oz)	84	1	0	tr	tr	tr	–	3	2
hamburger or hot dog whole wheat	1 (1.5 oz)	114	2	0	tr	1	1	–	3	4
hard	1 (2 oz)	167	2	0	tr	1	1	–	1	1
hoagie or submarine roll whole wheat	1 (4.7 oz)	359	6	0	1	3	2	–	10	11
mexican bolillo	1 (4.1 oz)	305	2	1	tr	1	tr	–	2	tr
oat bran	1 (1.2 oz)	78	2	0	tr	1	tr	–	1	2
oatmeal	1 (1.3 oz)	103	2	7	1	1	1	–	1	2
pumpernickel	1 (1.3 oz)	100	1	0	tr	tr	tr	–	2	tr
rye	1 med (1.3 oz)	103	1	0	tr	tr	tr	–	2	tr
sourdough	1 (1.6 oz)	130	1	0	tr	tr	tr	–	1	1
wheat	1 (1 oz)	76	2	0	tr	1	tr	–	1	tr
whole wheat	1 med (1.3 oz)	96	2	0	tr	1	tr	–	3	3
Arnold										
Wheat Hot Dog	1 (1.8 oz)	130	2	0	0	–	–	0	2	5
Martin's										
Potato	1 (1.9 oz)	130	2	0	0	0	0	0	3	7

FOOD	PORTION	CALS	TOTAL FAT	CHOL	SAT FAT	POLY FAT	MONO FAT	TRANS FAT	FIBER	SUGAR
Nature's Own										
Butter Hamburger Bun	1 (2 oz)	140	2	<5	1	0	0	0	1	2
Hot Dog Honey Wheat	1 (1.4 oz)	100	1	0	1	1	0	0	tr	2
Sandwich 100% Whole Wheat	1 (1.9 oz)	130	2	0	1	1	0	0	4	2
Pepperidge Farm										
Deli Flats Soft 100% Whole Wheat	1	100	2	0	0	0	0	0	5	3
Deli Flats Soft Honey Wheat	1	100	1	0	0	1	0	0	5	3
Dinner Classic	1	90	2	0	0	1	0	0	1	3
Hamburger 100% Whole Wheat	1	110	2	0	0	1	0	0	2	2
Hot Dog Top Sliced	1	150	3	0	1	2	1	0	<2	4
Sandwich Mini	1	100	2	0	0	1	0	0	1	3
Soft Hoagie	1	210	6	0	2	3	2	0	2	3
Stone Baked Artisan Ciabatta Sourdough	1	140	1	0	0	–	–	0	3	1
Stone Baked Artisan French Dinner	1	120	0	0	0	0	0	0	1	tr
Stone Baked Artisan Multi-Grain Dinner	1	120	1	0	0	1	0	0	3	5
REFRIGERATED										
crescent	1 (1 oz)	78	1	0	tr	1	tr	–	1	2
ROSE APPLE										
fresh	3.5 oz	32	tr	0	–	–	–	–	–	–
ROSE HIP										
fresh	1 oz	26	0	0	0	0	0	0	–	–
ROSELLE										
fresh	1 cup	28	tr	0	–	–	–	–	–	–
ROSEMARY										
dried	1 tsp	4	tr	0	tr	tr	tr	0	1	–
fresh	1 tbsp	1	tr	0	tr	tr	tr	0	tr	–
ROUGHY										
orange baked	3 oz	75	1	22	tr	tr	1	–	0	0

RUBS (see HERBS/SPICES)

FOOD	PORTION	CALS	TOTAL FAT	CHOL	SAT FAT	POLY FAT	MONO FAT	TRANS FAT	FIBER	SUGAR
RUTABAGA										
cooked mashed	1 cup	94	1	0	tr	tr	tr	0	4	14
cubed cooked	1 cup	66	tr	0	tr	tr	tr	0	3	10
SABLEFISH										
baked	3 oz	213	17	53	3	2	9	–	0	0
fillet baked	5.3 oz	378	30	95	6	4	16	–	0	0
smoked	1 oz	72	6	18	1	1	3	–	0	0
smoked	3 oz	218	17	55	4	2	9	–	0	0
SAFFLOWER										
seeds dried	1 oz	147	11	0	1	8	1	–	–	–
SAFFRON										
dried	1 tsp	2	tr	0	tr	tr	tr	0	tr	–
SAGE										
ground	1 tsp	2	tr	0	tr	tr	tr	0	tr	tr
SALAD (see also SALAD TOPPINGS)										
Dole										
American Blend	1½ cups (3 oz)	15	0	0	0	0	0	0	2	1
Butter Bliss	1½ cups (3 oz)	15	0	0	0	0	0	0	1	1
European Blend	1½ cups (3 oz)	15	0	0	0	0	0	0	1	1
Field Greens	1½ cups (3 oz)	20	0	0	0	0	0	0	2	1
Italian Blend	1½ cups (3 oz)	15	0	0	0	0	0	0	1	2
Kit Asian Island Crunch as prep	1½ cups (3.5 oz)	130	7	5	1	–	–	0	3	9
Seven Lettuces	1½ cups (3 oz)	20	0	0	0	0	0	0	1	1
Spring Mix	1½ cups (3 oz)	20	0	0	0	0	0	0	2	2
Very Veggie Blend	1½ cups (3 oz)	20	0	0	0	0	0	0	2	2
Eat Smart										
Asian Salad Kit as prep	1 serv (3 oz)	120	8	0	1	–	–	0	3	4
Broccoli Salad Kit as prep	1 serv (3 oz)	90	4	0	0	–	–	0	3	5
Chipotle Salad Kit as prep	1 serv (3 oz)	140	10	10	3	–	–	0	2	2
Mann's										
Rainbow	1 serv (3 oz)	25	0	0	0	0	0	0	2	2
Ready Pac										
All American	2 cups (3 oz)	15	0	0	0	0	0	0	1	2
American Blue Cheese Mix as prep	1¾ cups (3.5 oz)	110	8	10	2	–	–	0	1	2
Baby Romaine Blend	4½ cups (3 oz)	20	0	0	0	0	0	0	2	0

FOOD	PORTION	CALS	TOTAL FAT	CHOL	SAT FAT	POLY FAT	MONO FAT	TRANS FAT	FIBER	SUGAR
Baby Spinach Mix as prep	2 cups (3.5 oz)	140	3	0	0	–	–	0	2	12
Chef	1 pkg (7.7 oz)	270	20	55	7	–	–	0	2	5
Cobb	1 pkg (7.2 oz)	300	23	140	6	–	–	0	2	4
Garden	2 cups (3 oz)	15	0	0	0	0	0	0	1	2
Grand Asian Mix as prep	1¼ cups (3.5 oz)	130	6	0	1	3	2	0	2	11
Spinach Bacon	1 pkg (4.7 oz)	240	12	130	4	–	–	0	3	8
Spring Mix	4½ cups	20	0	0	0	0	0	0	2	0
Spring Mix Spinach	5 cups (3 oz)	20	0	0	0	0	0	0	2	1
Veggie Medley	2 cups (3 oz)	15	0	0	0	0	0	0	1	2
River Ranch										
American Blend	2 cups (3 oz)	15	0	0	0	0	0	0	1	2
Classic Garden	2 cups (3 oz)	15	0	0	0	0	0	0	1	2
Complete Caesar Salad Kit as prep	2 cups (3.5 oz)	150	11	5	2	–	–	0	2	2
Heritage Blend	4 cups (3 oz)	25	0	0	0	0	0	0	3	1
TAKE-OUT										
7-layer salad	2 cups	557	51	119	11	24	14	–	3	8
caesar	4 cups	734	61	173	11	7	40	–	7	6
chef salad w/o dressing	3 cups	535	32	280	16	3	10	–	–	–
cobb w/ dressing	4 cups	645	49	294	13	10	21	0	11	9
greek w/dressing	4 cups	424	29	475	14	3	10	–	4	8
mixed salad greens shredded	1 cup	9	tr	0	tr	tr	tr	0	1	tr
somen w/ lettuce egg fish pork	2 cups	550	17	429	5	3	7	–	4	4
spinach w/o dressing	4 cups	429	19	308	6	3	9	–	6	5
tossed w/ avocado w/o dressing	2 cups	90	6	0	1	1	4	0	5	4
tossed w/ chicken w/o dressing	3 cups	194	4	86	1	1	1	0	2	3
tossed w/ egg w/o dressing	2 cups	93	5	183	1	1	2	0	2	4
tossed w/ shrimp w/o dressing	1½ cups (8.3 oz)	106	2	179	1	tr	1	–	–	–
tossed w/ shrimp & egg w/o dressing	3 cups	185	5	430	1	1	1	0	2	3
tossed w/o dressing	2 cups	22	tr	0	tr	tr	tr	0	2	3
waldorf	1 cup	242	21	7	3	12	4	–	3	10
wilted lettuce w/ bacon dressing	1 cup	99	8	11	3	1	4	–	1	1

FOOD	PORTION	CALS	TOTAL FAT	CHOL	SAT FAT	POLY FAT	MONO FAT	TRANS FAT	FIBER	SUGAR
SALAD DRESSING (see also SALAD TOPPINGS)										
READY-TO-EAT										
french reduced calorie	1 tbsp	22	1	1	tr	1	tr	–	–	–
italian	1 tbsp (0.5 oz)	35	3	0	tr	2	1	tr	0	2
italian reduced fat	1 tbsp (0.5 oz)	15	1	0	tr	tr	tr	tr	0	1
russian reduced calorie	1 tbsp	23	1	1	tr	tr	tr	–	–	–
sesame seed	1 tbsp	68	7	0	1	4	2	–	–	–
thousand island reduced calorie	1 tbsp	24	2	2	tr	1	tr	–	–	–
Annie's Homegrown										
Cowgirl Ranch	2 tbsp (1 oz)	90	11	10	1	–	–	–	–	2
Vinaigrette Mango Fat Free	2 tbsp (1.1 oz)	20	0	0	0	0	0	0	–	5
Cains										
Caesar Fat Free	2 tbsp (1 oz)	30	0	0	0	0	0	0	0	2
Creamy Dill Cucumber Fat Free	2 tbsp (1 oz)	35	0	0	0	0	0	0	0	3
French	2 tbsp (1 oz)	120	11	0	2	–	–	0	0	4
French Light	2 tbsp (1 oz)	80	5	0	1	–	–	0	0	6
Italian Bellissimo	2 tbsp (2 oz)	150	16	0	3	–	–	0	0	1
Italian Fat Free	2 tbsp (1 oz)	15	0	0	0	0	0	0	0	2
Italian Light	2 tbsp (1 oz)	50	4	0	1	–	–	0	0	2
Peppercorn Ranch Fat Free	2 tbsp (1 oz)	45	0	0	0	0	0	0	0	3
Ranch	2 tbsp (1 oz)	180	19	5	3	–	–	0	0	1
Ranch Light	2 tbsp (1 oz)	80	6	5	1	–	–	0	0	2
Ranch w/ Bacon	2 tbsp (1 oz)	170	17	5	3	–	–	0	0	1
Vinaigrette Chianti	2 tbsp (1 oz)	130	12	0	2	–	–	0	0	3
Vinaigrette Citrus	2 tbsp (1 oz)	120	12	0	2	–	–	0	0	3
Vinaigrette White Balsamic	2 tbsp (1 oz)	130	10	0	2	–	–	0	0	7
David's Unforgettables										
Balsamic Vinaigrette Low Fat	1 tbsp (0.5 oz)	40	3	0	0	–	–	0	0	3
Balsamic Vinaigrette Original	1 tbsp (0.5 oz)	70	7	0	0	–	–	0	0	3
Follow Your Heart										
Oil Free Citrus Poppy Seed	2 tbsp (1 oz)	10	0	0	0	0	0	0	0	1
Organic Italian Vinaigrette	2 tbsp (1 oz)	90	10	0	2	–	–	0	0	1
Organic Miso Ginger	2 tbsp (1 oz)	80	7	0	1	–	–	0	1	3
Vegan High Omega Bleu Cheese	2 tbsp (1 oz)	140	15	0	0	–	–	0	0	0
Vegan High Omega Ranch	2 tbsp (1 oz)	140	15	0	2	4	9	0	0	0
Vegan Honey Mustard	2 tbsp (1 oz)	120	10	0	1	–	–	0	0	6

FOOD	PORTION	CALS	TOTAL FAT	CHOL	SAT FAT	POLY FAT	MONO FAT	TRANS FAT	FIBER	SUGA
Vegan Lemon Herb	2 tbsp (1 oz)	90	10	0	0	–	–	0	0	0
Vegan Thousand Island	2 tbsp (1 oz)	80	8	0	0	–	–	0	0	2
Gazebo Room										
Lite Greek	1 tbsp (0.5 oz)	40	4	0	1	–	–	0	0	0
Jake & Amos										
Bacon	2 tbsp (1 oz)	90	5	25	1	–	–	0	1	10
Ken's										
Light Vinaigrette Balsamic	2 tbsp (1 oz)	60	5	0	1	2	2	0	0	4
Maple Grove Farms										
Cranberry Balsamic Fat Free	2 tbsp (1 oz)	30	0	0	0	0	0	0	–	6
Honey Dijon Fat Free	2 tbsp (1 oz)	35	0	0	0	0	0	0	tr	8
Poppyseed Fat Free	2 tbsp (1 oz)	35	0	0	0	0	0	0	–	7
Strawberry Balsamic	1 tbsp (1 oz)	30	0	0	0	0	0	0	–	6
Vidalia Onion Fat Free	2 tbsp (1 oz)	20	0	0	0	0	0	0	–	4
Vinaigrette Balsamic Sugar Free	2 tbsp (1 oz)	5	0	0	0	0	0	0	–	–
Newman's Own										
Lighten Up Light Balsamic Vinaigrette	2 tbsp (1 oz)	45	4	0	1	–	–	0	0	2
OrganicVille										
Coleslaw Non Dairy	2 tbsp (1 oz)	70	5	0	1	–	–	0	0	6
French	2 tbsp (1 oz)	130	7	0	2	–	–	0	0	8
Miso Ginger	2 tbsp (1 oz)	100	10	0	2	–	–	0	0	tr
Pomegranate	2 tbsp (1 oz)	100	10	0	2	–	–	0	0	2
Ranch Non Dairy	2 tbsp (1 oz)	90	9	0	2	–	–	0	0	1
Thousand Island Non Dairy	2 tbsp (1 oz)	80	7	0	1	–	–	0	0	3
Sonoma Gourmet										
Blue Cheese	2 tbsp (1 oz)	170	18	10	2	–	–	0	0	0
Caesar	2 tbsp (1 oz)	130	14	5	1	–	–	0	0	0
Greek	2 tbsp (1 oz)	60	7	0	1	–	–	0	0	0
Raspberry	2 tbsp (1 oz)	60	6	0	1	–	–	0	0	0
Soy Vay										
Toasted Sesame	3 tbsp	190	15	0	3	–	–	0	0	9
Wishbone										
Buffalo Blue Cheese	2 tbsp (1 oz)	120	13	0	2	8	3	0	0	tr
Chunky Blue Cheese Fat Free	2 tbsp (1 oz)	30	0	0	0	0	0	0	tr	2
Guacamole Ranch	2 tbsp (1 oz)	130	13	0	2	8	3	0	0	1
Italian	2 tbsp (1 oz)	160	12	0	2	–	–	0	0	11
Ranch Light	2 tbsp (1 oz)	70	5	<5	1	3	1	0	0	2
Robusto Italian	2 tbsp (1 oz)	80	7	0	1	5	2	0	0	3

FOOD	PORTION	CALS	TOTAL FAT	CHOL	SAT FAT	POLY FAT	MONO FAT	TRANS FAT	FIBER	SUGAR
TAKE-OUT										
vinegar & oil	1 tbsp	72	8	0	2	4	2	–	–	–
SALAD TOPPINGS										
McCormick										
Salad Toppins	1.3 tbsp (7 g)	35	2	0	–	–	–	0	0	tr
Salad Toppins Garden Vegetable	1.3 tbsp (7 g)	35	2	0	–	–	–	0	0	tr
SALMON										
CANNED										
w/ bone	½ cup	106	5	39	1	1	2	0	0	0
Chicken Of The Sea										
Pink	¼ cup (2.2 oz)	90	5	40	1	–	–	0	0	0
Pink Skinless & Boneless	⅓ pkg (2 oz)	60	2	20	1	–	–	–	0	0
Pink Smoked Pacific	1 pkg (3 oz)	120	4	45	1	–	–	0	0	1
Red	¼ cup	110	7	40	2	–	–	0	0	0
Sea Fare Pacific										
Smoked Alaskan Red Sockeye	½ pkg (1.5 oz)	70	4	25	1	–	–	0	0	0
FRESH										
atlantic farmed baked	4 oz	233	14	71	3	5	5	0	0	0
coho wild poached	4 oz	209	9	65	2	3	3	0	0	0
pink baked	4 oz	169	5	76	1	2	1	0	0	0
sockeye baked	4 oz	245	12	99	2	3	6	0	0	0
FROZEN										
Gorton's										
Classic Grilled Fillets	1 (3 oz)	100	3	35	1	1	2	0	–	1
SMOKED										
lox	1 oz	33	1	7	tr	tr	1	0	0	0
TAKE-OUT										
guisado salmon stew	1 serv (7.4 oz)	320	16	66	3	6	6	0	3	3
roulette w/ spinach stuffing	1 serv (4 oz)	160	6	45	2	–	–	–	tr	0
salmon cake	1 (4.2 oz)	264	16	56	4	5	6	0	1	1
salmon loaf	1 slice (3.7 oz)	206	11	120	3	3	4	0	tr	2
SALSA										
black bean & corn	2 tbsp	15	0	0	0	0	0	0	tr	1
citrus	2 tbsp (1 oz)	10	0	0	0	0	0	0	0	2
peach	2 tbsp	15	0	0	0	0	0	0	0	4
tomatoless corn & chile	2 tbsp	45	0	0	0	0	0	0	tr	6

FOOD	PORTION	CALS	TOTAL FAT	CHOL	SAT FAT	POLY FAT	MONO FAT	TRANS FAT	FIBER
Frontera									
Chipotle Hot	2 tbsp (1 oz)	10	0	0	0	0	0	0	0
Corn & Poblano Medium	2 tbsp (1 oz)	10	0	0	0	0	0	0	0
Guajillo Medium	2 tbsp (1 oz)	10	1	0	0	0	0	0	1
Spanish Olive Mild	2 tbsp (1 oz)	10	1	0	0	0	0	0	0
Jake & Amos									
Black Bean	2 tbsp (1 oz)	15	0	0	0	0	0	0	0
Peach	2 tbsp (1 oz)	20	0	0	0	0	0	0	0
Margaritaville									
Medium	2 tbsp	10	0	0	0	0	0	0	tr
Peppadew Chipotle Garlic	1 oz	10	0	0	0	0	0	0	0
Peppadew Mild	1 oz	10	0	0	0	0	0	0	0
Newman's Own									
Mild	2 tbsp (1.1 oz)	10	0	0	0	0	0	0	tr
OrganicVille									
Medium	2 tbsp (1 oz)	15	0	0	0	0	0	0	0
Pineapple	2 tbsp (1 oz)	15	0	0	0	0	0	0	0
Ready Pac									
Pico De Gallo	2 tbsp (1 oz)	5	0	0	0	0	0	0	0
Tostitos									
All Natural Chunky Mild	2 tbsp (1.2 oz)	10	0	0	0	0	0	0	tr
Con Queso	2 tbsp	40	3	<5	1	–	–	0	tr
SALSIFY									
fresh sliced cooked	½ cup	46	tr	0	–	–	–	–	–
SALT/SEASONED SALT									
kosher	¼ tsp	0	0	0	0	0	0	0	0
salt	1 tsp (6 g)	0	0	0	0	0	0	0	0
salt	1 tbsp (0.6 oz)	0	0	0	0	0	0	0	0
sea salt coarse	1 tsp	0	0	0	0	0	0	0	0
sea salt fine	¼ tsp	0	0	0	0	0	0	0	0
David's									
Kosher Salt	¼ tsp (1.5 g)	0	0	0	0	0	0	0	0
Manischewitz									
Kosher	¼ tsp (1.5 g)	0	0	0	0	0	0	0	0
McCormick									
Grinder Garlic Sea Salt	¼ tsp	0	0	0	0	0	0	0	0
Grinder Sea Salt	¼ tsp	0	0	0	0	0	0	0	0

FOOD	PORTION	CALS	TOTAL FAT	CHOL	SAT FAT	POLY FAT	MONO FAT	TRANS FAT	FIBER	SUGAR
SANDWICHES										
Aunt Jemima										
Biscuit	1 (4 oz)	340	21	110	7	–	–	3	tr	2
Griddlecake Sausage Egg & Cheese	1 (4.4 oz)	350	20	150	7	–	–	–	tr	11
Sausage Egg & Cheese On French Toast	1 (4.7 oz)	310	18	205	7	–	–	–	tr	6
Farm Rich										
Philly Cheese Steak	2 (3 oz)	220	11	35	5	–	–	0	1	3
Sandwich Melts	2 (4.2 oz)	290	14	35	5	–	–	0	1	1
IHOP At Home										
Breakfast Sandwich Flatbread Apple Bacon	1 (3.1 oz)	250	13	90	5	–	–	0	2	2
Wrap Griddle 'N Sausage Blueberry	1 (1.5 oz)	150	10	20	4	–	–	0	0	2
Wrap Griddle 'N Sausage Original	1 (1.6 oz)	140	11	20	4	–	–	0	0	2
Lean Cuisine										
Casual Cuisine Panini Chicken Club	1 pkg (6 oz)	360	9	40	4	3	3	0	4	6
Casual Cuisine Panini Spinach Artichoke Chicken	1 pkg (6 oz)	320	9	25	4	2	3	0	5	5
Casual Cuisine Panini Steak Cheddar & Mushroom	1 pkg (6 oz)	340	9	30	4	2	3	0	5	5
Lifestyle Chefs										
Meal-In-A-Bun Channa Masala	1 (4.5 oz)	250	10	0	4	–	–	0	7	4
Meal-In-A-Bun Creamy Vegetable Medley	1 (4.5 oz)	260	12	10	5	–	–	0	5	3
Meal-In-A-Bun Herb Vegetable Melange	1 (4.5 oz)	270	14	0	6	–	–	0	6	4
Meal-In-A-Bun Peas Paneer	1 (4.5 oz)	260	13	5	5	–	–	0	6	3
Meal-In-A-Bun Thai Satay	1 (4.5 oz)	270	14	0	5	–	–	0	5	3
Lunchables										
Cracker Stackers Bologna & American	1 pkg	390	22	60	9	–	–	1	2	11
Cracker Stackers Ham & Cheddar	1 pkg	410	21	50	9	–	–	1	1	14
Sub Sandwich Ham + American	1 pkg	240	7	20	3	–	–	0	1	7

FOOD	PORTION	CALS	TOTAL FAT	CHOL	SAT FAT	POLY FAT	MONO FAT	TRANS FAT	FIBER
Sub Sandwich Turkey & Cheddar	1 pkg	230	6	15	2	–	–	0	1
Mom Made									
Munchie Turkey Sausage	1 (2.5 oz)	220	11	5	5	–	–	–	1
Munchies Chicken	1 (2.5 oz)	220	11	10	5	–	–	–	2
Saffron Road									
Crispy Samosas w/ Saag Paneer	⅓ pkg (2.75 oz)	160	7	5	2	–	–	0	2
Crispy Samosas w/ Vegetables	⅓ pkg (2.75 oz)	180	8	0	1	–	–	0	2
Smucker's									
Uncrustables Peanut Butter & Grape Jelly On Whole Wheat	1 (2 oz)	210	9	0	2	–	–	0	3
Uncrustables Peanut Butter & Strawberry Jam	1 (2 oz)	210	9	0	2	–	–	0	2
Uncrustables Peanut Butter On Wheat Bread	1 (2 oz)	210	9	0	2	–	–	0	3
Soul									
Wrap Butter Chicken	1 (7 oz)	390	15	25	2	–	–	0	1
Wrap Chicken Tikka Masala	1 (7 oz)	370	11	20	1	–	–	0	1
Wrap Chicken Vindaloo	1 (7 oz)	400	11	25	1	–	–	0	1
Wrap Vegetable Curry	1 (7 oz)	410	16	0	1	–	–	0	2
Vegetarian Plus									
Vegan Tuna Roll	1 serv (2.5 oz)	160	8	0	3	–	–	0	0
TAKE-OUT									
bacon & egg	1 (6.2 oz)	388	21	421	6	4	8	–	1
bacon lettuce & tomato w/ mayo	1 (5.8 oz)	344	17	21	4	7	5	–	3
beef barbecue w/ bun	1 (6.7 oz)	417	12	69	4	2	5	–	2
calzone beef & cheese	1 (14 oz)	1476	76	187	27	15	30	–	6
calzone cheese	1 (15 oz)	1632	93	254	44	13	30	–	5
chicken fillet	1 (6.4 oz)	515	29	60	9	8	10	–	–
chicken fillet w/ cheese	1 (8 oz)	632	39	78	12	10	14	–	–
chicken salad	1 (5 oz)	333	16	49	3	7	4	–	2
crab cake w/ bun	1	308	8	97	2	3	3	–	2
crispy chicken fillet w/ lettuce tomato & mayo	1 (7.7 oz)	537	26	64	5	12	8	–	3
croque monsieur	1 (12.4 oz)	765	46	152	26	–	–	–	2
egg salad	1 (5.6 oz)	485	35	329	7	15	10	–	1

FOOD	PORTION	CALS	TOTAL FAT	CHOL	SAT FAT	POLY FAT	MONO FAT	TRANS FAT	FIBER	SUGAR
french dip w/ roll	1 (6.8 oz)	357	13	54	5	2	5	–	1	4
fried egg	1 (3.4 oz)	226	9	206	2	2	3	–	1	3
grilled cheese	1 (2.9 oz)	290	16	22	6	3	6	–	1	4
gyro	1 (13.7 oz)	593	12	82	4	2	4	–	4	8
ham & egg	1 (4.4 oz)	272	11	222	3	2	4	0	2	3
ham w/ cheese lettuce & mayo	1 (5.4 oz)	369	18	57	7	3	7	–	2	4
hot turkey w/ gravy	1	389	10	88	3	3	3	–	2	2
peanut butter	1 (3.3 oz)	342	17	0	4	5	8	–	3	5
peanut butter & banana	1	617	14	0	3	4	6	0	4	11
peanut butter & jelly	1 (3.3 oz)	327	14	0	3	4	6	–	3	12
reuben w/ sauerkraut & cheese	1 (6.4 oz)	463	29	81	10	6	10	–	4	7
roast beef w/ gravy	1 (7.8 oz)	386	16	69	6	1	6	–	2	2
sloppy joe pork on bun	1 (6.5 oz)	318	9	50	3	2	4	–	2	6
tuna melt	1 (5.3 oz)	350	16	34	5	6	4	–	1	6
tuna salad w/ lettuce	1 (5.9 oz)	289	7	22	1	4	2	–	2	6
turkey w/ mayo	1 (5 oz)	329	11	67	3	5	3	–	1	2

SAPODILLA

FOOD	PORTION	CALS	TOTAL FAT	CHOL	SAT FAT	POLY FAT	MONO FAT	TRANS FAT	FIBER	SUGAR
fresh	1	140	2	0	–	–	–	–	–	–
fresh cut up	1 cup	199	3	0	–	–	–	–	–	–

SAPOTES

FOOD	PORTION	CALS	TOTAL FAT	CHOL	SAT FAT	POLY FAT	MONO FAT	TRANS FAT	FIBER	SUGAR
fresh	1	301	i	0	–	–	–	–	–	–

SARDINES
CANNED

FOOD	PORTION	CALS	TOTAL FAT	CHOL	SAT FAT	POLY FAT	MONO FAT	TRANS FAT	FIBER	SUGAR
atlantic in oil w/ bone	2	50	3	34	tr	1	1	–	0	0
atlantic in oil w/ bone	1 can (3.2 oz)	192	11	131	1	5	4	–	0	0
pacific in tomato sauce w/ bone	1 (1.3 oz)	68	5	23	1	2	1	–	0	0
pacific in tomato sauce w/ bone	1 can (13 oz)	658	44	225	11	16	14	–	0	0

Chicken Of The Sea

FOOD	PORTION	CALS	TOTAL FAT	CHOL	SAT FAT	POLY FAT	MONO FAT	TRANS FAT	FIBER	SUGAR
In Hot Sauce	1 can (3.75 oz)	120	3	70	1	–	–	–	1	0
In Oil Lightly Smoked	1 can (3.75 oz)	150	10	75	2	–	–	–	0	0
In Tomato Sauce	1 can (3.75 oz)	90	2	60	1	–	–	–	1	2
In Water	1 can (3.75 oz)	90	2	70	1	–	–	–	0	0

King Oscar

FOOD	PORTION	CALS	TOTAL FAT	CHOL	SAT FAT	POLY FAT	MONO FAT	TRANS FAT	FIBER	SUGAR
In Dijon Mustard	1 can (3.5 oz)	160	11	125	4	3	5	0	0	0

FOOD	PORTION	CALS	TOTAL FAT	CHOL	SAT FAT	POLY FAT	MONO FAT	TRANS FAT	FIBER	SUG
In Pure Spring Water Low Sodium	1 can (3.5 oz)	140	10	110	3	3	5	0	0	0
In Tomato Sauce	1 can (3.5 oz)	170	12	110	4	5	3	0	0	0
Skinless Boneless In Olive Oil drained	1 serv (3 oz)	210	15	130	3	8	4	0	0	0
Matiz										
In Olive Oil	½ pkg (2 oz)	120	7	0	1	–	–	0	0	0

SAUCE (see BARBECUE SAUCE, CURRY, GRAVY, SPAGHETTI SAUCE)

FOOD	PORTION	CALS	TOTAL FAT	CHOL	SAT FAT	POLY FAT	MONO FAT	TRANS FAT	FIBER	SUG
adobo fresco	2 tbsp	81	8	0	1	1	5	–	1	tr
bearnaise	1 oz	177	19	21	12	1	5	–	tr	–
cheese mix as prep w/ milk	1 cup	307	17	53	9	2	5	–	–	–
enchilada sauce green	¼ cup	46	4	11	2	tr	1	–	1	2
enchilada sauce red	¼ cup	79	8	22	4	1	2	–	1	1
fish sauce vietnamese nuoc mam	1 tbsp	6	0	0	0	0	0	0	0	–
hoisin	1 tbsp	35	1	0	–	–	–	–	tr	–
moroccan tagine	½ cup (4 oz)	70	3	0	0	–	–	–	1	10
mushroom mix as prep w/ milk	1 cup	228	10	34	5	1	3	–	–	–
oyster	1 tbsp	8	0	0	0	0	0	0	0	–
satay peanut sauce	1 oz	77	6	0	2	2	3	–	1	3
sour cream mix as prep w/ milk	1 cup	509	30	91	16	3	10	–	–	–
stroganoff mix as prep	1 cup	271	11	38	7	tr	3	–	–	–
sweet & sour mix as prep	1 cup	294	tr	0	tr	tr	tr	–	–	–
teriyaki	1 tbsp	15	0	0	0	0	0	0	–	–
teriyaki mix as prep	1 cup	131	1	0	tr	1	tr	–	–	–
white sauce mix as prep w/ milk	1 cup	241	13	34	6	2	5	–	–	–
Annie's Homegrown										
Organic Worcestershire	1 tsp (5 g)	5	0	0	0	0	0	0	–	1
Cains										
Tartar	2 tbsp (1 oz)	160	16	15	3	–	–	0	0	1
Chun's										
Sweet N' Sour	2 tbsp (1.2 oz)	45	0	0	0	0	0	0	0	9
Del Monte										
Chili Sauce	1 tbsp (0.6 oz)	20	0	0	0	0	0	0	–	4
Seafood Cocktail	¼ cup	100	0	0	0	0	0	0	0	22

FOOD	PORTION	CALS	TOTAL FAT	CHOL	SAT FAT	POLY FAT	MONO FAT	TRANS FAT	FIBER	SUGAR
Fischer & Wieser										
Bourbon Charred Pineapple	1 tbsp (0.7 oz)	35	0	0	0	0	0	0	0	8
Chipotle Original Roasted Raspberry	1 tbsp (0.7 oz)	40	0	0	0	0	0	0	1	9
Grilling Chipotle Plum	1 tbsp (0.7 oz)	40	0	0	0	0	0	0	–	10
Grilling Spicy Garlic Steak	1 tbsp (0.7 oz)	20	1	0	0	–	–	0	0	2
Habanero Mango Ginger	1 tbsp (0.7 oz)	40	0	0	0	0	0	0	–	9
Marinade All Purpose Vegetable & Meat	1 tbsp (0.7 oz)	35	3	0	0	–	–	0	0	2
Onion Glaze Sweet & Savory	1 tbsp (0.7 oz)	45	0	0	0	0	0	0	–	11
Roasted Blackberry Chipotle	1 tbsp (0.7 oz)	35	0	0	0	0	0	0	–	9
Soppin' Big Bold Red	1 tbsp (0.7 oz)	35	0	0	0	0	0	0	–	6
Frontera										
Hot Sauce Habanero	1 tsp	5	0	0	0	0	0	0	0	0
Hot Squeeze										
Original	2 tbsp (1 oz)	110	0	0	0	0	0	0	–	25
Loney's										
Bar-B-Q Chicken as prep	¼ cup (2.1 oz)	15	0	0	0	0	0	0	0	0
Manwich										
Sloppy Joe Original	¼ cup (2.2 oz)	40	0	0	0	0	0	0	2	6
Margaritaville										
ConQueso In Paradise	1 oz	45	3	10	2	–	–	0	0	1
Matiz										
Paella Sofrito	¼ cup	137	12	tr	2	–	–	0	1	5
McCormick										
Cocktail For Seafood Original	¼ cup (2.1 oz)	90	1	0	–	–	–	0	1	16
Seafood Sauce Asian	2 tbsp (1.2 oz)	50	2	0	–	–	–	0	0	4
Seafood Sauce Cajun Style	1 tbsp (1.1 oz)	15	0	0	0	0	0	0	0	3
Seafood Sauce Scampi	1 tbsp (1 oz)	160	17	0	–	–	–	0	0	1
Tartar Fat Free	2 tbsp (1.1 oz)	30	0	0	0	0	0	0	1	5
Tartar Original	2 tbsp (1 oz)	140	14	20	–	–	–	0	0	3
More Than Gourmet										
Bearnaise	1 pkg (1.8 oz)	120	12	75	9	–	–	0	tr	0
Demi-Glace Classic French	2 tsp (0.4 oz)	30	1	0	0	–	–	0	0	1
Hollandaise	1 pkg (1.8 oz)	120	12	60	9	–	–	0	0	tr
Red Wine Shallot	1 pkg (1.8 oz)	70	6	70	4	–	–	0	0	tr
White Wine	¼ cup (2.1 oz)	45	3	5	2	–	–	0	0	0
Old Bay										
Tartar Sauce	2 tbsp (1.1 oz)	130	12	15	–	–	–	–	0	–

FOOD	PORTION	CALS	TOTAL FAT	CHOL	SAT FAT	POLY FAT	MONO FAT	TRANS FAT	FIBER	SUG
OrganicVille										
Sesame Teriyaki	1 tbsp (0.5 oz)	25	1	0	0	–	–	0	0	3
Progresso										
Bruschetta	2 tbsp (1 oz)	10	1	0	0	–	–	0	0	1
Recipe Starters Cooking Sauce Creamy Parmesan Basil	½ cup	90	7	<5	2	3	1	0	0	0
Recipe Starters Cooking Sauce Creamy Portabella Mushroom	½ cup	90	6	<5	2	3	2	0	0	1
Recipe Starters Cooking Sauce Creamy Three Cheese	½ cup	90	7	10	3	2	1	0	0	tr
Saffron Road										
Simmer Sauce Moroccan Tagine	1 oz	50	2	<5	0	–	–	0	tr	6
Simmer Sauce Rogan Josh	1 oz	25	1	0	0	–	–	0	0	2
Simmer Sauce Tikka Masala	1 oz	35	2	<5	1	–	–	0	0	3
Saucy Susan										
Peach Apricot	2 tbsp (1.3 oz)	80	0	0	0	0	0	0	2	11
Soy Vay										
Hoisin Garlic Asian Glaze & Marinade	1 tbsp	40	1	0	0	–	–	0	0	7
Island Teriyaki	1 tbsp	30	1	0	0	–	–	0	0	4
Veri Veri Teriyaki	1 tbsp	35	1	0	0	–	–	0	0	5
Thai Kitchen										
Pineapple & Chili	2 tbsp (1 oz)	25	0	0	0	0	0	0	0	6
Premium Fish Sauce	1 tbsp (0.5 oz)	10	0	0	0	0	0	0	0	0
Sweet Red Chili	2 tbsp (1 oz)	70	0	0	0	0	0	0	0	14
Thai Chili & Ginger	2 tbsp (1 oz)	40	0	0	0	0	0	0	0	8
TAKE-OUT										
cucumber yogurt sauce	1½ tbsp	20	0	2	0	–	–	0	0	–
SAUERKRAUT										
canned	½ cup	22	tr	0	tr	tr	tr	–	–	–
Del Monte										
Sweet Bavarian	2 tbsp (1 oz)	15	0	0	0	0	0	0	0	3
Gedney										
Sauerkraut	½ cup (4 oz)	15	0	0	0	0	0	0	0	0
Hebrew National										
Sauerkraut	2 tbsp (1.1 oz)	5	0	0	0	0	0	0	–	–

FOOD	PORTION	CALS	TOTAL FAT	CHOL	SAT FAT	POLY FAT	MONO FAT	TRANS FAT	FIBER	SUGAR
SAUSAGE										
beef & pork	1 link (2.3 oz)	196	17	51	4	1	5	–	0	0
beef & pork w/ cheddar cheese	1 link (2.7 oz)	228	20	49	7	2	10	–	0	tr
bratwurst chicken cooked	1 (3 oz)	148	9	60	–	–	–	–	0	0
bratwurst pork cooked	1 link (2.5 oz)	226	19	44	7	2	9	–	0	2
brotwurst pork & beef	1 link (2.5 oz)	226	19	44	7	2	9	–	0	2
chipolata	3.5 oz	342	32	66	12	4	15	–	0	1
chorizo	1 link (2.1 oz)	273	23	53	8	2	11	–	0	0
free range chicken breakfast	2 links (2.7 oz)	110	6	45	1	–	–	–	0	1
italian pork cooked	1 (2.4 oz)	230	18	38	6	2	8	–	1	1
italian turkey smoked	1 (2 oz)	88	5	30	–	–	–	–	1	2
knockwurst pork & beef	1 (2.5 oz)	221	20	43	7	2	9	–	0	0
polish kielbasa	2 oz	127	10	39	3	1	5	–	0	0
pork cooked	2 links (1.7 oz)	163	14	40	4	2	6	–	0	0
smoked beef cooked	1 (1.4 oz)	134	12	29	–	–	–	–	–	–
venison patty	1 (1 oz)	84	8	15	3	tr	3	–	0	0
vienna canned	1 link (0.5 oz)	37	3	14	1	tr	2	–	0	0
vienna canned	1 can (4 oz)	260	22	98	8	1	11	–	0	0
Al Fresco										
Chicken Buffalo	1 (3 oz)	130	6	60	2	–	–	0	0	2
Chicken Hot Italian	1 (2.7 oz)	120	7	60	2	–	–	0	0	1
Chicken Roasted Garlic	1 (3 oz)	140	7	65	2	–	–	0	0	1
Chicken Smoked Andouille	1 (3 oz)	140	7	65	2	–	–	0	1	1
Chicken Spicy Chipotle	1 (2.7 oz)	120	6	60	2	–	–	0	0	1
Chicken Spinach & Feta	1 (3 oz)	130	7	65	3	–	–	0	–	0
Chicken Sweet Apple	1 (3 oz)	160	7	60	2	–	–	0	0	9
Chicken Wild Blueberry	1 (1.2 oz)	70	3	25	1	–	–	0	0	4
Banquet										
Brown'N Serve Turkey	3 (2.1 oz)	110	7	40	2	–	–	0	0	1
Coleman										
Bratwurst	1 (3 oz)	240	21	55	8	–	–	0	0	0
Chicken Spicy Chorizo	1 (3 oz)	150	8	65	3	–	–	0	0	0
Foster Farms										
Turkey Breakfast Links	2 (2 oz)	120	10	45	–	–	–	0	0	0
Hans All Natural										
Breakfast Links Skinless Chicken	2 (1.7 oz)	60	4	40	2	–	–	0	0	0
Chicken Spinach & Feta	1 (2.7 oz)	130	8	45	2	–	–	0	0	0

FOOD	PORTION	CALS	TOTAL FAT	CHOL	SAT FAT	POLY FAT	MONO FAT	TRANS FAT	FIBER	SU
Hebrew National										
Knockwurst Beef	1 (3 oz)	270	25	45	10	–	–	1	0	0
Murray's										
Chicken Cheese & Parsley	3 oz	130	7	85	2	–	–	0	0	0
Chicken Spinach & Garlic	3 oz	130	7	85	2	–	–	0	–	–
SAUSAGE DISHES										
TAKE-OUT										
italian sausage w/ peppers & onions	1 cup	210	11	70	–	–	–	–	–	–
SAUSAGE SUBSTITUTES										
meatless	1 patty (1.3 oz)	98	7	0	1	4	2	–	1	0
meatless	1 link (0.9 oz)	64	5	0	1	2	1	–	1	0
Harmony Valley										
Vegetarian Breakfast Sausage Mix as prep	1 (2 oz)	90	4	0	2	–	–	0	3	1
SAVORY										
ground	1 tsp	4	tr	0	tr	–	–	0	tr	–
SCALLOP										
raw	3 oz	75	1	28	tr	tr	tr	–	–	–
TAKE-OUT										
breaded & fried	2 lg	67	3	19	1	1	1	–	–	–
SCONE										
TAKE-OUT										
apricot	1	232	7	34	–	–	–	–	–	–
blueberry	1 (3 oz)	270	9	10	4	–	–	–	2	7
orange poppy	1 (3 oz)	260	6	30	4	–	–	–	2	12
raisin	1 (3 oz)	270	8	10	3	–	–	–	2	12
SEA BASS (see BASS)										
SEA CUCUMBER										
dried	1 oz	74	1	17	–	–	–	–	0	–
fresh	1 oz	20	tr	14	–	–	–	–	0	–
SEA TROUT (see TROUT)										
SEAWEED										
agar dried	1 oz	92	tr	0	tr	tr	tr	0	2	1
agar fresh	⅛ cup (0.4 oz)	3	0	0	0	0	0	0	0	tr

FOOD	PORTION	CALS	TOTAL FAT	CHOL	SAT FAT	POLY FAT	MONO FAT	TRANS FAT	FIBER	SUGAR
furikake	1 tbsp (5 g)	15	1	1	0	0	0	–	0	–
hijiki rehydrated	1 tbsp (3 g)	1	0	0	0	0	0	0	0	0
hijiki dried	1 tbsp	9	0	0	0	0	0	0	1	–
irishmoss fresh	⅛ cup (0.4 oz)	5	tr	0	tr	tr	tr	0	tr	tr
kelp dried	¼ cup (4 g)	11	tr	0	tr	tr	tr	0	tr	tr
kelp fresh	⅛ cup (0.4 oz)	4	tr	0	tr	tr	tr	0	tr	tr
kelp strip	1 (0.5 g)	1	tr	0	tr	tr	tr	0	0	tr
konbu dried	1 piece (5 g)	11	0	0	0	0	0	0	1	–
konbu fresh	1 oz	12	0	0	0	tr	tr	–	–	–
laver fresh	⅛ cup (0.4 oz)	4	tr	0	tr	tr	tr	0	0	tr
nori fresh	1 oz	10	tr	0	tr	tr	tr	–	–	–
nori sheet dried	1 (8 x 8 in)	5	0	0	0	0	0	0	1	–
ogo fresh	1 cup (2.8 oz)	24	0	0	0	0	0	0	0	–
pickled	¼ cup (1.3 oz)	58	tr	0	tr	tr	tr	0	tr	13
seahair dried	1 tbsp	13	0	0	0	0	0	0	tr	–
seaweed w/ soy sauce	½ cup (1.7 oz)	21	tr	0	tr	tr	tr	0	tr	tr
spirulina dried	¼ cup (1 oz)	81	2	0	1	1	tr	0	1	1
spirulina fresh	1 oz	8	tr	0	tr	tr	tr	0	–	–
steamed	½ cup (1.4 oz)	15	tr	0	tr	tr	tr	0	tr	tr
tangle fresh	1 oz	12	tr	0	tr	tr	tr	–	–	–
wakame fresh	⅛ cup (0.4 oz)	4	tr	0	tr	tr	tr	0	0	tr
wakame rehydrated	1 tbsp (3 g)	1	0	0	0	0	0	0	0	0
Annie Chun's										
Roasted Snacks Sesame	1 pkg (1.5 g)	5	0	0	0	0	0	0	0	0
Sea's Gift										
Roasted	1 pkg (5 g)	30	2	0	0	–	–	0	1	0
Roasted Snack Organic	1 pkg (5 g)	30	2	0	0	–	–	0	1	0
Roasted Snack Wasabi	1 pkg (5 g)	30	2	0	0	–	–	0	1	0
Sweet Snack	1 pkg (6 g)	35	3	0	0	–	–	0	1	tr
SEEDS										
SaviSeed										
Cocoa Kissed	⅕ pkg (1 oz)	170	13	0	4	–	–	0	4	5
Karmalized	⅕ pkg (1 oz)	160	11	0	1	–	–	0	3	8
Oh Natural	⅕ pkg (1 oz)	190	15	0	1	–	–	0	5	0
SEITAN (see WHEAT)										
SEMOLINA										
dry	1 cup (5.9 oz)	601	2	0	tr	1	tr	–	7	–

FOOD	PORTION	CALS	TOTAL FAT	CHOL	SAT FAT	POLY FAT	MONO FAT	TRANS FAT	FIBER	SUGAR
SESAME										
seeds	1 tsp	16	2	0	–	–	–	–	–	–
sesame butter	1 tbsp	95	8	0	1	4	3	–	1	–
sesame crunch candy	20 pieces (1.2 oz)	181	12	0	2	5	4	–	–	–
sesame crunch candy	1 oz	146	9	0	1	4	4	–	–	–
tahini from roasted & toasted kernels	1 tbsp	89	8	0	1	4	3	–	–	–
tahini from stone ground kernels	1 tbsp	86	7	0	1	3	3	–	–	–
tahini from unroasted kernels	1 tbsp	85	8	0	1	3	3	–	–	–
Oskri										
Organic Sesame Bars	1 (1.9 oz)	217	6	0	0	–	–	0	1	20
SESBANIA										
flower	1 (3 g)	1	0	0	0	0	0	0	–	–
flowers	1 cup (0.7 oz)	5	tr	0	–	–	–	0	–	–
flowers cooked	1 cup	23	tr	0	–	–	–	0	–	–
SHAD										
cooked	1 oz	55	3	121	1	1	1	0	0	tr
SHALLOTS (see ONION)										
SHARK										
raw	3 oz	111	4	43	1	1	1	–	0	0
TAKE-OUT										
batter-dipped & fried	3 oz	194	12	50	3	3	5	–	–	–
SHELLFISH (see individual names, SHELLFISH SUBSTITUTES)										
SHELLFISH SUBSTITUTES										
crab imitation	1 cup (4.4 oz)	144	1	60	tr	tr	tr	–	tr	0
scallop imitation	3 oz	84	tr	18	–	–	–	–	–	–
shrimp imitation surimi	3 oz	86	1	31	tr	1	tr	–	0	–
surimi	3 oz	84	1	25	–	–	–	–	–	–
Louis Kemp										
Crab Delights Flake Style	½ cup (3 oz)	90	0	5	0	–	–	0	0	3
Crab Delights Leg Style	½ cup (3 oz)	90	0	5	0	–	–	0	0	3
Crab Delights Snack Delights	1 stick (1.5 oz)	35	0	<5	0	–	–	0	0	2
Lobster Delights Chunk Style	½ cup (3 oz)	90	0	5	0	–	–	0	0	3

FOOD	PORTION	CALS	TOTAL FAT	CHOL	SAT FAT	POLY FAT	MONO FAT	TRANS FAT	FIBER	SUGAR
TAKE-OUT										
crab salad	1 cup	395	26	77	4	14	6	–	1	1
SHELLIE BEANS										
canned	½ cup	37	tr	0	tr	tr	tr	–	–	–
SHERBET										
orange	½ gal	2158	31	113	19	1	9	–	–	–
orange	1 bar (2.75 fl oz)	91	1	3	1	tr	tr	–	–	–
orange	½ cup (4 fl oz)	132	2	5	1	tr	1	–	–	–
SHRIMP (*see also* ASIAN FOOD, EGG ROLLS)										
CANNED										
canned drained	10 (1.1 oz)	32	tr	81	tr	tr	tr	–	0	0
canned drained	1 cup (4.5 oz)	128	2	323	tr	1	tr	–	0	0
chinese shrimp paste	1 tbsp	46	0	9	0	0	0	0	tr	8
Chicken Of The Sea										
Medium	½ can (2 oz)	45	1	145	0	–	–	–	0	1
Small	½ can (2 oz)	45	1	145	0	–	–	–	0	1
Tiny	½ can (2 oz)	45	1	145	0	–	–	–	0	1
DRIED										
dried	10 (5 g)	13	tr	32	tr	tr	tr	–	0	0
dried	1 oz	72	1	181	tr	tr	tr	–	0	0
FRESH										
broiled jumbo	3 (1 oz)	44	1	55	tr	1	tr	–	0	0
broiled small	3 (0.4 oz)	18	1	22	tr	tr	tr	–	0	0
broiled tiny popcorn	3 (3 g)	4	tr	5	tr	tr	tr	–	0	0
prawn broiled	3 (0.6 oz)	27	1	33	tr	tr	tr	–	0	0
steamed jumbo	3 (1 oz)	41	1	59	tr	tr	tr	0	0	0
steamed large	3 (0.6 oz)	25	tr	36	tr	tr	tr	–	0	0
steamed medium	3 (0.5 oz)	21	tr	30	tr	tr	tr	–	0	0
Chicken Of The Sea										
Ring w/ Cocktail Sauce	⅓ pkg (3 oz)	100	1	130	0	–	–	–	0	3
FROZEN										
Chicken Of The Sea										
Tempura w/ Soy Dipping Sauce	3	200	13	50	3	–	–	–	0	1
Margaritaville										
Island Lime	6 (4 oz)	240	11	115	3	–	–	0	0	2
Jammin' Jerk	7 (4 oz)	210	10	120	6	–	–	0	1	–
Plum Crazy + Sauce	7 + 2 oz sauce	270	12	55	2	–	–	–	1	13

FOOD	PORTION	CALS	TOTAL FAT	CHOL	SAT FAT	POLY FAT	MONO FAT	TRANS FAT	FIBER	SUG
Shrimp Burgers										
Cajun	1 (4 oz)	160	3	185	1	–	–	0	0	0
Original	1 (4 oz)	160	3	180	1	–	–	0	0	0
Teriyaki	1 (4 oz)	150	3	175	1	–	–	0	0	2
TAKE-OUT										
battered jumbo	3 (3 oz)	268	17	95	3	6	6	tr	1	1
battered large	3 (1.8 oz)	152	9	54	2	3	4	tr	1	tr
battered medium	3 (1.2 oz)	98	5	35	1	2	2	tr	tr	tr
battered small	3 (0.6 oz)	54	3	19	1	1	1	tr	tr	tr
battered tiny popcorn	3 (6 g)	18	1	6	tr	tr	tr	tr	tr	tr
breaded & fried	1 lg (0.6 oz)	44	3	30	0	1	1	–	0	–
cocktail w/ cocktail sauce	4 shrimp (3.2 oz)	78	1	114	tr	tr	tr	–	2	3
creole w/o rice	1 cup (8.6 oz)	335	13	293	3	4	5	–	2	3
gingered	4	80	tr	140	tr	–	–	–	–	–
jambalaya w/ rice	1 cup (8.5 oz)	294	9	262	2	3	4	–	2	2
scampi	1 cup	310	22	246	13	2	6	–	0	tr
shish kabob w/ vegetables	1 (7.1 oz)	184	5	184	1	2	1	–	2	5
shrimp cake	1 (4.2 oz)	238	13	194	3	4	5	–	1	1
shrimp egg patty torta de cameron seco	2 (1.3 oz)	152	11	171	2	4	4	–	tr	1
shrimp in garlic sauce	1 cup (7.4 oz)	649	54	267	9	11	32	–	tr	1
shrimp newburg	1 cup (8.6 oz)	605	50	417	30	3	14	–	tr	tr
shrimp salad	1 cup (6.4 oz)	258	16	291	2	9	4	–	1	2
shrimp w/ crab stuffing	3 (1.7 oz)	94	5	76	1	1	2	–	tr	tr
tempura	1 (0.9 oz)	65	4	43	1	2	2	–	0	–
toast fried	3 pieces (2.5 oz)	219	14	35	2	6	5	–	2	2
SMELT										
rainbow cooked	3 oz	106	3	76	tr	1	1	–	0	0
rainbow raw	3 oz	83	2	60	tr	1	1	–	0	0
SMOOTHIES (*see also* FRUIT DRINKS, YOGURT DRINKS)										
Arizona										
Smoothie Mix Orchard Peach as prep	8 oz	150	0	0	0	0	0	0	0	38
Chia\Vie										
Acerola-Pina	1 bottle (10.4 oz)	160	3	0	0	–	–	0	4	27

FOOD	PORTION	CALS	TOTAL FAT	CHOL	SAT FAT	POLY FAT	MONO FAT	TRANS FAT	FIBER	SUGAR
Banapple-Berry	1 bottle (10.4 oz)	170	4	0	1	–	–	0	5	26
Cogo										
Coconut Milk Cappuccino	1 bottle (7.5 oz)	130	3	0	3	–	–	0	4	14
Coconut Milk Mango	1 bottle (7.5 oz)	120	3	0	2	–	–	0	4	16
Coconut Milk Strawberry	1 bottle (7.5 oz)	130	3	0	2	–	–	0	4	15
Coconut Milk Vanilla	1 bottle (7.5 oz)	110	4	0	3	–	–	0	4	9
Del Monte										
Ready-To-Blend Pomegranate Peach Pear	1 serv (6 oz)	125	0	0	0	0	0	0	4	22
Ready-To-Blend Strawberry Peach	1 serv (6 oz)	120	0	0	0	0	0	0	4	21
Ready-To-Blend Strawberry Peach Lite	1 serv (6 oz)	80	0	0	0	0	0	0	4	15
Dole										
Shakers Mixed Berry not prep	1 pkg (4 oz)	100	2	10	1	–	–	0	3	13
Jamba Juice										
Mango-A-Go-Go not prep	½ pkg (4 oz)	70	0	0	0	0	0	0	1	15
Razzmatazz not prep	½ pkg (4 oz)	60	0	0	0	0	0	0	2	10
Strawberries Wild not prep	½ pkg (4 oz)	60	0	0	0	0	0	0	1	11
Main St. Cafe										
Protein Smoothie Mixed Berry	1 bottle (11 oz)	270	2	15	2	–	–	0	1	42
Protein Smoothie Peach	1 bottle (11 oz)	260	2	15	2	–	–	0	1	43
Protein Smoothie Strawberry	1 bottle (11 oz)	280	2	15	2	–	–	0	1	48
Oatworks										
Oat & Fruit Mango & Peach	1 bottle (10.8 oz)	150	0	0	0	0	0	0	2	31
Oat & Fruit Pomegranate & Blueberry	1 bottle (10.8 oz)	160	0	0	0	0	0	0	2	32
Simpli										
OatShake Tropical Fruits	1 (8.4 oz)	160	2	0	1	–	–	0	8	23

FOOD	PORTION	CALS	TOTAL FAT	CHOL	SAT FAT	POLY FAT	MONO FAT	TRANS FAT	FIBER	SUGAR
Yasso										
Greek Yogurt Mango Pineapple as prep	8 oz	120	0	6	0	0	0	0	4	13
Greek Yogurt Mixed Berry as prep	8 oz	110	0	0	0	0	0	0	4	9
Yoplait										
Mixed Berry as prep	1 serv (12 oz)	160	2	6	1	–	–	0	1	14
Strawberry Banana Orange as prep	1 serv (12 oz)	170	2	6	1	–	–	0	1	14
SNACKS										
cheese puffs	1 oz	122	3	0	1	2	1	–	3	2
oriental mix	1 oz	155	12	0	–	–	–	–	–	–
Annie's Homegrown										
Organic Cheddar Snack Mix	40 pieces (1 oz)	140	5	0	1	–	–	0	0	1
Organic Pizza Snack Mix	½ cup (1 oz)	140	5	0	1	–	–	0	0	1
Bachman										
Baked Cheese Curls	23 (1 oz)	140	7	0	1	–	–	0	0	2
Onion Rings	½ pkg (1 oz)	130	6	0	1	–	–	0	1	1
Cheetos										
Baked Crunchy	34 (1 oz)	130	5	0	1	3	2	0	tr	tr
Corn BBQ	29 (1 oz)	150	10	0	2	–	–	0	1	tr
Natural White Cheddar	1 oz	150	9	0	2	–	–	0	tr	1
Puffs	13 (1 oz)	160	10	0	2	–	–	0	0	1
Chester's										
Puffcorn Butter	1 oz	160	11	0	2	–	–	0	tr	0
Snack Mix Crazy Cheddar	1¼ cups (1 oz)	140	7	0	1	–	–	0	1	tr
DrSears										
Popumz BBQ	1 pkg (0.74 oz)	70	2	0	0	–	–	0	2	1
Popumz Caramel Drizzle	1 pkg (0.75 oz)	90	3	0	2	–	–	0	2	5
Popumz Cheddar	1 pkg (0.74 oz)	80	3	5	1	–	–	0	2	1
Popumz Cool Ranch	1 pkg (0.74 oz)	80	2	0	0	–	–	0	2	2
Popumz Vanilla Drizzle	1 pkg (0.74 oz)	90	3	0	2	–	–	0	2	5
Funyuns										
Onion Rings	13 (1 oz)	140	7	0	1	–	–	0	tr	tr
Garden Of Eatin'										
Puffs Baked Cheddar	32 (1 oz)	150	10	<5	1	–	–	0	1	1
Hawaiian Snacks										
Sweet Maui Onion Rings	27 (1 oz)	130	6	5	1	–	–	0	tr	3

FOOD	PORTION	CALS	TOTAL FAT	CHOL	SAT FAT	POLY FAT	MONO FAT	TRANS FAT	FIBER	SUGAR
Hi I'm Skinny Sticks										
Multi Grain Cheddar	34 (1 oz)	130	6	0	1	–	–	0	1	2
Multi Grain Sea Salt	34 (1 oz)	130	6	0	1	–	–	0	1	1
Multi Grain Sweet Onion	34 (1 oz)	120	6	0	1	–	–	0	1	2
Multi Grain Sweet Potato	34 (1 oz)	120	7	0	1	–	–	0	1	5
Multi Grain Tangy BBQ	34 (1 oz)	130	6	0	1	–	–	0	1	2
Multi Grain Veggie Tortilla	34 (1 oz)	130	7	0	1	–	–	0	2	0
I Heart Keenwah										
Quinoa Cluster Almond	7 to 8 (1 oz)	130	5	0	0	–	–	0	tr	7
Quinoa Cluster Chocolate Sea Salt	7 (1 oz)	130	5	0	1	–	–	0	1	8
Quinoa Cluster Cranberry Cashew	¼ pkg (1 oz)	120	4	0	1	–	–	0	tr	9
Quinoa Cluster Ginger Peanut	7 to 8 (1 oz)	120	4	0	1	–	–	0	tr	10
Munchies										
Snack Mix Totally Ranch	¾ cup (1 oz)	140	7	0	1	3	3	0	2	1
Quaker										
Fiber Crisps Wild Blueberry	13 (1 oz)	110	2	0	0	–	–	0	3	6
Sabritones										
Puffed Wheat Chili & Lime	23 pieces (1 oz)	150	10	0	3	–	–	–	1	0
SNAIL										
cooked	3 oz	233	1	110	tr	tr	tr	–	–	–
raw	3 oz	117	tr	55	tr	tr	tr	–	–	–
TAKE-OUT										
escargot cooked	5	25	0	15	0	0	0	0	0	–
SNAPPER										
cooked	3 oz	109	1	40	tr	1	tr	–	0	0
cooked	1 fillet (6 oz)	217	3	80	1	1	1	–	0	0
raw	3 oz	85	1	31	tr	tr	tr	–	0	0
SODA										
club	12 oz	0	0	0	0	0	0	0	0	0
cola	12 oz	151	tr	0	–	–	–	–	–	–
cream	12 oz	191	0	0	0	0	0	0	–	–
diet cola	12 oz	2	0	0	0	0	0	0	–	–
ginger ale	12 oz	124	0	0	–	–	–	0	–	–
grape	12 oz	161	0	0	0	0	0	0	–	–

FOOD	PORTION	CALS	TOTAL FAT	CHOL	SAT FAT	POLY FAT	MONO FAT	TRANS FAT	FIBER	SUG
lemon lime	12 oz	149	0	0	0	0	0	0	–	–
orange	12 oz	177	0	0	0	0	0	0	–	–
pepper type	12 oz	151	tr	0	–	–	–	–	–	–
quinine	12 oz	125	0	0	0	0	0	0	–	–
root beer	12 oz	152	0	0	0	0	0	0	–	–
shirley temple	1 serv	159	0	0	0	0	0	0	0	–
tonic water	12 oz	125	0	0	0	0	0	0	–	–
CasCal										
Crisp White	1 can (12 oz)	70	0	0	0	0	0	0	–	11
Ripe Rouge	1 can (12 oz)	60	0	0	0	0	0	0	–	10
Fresh Ginger										
Ginger Ale Jasmine Green Tea	1 bottle (12 oz)	160	0	0	0	0	0	0	0	37
Ginger Ale Original	1 bottle (12 oz)	160	0	0	0	0	0	0	0	37
Ginger Ale Pomegranate w/ Hibiscus	1 bottle (12 oz)	160	0	0	0	0	0	0	0	37
Gus										
Dry Valencia Orange	1 bottle (12 oz)	95	0	0	0	0	0	0	–	24
In The Raw										
Cola	1 bottle (12 oz)	150	0	0	0	0	0	0	–	37
Joia										
Grapefruit Chamomile & Cardamon	1 bottle (12 oz)	110	0	0	0	0	0	0	–	28
Lime Hibiscus & Clove	1 bottle (12 oz)	120	0	0	0	0	0	0	–	28
Pineapple Coconut & Nutmeg	1 bottle (12 oz)	110	0	0	0	0	0	0	–	26
Minta										
Diet	1 bottle (12 oz)	5	0	0	0	0	0	0	–	0
Original	1 bottle (12 oz)	120	0	0	0	0	0	0	–	30
OrganicVille										
Carbonate Beverage	1 bottle (12 oz)	140	0	0	0	0	0	0	0	34
Spindrift										
Sparkling Blackberry	8 oz	70	0	0	0	0	0	0	0	17
Sparkling Cranberry Raspberry	8 oz	60	0	0	0	0	0	0	0	16
Sparkling Grapefruit	8 oz	80	0	0	0	0	0	0	0	21
Sparkling Mango Orange	8 oz	80	0	0	0	0	0	0	0	21
Stewart's										
Birch Beer	1 bottle	170	0	0	0	0	0	0	–	42

FOOD	PORTION	CALS	TOTAL FAT	CHOL	SAT FAT	POLY FAT	MONO FAT	TRANS FAT	FIBER	SUGAR
Sunkist										
Grape	8 oz	120	0	0	0	0	0	0	-	30
Orange	8 oz	110	0	0	0	0	0	0	-	29
Pineapple	8 oz	130	0	0	0	0	0	0	-	34
Taylor's Tonics										
Chai Cola	1 bottle (12 oz)	135	0	0	0	0	0	0	-	32
Cola Azteca	1 bottle (12 oz)	95	0	0	0	0	0	0	-	28
Mate Majito Mint & Lime	1 bottle (12 oz)	98	0	0	0	0	0	0	-	28
The Pop Shoppe										
Cola	1 bottle (12 oz)	180	0	0	0	0	0	0	-	45
Cream	1 bottle (12 oz)	190	0	0	0	0	0	0	-	46
Lime Ricky	1 bottle (12 oz)	150	0	0	0	0	0	0	-	37
Pineapple	1 bottle (12 oz)	240	0	0	0	0	0	0	-	58
Welch's										
Sparkling Grape	1 bottle (20 oz)	330	0	0	0	0	0	0	-	78
Sparkling Strawberry	1 can (8 oz)	120	0	0	0	0	0	0	-	34
Zevia										
All Flavors	1 can (12 oz)	0	0	0	0	0	0	0	0	0
SOLE										
cooked	1 fillet (4.5 oz)	148	2	86	tr	1	tr	-	0	0
cooked	3 oz	99	1	58	tr	tr	tr	-	0	0
TAKE-OUT										
breaded & fried	3.2 oz	211	11	31	3	6	2	-	0	0
SORGHUM										
sorghum	1 cup (6.7 oz)	651	6	0	1	3	2	-	-	-
SOUFFLE										
Garden Lites										
Butternut Squash Souffle	1 pkg (7 oz)	180	5	55	1	-	-	0	3	18
Pizza Souffle	1 pkg (7 oz)	200	4	5	2	-	-	0	3	6
Roasted Vegetable	1 pkg (7 oz)	140	2	0	0	-	-	0	4	8
Southwestern Souffle	1 pkg (7 oz)	180	3	0	0	-	-	0	4	4
Spinach Souffle	1 pkg (7 oz)	140	2	0	0	-	-	0	4	6
Zucchini Souffle	1 pkg (7 oz)	140	2	0	0	-	-	0	3	6
TAKE-OUT										
cheese	1 cup	194	15	134	6	2	6	-	tr	3
chicken	1 cup (5.6 oz)	278	18	218	5	4	8	-	tr	4
corn	1 cup	257	11	152	3	3	4	-	3	11

FOOD	PORTION	CALS	TOTAL FAT	CHOL	SAT FAT	POLY FAT	MONO FAT	TRANS FAT	FIBER	SUGAR
lime chilled	1 cup	388	18	306	3	4	9	–	2	45
seafood	1 cup	245	15	231	4	4	6	–	tr	4
spinach	1 cup	124	8	97	2	2	3	–	1	3

SOUP
CANNED
Campbell's

FOOD	PORTION	CALS	TOTAL FAT	CHOL	SAT FAT	POLY FAT	MONO FAT	TRANS FAT	FIBER	SUGAR
100% Natural Creole Chicken w/ Red Beans & Rice	1 cup (8.4 oz)	130	3	30	2	–	–	0	2	4
100% Natural Harvest Tomato w/ Basil	1 cup (8.4 oz)	100	0	0	0	0	0	0	2	15
100% Natural Light Vegetable & Pasta	1 cup (8.4 oz)	60	0	0	0	0	0	0	4	3
100% Natural Southwest White Chicken Chili	1 cup (8.4 oz)	140	2	10	1	0	0	0	5	3
98% Fat Free Cream Of Chicken as prep	1 cup	70	3	5	1	1	1	0	1	0
Chunky Creamy Chicken & Dumplings	1 cup (8.4 oz)	170	8	30	2	–	–	0	3	3
Chunky Italian Wedding	1 cup (8.4 oz)	130	3	15	1	1	1	0	3	6
Chunky Split Pea & Ham	1 cup (8.4 oz)	170	3	10	1	1	1	0	5	4
Go Soup Creamy Red Pepper w/ Smoked Gouda	1 cup	220	15	60	9	–	–	1	2	8
Go Soup Moroccan Style Chicken w/ Chickpeas	1 cup	160	2	25	0	–	–	0	6	11
Gourmet Bisques Thai Tomato Coconut	1 cup	200	9	15	8	–	–	0	3	17
Gourmet Bisques Tomato Roasted Garlic Bacon	1 cup	240	10	35	6	–	–	0	3	25
Healthy Kids Goldfish Pasta as prep	1 cup	80	2	5	1	1	1	0	1	1
Italian Wedding Light as prep	1 cup (8.4 oz)	80	2	5	1	0	1	0	2	2
Slow Kettle Burgundy Beef Stew w/ Baby Bella Mushrooms & Roasted Garlic	1 cup (8.4 oz)	160	4	20	2	–	–	0	4	5
Slow Kettle Portobello Mushroom & Madeira Bisque w/ Shallots	1 cup (8.4 oz)	230	17	25	6	–	–	0	4	7

FOOD	PORTION	CALS	TOTAL FAT	CHOL	SAT FAT	POLY FAT	MONO FAT	TRANS FAT	FIBER	SUGAR
Slow Kettle Southwest Chicken Chile w/ Black Beans & Sweet Corn	1 cup (8.4 oz)	190	2	20	1	–	–	0	7	6
Slow Kettle Tuscan Chicken & White Bean w/ Asiago Cheese Thyme & Rosemary	1 cup (8.4 oz)	140	3	15	1	–	–	0	4	4
Sun-Ripened Yellow Tomato as prep	1 cup	100	1	5	0	0	0	0	1	13
College Inn										
Beef Broth 99% Fat Free	1 cup (8.4 oz)	25	1	0	0	–	–	0	0	0
Beef Broth Fat Free Lower Sodium	1 cup (8.4 oz)	15	0	0	0	0	0	0	0	0
Bold Stock Rotisserie Chicken	1 cup (8.4 oz)	30	0	0	0	0	0	0	0	1
Bold Stock Tender Beef	1 cup (8.4 oz)	45	0	0	0	0	0	0	0	2
Chicken Broth 99% Fat Free	1 cup (8.5 oz)	15	1	0	0	–	–	0	0	1
Chicken Broth Light & Fat Free 50% Less Sodium	1 cup (8.4 oz)	5	0	0	0	0	0	0	0	0
Chicken Broth w/ Roasted Garlic	1 cup (8.5 oz)	20	0	0	0	0	0	0	0	1
Chicken Broth w/ Roasted Vegetables & Herbs	1 cup (8.5 oz)	20	0	0	0	0	0	0	0	1
Culinary Broth Thai Coconut Curry	1 cup (8.4 oz)	20	1	0	0	–	–	–	0	4
Culinary Broth Wine & Herbs	1 cup (8.4 oz)	5	1	0	0	–	–	0	1	1
Garden Vegetable Broth	1 cup (8.4 oz)	25	1	0	0	–	–	0	0	4
Turkey Broth	1 cup (8.4 oz)	20	1	0	0	–	–	0	0	0
Dr. McDougall's										
Chunky Tomato Gluten Free	1 cup (8.6 oz)	90	0	0	0	0	0	0	3	8
Lentil	1 cup (8.6 oz)	115	1	0	0	–	–	0	8	1
Organic Black Bean Lower Sodium	1 cup (8.6 oz)	150	1	0	0	–	–	0	6	3
Organic Tortilla	1 cup (8.6 oz)	100	1	0	0	–	–	0	4	2
Split Pea	1 cup (8.6 oz)	110	0	0	0	0	0	0	8	1
Frontera										
Gourmet Mexican Classic Tortilla	1 cup (8.6 oz)	80	2	0	0	0	0	0	3	5
Gourmet Mexican Roasted Vegetable	1 cup (8.6 oz)	80	2	0	0	0	1	0	2	5
Healthy Choice										
Bean & Ham	1 cup (8.7 oz)	180	3	10	1	–	–	0	6	3

FOOD	PORTION	CALS	TOTAL FAT	CHOL	SAT FAT	POLY FAT	MONO FAT	TRANS FAT	FIBER	SUGAR
Chicken & Dumplings	1 cup (8.8 oz)	150	3	25	1	–	–	0	3	2
Chicken w/ Rice	1 cup (8.4 oz)	110	2	10	1	–	–	0	2	tr
Garden Vegetable	1 cup (8.6 oz)	130	1	5	0	–	–	0	5	4
Italian Wedding	1 cup (8.6 oz)	120	3	10	1	–	–	0	3	1
New England Clam Chowder	1 cup (8.4 oz)	110	2	10	1	–	–	0	3	3
Split Pea & Ham	1 cup (8.8 oz)	160	3	10	1	–	–	0	6	3
Tomato Basil	1 cup (8.8 oz)	100	0	0	0	0	0	0	3	10
Manischewitz										
Borscht Low Calorie	¾ cup (6.2 oz)	15	0	0	0	0	0	0	tr	2
Borscht Reduced Sodium	¾ cup (6.2 oz)	50	0	0	0	0	0	0	tr	11
Borscht w/ Shredded Beets	¾ cup (6.2 oz)	50	0	0	0	0	0	0	tr	11
Matzo Ball Chicken	1 cup (8.4 oz)	120	5	40	2	–	–	0	1	2
Matzo Ball Chicken Reduced Sodium	1 cup (8.4 oz)	120	5	40	2	–	–	0	1	2
Marie Callender's										
Classic Chicken & Rice	1 cup (7.8 oz)	80	3	10	1	1	1	0	1	tr
Homestyle Vegetable	1 cup (7.8 oz)	80	1	0	0	0	1	0	3	4
More Than Gourmet										
Roasted Duck & Chicken Stock	2 tsp (0.4 oz)	40	3	<5	1	–	–	0	0	0
Seafood & Shrimp Stock	2 tsp (0.4 oz)	15	0	25	0	0	0	0	0	1
Venison Stock	2 tsp (0.4 oz)	25	0	0	0	–	–	0	0	0
New England Country Soup										
Caribbean Black Bean	1 cup (8.8 oz)	210	3	0	0	–	–	0	8	4
Chicken Pomodoro	1 cup (8.6 oz)	140	6	15	2	–	–	0	2	3
Nana's Chicken	1 cup (8.6 oz)	120	4	10	1	–	–	0	4	2
Sweet Chicken Curry	1 cup (8.8 oz)	160	4	20	1	–	–	0	3	9
Yankee White Bean	1 cup (9.3 oz)	380	9	35	5	–	–	0	12	4
Pacific Foods										
Beef Broth Organic	1 cup (8 oz)	20	1	5	0	–	–	0	0	1
Butternut Squash Organic	1 cup (8 oz)	90	2	0	0	–	–	0	3	4
Cashew Carrot Ginger Bisque	1 cup (8.4 oz)	130	5	0	4	–	–	0	4	8
Chicken Broth Free Range	1 cup (8 oz)	10	0	0	0	0	0	0	0	1
Chicken Broth Free Range Low Sodium Organic	1 cup (8 oz)	15	0	0	0	0	0	0	0	0
Cream Of Celery	1 cup (8.6 oz)	70	3	10	2	–	–	0	0	1
Curried Red Lentil	1 cup (8 oz)	140	5	0	4	–	–	0	5	8
French Onion Organic	1 cup (8 oz)	30	1	0	1	–	–	0	0	3

FOOD	PORTION	CALS	TOTAL FAT	CHOL	SAT FAT	POLY FAT	MONO FAT	TRANS FAT	FIBER	SUGAR
Minestrone w/ Chicken Meatballs	1 cup (8.8 oz)	130	4	10	1	–	–	0	3	3
Mushroom Broth Organic	1 cup (8 oz)	5	0	0	0	0	0	0	0	0
Pho Beef Broth Organic	1 cup (8 oz)	35	0	5	0	–	–	0	0	5
Pho Vegetarian Soup Base Organic	1 cup (8 oz)	25	0	0	0	0	0	0	0	5
Poblano Pepper & Corn Chowder	1 cup (8.7 oz)	190	10	35	6	–	–	0	1	2
Red Pepper & Tomato Light Sodium Organic	1 cup (8 oz)	110	2	10	2	–	–	0	1	12
Rosemary Potato Chowder	1 cup (8.7 oz)	230	8	30	5	–	–	0	2	0
Thai Sweet Potato	1 cup (8.6 oz)	160	6	0	4	–	–	0	3	3
Tomato Light Sodium Organic	1 cup (8 oz)	100	2	10	2	–	–	0	1	12
Vegetable Broth Organic	1 cup (8 oz)	15	0	0	0	0	0	0	1	2
Progresso										
High Fiber Chicken Tuscany	1 cup (8.7 oz)	130	3	15	2	0	1	0	7	2
High Fiber Creamy Tomato Basil	1 cup (8.8 oz)	130	4	5	1	2	1	0	7	13
Light Chicken Noodle	1 cup (8.3 oz)	70	2	15	1	0	1	0	1	1
Light Vegetable & Noodle	1 cup (8.7 oz)	60	1	5	0	0	0	0	4	2
Reduced Sodium Chicken Gumbo	1 cup (8.7 oz)	110	2	10	1	1	1	0	4	3
Rich & Hearty Chicken & Homestyle Noodles	1 cup (8.6 oz)	100	3	25	1	1	1	0	1	2
Traditional Chicken Noodle	1 cup (8.3 oz)	100	3	20	1	1	1	0	1	1
Saffron Road										
Chicken Broth Artisan Roasted	1 cup (8.4 oz)	20	1	0	0	–	–	0	0	0
Spoonful Of Comfort										
Chicken Soup	1 serv (8 oz)	80	2	20	0	–	–	0	1	1
Tabatchnick										
Garden Fresh Vegetable Broth	⅔ cup (5.5 oz)	10	0	0	0	0	0	0	0	1
Wisconsin Cheddar Cheese	⅔ cup (5.5 oz)	150	11	0	3	–	–	4	0	2
FROZEN										
Kettle Cuisine										
Thai Curry Chicken Gluten Free Dairy Free	1 pkg (10 oz)	330	11	25	8	–	–	0	4	2

FOOD	PORTION	CALS	TOTAL FAT	CHOL	SAT FAT	POLY FAT	MONO FAT	TRANS FAT	FIBER	SUGAR
Tabatchnick										
Cabbage	1 serv (7.5 oz)	90	1	0	0	–	–	0	1	11
Chicken Broth w/ Noodles & Dumplings	1 serv (7.25 oz)	150	6	65	1	–	–	0	tr	1
Corn Chowder	1 serv (7.5 oz)	130	5	10	2	–	–	0	2	4
Organic Vegetarian Chili	1 serv (7.5 oz)	180	4	0	0	–	–	0	8	3
Soup Singles Split Pea	1 bowl (10.9 oz)	210	1	0	0	–	–	0	20	1
Split Pea	1 serv (7.5 oz)	140	0	0	0	0	0	0	13	0
Vegetable	1 serv (7.5 oz)	90	2	0	0	–	–	0	4	3
Vegetable Low Sodium	1 serv (7.5 oz)	90	2	0	0	–	–	0	4	3
Wilderness Wild Rice	1 serv (7.5 oz)	80	1	0	0	–	–	0	1	1
Yankee Bean	1 serv (7.5 oz)	180	2	0	0	–	–	0	10	2
MIX										
beef broth cube	1 cube	6	tr	tr	tr	tr	tr	–	–	–
chicken broth cube	1 cube (4.8 g)	9	tr	1	tr	tr	tr	–	–	–
Annie Chun's										
Ramen Soy Ginger as prep	1 pkg (4.9 oz)	230	1	0	0	–	–	0	1	tr
Ramen Spring Vegetable as prep	1 pkg (4.9 oz)	230	1	0	0	–	–	0	2	2
Dr. McDougall's										
Black Bean & Lime not prep	1 pkg (3.3 oz)	340	2	0	0	–	–	0	28	4
Chicken Noodle Light Sodium not prep	1 pkg (1.4 oz)	140	1	0	0	–	–	0	2	2
Chinese Chicken Noodle Light Sodium not prep	1 pkg (1.4 oz)	140	1	0	0	–	–	0	2	2
Minestrone & Pasta not prep	1 pkg (2.3 oz)	200	1	0	0	–	–	0	8	2
Tamale w/ Baked Chips not prep	1 pkg (2.4 oz)	200	2	0	0	–	–	0	6	2
Tortilla w/ Baked Chips not prep	1 pkg (2 oz)	200	2	0	0	–	–	0	6	2
White Bean & Pasta Light Sodium not prep	1 pkg (1.8 oz)	170	1	0	0	–	–	0	8	2
Herb Ox										
Beef Cubes	1 (3.5 g)	5	0	0	0	0	0	0	0	0
Beef Instant	1 pkg (4 g)	5	0	0	0	0	0	0	0	0
Chicken Cubes	1 (4 g)	5	0	0	0	0	0	0	0	0
Chicken Instant	1 pkg (3.5 g)	5	0	0	0	0	0	0	0	0
Chicken Instant Sodium Free	1 pkg (4 g)	10	0	0	0	0	0	0	0	1

FOOD	PORTION	CALS	TOTAL FAT	CHOL	SAT FAT	POLY FAT	MONO FAT	TRANS FAT	FIBER	SUGAR
TAKE-OUT										
ban mien fish head	1 serv (10 oz)	277	10	59	4	1	4	–	4	2
beef stew soup	1 cup (8.8 oz)	221	5	60	2	tr	2	–	–	–
bird's nest	1 cup (8.6 oz)	112	3	27	1	tr	1	–	0	1
black bean turtle soup	1 cup (6.5 oz)	240	1	0	tr	tr	tr	–	10	1
broccoli cheese	1 cup	165	9	14	3	2	3	–	2	7
brunswick stew soup	1 cup (8.5 oz)	232	6	71	2	2	2	–	–	–
caldo de res beef soup	1 cup	143	5	22	2	tr	2	–	2	3
chinese velvet corn	1¼ cups	135	0	1	0	–	–	–	–	–
corn & cheese chowder	¾ cup	215	12	66	7	2	3	–	3	–
duck soup	1 cup (8.6 oz)	412	37	88	12	5	17	–	tr	tr
egg drop	1 cup	73	4	102	1	1	2	–	0	tr
gazpacho	1 cup	46	tr	0	–	–	–	–	–	–
greek lemon	¾ cup	63	2	83	1	tr	1	–	2	–
hot & sour	1 serv (14 oz)	173	9	79	3	2	4	–	3	3
matzo ball soup	1 cup	118	5	63	1	1	2	–	1	tr
minestrone	1 cup	233	13	9	4	2	7	–	4	4
miso w/ tofu	1 cup	84	3	0	1	1	1	–	2	2
onion soup gratinee	1 serv	492	27	77	16	–	–	–	4	6
oxtail	1 cup	68	2	2	1	tr	1	–	1	2
pasta e fagioli	1 cup (8.8 oz)	194	5	3	1	1	3	–	–	–
ratatouille	1 cup (7.5 oz)	266	25	0	3	2	18	–	–	–
seaweed	1 cup (8 oz)	80	3	14	1	1	1	–	1	1
shark fin	1 bowl (10 oz)	164	9	84	2	–	–	–	0	–
shrimp bisque	1 cup	263	14	129	4	3	5	–	tr	10
shrimp gumbo	1 cup (8.6 oz)	163	7	73	1	2	3	–	3	5
sopa de albondigas	1 cup	171	11	50	4	1	4	–	1	3
thai lemon grass	1 bowl	100	4	65	–	–	–	–	–	–
vietnamese pho beef noodle	1 serv (7.8 oz)	480	12	46	5	–	–	–	1	2
wonton soup	1 cup	183	7	53	2	1	3	0	1	tr
yookgaejang korean beef	1 cup (8.4 oz)	94	6	50	2	1	3	–	1	–
zupa koprowa polish dill soup	1 bowl	54	2	55	–	–	–	–	–	–
SOUR CREAM										
fat free	1 tbsp	12	0	1	0	0	0	0	0	tr
fat free	½ cup (4.5 oz)	95	0	12	0	0	0	0	0	1
reduced fat	1 tbsp (0.5 oz)	29	2	6	1	tr	1	–	0	tr
reduced fat	½ cup (4.4 oz)	224	17	43	11	1	5	–	0	tr
sour cream	1 tbsp (0.4 oz)	23	2	6	1	tr	1	–	0	tr
sour cream	½ cup (4 oz)	222	23	60	13	1	6	–	0	3

FOOD	PORTION	CALS	TOTAL FAT	CHOL	SAT FAT	POLY FAT	MONO FAT	TRANS FAT	FIBER	SUGAR
Friendship										
Light	2 tbsp (1 oz)	40	3	10	2	0	1	0	0	2
Green Valley										
Sour Cream	2 tbsp	100	10	35	7	–	–	0	0	1
SOUR CREAM SUBSTITUTES										
imitation	½ cup (4 oz)	239	22	0	20	tr	1	–	0	8
Follow Your Heart										
Vegan	1 oz	50	5	0	2	–	–	0	2	0
Tofutti										
Better Than Sour Cream	2 tbsp (1 oz)	85	5	0	2	–	–	0	0	2
SOURSOP										
fresh	1	416	2	0	–	–	–	–	–	–
fresh cut up	1 cup	150	1	0	–	–	–	–	–	–
SOY (see also CHEESE SUBSTITUTES, ICE CREAM AND FROZEN DESSERTS, MILK SUBSTITUTES, MISO, SMOOTHIES, SOY SAUCE, SOYBEANS, TEMPEH, TOFU, YOGURT FROZEN)										
natto	½ cup (3.1 oz)	187	10	0	1	5	2	–	5	4
SOY DRINKS (see also MILK SUBSTITUTES, SMOOTHIES)										
SOY SAUCE										
shoyu	1 tbsp	9	tr	0	tr	tr	tr	–	–	–
soy sauce	1 tbsp	7	tr	0	tr	tr	tr	–	–	–
tamari	1 tbsp	11	tr	0	tr	tr	tr	–	–	–
Lee Kum Kee										
Less Sodium	1 tbsp (0.5 oz)	10	0	0	0	0	0	0	–	1
Soy Vay										
Wasabi Teriyaki	1 tbsp	35	1	0	0	–	–	0	0	5
SOYBEANS										
dried cooked	1 cup	298	15	0	2	9	3	–	–	–
dry roasted	½ cup	387	19	0	3	10	4	–	–	–
green cooked	½ cup	127	6	0	1	–	–	–	4	–
roasted	½ cup	405	22	0	3	12	5	–	–	–
roasted & toasted	1 cup	490	26	0	3	14	6	–	–	–
roasted & toasted salted	1 cup	490	26	0	3	14	6	–	–	–
sprouts raw	½ cup	43	2	0	tr	1	1	–	–	–
sprouts steamed	½ cup	38	2	0	tr	1	tr	–	–	–
sprouts stir fried	1 cup	125	7	0	1	4	2	–	–	–
Crunchies										
Freeze Dried Edamame	⅜ cup (1 oz)	124	6	0	1	–	–	0	3	2

FOOD	PORTION	CALS	TOTAL FAT	CHOL	SAT FAT	POLY FAT	MONO FAT	TRANS FAT	FIBER	SUGAR
Freeze Dried Edamame Grilled	⅜ cup (0.9 oz)	84	1	0	0	–	–	0	1	1
Freeze Dried Edamame Salted	¼ cup (0.9 oz)	90	4	0	0	–	–	0	3	0
South Beach										
Dark Chocolate Covered	1 pkg (0.71 oz)	100	6	0	3	–	–	0	2	6
Sunrich Naturals										
Edamame Fiesta Blend frzn	½ cup (3 oz)	90	3	0	0	–	–	0	3	1
Edamame In The Shell frzn	½ cup (3 oz)	120	5	0	1	–	–	0	4	3
Soy Honey Nutz	1 pkg (1 oz)	130	6	0	1	–	–	0	4	3

SPAGHETTI (*see* PASTA, PASTA DINNERS, PASTA SALAD, SPAGHETTI SAUCE)

SPAGHETTI SAUCE
JARRED

FOOD	PORTION	CALS	TOTAL FAT	CHOL	SAT FAT	POLY FAT	MONO FAT	TRANS FAT	FIBER	SUGAR
marinara sauce	1 cup	171	8	0	tr	tr	tr	–	–	–
spaghetti sauce	1 cup	272	12	0	2	3	6	–	–	–
Barilla										
Toscana Tuscan Herb	½ cup (4.4 oz)	70	2	0	0	–	–	0	3	6
Bella Sun Luci										
Sun Dried Tomato Pesto w/ Whole Pine Nuts	¼ cup (1.9 oz)	270	27	<5	3	–	–	0	1	5
Del Monte										
Garlic & Onion	½ cup (4.4 oz)	70	1	0	0	–	–	0	2	6
DelGrosso										
Aunt Cindy's Roasted Garlic Gala	½ cup (4.2 oz)	90	6	0	1	–	–	0	2	5
Hunt's										
Pasta Sauce Four Cheese	½ cup (4.4 oz)	60	1	0	0	–	–	0	3	5
Pasta Sauce Garlic & Herb	½ cup (4.4 oz)	40	1	0	0	–	–	0	3	4
Pasta Sauce Meat	½ cup (4.4 oz)	60	1	0	0	–	–	0	3	6
Pasta Sauce Mushroom	½ cup (4.4 oz)	50	1	0	0	–	–	0	3	6
Tomato Sauce	¼ cup (2.2 oz)	20	0	0	0	0	0	0	1	2
Tomato Sauce No Salt Added	¼ cup (2.2 oz)	20	0	0	0	0	0	0	1	3
Traditional Pasta Sauce	½ cup (4.4 oz)	50	1	0	0	–	–	0	3	5
Manischewitz										
Tomato & Mushroom	¼ cup (2.2 oz)	40	2	0	1	–	–	0	1	3
Mom's										
Artichoke Heart & Asiago Cheese	½ cup (4.2 oz)	90	6	5	2	–	–	0	3	3
Fresh Garlic Basil	½ cup (4.2 oz)	30	3	0	0	–	–	0	2	4

FOOD	PORTION	CALS	TOTAL FAT	CHOL	SAT FAT	POLY FAT	MONO FAT	TRANS FAT	FIBER	SUGAR
Martini	½ cup (4.2 oz)	120	4	20	0	–	–	0	1	3
Puttanesca	½ cup (4.2 oz)	90	6	5	2	–	–	0	2	5
OrganicVille										
Marinara	½ cup (4 oz)	50	1	0	0	–	–	0	2	3
Mushroom	½ cup (4 oz)	45	1	0	0	–	–	0	2	3
Pizza Sauce	½ cup (2 oz)	25	1	0	tr	–	–	0	1	2
Progresso										
Lobster Sauce	½ cup (4.3 oz)	100	7	5	1	–	–	0	2	3
Pesto Arrabiata	2 tbsp (1 oz)	140	11	5	2	–	–	0	2	2
Pesto Basil & Roasted Garlic	2 tbsp (1 oz)	130	13	0	2	–	–	0	0	0
Red Clam w/ Tomato & Basil	½ cup (4.4 oz)	60	1	10	0	–	–	0	1	4
White Clam w/ Garlic & Herb	½ cup (4.4 oz)	120	10	5	2	–	–	0	1	1
Racconto										
Essentials Heart Health Roasted Garlic	½ cup (4.4 oz)	90	5	0	1	–	–	0	2	5
Randazzo's										
Alfredo	¼ cup (2.2 oz)	200	20	65	13	–	–	0	0	1
Fra Diavolo	½ cup (4.4 oz)	90	4	0	1	–	–	0	4	4
Puttanesca	½ cup (4.4 oz)	100	6	0	1	–	–	0	4	4
Vodka	½ cup (4.4 oz)	230	20	65	11	–	–	0	3	3
Sonoma Gourmet										
Fennel Romano	½ cup (4.4 oz)	70	4	0	1	–	–	0	2	4
Puttanesca	½ cup (4.4 oz)	70	5	0	1	–	–	0	2	4
Red Clam	½ cup (4.4 oz)	60	4	5	0	–	–	0	2	3
Vodka Cream	½ cup (4.4 oz)	100	6	10	2	–	–	0	1	3
Victoria										
Bolognese	½ cup (4 oz)	120	8	10	2	–	–	0	tr	4
Italian w/ Imported Cheeses	½ cup (4 oz)	150	12	20	2	–	–	0	2	3
Marinara	½ cup (4 oz)	70	4	0	1	–	–	0	2	3
Pesto	¼ cup (2 oz)	380	37	17	7	–	–	0	2	1
Sicilian Caponata Eggplant	½ cup (4 oz)	70	4	0	1	–	–	0	2	3
Tomato Basil	½ cup (4 oz)	70	4	0	1	–	–	0	2	3
White Clam Sauce	½ cup (4.4 oz)	140	9	20	2	–	–	0	0	0
MIX										
Loney's										
Carbonara as prep	¼ cup (2.1 oz)	33	3	9	2	–	–	0	0	0
Rose as prep	¼ cup (2.1 oz)	29	3	0	0	–	–	0	0	1
REFRIGERATED										
Buitoni										
Alfredo	¼ cup (2.1 oz)	140	12	30	7	–	–	0	0	2

FOOD	PORTION	CALS	TOTAL FAT	CHOL	SAT FAT	POLY FAT	MONO FAT	TRANS FAT	FIBER	SUGAR
Alfredo Light	¼ cup (2.1 oz)	90	6	15	4	–	–	0	0	1
Marinara	½ cup (4.4 oz)	70	3	0	0	–	–	0	2	6
Pesto	¼ cup (2.2 oz)	270	23	10	4	–	–	0	1	4
Pesto Basil Reduced Fat	¼ cup (2.2 oz)	230	17	10	3	–	–	0	2	6
Vodka Sauce	½ cup (4.2 oz)	90	6	15	4	–	–	0	1	3

SPANISH FOOD
FRESH
Texas Tamale Company

FOOD	PORTION	CALS	TOTAL FAT	CHOL	SAT FAT	POLY FAT	MONO FAT	TRANS FAT	FIBER	SUGAR
Tamales Beef	2 (3 oz)	160	12	25	3	–	–	0	2	0
Tamales Chicken	2 (3 oz)	130	7	15	1	–	–	0	1	1
Tamales Spinach	2 (3 oz)	140	8	20	4	–	–	0	0	0

FROZEN
Dr. Praeger's

Burrito Bites	2 (2 oz)	130	3	0	0	–	–	0	4	1

Farm Rich

Quesadillas	2 (3.1 oz)	200	10	25	5	–	–	0	1	1

Lean Cuisine

Simple Favorites Chicken Enchilada Suiza	1 pkg (9 oz)	290	5	20	2	1	1	0	3	8

Mom Made

Fiesta Rice	1 pkg (7 oz)	200	1	0	0	–	–	0	5	2
Munchie Bean Burrito	1 (2.5 oz)	140	9	10	4	–	–	0	1	1

Pjs Organics

Burrito Breakfast	1 (6 oz)	310	7	30	1	–	–	0	2	1
Burrito Five Layer	1 (6 oz)	390	11	30	4	–	–	0	4	1
Burrito Skinny	1 (6 oz)	310	2	15	0	–	–	0	4	0
Burrito Traditional Chicken	1 (6 oz)	380	8	25	2	–	–	0	4	1

READY-TO-EAT

taco shell corn	1 (6.5 inch)	98	5	0	1	2	2	–	2	tr
taco shell flour	1 (7 inch)	173	9	0	2	1	5	–	1	tr

Garden Of Eatin'

Taco Shells Yellow Corn	2 (0.9 oz)	140	7	0	1	–	–	0	1	0

TAKE-OUT

arroz con coco	1 cup	532	38	4	33	1	2	–	4	5
burrito w/ beans	1 med (5 oz)	295	8	6	2	2	4	–	7	1
burrito w/ beans & rice	1 (3.5 oz)	221	5	2	1	1	2	–	4	tr
burrito w/ beef	1 sm (3.4 oz)	297	13	49	5	1	6	–	1	tr
burrito w/ beef & beans	1 med (5 oz)	331	13	34	4	2	6	–	6	1

FOOD	PORTION	CALS	TOTAL FAT	CHOL	SAT FAT	POLY FAT	MONO FAT	TRANS FAT	FIBER	SUGAR
burrito w/ beef beans & cheese	1 med (5 oz)	379	19	57	9	2	7	–	5	1
burrito w/ chicken & beans	1 med (5 oz)	295	9	37	2	2	4	–	5	1
burrito w/ pork & beans	1 med (5 oz)	320	12	34	4	2	5	–	6	1
chiles rellenos meat & cheese filled	1 (5 oz)	213	16	109	5	4	6	0	2	3
chimichanga w/ bean cheese lettuce & tomato	1 (4.1 oz)	271	18	17	5	4	7	–	3	2
chimichanga w/ beef & rice	1 (10 oz)	634	36	35	8	10	16	–	5	5
chimichanga w/ beef beans lettuce & tomato	1 (4.1 oz)	254	15	15	3	4	7	–	3	2
chimichanga w/ beef cheese lettuce & tomato	1 (4.1 oz)	337	24	37	8	5	10	–	1	1
chimichanga w/ chicken sour cream lettuce & tomato	1 (4 oz)	277	20	30	6	5	8	–	1	1
empanada fruit filled	1 (3.8 oz)	452	25	0	6	8	10	–	2	25
empanada meat & vegetable	1 (7.8 oz)	881	61	40	15	16	24	–	3	1
empanada sweet potato	1 (7.8 oz)	546	23	56	6	7	9	–	4	22
enchilada w/ beans	1 (4.1 oz)	179	6	4	1	2	2	–	6	2
enchilada w/ beans & cheese	1 (4.6 oz)	233	11	21	5	2	4	–	5	2
enchilada w/ beef	1 (4 oz)	214	10	30	3	2	4	–	3	2
enchilada w/ beef & beans	1 (4 oz)	195	8	15	2	2	3	–	4	2
frijoles	1 cup	278	2	0	tr	1	tr	–	9	6
frijoles w/ cheese	1 cup	225	8	37	4	1	3	–	–	–
nachos w/ beans & cheese	1 serv (9.4 oz)	616	33	56	13	5	13	–	13	2
nachos w/ beef beans cheese & sour cream	1 serv (19 oz)	1620	97	171	37	9	43	–	19	4
paella	1 serv (7 oz)	308	16	92	3	4	9	–	3	–
pupusa meat filled	1 (3.6 oz)	187	6	20	2	1	2	–	3	1
quesadilla w/ cheese	1 (5 oz)	498	28	60	14	4	9	–	3	1
quesadilla w/ meat & cheese	1 (6.5 oz)	605	35	98	16	4	12	–	2	1
taco de jueye w/ crab meat	1 (4.2 oz)	266	14	79	5	2	7	–	2	1
taco w/ beans lettuce tomato & salsa	1 (2.8 oz)	117	5	2	1	2	2	–	4	1
taco w/ chicken lettuce tomato & salsa	1 (2.5 oz)	114	5	22	1	2	2	–	1	1
taco w/ fish lettuce tomato & salsa	1 (2.7 oz)	101	4	39	1	1	1	–	1	1

FOOD	PORTION	CALS	TOTAL FAT	CHOL	SAT FAT	POLY FAT	MONO FAT	TRANS FAT	FIBER	SUGAR
tostada w/ beef lettuce tomato & salsa	1 (2.7 oz)	143	8	21	2	1	3	–	2	1

SPICES (see individual names, HERBS/SPICES)

SPINACH
CANNED
drained	1 cup	49	1	0	tr	tr	tr	0	5	1

Del Monte
Leaf No Salt Added	½ cup (4 oz)	30	0	0	0	0	0	0	2	0
Whole Leaf	½ cup (4 oz)	30	0	0	0	0	0	0	2	0

FRESH
baby raw	2 cups	20	0	0	0	0	0	0	3	0
cooked	1 cup	41	tr	0	tr	tr	tr	0	4	1
malabar cooked	1 cup	10	tr	0	–	–	–	–	1	–
mustard cooked	1 cup	29	tr	0	–	–	–	0	4	–
new zealand cooked	1 cup	22	tr	0	tr	tr	tr	–	–	–
raw	1 cup	7	tr	0	tr	tr	tr	–	1	tr

Dole
Baby Spinach	1½ cups (3 oz)	20	0	0	0	0	0	0	2	0

Ready Pac
Microwave Spinach as prep	½ cup (3 oz)	20	0	0	0	0	0	0	1	0

River Ranch
Baby Spinach	3 cups (3 oz)	20	0	0	0	0	0	0	3	0

FROZEN
chopped cooked	1 cup	30	tr	0	tr	tr	tr	0	4	tr

Seabrook Farms
Creamed	½ cup (4.4 oz)	100	5	10	2	–	–	0	2	3

Tabatchnick
Creamed	1 serv (3.7 oz)	40	1	5	1	–	–	0	1	1

Tandoor Chef
Palak Saag Paneer	1 pkg (6 oz)	240	18	15	6	–	–	0	3	4
Samosa Palak Paneer	2 (2 oz)	176	12	6	2	–	–	0	0	0

TAKE-OUT
indian saag	1 serv	28	2	0	tr	–	–	–	1	–
spanakopita spinach pie	1 serv (3 oz)	148	11	60	5	1	4	–	1	1

SPINACH JUICE
juice	7 oz	14	0	0	0	0	0	0	–	–

SPORTS DRINKS (see ENERGY DRINKS)

FOOD	PORTION	CALS	TOTAL FAT	CHOL	SAT FAT	POLY FAT	MONO FAT	TRANS FAT	FIBER	SUG
SPROUTS										
kidney bean	½ cup	27	tr	0	tr	tr	tr	–	–	–
lentil sprouts	½ cup	40	tr	0	tr	tr	tr	–	–	–
mung bean	½ cup	16	tr	0	tr	tr	tr	–	–	–
mung bean canned	½ cup	8	tr	0	tr	tr	tr	–	–	–
mung bean cooked	½ cup	13	tr	0	tr	tr	tr	–	–	–
pea	½ cup (2.1 oz)	74	tr	0	tr	tr	tr	0	–	–
radish	½ cup	8	tr	0	tr	tr	tr	–	–	–
TAKE-OUT										
mung bean stir fried	½ cup	31	tr	0	tr	tr	tr	–	–	–
SQUAB										
boneless baked	1 (4 oz)	242	14	129	4	3	6	0	0	0
SQUASH (see also SQUASH SEEDS, ZUCCHINI)										
CANNED										
crookneck sliced	½ cup	14	tr	0	tr	tr	tr	–	–	–
FRESH										
acorn cooked mashed	½ cup	41	tr	0	tr	tr	tr	–	3	–
acorn cubed baked	½ cup	57	tr	0	tr	tr	tr	–	2	–
butternut baked	½ cup	41	tr	0	tr	tr	tr	–	2	–
crookneck sliced cooked	½ cup	18	tr	0	tr	tr	tr	–	1	–
hubbard baked	½ cup	51	tr	0	tr	tr	tr	–	3	–
hubbard cooked mashed	½ cup	35	tr	0	tr	tr	tr	–	3	–
scallop sliced cooked	½ cup	14	tr	0	tr	tr	tr	–	1	–
spaghetti cooked	½ cup	23	tr	0	tr	tr	tr	–	2	–
Mann's										
Butternut Cubes (3 oz)	1 serv	40	0	0	0	0	0	0	2	2
Plainville Farm										
Butternut Peeled (3 oz)	½ cup	40	0	0	0	0	0	0	1	5
FROZEN										
butternut cooked mashed	½ cup	47	tr	0	tr	tr	tr	–	3	–
crookneck sliced cooked	½ cup	24	tr	0	tr	tr	tr	–	–	–
TAKE-OUT										
fritter	1 (0.8 oz)	81	5	15	1	1	2	0	1	1
squash pie	1 slice (5.4 oz)	291	12	66	4	3	5	0	2	24
SQUASH SEEDS										
kernels dried	¼ cup (1.1 oz)	180	16	0	3	7	5	tr	2	tr
kernels roasted	¼ cup (1 oz)	169	14	0	3	6	5	tr	2	tr
kernels roasted w/ salt	¼ cup (1 oz)	169	14	0	3	6	5	tr	2	tr

FOOD	PORTION	CALS	TOTAL FAT	CHOL	SAT FAT	POLY FAT	MONO FAT	TRANS FAT	FIBER	SUGAR
whole roasted w/ salt	¼ cup (0.5 oz)	71	3	0	1	1	1	–	3	–
whole roasted w/o salt	¼ cup (0.5 oz)	71	3	0	1	1	1	–	3	–
SQUID										
baked	1 cup	192	6	393	1	2	2	0	0	0
canned in its own ink	1 can (4 oz)	122	2	308	tr	1	tr	0	0	0
dried	1 sm (1.5 oz)	147	2	371	1	1	tr	0	0	0
pickled	1 oz	26	tr	63	tr	tr	tr	0	0	tr
steamed	1 cup	147	2	374	1	1	tr	0	0	0
Margaritaville										
Captain's Calamari Rings + Sauce	3 + 2 tbsp sauce	320	21	100	4	–	–	0	1	3
TAKE-OUT										
arroz con calamares	1 cup	400	17	150	2	2	12	–	1	2
calamari breaded & fried	1 cup	296	12	378	3	4	5	–	1	1
SQUIRREL										
roasted	3 oz	147	4	103	tr	1	1	–	0	0
STARFRUIT										
fresh	1	42	tr	0	–	–	–	–	–	–
STRAWBERRIES										
canned in heavy syrup	½ cup	117	tr	0	tr	tr	tr	0	2	28
fresh halves	1 cup	49	tr	0	tr	tr	tr	0	3	7
fresh whole	1 pint	114	1	0	tr	1	tr	0	7	17
fresh whole	1 cup	46	tr	0	tr	tr	tr	0	3	7
frzn sweetened sliced	½ cup	122	tr	0	tr	tr	tr	0	2	31
frzn sweetened whole	1 cup	199	tr	0	tr	tr	tr	0	5	48
frzn whole unsweetened	1 cup	77	tr	0	tr	tr	tr	0	5	10
organic fresh whole	8 med	45	0	0	0	0	0	0	4	8
Crunchies										
Freeze Dried	¼ cup (6 g)	20	0	0	0	0	0	0	1	3
Crunchy N'Yummy										
Organic Freeze Dried	1 pkg (1 oz)	60	0	0	0	0	0	0	3	0
Dole										
Sliced frzn	1 pkg (3 oz)	35	0	0	0	0	0	0	2	4
Squish'ems	1 pkg	70	0	0	0	0	0	0	1	15
Whole Fresh	1 cup (5.2 oz)	45	0	0	0	0	0	0	3	7
Whole frzn	1 cup (4.9 oz)	50	0	0	0	0	0	0	3	61

FOOD	PORTION	CALS	TOTAL FAT	CHOL	SAT FAT	POLY FAT	MONO FAT	TRANS FAT	FIBER	SUG
STUFFING/DRESSING										
Mrs. Cubbison's										
Corn Bread not prep	½ cup (1.2 oz)	130	1	0	0	–	–	0	2	2
Focaccia not prep	½ cup (1 oz)	110	2	0	0	–	–	0	4	3
Multi-Grain Cranberry not prep	⅓ cup (1 oz)	110	3	0	0	–	–	0	1	3
Pepperidge Farm										
Cornbread	¾ cup	170	2	0	0	–	–	0	2	2
Country Style	¾ cup	140	1	0	0	–	–	0	2	2
Herb Seasoned	¾ cup	170	2	0	1	–	–	0	3	2
TAKE-OUT										
bread	1 cup	352	17	0	3	5	8	–	2	5
cornbread	½ cup	179	9	0	2	3	4	–	3	0
kishke stuffed derma	1 piece (1.3 oz)	166	12	13	6	1	5	–	1	tr
oyster	1 cup	304	18	23	4	5	8	0	2	3
sausage	½ cup	292	11	12	2	1	2	–	1	–
STURGEON										
broiled	3 oz	115	4	65	1	1	2	0	0	0
smoked	1 oz	49	1	23	tr	tr	1	0	0	0
TAKE-OUT										
breaded & fried	4 oz	252	15	85	3	4	7	0	1	1
SUCKER										
white baked	3 oz	101	3	45	tr	1	1	–	0	0
SUGAR (see also FRUCTOSE, SYRUP)										
brown organic	1 tsp	17	0	0	0	0	0	0	0	4
brown packed	1 cup (7.7 oz)	828	0	0	0	0	0	0	–	214
brown unpacked	1 cup (5.1 oz)	547	0	0	0	0	0	0	0	140
cinnamon sugar	1 tsp	16	tr	0	tr	tr	tr	–	tr	4
cube	1 (2 g)	9	0	0	0	0	0	0	0	2
maple	1 piece (1 oz)	99	tr	0	tr	tr	tr	–	0	24
powdered	1 tbsp (0.3 oz)	31	0	0	0	0	0	0	–	8
powdered unsifted	1 cup (4.2 oz)	467	tr	0	–	–	–	–	–	115
raw	1 pkg (5 g)	19	0	0	0	0	0	0	0	5
sugarcane stem	3 oz	54	0	0	0	0	0	0	3	–
white	1 tbsp (0.4 oz)	49	0	0	0	0	0	0	0	13
white	1 tsp (4 g)	15	0	0	0	0	0	0	–	4
white	1 pkg (3 g)	12	0	0	0	0	0	0	0	3
white	1 cup (7 oz)	773	0	0	0	0	0	0	–	200

FOOD	PORTION	CALS	TOTAL FAT	CHOL	SAT FAT	POLY FAT	MONO FAT	TRANS FAT	FIBER	SUGAR
Coconut World										
Coconut Sugar	1 tsp (3 g)	10	0	0	0	0	0	0	0	3
Domino										
White	1 tsp	15	0	0	0	0	0	0	–	–
In The Raw										
Granulated	1 pkg (5 g)	20	0	0	0	0	0	0	–	5
Liquid Cane	1 tsp (6 g)	20	0	0	0	0	0	0	0	5
Maple Grove Farms										
Granulated Maple	1 tsp (4 g)	15	0	0	0	0	0	0	–	3
SUGAR SUBSTITUTES										
Fibrelle										
Fiber-Rich Sweetener	1 tsp (4 g)	5	0	0	0	0	0	0	2	0
Ideal										
Brown	1 tsp (1.5 g)	0	0	0	0	0	0	0	0	0
Confectionary	¼ cup (1 oz)	86	0	0	0	0	0	0	0	0
Packets	1 (1.5 g)	0	0	0	0	0	0	0	0	0
White Granulated	1 tsp (1.5 g)	0	0	0	0	0	0	0	0	0
In The Raw										
Monk Fruit	1 pkg (0.8 g)	0	0	0	0	0	0	0	–	0
Stevia	1 pkg (1 g)	0	0	0	0	0	0	0	–	0
Nevella										
No Calorie Sweetener	1 tsp (0.5 g)	0	0	0	0	0	0	0	0	0
Pyure										
Organic Stevia	1 pkg (1 g)	0	0	0	0	0	0	0	1	0
Splenda										
Nectresse	1 pkg (2.4 g)	0	0	0	0	0	0	0	–	tr
No Calorie Sweetener w/ Antioxidants	1 pkg	0	0	0	0	0	0	0	–	0
No Calorie Sweetener w/ B Vitamins	1 pkg	0	0	0	0	0	0	0	0	0
No Calorie Sweetener w/ Fiber	1 pkg	0	0	0	0	0	0	0	1	0
Swerve										
Sweetener	1 tsp (5 g)	0	0	0	0	0	0	0	–	0
Whey Low										
Gold	1 tsp (4 g)	4	0	0	0	0	0	0	0	4
Granular	1 tsp (4 g)	4	0	0	0	0	0	0	0	4
Maple	¼ cup (2 oz)	57	0	0	0	0	0	0	0	14
Powder	1 tsp (4 g)	4	0	0	0	0	0	0	0	4

FOOD	PORTION	CALS	TOTAL FAT	CHOL	SAT FAT	POLY FAT	MONO FAT	TRANS FAT	FIBER	SUG
SUGAR-APPLE										
fresh	1	146	tr	0	–	–	–	–	–	–
fresh cut up	1 cup	236	1	0	–	–	–	–	–	–
SUNCHOKE										
fresh raw sliced	½ cup	57	tr	0	0	tr	tr	–	–	–
SUNFISH										
pumpkinseed baked	3 oz	97	1	73	tr	tr	tr	–	0	0
SUNFLOWER										
seeds dry roasted w/ salt	¼ cup	186	16	0	2	11	3	0	3	1
seeds dry roasted w/o salt	¼ cup	186	16	0	2	11	3	0	4	1
seeds w/ hulls dried	¼ cup	66	6	0	1	4	1	0	1	tr
David										
Kernels	¼ cup (1.1 oz)	190	15	0	2	8	5	0	3	tr
Seeds Reduced Sodium w/o Shell	¼ cup (1.1 oz)	190	14	0	2	5	7	0	3	tr
Seeds w/o Shell	¼ cup (1.1 oz)	190	15	0	2	8	4	0	4	tr
Frito Lay										
Seeds	1 oz	190	16	0	2	9	6	0	3	tr
Kaia Foods										
Seeds Sprouted Cocoa Mole	⅙ pkg (1 oz)	80	6	0	1	–	–	0	2	3
Sprouted Seeds Sweet Curry	⅙ pkg (1 oz)	80	6	0	1	–	–	0	2	2
Planters										
Kernels	1 oz	160	14	0	2	–	–	0	3	1
Seeds Roasted & Salted	¾ cup (1 oz)	160	14	0	2	–	–	0	3	0
Somersaults										
Snacks Pacific Sea Salt	14 (1.1 oz)	150	8	0	1	–	–	0	3	1
South Beach										
Dark Chocolate Covered	1 pkg (0.67 oz)	100	8	0	3	–	–	0	1	6
Spitz										
Seeds Salted	⅓ pkg (1 oz)	180	15	0	2	10	3	0	3	tr
Sunrich Naturals										
Kernels Cocoa Sunnies	1 pkg (2 oz)	280	16	0	2	–	–	0	4	13
Kernels Honey Roasted	1 pkg (1 oz)	170	14	0	2	–	–	0	2	3
Kernels Lightly Salted	1 pkg (1 oz)	170	16	0	2	–	–	0	2	1
SUSHI										
TAKE-OUT										
california roll	1 (1.2 oz)	48	1	17	tr	tr	tr	–	tr	1
crabmeat mayonnaise	1 (1.2 oz)	60	2	3	tr	1	1	–	tr	–

FOOD	PORTION	CALS	TOTAL FAT	CHOL	SAT FAT	POLY FAT	MONO FAT	TRANS FAT	FIBER	SUGAR
futomaki roll	1 (1.8 oz)	73	1	22	tr	tr	tr	–	1	3
ikura salmon roe & cucumber	1 (1.1 oz)	50	1	22	tr	tr	1	–	1	1
inari	1 sm (1.2 oz)	46	1	0	0	0	0	–	0	–
kappa cucumber roll	1 (1.1 oz)	43	0	0	0	0	0	–	tr	2
kim bap	1 (1.2 oz)	56	2	10	0	1	1	–	0	–
nigiri	1 (0.7 oz)	27	0	6	0	0	0	–	0	–
prawn cooked	1 (1.1 oz)	36	0	0	0	0	0	–	1	–
preserved radish roll	1 (0.3 oz)	9	0	0	0	0	0	–	tr	0
saba raw mackerel	1 (0.8 oz)	33	1	2	1	0	tr	–	tr	1
salmon slice	1 (1.2 oz)	59	1	3	1	tr	tr	–	tr	1
sashimi ahi	1 slice (0.3 oz)	10	0	4	0	0	0	0	0	0
scallop cooked	1 (1.1 oz)	43	tr	10	tr	tr	tr	–	tr	–
seasoned baby octopus	1 (1.2 oz)	55	tr	19	tr	tr	–	–	tr	1
seasoned jellyfish	1 (1.2 oz)	58	1	1	tr	tr	tr	–	tr	2
seaweed roll	1 (1.1 oz)	43	1	1	tr	tr	tr	–	1	1
sweet beancurd	1 (1.2 oz)	64	2	0	tr	1	1	–	1	3
tekka tuna maki	1 (0.6 oz)	25	0	0	0	0	0	0	0	–
torigai cockle	1 piece (1.1 oz)	41	0	0	0	0	0	–	tr	–
tuna roll	1 (0.6 oz)	19	0	0	0	0	0	–	tr	0
unagi grilled eel	1 (1 oz)	54	2	9	1	tr	1	–	1	1
vegetable roll	1 (1.2 oz)	27	1	0	tr	tr	tr	–	–	tr
vinegared ginger	⅓ cup (1.6 oz)	48	tr	0	tr	tr	tr	–	–	4
wasabi	2 tsp (0.3 oz)	5	tr	0	0	0	0	–	–	–
yellowtail roll	1 (0.6 oz)	25	1	0	tr	tr	tr	–	–	tr

SWAMP CABBAGE

FOOD	PORTION	CALS	TOTAL FAT	CHOL	SAT FAT	POLY FAT	MONO FAT	TRANS FAT	FIBER	SUGAR
chopped cooked w/o salt	1 cup	20	tr	0	tr	tr	tr	0	2	–

SWEET POTATO (see also YAM)

FOOD	PORTION	CALS	TOTAL FAT	CHOL	SAT FAT	POLY FAT	MONO FAT	TRANS FAT	FIBER	SUGAR
baked w/ skin w/o salt	1 lg (6.3 oz)	162	tr	0	tr	tr	tr	0	6	12
baked w/ skin w/o salt	1 med (4 oz)	103	tr	0	tr	tr	tr	0	4	7
canned in syrup	½ cup	106	tr	0	tr	tr	tr	0	3	6
canned mashed	½ cup	129	tr	0	tr	tr	tr	0	2	7
leaves cooked w/o salt	1 cup (2.2 oz)	26	tr	0	tr	tr	tr	0	1	4
paste dulce de calabaza	1 oz	82	tr	0	tr	tr	tr	0	tr	20
Jake & Amos										
Sweet Potato Butter	1 tbsp (0.5 oz)	25	0	0	0	0	0	0	0	3
Mann's										
Fresh Cubes	1 serv (3 oz)	60	0	0	0	0	0	0	3	3
Fries Fresh	1 serv (3 oz)	60	0	0	0	0	0	0	3	3

FOOD	PORTION	CALS	TOTAL FAT	CHOL	SAT FAT	POLY FAT	MONO FAT	TRANS FAT	FIBER	SUG
TAKE-OUT										
candied	1 serv (3.7 oz)	151	3	8	1	tr	1	–	3	–
white fried batata blanca frita	1 serv (8 oz)	792	29	0	7	8	11	–	19	2
SWEETBREAD (PANCREAS)										
beef braised	3 oz	230	15	223	5	3	5	0	0	0
lamb braised	3 oz	199	13	340	6	1	5	0	0	0
pork braised	3 oz	186	9	268	3	2	3	0	0	0
SWISS CHARD										
cooked	½ cup	18	tr	0	–	–	–	–	–	–
raw chopped	½ cup	3	tr	0	–	–	–	–	–	–
SWORDFISH										
cooked	3 oz	132	4	43	1	1	2	–	0	0
raw	3 oz	103	3	33	1	1	1	–	0	0
SYRUP										
agave	¼ cup (2 oz)	170	tr	0	–	–	–	0	0	5
corn dark & light	¼ cup	240	tr	0	0	0	0	–	0	65
maple	1 tbsp	52	0	0	–	–	–	0	–	12
maple	1 cup (11.1 oz)	824	1	0	–	–	–	–	–	191
raspberry	1 oz	76	0	0	0	0	0	0	–	–
sorghum	1 cup (11.6 oz)	957	0	0	0	0	0	–	0	247
sorghum	1 tbsp (0.7 oz)	61	0	0	0	0	0	–	0	16
sugar syrup	¼ cup	76	0	0	0	0	0	0	0	20
Domino										
Agave Nectar Organic Light or Amber	1 tbsp (0.7 oz)	60	0	0	0	0	0	0	–	16
In The Raw										
Agave	1 tbsp (0.7 oz)	60	0	0	0	0	0	0	–	15
Karo										
Corn Syrup Light	2 tbsp (1 oz)	120	0	0	0	0	0	0	–	10
Lundberg										
Organic Sweet Dreams Brown Rice	2 tbsp (1.5 oz)	150	0	0	0	0	0	0	0	22
Maple Grove Farms										
Apricot	¼ cup (2.1 oz)	170	0	0	0	0	0	0	–	40
Butter Flavor Sugar Free	¼ cup (2.1 oz)	30	0	0	0	0	0	0	–	0
Red Raspberry	¼ cup (2.1 oz)	230	0	0	0	0	0	0	–	45

FOOD	PORTION	CALS	TOTAL FAT	CHOL	SAT FAT	POLY FAT	MONO FAT	TRANS FAT	FIBER	SUGAR
Nature's Agave										
Agave Nectar Organic Amber Clear or Raw	1 tbsp (0.7 oz)	60	0	0	0	0	0	0	–	16
Smucker's										
Blackberry	¼ cup (2.1 oz)	200	0	0	0	0	0	0	–	44
Blueberry Sugar Free	¼ cup (2.1 oz)	25	0	0	0	0	0	0	1	0
Plate Scrapers Caramel	2 tbsp (1.4 oz)	100	0	0	0	0	0	0	0	20
Plate Scrapers Raspberry	2 tbsp (1.3 oz)	100	0	0	0	0	0	0	0	17
Plate Scrapers Vanilla	2 tbsp (1.4 oz)	110	1	0	0	–	–	0	0	19
Pure Maple	¼ cup (2.1 oz)	210	0	0	0	0	0	0	–	47
Red Raspberry	¼ cup (2.1 oz)	200	0	0	0	0	0	0	–	44
TAHINI (see SESAME)										
TAMARIND										
dried sweetened pulpitas	1 piece (0.8 oz)	56	tr	0	tr	tr	tr	0	1	14
dried sweetened pulpitas	½ cup	279	1	0	tr	tr	tr	0	5	68
fresh	1 (2 g)	5	tr	0	tr	tr	tr	0	tr	0
fresh cut up	1 cup	143	tr	0	tr	tr	tr	0	3	34
TAMARIND JUICE										
nectar	1 cup	143	tr	0	–	–	–	0	1	32
TANGERINE										
CANNED										
in light syrup	1 cup	154	tr	0	tr	tr	tr	0	2	39
juice pack	1 cup	92	tr	0	tr	tr	tr	0	2	22
FRESH										
fresh	1 lg (4.2 oz)	64	tr	0	tr	tr	tr	0	2	13
fresh	1 med (3.1 oz)	47	tr	0	tr	tr	tr	0	2	9
fresh	1 sm (2.7 oz)	40	tr	0	tr	tr	tr	0	1	8
sections	1 cup	103	1	0	tr	tr	tr	0	4	21
Sunkist										
Fresh	1 med (3.8 oz)	50	0	0	0	0	0	0	2	9
TANGERINE JUICE										
canned sweetened	1 cup	124	1	0	tr	tr	tr	0	1	29
fresh	1 cup	106	tr	0	tr	tr	tr	0	1	24
Italian Volcano										
Organic	8 oz	113	1	0	–	–	–	0	–	23
TAPIOCA										
pearl dry	¼ cup (1.3 oz)	136	tr	0	tr	tr	tr	0	tr	1

FOOD	PORTION	CALS	TOTAL FAT	CHOL	SAT FAT	POLY FAT	MONO FAT	TRANS FAT	FIBER	SUGAR
TARO										
chips	10 (0.8 oz)	115	6	0	1	3	1	–	–	–
leaves cooked	½ cup	18	tr	0	tr	tr	tr	–	–	–
raw sliced	½ cup	56	tr	0	tr	tr	tr	–	–	–
shoots sliced cooked	½ cup	10	tr	0	tr	tr	tr	–	–	–
sliced cooked	½ cup (2.3 oz)	94	tr	0	tr	tr	tr	–	–	–
tahitian sliced cooked	½ cup	30	tr	0	tr	tr	tr	–	–	–
TARRAGON										
dried crumbled	1 tsp	2	tr	0	tr	tr	tr	0	0	–
ground	1 tsp	5	tr	0	tr	tr	tr	0	tr	–
TEA/HERBAL TEA (see also ICED TEA)										
HERBAL										
chamomile brewed	1 cup	2	tr	0	tr	tr	tr	–	0	0
Bambusland										
Bamboo Tea Blueberry as prep	1 tea bag	0	0	0	0	0	0	0	0	0
Bamboo Tea Organic	1 tea bag	0	0	0	0	0	0	0	0	0
Bigelow										
Cozy Chamomile	1 tea bag	0	0	0	0	0	0	0	0	0
Celestial Seasonings										
Chamomile Honey Vanilla as prep	1 cup (8 oz)	0	0	0	0	0	0	0	0	0
Nature's Guru										
Cardamon Chai Sweetened Instant	1 pkg (0.9 oz)	35	1	0	0	0	0	0	0	7
Lemongrass Sweetened Instant	1 pkg	65	0	0	0	0	0	0	0	7
REGULAR										
brewed tea	1 cup (6 oz)	2	0	0	0	0	0	0	0	–
Lipton										
Green Tea as prep	1 cup (8 oz)	0	0	0	0	0	0	0	0	0
Green Tea Cranberry Pomegranate	1 tea bag	0	0	0	0	0	0	0	0	0
Green Tea Decaffeinated as prep	1 tea bag	0	0	0	0	0	0	0	0	0
Tetley										
Classic Black as prep	1 tea bag	0	0	0	0	0	0	0	0	0
TAKE-OUT										
chai spiced latte	1 cup	130	3	0	1	–	–	–	0	18

FOOD	PORTION	CALS	TOTAL FAT	CHOL	SAT FAT	POLY FAT	MONO FAT	TRANS FAT	FIBER	SUGAR
TEMPEH										
tempeh	½ cup (2.9 oz)	160	9	0	2	3	2	–	–	–
TESTICLES										
prairie oysters cooked	1 pair (6.8 oz)	241	6	673	2	1	2	0	0	0
THYME										
dried crumbled	1 tsp	3	tr	0	tr	tr	tr	0	tr	tr
fresh	1 tsp	1	tr	0	tr	tr	tr	0	tr	–
ground	1 tsp	4	tr	0	tr	tr	tr	0	1	tr
TILAPIA										
Beacon Light										
Boneless Fillet Farm Raised	1 (3 oz)	85	1	50	0	–	–	0	0	0
Gorton's										
Grilled Fillets Roasted Garlic & Butter	1 (3 oz)	80	3	50	1	1	1	0	–	–
TAKE-OUT										
battered & fried	1 fillet (4 oz)	206	9	109	2	3	4	–	tr	tr
breaded & fried	1 fillet (4 oz)	300	14	142	3	4	6	0	1	2
broiled w/o fat	1 fillet (3.5 oz)	128	3	57	1	1	1	0	0	0
TOFU										
firm	½ cup	183	11	0	2	6	2	–	2	–
firm	¼ block (3 oz)	118	7	0	1	4	2	–	1	–
fresh fried	1 piece (0.5 oz)	35	3	0	tr	1	1	–	tr	–
fuyu salted & fermented	1 block (⅓ oz)	13	1	0	tr	tr	tr	–	tr	–
koyadofu dried frozen	1 piece (½ oz)	82	5	0	1	3	1	–	tr	–
okara	½ cup	47	1	0	tr	tr	tr	–	1	–
regular	½ cup	94	6	0	1	3	1	–	1	–
regular	¼ block (4 oz)	88	6	0	1	3	1	–	1	–
Azumaya										
Extra Firm	3 oz	70	4	0	0	2	1	0	1	0
Lite Extra Firm	⅕ pkg (2.8 oz)	60	2	0	0	–	–	0	1	0
Silken	⅕ pkg (3.2 oz)	40	2	0	0	–	–	–	tr	0
Nasoya										
Extra Firm	⅕ pkg (2.8 oz)	80	4	0	1	3	1	0	1	0
Silken	⅕ pkg (3.2 oz)	160	1	0	0	1	1	0	0	0
Sprouted	3 oz	160	6	0	1	4	2	0	1	1
TAKE-OUT										
breaded deep fried w/ soy sauce japanese style	1 piece (0.4 oz)	15	1	1	tr	tr	tr	–	tr	0

FOOD	PORTION	CALS	TOTAL FAT	CHOL	SAT FAT	POLY FAT	MONO FAT	TRANS FAT	FIBER	SUGAR
soy sauce marinated & grilled	1 serv (4 oz)	181	11	0	2	–	–	–	1	–
stir-fried w/ vegetables	1 cup (7.6 oz)	186	10	0	1	4	4	–	3	–

TOMATILLO

FOOD	PORTION	CALS	TOTAL FAT	CHOL	SAT FAT	POLY FAT	MONO FAT	TRANS FAT	FIBER	SUGAR
fresh	1 (1.2 oz)	11	tr	0	tr	tr	tr	0	1	1
fresh chopped	½ cup (2.3 oz)	21	1	0	tr	tr	tr	0	1	3

TOMATO
CANNED

FOOD	PORTION	CALS	TOTAL FAT	CHOL	SAT FAT	POLY FAT	MONO FAT	TRANS FAT	FIBER	SUGAR
green pickled	½ cup (2.5 oz)	26	tr	0	tr	tr	tr	0	1	5
green whole pickled	1 (2.6 oz)	27	tr	0	tr	tr	tr	0	1	5
paste	¼ cup (2.3 oz)	54	tr	0	tr	tr	tr	0	3	8
paste	1 can (6 oz)	139	1	0	tr	tr	tr	0	7	21
paste no salt added	1 can (6 oz)	139	1	0	tr	tr	tr	0	7	21
puree	1 cup (8.8 oz)	95	1	0	tr	tr	tr	0	5	12
puree	1 can (28 oz)	312	2	0	tr	tr	1	0	16	40
puree w/o salt	1 can (28 oz)	312	2	0	tr	1	1	0	16	40
sauce	1 cup (8.6 oz)	59	tr	0	tr	tr	tr	–	4	10
stewed	1 cup (8.9 oz)	66	tr	0	tr	tr	tr	0	3	9

Bella Sun Luci

FOOD	PORTION	CALS	TOTAL FAT	CHOL	SAT FAT	POLY FAT	MONO FAT	TRANS FAT	FIBER	SUGAR
Bruschetta w/ Italian Basil	¼ cup (1.9 oz)	190	17	<5	3	–	–	0	2	4
Sun Dried Halves w/ Italian Herbs	1 tbsp (0.7 oz)	70	5	0	1	–	–	0	1	3
Sun Dried Julienne Cut w/ Italian Herbs	1 tbsp (0.7 oz)	70	5	0	1	–	–	0	1	3

Del Monte

FOOD	PORTION	CALS	TOTAL FAT	CHOL	SAT FAT	POLY FAT	MONO FAT	TRANS FAT	FIBER	SUGAR
Diced Organic	½ cup (4.4 oz)	20	0	0	0	0	0	0	1	2
Diced Peeled	½ cup (4.2 oz)	25	0	0	0	0	0	0	1	3
Diced Peeled No Salt Added	½ cup (4.4 oz)	25	0	0	0	0	0	0	2	4
Diced Petite No Salt Added	½ cup (4.4 oz)	25	0	0	0	0	0	0	2	4
Diced w/ Basil Garlic & Oregano Organic	½ cup (4.4 oz)	45	0	0	0	0	0	0	1	5
Diced w/ Mushrooms & Garlic	½ cup (4.4 oz)	45	0	0	0	0	0	0	1	6
Diced Zesty Chili	½ cup (4.5 oz)	30	0	0	0	0	0	0	2	6
Petite Cut Garlic & Olive Oil	½ cup (4.4 oz)	40	1	0	0	–	–	0	1	6
Wedges	½ cup (4.4 oz)	35	0	0	0	0	0	0	1	4

Hunt's

FOOD	PORTION	CALS	TOTAL FAT	CHOL	SAT FAT	POLY FAT	MONO FAT	TRANS FAT	FIBER	SUGAR
Crushed	½ cup (4.2 oz)	45	0	0	0	0	0	0	3	4
Diced	½ cup (4.2 oz)	30	0	0	0	0	0	0	2	3

FOOD	PORTION	CALS	TOTAL FAT	CHOL	SAT FAT	POLY FAT	MONO FAT	TRANS FAT	FIBER	SUGAR
Diced Fire Roasted	½ cup (4.3 oz)	30	0	0	0	0	0	0	2	3
Diced In Sauce	½ cup (4.3 oz)	35	0	0	0	0	0	0	2	3
Diced No Salt Added	½ cup (4.2 oz)	30	0	0	0	0	0	0	2	3
Diced Petite	½ cup (4.2 oz)	30	0	0	0	0	0	0	2	2
Diced w/ Roasted Garlic	½ cup (4.2 oz)	35	0	0	0	0	0	0	2	4
Stewed	½ cup (4.2 oz)	45	0	0	0	0	0	0	2	6
Stewed No Salt Added	½ cup (4.2 oz)	40	0	0	0	0	0	0	2	5
Whole	½ cup (4.2 oz)	25	0	0	0	0	0	0	2	3
Whole No Salt Added	½ cup (4.2 oz)	30	0	0	0	0	0	0	2	3
Redpack										
Crushed w/ Basil Garlic & Oregano	¼ cup (2.1 oz)	20	0	0	0	0	0	0	1	1
Rienzi										
Italian Cherry Tomatoes No Salt Added	⅓ can (4.5 oz)	30	0	0	0	0	0	0	1	4
Ro-Tel										
Original	½ cup (4.4 oz)	20	0	0	0	0	0	0	1	3
DRIED										
sun dried	¼ cup (0.5 oz)	35	tr	0	tr	tr	tr	0	2	5
sun dried	1 piece (2 g)	5	tr	0	tr	tr	tr	0	tr	1
sun dried in oil drained	1 piece (3 g)	6	tr	0	tr	tr	tr	0	tr	–
sun dried in oil drained	¼ cup (1 oz)	59	4	0	1	1	2	0	2	–
tomato powder	1 oz	85	tr	0	tr	tr	tr	0	5	12
Bella Sun Luci										
Sun Dried w/ Italian Basil	1/7 pkg (0.5 oz)	35	0	0	0	0	0	0	1	4
Sun Dried w/ Zesty Peppers	1/7 pkg (0.5 oz)	35	0	0	0	0	0	0	1	4
FRESH										
bruschetta	¼ cup	50	3	0	0	–	–	–	tr	4
cherry	½ cup (2.6 oz)	13	tr	0	tr	tr	tr	0	1	2
cherry	1 (0.6 oz)	3	tr	0	tr	tr	tr	0	tr	tr
grape tomatoes	20	30	0	0	0	0	0	0	1	4
green	1 sm (3.2 oz)	21	tr	0	tr	tr	tr	0	1	4
green	1 lg (6.4 oz)	42	tr	0	tr	tr	tr	0	2	7
green	1 med (4.3 oz)	28	tr	0	tr	tr	tr	0	1	5
green chopped	1 cup (6.3 oz)	41	tr	0	tr	tr	tr	0	2	7
orange	1 (4 oz)	18	tr	0	tr	tr	tr	0	1	–
orange chopped	1 cup (5.5 oz)	25	tr	0	tr	tr	tr	0	1	–
plum	1 (2.2 oz)	11	tr	0	tr	tr	tr	0	1	2
red	1 lg (6.4 oz)	33	tr	0	tr	tr	tr	0	2	5
red	1 sm (3.2 oz)	16	tr	0	tr	tr	tr	0	1	2

FOOD	PORTION	CALS	TOTAL FAT	CHOL	SAT FAT	POLY FAT	MONO FAT	TRANS FAT	FIBER	SUGAR
red	1 med (4.3 oz)	22	tr	0	tr	tr	tr	0	2	3
red chopped	½ cup (3.2 oz)	16	tr	0	tr	tr	tr	0	1	2
red slice	1 lg (0.9 oz)	5	tr	0	tr	tr	tr	0	tr	1
roma	1 (2.2 oz)	11	tr	0	tr	tr	tr	0	1	2
yellow	1 (7.4 oz)	32	1	0	tr	tr	tr	0	2	–
yellow chopped	½ cup (2.4 oz)	10	tr	0	tr	tr	tr	0	1	–
Ready Pac										
Bruschetta	2 tbsp (1.6 oz)	70	7	0	1	–	–	0	1	1
TAKE-OUT										
aspic	½ cup (4 oz)	32	tr	0	tr	tr	tr	0	tr	5
broiled slices	2 (2.9 oz)	18	tr	0	tr	tr	tr	–	1	3
broiled whole	1 med (3.7 oz)	23	tr	0	tr	tr	tr	–	2	3
bruschetta on toasted italian bread	1 slice	106	3	0	0	–	–	–	tr	2
fried slices	2 (2.5 oz)	122	9	17	1	4	4	–	1	2
scalloped	½ cup (4 oz)	99	5	0	1	2	1	–	1	5
stewed	½ cup (1.8 oz)	40	1	0	tr	tr	1	–	1	–
stuffed w/ rice	1 (5.2 oz)	110	3	0	1	1	1	–	2	3
stuffed w/ rice & meat	1 (5.2 oz)	142	6	18	2	1	3	–	2	3
TOMATO JUICE										
tomato juice	1 cup (8.5 oz)	41	tr	0	tr	tr	tr	0	1	9
tomato juice w/o added salt	1 cup (8.5 oz)	41	tr	0	tr	tr	tr	0	1	9
TONGUE										
beef simmered	3 oz	241	19	112	7	1	9	0	0	0
lamb braised	3 oz	234	17	161	7	1	9	0	0	0
pork braised	3 oz	230	16	124	5	2	7	0	0	0
veal braised	3 oz	172	9	202	4	tr	4	0	0	0
TORTILLA										
corn	1 (6 in diam)	56	1	0	tr	tr	tr	–	1	–
corn w/o salt	1 (6 in diam)	56	1	0	tr	tr	tr	–	1	–
flour w/o salt	1 (8 in diam)	114	3	0	tr	1	1	–	1	–
Garden Of Eatin'										
Organic Whole Wheat	1 (1.6 oz)	110	1	0	0	–	–	0	3	0
Shells Blue Corn	2 (0.9 oz)	140	7	0	1	–	–	0	1	0
La Tortilla Factory										
Corn Chipotle	1 (1.4 oz)	90	1	0	0	–	–	0	1	0
Smart & Delicious 100 Calorie 100% Whole Wheat	1 (2 oz)	100	2	0	0	–	–	0	8	3

FOOD	PORTION	CALS	TOTAL FAT	CHOL	SAT FAT	POLY FAT	MONO FAT	TRANS FAT	FIBER	SUGAR
Smart & Delicious 100 Calorie Traditional	1 (2 oz)	100	2	0	0	–	–	0	8	0
Smart & Delicious Low Carb Whole Wheat	1 (2.2 oz)	80	3	0	0	1	2	0	12	1
White Corn	1 (1.4 oz)	90	1	0	0	–	–	0	1	0

TORTILLA CHIPS (see CHIPS)

TRAIL MIX
Emerald
Breakfast On The Go Berry Nut Blend	1 pkg (1.5 oz)	180	9	0	2	–	–	0	3	16
Breakfast On The Go Breakfast Nut Blend	1 pkg (1.5 oz)	180	7	0	2	–	–	0	3	20
Breakfast On The Go Smores Nut Blend	1 pkg (1.5 oz)	200	10	0	3	–	–	0	2	14

Frito Lay
Nut & Fruit	1 oz	150	9	0	2	–	–	0	2	7
Original	3 tbsp	160	9	0	2	–	–	0	2	11

Planters
Daybreak Blend Berry & Almond	⅓ pkg (1.5 oz)	180	7	0	1	–	4	–	3	19
Energy Go-Paks	1 (1.5 oz)	250	20	0	3	–	8	0	3	6
Fruit & Nut	⅙ pkg (1 oz)	140	9	0	3	–	4	0	2	10
Nut & Chocolate	1 oz	150	9	0	3	–	5	0	2	12
Sweet & Nutty	⅓ pkg (1.1 oz)	160	10	0	2	–	5	0	2	11

SunRidge Farms
Mountain Rainbow Mix	¼ cup (1 oz)	150	9	0	3	–	–	0	2	12

TREE FERN
chopped cooked	½ cup	28	tr	0	–	–	–	–	–	–

TRIPE
beef simmered	3 oz	80	3	133	1	tr	1	tr	0	0

TAKE-OUT
mondongo w/ potatoes	1 cup	300	11	148	3	3	4	–	6	5

TRITICALE
dry	½ cup (3.4 oz)	323	2	0	tr	1	tr	–	–	–

TROUT
baked	3 oz	162	7	63	1	2	4	–	0	0

FOOD	PORTION	CALS	TOTAL FAT	CHOL	SAT FAT	POLY FAT	MONO FAT	TRANS FAT	FIBER	SUGAR
rainbow cooked	3 oz	129	4	62	1	1	1	–	0	0
seatrout baked	3 oz	113	4	90	1	1	1	–	0	0

TRUFFLES
fresh	0.5 oz	4	tr	0	–	–	–	–	2	–

TUNA
CANNED
light in oil	1 can (6 oz)	399	14	30	3	5	5	–	0	0
light in oil	3 oz	169	7	15	1	2	3	–	0	0
light in water	3 oz	99	1	25	tr	tr	tr	–	0	0
light in water	1 can (5.8 oz)	192	1	49	tr	1	tr	–	0	0
white in oil	3 oz	158	7	26	–	–	–	–	0	0
white in oil	1 can (6.2 oz)	331	14	55	–	–	–	–	0	0
white in water	1 can (6 oz)	234	4	72	1	2	1	–	0	0
white in water	3 oz	116	2	35	1	1	1	–	0	0

Arroyabe
Bonito In Olive Oil	2 oz	109	5	0	–	–	0	0	0	0

Chicken Of The Sea
Albacore Solid White In Oil	2 oz	90	4	25	1	–	–	–	0	0
Albacore Solid White In Water	2 oz	80	4	25	0	–	–	0	0	0
Albacore Chunk White In Water	½ can (2.5 oz)	50	1	25	0	–	–	–	0	0
Chunk Light 50% Less Sodium	2 oz	180	1	25	0	–	–	–	0	0
Chunk Light In Oil	2 oz	100	6	25	1	–	–	–	0	0
Chunk Light In Water	2 oz	50	1	25	0	–	–	–	0	0
Chunk White In Water Very Low Sodium	2 oz	50	1	25	0	–	–	0	0	0

Genova
Tonno In Olive Oil	2 oz	110	6	25	1	–	–	–	0	0

Progresso
Light Olive Oil drained	¼ cup (2 oz)	120	6	35	2	–	–	–	0	0

FRESH
bluefin cooked	3 oz	157	5	42	1	2	2	–	0	0
bluefin raw	3 oz	122	4	32	1	1	1	–	0	0
skipjack baked	3 oz	112	1	51	tr	tr	tr	–	0	0
yellowfin baked	3 oz	118	1	49	tr	tr	tr	–	0	0

FOOD	PORTION	CALS	TOTAL FAT	CHOL	SAT FAT	POLY FAT	MONO FAT	TRANS FAT	FIBER	SUGAR
SHELF-STABLE										
Sea Fare Pacific										
Albacore Wild Caught Jalapeno	⅓ pkg (2 oz)	160	13	15	3	3	–	0	0	0
Albacore Wild Caught Salt Free	⅓ pkg (2 oz)	100	6	20	2	2	–	0	0	0
Albacore Wild Caught Sea Salt	⅓ pkg (2 oz)	100	6	20	2	2	–	0	0	0
Albacore Wild Caught Smoked	⅓ pkg (2 oz)	100	6	10	2	3	–	0	0	0
TAKE-OUT										
tuna salad	1 cup	383	19	27	3	8	6	–	–	–

TURKEY (see also JERKY, TURKEY DISHES, TURKEY SUBSTITUTES)

FOOD	PORTION	CALS	TOTAL FAT	CHOL	SAT FAT	POLY FAT	MONO FAT	TRANS FAT	FIBER	SUGAR
CANNED										
w/ broth	1 cup	220	9	89	3	2	3	–	0	0
Spam										
Oven Roasted	2 oz	80	5	35	2	–	–	–	0	0
FRESH										
breast roasted pre-basted w/ skin	3.5 oz	126	3	42	1	1	1	–	0	0
breast roasted w/o skin	4 oz	166	2	90	1	1	1	tr	0	0
breast w/ skin w/o bone roasted	4 oz	200	6	101	2	2	2	tr	0	0
dark meat w/ skin w/o bone roasted	3.5 oz	175	8	114	2	3	2	–	0	0
dark meat w/o skin roasted	1 cup (5 oz)	262	10	119	3	3	2	–	0	0
dark meat w/o skin w/o bone roasted	4 oz	196	7	145	2	2	2	tr	0	0
ground cooked	3 oz	193	11	84	3	3	4	–	0	0
leg w/ skin roasted	1 (19 oz)	1136	54	464	17	15	16	–	0	0
light meat w/ skin w/o bone half turkey roasted	2.3 lbs	2069	87	794	25	21	30	–	0	0
neck meat only simmered	3 oz	128	6	109	2	2	2	–	0	0
skin roasted	1 oz	129	11	50	3	3	4	tr	0	0
tail cooked	1 (2 oz)	197	16	53	5	4	6	–	0	0
w/o skin meat only roasted	4 oz	188	1	29	tr	tr	tr	tr	0	0
w/o skin meat only roasted	1 cup (5 oz)	238	7	107	2	2	1	–	0	0
whole w/ skin w/o bone roasted	4 oz	214	8	124	2	2	3	tr	0	0

FOOD	PORTION	CALS	TOTAL FAT	CHOL	SAT FAT	POLY FAT	MONO FAT	TRANS FAT	FIBER	SUGAR
wing w/ skin roasted	1 (6.5 oz)	426	23	151	6	5	9	–	0	0
wing w/o skin roasted	1 (5.2 oz)	237	5	147	2	1	1	–	0	0
Empire										
Ground	4 oz	220	16	85	5	–	–	0	0	0
Foster Farms										
Breast Cutlets	4 oz	120	1	45	–	–	–	0	0	0
Necks	4 oz	150	6	90	–	–	–	0	0	0
Tails	4 oz	380	36	35	–	–	–	0	0	0
Shady Brook										
Breast Tenderloin Lemon Garlic	4 oz	130	4	55	0	–	–	0	0	1
Breast Tenderloin Rotisserie	4 oz	130	4	50	0	–	–	0	0	1
Tenderloins Turkey Breast Homestyle	4 oz	130	3	50	0	–	–	0	0	0
FROZEN										
roast boneless seasoned light & dark meat roasted	3.5 oz	155	6	53	2	2	1	–	0	0
sticks breaded fried	1 (2.2 oz)	179	11	41	3	3	4	–	–	–
READY-TO-EAT										
bologna	1 slice (1 oz)	59	4	21	1	1	2	–	tr	1
breast	1 slice (0.7 oz)	22	tr	9	tr	tr	tr	0	tr	1
ham	1 slice (1 oz)	35	1	20	tr	tr	1	–	tr	tr
pastrami	2 oz	70	2	39	1	1	1	–	tr	2
salami	1 slice (1 oz)	48	3	21	1	1	1	0	0	tr
Boar's Head										
Breast Hickory Smoked Black Forest	2 oz	60	1	25	0	0	0	0	0	0
Foster Farms										
Breast Honey Roasted	1 slice (1 oz)	25	0	10	0	0	0	0	0	1
Breast Oven Roasted	1 slice (1 oz)	30	0	10	0	0	0	0	0	0

TURKEY DISHES
CANNED
Dinty Moore

FOOD	PORTION	CALS	TOTAL FAT	CHOL	SAT FAT	POLY FAT	MONO FAT	TRANS FAT	FIBER	SUGAR
Turkey Stew	½ can	140	3	20	1	–	–	–	2	3
TAKE-OUT										
boneless breast w/ cranberry apple stuffing	1 serv (5 oz)	260	9	80	2	–	–	–	1	2
turkey a la king	1 cup (8.5 oz)	465	34	190	12	7	13	–	1	4
turkey creole w/o rice	1 cup	189	4	69	1	1	2	–	2	5

FOOD	PORTION	CALS	TOTAL FAT	CHOL	SAT FAT	POLY FAT	MONO FAT	TRANS FAT	FIBER	SUGAR
turkey croquette	1 (2 oz)	158	9	28	2	3	4	–	tr	2
turkey divan	1 cup	321	14	135	6	2	5	–	3	2
turkey fricassee	1 cup	322	18	85	5	4	8	–	tr	tr
turkey meatloaf	1 lg slice (5 oz)	243	9	122	3	2	3	–	1	3
turkey salad	1 cup	417	32	100	6	15	9	–	1	1
turkey tetrazzini	1 cup	369	18	49	6	3	6	–	2	2

TURKEY SUBSTITUTES
Quorn
Turk'y Burger	1 (2.5 oz)	90	4	5	1	1	3	0	2	0

TURMERIC
ground	1 tsp	8	tr	0	tr	tr	tr	0	tr	tr

TURNIPS
canned greens	½ cup	17	tr	0	tr	tr	tr	–	–	–
cooked mashed	½ cup (4.2 oz)	47	tr	0	tr	tr	tr	–	–	–
cubed cooked	½ cup (3 oz)	33	tr	0	tr	tr	tr	–	–	–
fresh greens chopped cooked	½ cup	15	tr	0	tr	tr	tr	–	2	–
frzn greens cooked	½ cup	24	tr	0	tr	tr	tr	–	2	–
greens raw chopped	½ cup	7	tr	0	tr	tr	tr	–	1	–
raw cubed	½ cup (2.4 oz)	25	tr	0	tr	tr	tr	–	–	–

VANILLA
vanilla extract	1 tsp (4.2 g)	12	0	0	0	0	0	0	0	1
vanilla extract	1 tbsp (0.5 oz)	37	tr	0	tr	tr	tr	0	0	2
vanilla extract alcohol free	1 tsp (4.2 g)	2	0	0	0	0	0	0	0	1

Nielsen-Massey
Madagascar Bourbon Extract	1 tsp	11	tr	tr	tr	tr	tr	0	tr	tr

VEAL (see also VEAL DISHES)
australian rib roast lean & fat not prep	3.5 oz	201	13	60	6	1	5	1	0	0
breast braised	3 oz	226	14	96	6	1	7	0	0	0
chop breaded fried	1 med (6.5 oz)	290	12	142	4	2	4	0	tr	0
chop cooked	1 med (6.5 oz)	230	13	109	6	1	5	0	0	0
cubed braised	3 oz	160	4	123	1	tr	1	0	0	0
cutlet cooked	3 oz	141	4	83	1	tr	1	0	0	0
ground broiled	3 oz	146	6	88	3	tr	2	0	0	0
leg roasted	3 oz	136	4	88	2	tr	1	0	0	0

FOOD	PORTION	CALS	TOTAL FAT	CHOL	SAT FAT	POLY FAT	MONO FAT	TRANS FAT	FIBER	SUGAR
loin roasted	3 oz	184	10	88	4	1	4	0	0	0
patty breaded fried	1 (2.8 oz)	211	13	80	4	1	6	0	tr	1
shank braised	3 oz	162	5	105	2	tr	2	0	0	0

VEAL DISHES
TAKE-OUT

FOOD	PORTION	CALS	TOTAL FAT	CHOL	SAT FAT	POLY FAT	MONO FAT	TRANS FAT	FIBER	SUGAR
cordon bleu	1 serv (8 oz)	490	35	172	19	2	12	0	1	2
marengo	1 serv (8.8 oz)	274	9	118	3	3	3	0	1	3
marsala	1 slice + sauce (3.4 oz)	268	19	69	9	1	8	0	tr	2
paprikash	1 serv (8.6 oz)	280	12	138	5	2	4	0	1	1
parmigiana	1 serv (6.4 oz)	362	21	146	8	4	7	0	2	3
picatta	1 piece + sauce (3.5 oz)	154	9	72	5	1	3	0	tr	tr
scallopini	1 slice + sauce (3.4 oz)	238	17	64	5	3	7	0	tr	1
stew	1 serv (8.8 oz)	192	6	50	3	1	2	0	3	4

VEGETABLE JUICE (see also individual vegetable names, FRUIT DRINKS)

FOOD	PORTION	CALS	TOTAL FAT	CHOL	SAT FAT	POLY FAT	MONO FAT	TRANS FAT	FIBER	SUGAR
low sodium tomato & vegetable juice	1 cup	53	tr	0	tr	tr	tr	0	2	9
vegetable juice cocktail	8 oz	46	tr	0	tr	tr	tr	0	2	8
V8										
100% Juice Low Sodium	8 oz	50	0	0	0	0	0	0	2	7
Original Hint Of Black Pepper	8 oz	50	0	0	0	0	0	0	2	7
Vegetable Juice Original	8 oz	50	0	0	0	0	0	0	2	8

VEGETABLES MIXED
CANNED

FOOD	PORTION	CALS	TOTAL FAT	CHOL	SAT FAT	POLY FAT	MONO FAT	TRANS FAT	FIBER	SUGAR
mixed vegetables	½ cup	39	tr	0	tr	tr	tr	–	–	–
peas & carrots	½ cup (4.5 oz)	48	tr	0	tr	tr	tr	0	3	–
peas & onions	½ cup (2.1 oz)	31	tr	0	tr	tr	tr	0	1	–
succotash	½ cup	102	1	0	tr	tr	tr	–	–	–
Butter Kernel										
Mixed	½ cup (4.4 oz)	45	0	0	0	0	0	0	2	3
Del Monte										
Mixed Vegetables w/ Potatoes	½ cup (4.3 oz)	45	0	0	0	0	0	0	2	3
Peas And Carrots	½ cup (4.5 oz)	60	0	0	0	0	0	0	4	4
Victoria										
Fancy Giardiniera	¼ cup (1 oz)	5	0	0	0	0	0	0	0	0
Italian Antipasto	¼ jar (2 oz)	130	12	0	0	–	–	0	1	0

FOOD	PORTION	CALS	TOTAL FAT	CHOL	SAT FAT	POLY FAT	MONO FAT	TRANS FAT	FIBER	SUGAR
DRIED										
Crunchies										
Freeze Dried Power Veggies Buttered	½ cup (0.7 oz)	110	3	0	0	–	–	0	4	6
Freeze Dried Power Veggies Herb Spiced	½ cup (0.7 oz)	110	3	0	0	–	–	0	5	6
Freeze Dried Roasted Veggies	⅝ cup (1 oz)	100	1	0	0	–	–	0	2	10
Freeze Dried Roasted Veggies BBQ	½ cup (0.8 oz)	100	2	0	0	–	–	0	4	7
FRESH										
Dole										
Stir Fry Medley	1 cup (3 oz)	30	0	0	0	0	0	0	2	3
Vegetable Medley	3 oz	30	0	0	0	0	0	0	2	2
Eat Smart										
Broccoli & Carrots	1 serv (3 oz)	30	0	0	0	0	0	0	2	2
Harvest Blend	1 serv (3 oz)	30	0	0	0	0	0	0	2	1
Vegetable Medley	1 serv (3 oz)	25	0	0	0	0	0	0	2	3
Mann's										
Broccoli & Carrots	1 serv (3 oz)	25	0	0	0	0	0	0	2	3
Broccoli & Cauliflower	1 serv (3 oz)	25	0	0	0	0	0	0	2	2
California Stir Fry	1 serv (3 oz)	30	0	0	0	0	0	0	2	3
Low Mein Stir Fry	1 serv (3 oz)	80	1	0	0	–	–	0	2	5
Medley	1 serv (3 oz)	25	0	0	0	0	0	0	2	3
Ready Pac										
Carrots & Celery w/ Ranch Dressing	1 pkg (7 oz)	250	21	15	2	–	–	0	3	8
Ready Fixin's Chop Suey	1½ cups (3 oz)	15	0	0	0	0	0	0	1	1
FROZEN										
mixed vegetables cooked	½ cup	54	tr	0	tr	tr	tr	–	2	–
peas & carrots cooked	½ cup (2.8 oz)	38	tr	0	tr	tr	tr	0	3	3
peas & carrots creamed	½ cup (4.3 oz)	111	6	4	2	2	2	–	2	5
succotash cooked	½ cup	79	1	0	tr	tr	tr	–	–	–
Lisa's Organics										
California In Balsamic Glaze	½ pkg (4 oz)	35	0	0	0	0	0	0	2	4
Southwest In Ranchero Sauce	½ pkg (4 oz)	60	1	0	0	–	–	0	2	4
Tandoor Chef										
Vegetable Korma	1 pkg (9.9 oz)	330	11	0	3	–	–	0	8	4

FOOD	PORTION	CALS	TOTAL FAT	CHOL	SAT FAT	POLY FAT	MONO FAT	TRANS FAT	FIBER	SUGAR
TAKE-OUT										
buddha's delight	1 serv (16 oz)	174	5	35	1	–	–	–	3	8
fukujinzuke japanese pickled vegetables	1 tbsp (6 g)	8	0	0	0	0	0	0	0	–
pakoras	4 (1.7 oz)	57	2	0	tr	1	1	–	2	1
ratatouille	1 serv (3.5 oz)	96	7	0	1	1	4	–	4	7
samosa	1 (2.4 oz)	206	11	12	5	1	5	tr	2	1
stir fry mixed vegetables	1 serv (4 oz)	66	5	0	1	2	1	–	2	2
succotash	½ cup	111	1	0	tr	tr	tr	–	–	–
VENISON (see also JERKY)										
cubed stewed	1 cup (5 oz)	266	6	157	3	tr	1	–	0	0
hamburger grilled	1 (3.3 oz)	174	8	91	4	tr	2	–	0	0
loin steak lean only broiled	1 (2 oz)	81	1	43	tr	tr	tr	–	0	0
shoulder lean only braised	3 oz	162	3	96	2	tr	1	–	0	0
tenderloin roasted	3 oz	127	2	75	1	tr	tr	–	0	0
top round lean only broiled	3 oz	129	2	72	1	tr	tr	–	0	0
TAKE-OUT										
meatloaf	1 lg slice (5 oz)	238	10	125	4	1	2	–	1	2
stew w/ potatoes & vegetables	1 cup (8.8 oz)	179	2	48	1	tr	tr	–	4	5
VINEGAR										
balsamic	1 tbsp	14	0	0	0	0	0	0	–	2
cider	1 tbsp	3	0	0	0	0	0	0	0	tr
red wine	1 tbsp	3	0	0	0	0	0	0	0	0
white	1 tbsp	3	0	0	0	0	0	0	0	tr
Gedney										
Apple Cider	1 tbsp (0.5 oz)	3	0	0	0	0	0	0	0	0
Distilled White	1 tbsp (0.5 oz)	3	0	0	0	0	0	0	0	0
Heinz										
Apple Cider	1 tbsp (0.5 oz)	0	0	0	0	0	0	0	0	0
Malt	1 tbsp (0.5 oz)	0	0	0	0	0	0	0	0	0
Red Wine	1 tbsp (1 oz)	0	0	0	0	0	0	0	0	0
Tarragon	1 tbsp (0.5 oz)	0	0	0	0	0	0	0	0	0
White	1 tbsp (0.5 oz)	0	0	0	0	0	0	0	0	0
Spectrum										
Apple Cider Organic	1 tbsp (0.5 oz)	7	0	0	0	0	0	0	0	0
Brown Rice Organic	1 tbsp (0.5 oz)	10	0	0	0	0	0	0	0	0
Golden Balsamic Organic	1 tbsp (0.5 oz)	6	0	0	0	0	0	0	0	2
Red Wine Organic	1 tbsp (0.5 oz)	0	0	0	0	0	0	0	0	0

FOOD	PORTION	CALS	TOTAL FAT	CHOL	SAT FAT	POLY FAT	MONO FAT	TRANS FAT	FIBER	SUGAR
Victoria										
Balsamic	1 tbsp (0.5 oz)	5	0	0	0	0	0	0	0	0
WAFFLES										
FROZEN										
Aunt Jemima										
Blueberry	2 (2.5 oz)	170	5	<5	1	–	–	0	tr	5
Buttermilk	2 (2.5 oz)	190	5	<5	1	–	–	–	tr	3
Homestyle	2 (2.5 oz)	160	5	<5	1	–	–	–	tr	2
Low Fat	2 (2.5 oz)	160	3	<5	0	–	–	0	tr	2
Eggo										
Blueberry	2 (2.5 oz)	190	6	10	2	–	–	0	tr	6
Cinnamon Toast	3 sets (3.3 oz)	300	11	10	3	–	–	0	1	17
FiberPlus Calcium Buttermilk	2 (2.5 oz)	160	6	15	2	2	2	0	9	3
Homestyle Low Fat	2 (2.5 oz)	160	3	15	1	–	–	0	tr	4
Nutri-Grain Honey Oat	2 (2.5 oz)	190	6	0	2	–	–	0	3	7
Nutri-Grain Whole Wheat	2 (2.5 oz)	170	6	0	2	3	2	0	3	3
Original	2 (2.5 oz)	210	8	20	2	–	–	0	tr	4
Thick & Fluffy Original	1 (2 oz)	160	7	0	2	4	2	0	tr	3
Frozen Guru										
Flour-Free Coconut Chia	2 (2.3 oz)	125	4	0	2	–	–	0	6	2
Flour-Free Sweet Banana	2 (2.3 oz)	115	3	0	1	–	–	0	5	4
Nature's Path										
Buckwheat Wild Blueberry Organic	2 (2.5 oz)	190	7	0	1	4	2	0	1	5
Hemp Plus Organic	2 (2.5 oz)	200	8	0	1	5	2	0	5	5
Maple Cinn Organic	2 (2.5 oz)	180	6	0	1	3	1	0	4	6
Pomegran Plus Organic	2 (2.5 oz)	160	4	0	1	–	–	0	4	5
Smucker's										
Snack'n Waffles Blueberry	1 (2 oz)	230	8	20	2	–	–	0	2	16
Snack'n Waffles Maple	1 (2 oz)	220	8	25	3	–	–	0	2	15
Van's										
Belgian	2 (2.7 oz)	210	9	0	1	–	–	0	1	5
Lite	2 (2.7 oz)	140	2	0	0	–	–	0	2	4
Minis	8 (1.9 oz)	140	4	0	0	–	–	0	tr	4
Organic w/ Vitamin Boost	2 (2.7 oz)	200	8	0	1	–	–	0	6	3
Wheat Gluten Free	2 (3 oz)	230	7	0	1	–	–	0	2	4
Whole Grain	2 (2.8 oz)	190	7	0	1	–	–	0	6	5
MIX										
plain as prep 7 in diam	1 (2.6 oz)	218	11	52	2	5	3	0	–	–

FOOD	PORTION	CALS	TOTAL FAT	CHOL	SAT FAT	POLY FAT	MONO FAT	TRANS FAT	FIBER	SUGAR
READY-TO-EAT										
Mrs. Huber										
Fresh Egg Waffles	1 (1 oz)	100	5	10	0	–	–	0	0	7
TAKE-OUT										
belgian	1 (4.7 oz)	412	13	19	3	2	7	0	3	6
blueberry 9 in sq	1 (7 oz)	556	16	24	3	3	9	0	5	12
round 10 in diam	1 (6.8 oz)	598	18	27	4	4	10	0	5	9
square 9 in	1 (7 oz)	620	19	28	4	4	10	0	5	9
whole wheat 9 in sq	1 (7 oz)	534	22	188	6	6	9	0	5	15
WALNUTS										
black chopped	¼ cup	193	18	0	1	11	5	–	2	tr
english chopped	¼ cup	191	19	0	2	14	3	0	2	1
english ground	¼ cup	131	13	0	1	9	2	0	1	1
english halves	14 (1 oz)	185	18	0	2	13	3	–	2	1
english in shell	7 (1 oz)	183	18	0	2	13	3	0	2	1
honey roasted	¼ cup	172	16	0	2	11	2	0	2	4
Planters										
Halves	1 oz	190	18	0	2	–	3	0	2	1
Recipe Ready Pieces	½ pkg (1 oz)	210	19	0	2	–	–	–	2	1
Sanguinetti Family Farms										
Red Walnuts Halves	14 (1 oz)	190	18	0	2	13	3	0	2	–
Sante										
Candied	¼ cup (1 oz)	200	17	0	2	11	4	0	2	8
WASABI (see HORSERADISH)										
• WATER										
ice cubes	3	0	0	0	0	0	0	0	0	0
tap water	8 oz	0	0	0	0	0	0	0	0	0
Aquafina										
Pure Water	8 oz	0	0	0	0	0	0	0	0	0
Arizona										
Rescue Relax	8 oz	25	0	0	0	0	0	0	–	6
Vapor	8 oz	0	0	0	0	0	0	0	0	0
EX										
Aqua Vitamins Raspberry	1 bottle (16.9 oz)	110	0	0	0	0	0	0	–	27
Mash										
Water Drink Grapefruit Citrus Zing	8 oz	40	0	0	0	0	0	0	–	10

FOOD	PORTION	CALS	TOTAL FAT	CHOL	SAT FAT	POLY FAT	MONO FAT	TRANS FAT	FIBER	SUGAR
Water Drink Ripe Mango Blood Orange	8 oz	40	0	0	0	0	0	0	–	10
Pellegrino										
Mineral Water	8 oz	0	0	0	0	0	0	0	0	0
SoBe										
Lifewater Blood Orange Mango	1 bottle (20 oz)	0	0	0	0	0	0	0	–	0
Lifewater w/ Coconut Water	1 bottle (20 oz)	80	0	0	0	0	0	0	5	20
Sparkling Ice										
All Flavors	1 bottle (16 oz)	0	0	0	0	0	0	0	0	0
Victoria's Kitchen										
Almond Water	8 oz	55	0	0	0	0	0	0	0	15
WATER CHESTNUTS										
chinese sliced canned	½ cup	35	tr	0	–	–	–	–	–	–
fresh sliced	½ cup	66	tr	0	–	–	–	–	–	–
WATERCRESS										
cooked w/o fat	1 cup	15	tr	0	tr	tr	tr	0	1	tr
raw chopped	1 cup	4	tr	0	tr	tr	tr	0	tr	tr
WATERMELON										
cut up	1 cup	46	tr	0	tr	tr	tr	0	1	10
seeds dried	¼ cup	150	13	0	3	8	2	0	–	–
wedge	1 lg (20 oz)	172	1	0	tr	tr	tr	0	2	35
wedge	1 med (10 oz)	86	tr	0	tr	tr	tr	0	1	18
wedge	1 sm (2.5 oz)	21	tr	0	tr	tr	tr	0	tr	4
whole melon	1 (9 lb)	1227	6	0	1	2	2	0	16	254
Jake & Amos										
Pickled Sweet Rind	2 tbsp (1 oz)	70	0	0	0	0	0	0	0	12
WATERMELON JUICE										
juice	8 oz	71	tr	0	tr	tr	tr	0	1	15
Arizona										
Fruit Juice Cocktail	8 oz	100	0	0	0	0	0	0	0	24
Izze										
Esque Sparkling Watermelon	1 bottle (12 oz)	50	0	0	0	0	0	0	–	14
Minute Maid										
Flavored Drink	8 oz	100	0	0	0	0	0	0	–	26
WHALE										
beluga dried	1 oz	93	2	35	tr	tr	1	–	0	0
beluga raw	3.5 oz	111	1	80	tr	tr	tr	–	0	0

FOOD	PORTION	CALS	TOTAL FAT	CHOL	SAT FAT	POLY FAT	MONO FAT	TRANS FAT	FIBER	SUGAR
WHEAT										
sprouted	1 cup (3.8 oz)	214	1	0	tr	tr	tr	–	1	–
WHEAT GERM										
plain	¼ cup	108	3	0	1	2	tr	0	4	2
Mother's										
Wheat Germ	2 tbsp (0.5 oz)	50	1	0	0	1	0	0	2	1
WHEY										
acid dry	1 tbsp	10	tr	0	tr	tr	tr	0	0	2
sweet dry	1 tbsp	26	tr	0	tr	tr	tr	0	0	6
sweet fluid	½ cup	33	tr	2	tr	tr	tr	0	0	6
Bodylogix										
Natural Whey	1 scoop (1 oz)	120	1	30	1	–	–	0	0	1
Premier										
100% Whey Isolate	2 scoops (1.5 oz)	160	2	5	1	–	–	0	2	1
WHIPPED TOPPINGS										
dairy fat free pressurized	¼ cup (0.6 oz)	24	1	0	tr	tr	tr	–	tr	3
nondairy fat free frzn	¼ cup (0.7 oz)	28	1	3	1	tr	tr	–	tr	3
nondairy frzn	¼ cup (0.7 oz)	60	5	0	4	tr	tr	–	0	4
nondairy lowfat frzn	¼ cup (0.7 oz)	42	2	0	2	tr	tr	–	0	4
nondairy pressurized	¼ cup (0.6 oz)	46	4	0	3	tr	tr	–	0	3
Reddiwip										
Chocolate	2 tbsp (5 g)	15	1	<5	1	–	–	0	0	tr
Fat Free	2 tbsp (5 g)	5	0	0	0	0	0	0	0	tr
Soyatoo										
Rice Whip	2 tbsp (6 g)	10	1	0	1	–	–	0	0	1
Soy Whip	2 tbsp (6 g)	10	1	0	1	–	–	0	0	1
Truwhip										
Whipped Topping	2 tbsp (0.4 oz)	30	2	0	2	–	–	0	0	2
WHITE BEANS										
canned	1 cup (9.2 oz)	299	1	0	tr	tr	tr	–	13	1
dried small cooked w/o salt	1 cup (6.3 oz)	254	1	0	tr	tr	tr	–	19	–
Bush's										
White Beans	½ cup (4.6 oz)	80	0	0	0	0	0	0	7	0
WHITEFISH										
baked	3 oz	146	6	65	1	2	2	–	0	0
fillet grilled no added fat	1 (5.4 oz)	265	12	119	2	4	4	–	0	0
smoked boneless	1 oz	31	tr	9	tr	tr	tr	–	0	0

FOOD	PORTION	CALS	TOTAL FAT	CHOL	SAT FAT	POLY FAT	MONO FAT	TRANS FAT	FIBER	SUGAR
WHITING										
broiled w/o fat	3 oz	99	1	71	tr	tr	tr	–	0	0
fillet broiled w/o fat	1 (2.5 oz)	84	1	60	tr	tr	tr	–	0	0
fillet steamed w/o fat	1 (2.6 oz)	84	1	63	tr	tr	tr	–	0	0
TAKE-OUT										
fillet battered & fried	1 (3.1 oz)	157	7	66	1	2	3	–	tr	tr
fillet breaded & fried	1 (3.1 oz)	191	10	75	2	3	4	–	tr	1
WILD RICE										
cooked	1 cup (5.8 oz)	166	1	0	tr	tr	tr	0	3	1
Gourmet House										
Cracked as prep	1 cup	170	0	0	0	0	0	0	2	0
Quick Cooking not prep	½ cup	170	0	0	0	0	0	0	2	0
Thai Jasmine as prep	¾ cup	160	0	0	0	0	0	0	0	0
WINE										
chianti	1 serv (5 oz)	125	0	0	0	0	0	0	0	1
chinese cooking	1 bottle (15 oz)	559	0	0	0	0	0	0	0	0
cooking	¼ cup (2 oz)	29	0	0	0	0	0	0	0	1
haiku	1 serv	93	0	0	0	0	0	0	0	–
japanese plum	3 oz	139	tr	0	–	–	–	–	0	–
japanese sake	2 oz	78	0	0	0	0	0	0	0	0
kir	1 serv	78	0	0	0	0	0	0	0	–
nonalcoholic	1 serv (5 oz)	9	0	0	0	0	0	0	0	2
port	1 serv (3.5 oz)	165	0	0	0	0	0	0	0	8
red barbera	1 serv (5 oz)	125	0	0	0	0	0	0	–	–
red burgundy	1 serv (5 oz)	127	0	0	0	0	0	0	–	–
red cabernet franc	1 serv (5 oz)	122	0	0	0	0	0	0	–	–
red claret	1 serv (5 oz)	122	0	0	0	0	0	0	–	–
red gamay	1 serv (5 oz)	115	0	0	0	0	0	0	–	–
red lemberger	1 serv (5 oz)	118	0	0	0	0	0	0	–	–
red mourvedre	1 serv (5 oz)	129	0	0	0	0	0	0	–	–
red pinot noir	1 serv (5 oz)	121	0	0	0	0	0	0	–	–
red sangiovese	1 serv (5 oz)	126	0	0	0	0	0	0	–	–
red sauvignon cabernet	1 serv (5 oz)	122	0	0	0	0	0	0	–	–
red syrah	1 serv (5 oz)	122	0	0	0	0	0	0	–	–
red zinfandel	1 serv (5 oz)	129	0	0	0	0	0	0	–	–
sake screwdriver	1 serv	175	tr	0	tr	–	–	–	tr	–
sangria	1 serv	88	tr	0	0	–	–	–	tr	–
sangria blanco	1 serv	155	tr	0	tr	–	–	–	3	–

FOOD	PORTION	CALS	TOTAL FAT	CHOL	SAT FAT	POLY FAT	MONO FAT	TRANS FAT	FIBER	SUGAR
sherry	2 oz	84	0	0	0	0	0	0	–	–
vermouth dry	3.5 oz	105	0	0	0	0	0	0	–	–
vermouth sweet	3.5 oz	167	0	0	0	0	0	0	–	–
wassail wine	1 serv	142	tr	0	tr	–	–	–	2	–
white	1 serv (5 oz)	121	0	0	0	0	0	0	0	1
white chardonnay	1 serv (5 oz)	123	0	0	0	0	0	0	0	1
white chenin blanc	1 serv (5 oz)	118	0	0	0	0	0	0	–	–
white fume blanc	1 serv (5 oz)	121	0	0	0	0	0	0	–	–
white gewurztaminer	1 serv (5 oz)	119	0	0	0	0	0	0	–	–
white muller thurgau	1 serv (5 oz)	112	0	0	0	0	0	0	–	–
white muscat	1 serv (5 oz)	123	0	0	0	0	0	0	–	–
white pinot blanc	1 serv (5 oz)	119	0	0	0	0	0	0	–	–
white pinot grigio	1 serv (5 oz)	122	0	0	0	0	0	0	–	–
white riesling	1 serv (5 oz)	128	0	0	0	0	0	0	–	–
white sauvignon blanc	1 serv (5 oz)	119	0	0	0	0	0	0	–	–
white semillon	1 serv (5 oz)	121	0	0	0	0	0	0	–	–
wine cooler	1 (7 oz)	116	tr	0	tr	tr	tr	0	0	11
wine spritzer	1 serv (7 oz)	73	0	0	0	0	0	0	0	1
Kedem										
Cooking Red	2 tbsp (1 oz)	30	0	0	0	0	0	0	–	–
Cooking Sherry	2 tbsp (1 oz)	40	0	0	0	0	0	0	–	1
Cooking Wine Marsala	2 tbsp (1 oz)	40	0	0	0	0	0	0	–	1

WINGED BEANS

FOOD	PORTION	CALS	TOTAL FAT	CHOL	SAT FAT	POLY FAT	MONO FAT	TRANS FAT	FIBER	SUGAR
dried cooked w/o salt	1 cup	253	10	0	1	3	4	0	3	–

WRAPS (see BREAD, SANDWICHES)

YAM (see also SWEET POTATO)
FRESH

FOOD	PORTION	CALS	TOTAL FAT	CHOL	SAT FAT	POLY FAT	MONO FAT	TRANS FAT	FIBER	SUGAR
mountain yam hawaii cooked w/o salt	1 cup	119	tr	0	tr	tr	tr	0	–	–
yam cooked w/o salt	1 cup	158	tr	0	tr	tr	tr	0	5	1

YARDLONG BEANS

FOOD	PORTION	CALS	TOTAL FAT	CHOL	SAT FAT	POLY FAT	MONO FAT	TRANS FAT	FIBER	SUGAR
sliced cooked w/o salt	1 cup	49	tr	0	tr	tr	tr	0	–	–

YAUTIA (see MALANGA)

YEAST

FOOD	PORTION	CALS	TOTAL FAT	CHOL	SAT FAT	POLY FAT	MONO FAT	TRANS FAT	FIBER	SUGAR
baker's compressed	1 cake (0.6 oz)	18	tr	0	tr	tr	tr	0	1	0
baker's dry	1 tbsp	35	1	0	tr	tr	tr	0	3	0

FOOD	PORTION	CALS	TOTAL FAT	CHOL	SAT FAT	POLY FAT	MONO FAT	TRANS FAT	FIBER	SUGAR
baker's dry	1 pkg (7 g)	21	tr	0	tr	tr	tr	0	2	0
brewer's dry	1 tbsp	35	1	0	tr	tr	tr	0	3	0

YELLOW BEANS

fresh cooked w/o salt	1 cup	44	tr	0	tr	tr	tr	0	4	2
fresh raw	1 cup	34	tr	0	tr	tr	tr	0	4	–

Del Monte

Cut Golden Wax Beans	½ cup (4.2 oz)	20	0	0	0	0	0	0	2	1

YELLOWTAIL

baked	4 oz	199	7	75	–	–	–	0	0	0

YOGURT (see also YOGURT DRINKS, YOGURT FROZEN)

plain lowfat	8 oz	143	4	14	2	tr	1	0	0	16
plain nonfat	8 oz	127	tr	5	tr	tr	tr	0	0	17
plain whole milk	8 oz	138	7	30	5	tr	2	0	0	11
tofu yogurt	1 cup	246	5	0	1	3	1	–	1	3

Activia

Breakfast Blends Apple Cinnamon	1 pkg (6 oz)	190	3	20	2	–	–	0	–	25
Breakfast Blends Banana Bread	1 pkg (6 oz)	190	3	20	2	–	–	0	–	26
Breakfast Blends Maple Brown Sugar	1 pkg (6 oz)	190	3	20	2	–	–	0	–	26
Breakfast Blends Vanilla	1 pkg (6 oz)	190	3	20	2	–	–	0	–	26
Harvest Picks Strawberry	1 pkg (4 oz)	110	4	10	3	–	–	0	–	15
Strawberry	1 pkg (4 oz)	120	2	5	1	–	–	0	0	19
Strawberry Light	1 pkg (4 oz)	70	0	<5	0	0	0	0	2	8

Alpina

Restart All Fruit Flavors	1 pkg (6 oz)	180	3	10	2	–	–	0	1	19

Chobani

0% Blueberry	1 pkg (6 oz)	140	0	0	0	0	0	0	tr	20
0% Honey	1 pkg (6 oz)	150	0	0	0	0	0	0	0	20
0% Peach	1 pkg (6 oz)	140	0	0	0	0	0	0	tr	19
0% Pear	1 pkg (6 oz)	140	0	0	0	0	0	0	tr	19
0% Plain	1 pkg (6 oz)	100	0	0	0	0	0	0	0	7
0% Pomegranate	1 pkg (6 oz)	140	0	0	0	0	0	0	0	19
0% Raspberry	1 pkg (6 oz)	140	0	0	0	0	0	0	1	19
0% Strawberry	1 pkg (6 oz)	140	0	0	0	0	0	0	tr	19
0% Vanilla	1 pkg (6 oz)	120	0	0	0	0	0	0	0	13
2% Mango	1 pkg (6 oz)	160	3	5	2	–	–	0	0	20

FOOD	PORTION	CALS	TOTAL FAT	CHOL	SAT FAT	POLY FAT	MONO FAT	TRANS FAT	FIBER	SUG
2% Plain	1 pkg (6 oz)	130	4	10	2	–	–	0	0	7
Bite Coffee w/ Dark Chocolate Chips	1 pkg (3.5 oz)	100	1	5	1	–	–	0	0	12
Bite Fig w/ Orange Zest	1 pkg (3.5 oz)	100	2	<5	1	–	–	0	tr	12
Champions Tube All Flavors	1 (2.25 oz)	70	1	0	1	–	–	0	0	8
Flip Almond Coco Loco	1 pkg (5.3 oz)	230	10	<10	5	–	–	0	2	22
Flip Key Line Crumble	1 pkg (5.3 oz)	170	3	0	1	–	–	0	0	19
Flip Vanilla Golden Crunch	1 pkg (5.3 oz)	150	2	0	0	–	–	0	0	14
Ehrmann										
Bavarian Lowfat Cherry	1 pkg	140	2	5	1	–	–	0	0	24
Bavarian Lowfat Peach	1 pkg	140	2	5	1	–	–	0	0	24
Bavarian Lowfat Strawberry	1 pkg	140	2	5	1	–	–	0	0	24
Emmi										
Apricot Low-fat	1 pkg (6 oz)	170	3	15	2	–	–	0	0	25
Green Apple Low-fat	1 pkg (6 oz)	170	3	15	2	–	–	0	0	26
Pink Grapefruit Low-fat	1 pkg (6 oz)	170	3	15	2	–	–	0	0	26
Plain Low-fat	1 pkg (6 oz)	170	3	15	2	–	–	0	0	10
Fage										
Total Cherry	1 pkg (5.3 oz)	170	6	15	5	–	–	0	0	16
Total Peach	1 pkg (5.3 oz)	170	6	15	5	–	–	0	0	16
Total Plain	1 pkg (5.3 oz)	190	10	25	7	–	–	0	0	8
Total Strawberry	1 pkg (5.3 oz)	170	6	15	5	–	–	0	0	16
Total 0% Cherry	1 pkg (5.3 oz)	130	0	0	0	0	0	0	0	16
Total 0% Cherry Pomegranate	1 pkg (5.3 oz)	130	0	0	0	0	0	0	0	16
Total 0% Honey	1 pkg (5.3 oz)	120	0	0	0	0	0	0	0	16
Total 0% Mango Guanabana	1 pkg (5.3 oz)	120	0	0	0	0	0	0	0	17
Total 0% Peach	1 pkg (5.3 oz)	120	0	0	0	0	0	0	0	16
Total 0% Plain	1 pkg (5.3 oz)	100	0	0	0	0	0	0	0	7
Total 2% Cherry	1 pkg (5.3 oz)	140	3	5	2	–	–	0	0	16
Total 2% Plain	1 pkg (5.3 oz)	150	4	10	3	–	–	0	0	8
Total 2% Strawberry	1 pkg (5.3 oz)	140	3	5	2	–	–	0	0	16
Green Valley										
Organic Lactose Free Blueberry	1 pkg (6 oz)	140	2	10	1	–	–	0	0	16
Organic Lactose Free Honey	1 pkg (6 oz)	140	2	10	2	–	–	0	0	14
Organic Lactose Free Plain	1 pkg (6 oz)	100	3	10	2	–	–	0	0	4
Organic Lactose Free Vanilla	1 pkg (6 oz)	120	3	10	2	–	–	0	0	9
Karoun										
Plain Lowfat	1 cup (8 oz)	180	5	25	3	–	–	0	0	15
Plain Whole Milk	1 cup (8 oz)	210	12	50	7	–	–	0	0	14

FOOD	PORTION	CALS	TOTAL FAT	CHOL	SAT FAT	POLY FAT	MONO FAT	TRANS FAT	FIBER	SUGAR
Muller										
Corner Choco Balls	1 pkg (5.3 oz)	210	5	15	4	–	–	0	0	26
Corner Crispy Crunch	1 pkg (5.3 oz)	200	4	15	2	–	–	0	0	24
Corner Strawberry	1 pkg (5.3 oz)	140	2	10	1	–	–	0	0	23
FruitUp Luscious Lemon	1 pkg (5.3 oz)	150	2	10	1	–	–	0	0	24
FruitUp Peach Passion Fruit	1 pkg (5.3 oz)	140	2	10	1	–	–	0	0	23
FruitUp Radiant Raspberry	1 pkg (5.3 oz)	150	2	10	1	–	–	0	0	23
Greek Corner Caramelized Almonds	1 pkg (5.3 oz)	220	9	15	2	–	–	0	1	18
Greek Corner Honeyed Apricots	1 pkg (5.3 oz)	130	2	15	1	–	–	0	0	17
Olympus										
Greek Strained Strawberry 1% Lowfat	1 pkg (6 oz)	155	15	3	1	–	–	0	tr	22
Stonyfield Farm										
0% Fat Chocolate Underground	1 pkg (6 oz)	150	0	<5	0	0	0	0	1	29
0% Fat Fruit On The Bottom Blueberry	1 pkg (6 oz)	120	0	0	0	0	0	0	0	20
0% Fat Fruit On The Bottom Pomegranate Raspberry	1 pkg (6 oz)	120	0	0	0	0	0	0	0	22
0% Fat Fruit On The Bottom Strawberry	1 pkg (6 oz)	110	0	0	0	0	0	0	0	21
0% Fat Smooth & Creamy Black Cherry	1 pkg (6 oz)	100	0	<5	0	0	0	0	0	17
0% Fat Smooth & Creamy French Vanilla	1 pkg (6 oz)	100	0	<5	0	0	0	0	0	17
0% Fat Smooth & Creamy Key Lime	1 pkg (6 oz)	100	0	<5	0	0	0	0	0	16
0% Fat Smooth & Creamy Lemon	1 pkg (6 oz)	100	0	<5	0	0	0	0	0	17
0% Fat Smooth & Creamy Peach	1 pkg (6 oz)	100	0	<5	0	0	0	0	0	17
0% Fat Smooth & Creamy Plain	1 pkg (6 oz)	80	0	0	0	0	0	0	0	11
0% Fat Smooth & Creamy Pomegranate Berry	1 pkg (6 oz)	100	0	<5	0	0	0	0	0	16
0% Fat Smooth & Creamy Strawberry	1 pkg (6 oz)	100	0	<5	0	0	0	0	0	17

FOOD	PORTION	CALS	TOTAL FAT	CHOL	SAT FAT	POLY FAT	MONO FAT	TRANS FAT	FIBER	SUG
Straus										
Organic Blueberry Pomegranate	1 cup (8 oz)	220	6	30	4	–	–	0	0	25
Organic Cinnamon Nonfat	1 cup (8 oz)	190	0	10	0	0	0	0	1	26
Organic Maple Whole Milk	1 cup (8 oz)	210	6	35	4	–	–	0	0	23
Organic Plain Lowfat	1 cup (8 oz)	150	2	15	1	–	–	0	0	10
Organic Plain Nonfat	1 cup (8 oz)	120	0	10	0	0	0	0	1	10
Organic Vanilla Nonfat	1 cup (8 oz)	190	0	10	0	0	0	0	0	25
WholeSoy & Co.										
Apricot Mango	1 pkg (6 oz)	160	4	0	0	–	–	0	2	19
Cherry	1 pkg (6 oz)	170	4	0	0	–	–	0	2	19
Lemon	1 pkg (6 oz)	160	4	0	0	–	–	0	2	18
Plain	1 pkg (6 oz)	150	5	0	1	–	–	0	1	13
Strawberry	1 pkg (6 oz)	160	4	0	0	–	–	0	2	21
Vanilla	1 pkg (6 oz)	160	4	0	1	–	–	0	1	18
Yoplait										
GoGurt Strawberry Ripetide & Sponge Berry	1 pkg (2.2 oz)	70	1	<5	0	–	–	0	0	10
Simplait Blackberry	1 pkg (6 oz)	200	7	30	5	–	–	0	–	24
Simplait Vanilla	1 pkg (6 oz)	200	7	30	5	–	–	0	–	24
YOGURT DRINKS *(see also* KEFIR, SMOOTHIES*)*										
lassi	7 oz	78	5	19	3	tr	1	–	0	8
Gopi										
Lassi	8 oz	126	10	37	6	–	–	0	0	4
Karoun										
Yogurt Drink	8 oz	126	10	37	6	–	–	0	0	4
Lifeway										
Lassi Mango	8 oz	160	2	10	2	–	–	0	3	21
YOGURT FROZEN										
chocolate soft serve	1 cup	230	9	7	5	tr	3	0	3	–
vanilla soft serve	1 cup	236	8	3	5	tr	2	0	0	35
Ben & Jerry's										
Greek Banana Peanut Butter	½ cup (3.5 oz)	210	8	25	3	–	–	0	tr	26
Greek Blueberry Vanilla Graham	½ cup (3.5 oz)	200	7	25	3	–	–	0	0	23
Greek Raspberry Fudge Chunk	½ cup (3.4 oz)	200	7	25	5	–	–	0	tr	25
Greek Strawberry Shortcake	½ cup (3.5 oz)	180	5	30	3	–	–	0	0	23

FOOD	PORTION	CALS	TOTAL FAT	CHOL	SAT FAT	POLY FAT	MONO FAT	TRANS FAT	FIBER	SUGAR
Healthy Choice										
Blueberry	1 pkg (4 oz)	100	2	10	1	–	–	0	1	13
Raspberry	1 pkg (4 oz)	100	2	5	1	–	–	0	1	13
Strawberry	1 pkg (4 oz)	100	2	10	1	–	–	0	tr	12
Vanilla Bean	1 pkg (4 oz)	100	2	10	1	–	–	0	1	12
Lifeway										
Probugs Frozen Kefir Pop Goo-Berry Pie	1 (1.9 oz)	70	1	5	0	–	–	0	–	12
Probugs Frozen Kefir Pop Orange Creamy Crawler	1 (1.9 oz)	70	1	5	0	–	–	0	–	12
Probugs Frozen Kefir Pop Strawnana Split	1 (1.9 oz)	70	1	5	0	–	–	0	0	12
Yasso										
Greek Yogurt Bar Raspberry	1 (2.6 oz)	70	0	5	0	0	0	0	0	12
Greek Yogurt Bar Strawberry	1 (2.6 oz)	70	0	5	0	0	0	0	0	11
ZUCCHINI										
baby raw	1 (0.5 oz)	3	tr	0	tr	tr	tr	0	tr	–
canned italian style	1 cup	66	tr	0	tr	tr	tr	0	–	–
fresh	1 sm (4.1 oz)	19	tr	0	tr	tr	tr	0	1	2
pickled	¼ cup	16	tr	0	tr	tr	tr	0	1	3
raw sliced	1 cup	19	tr	0	tr	tr	tr	0	1	2
sliced cooked w/o salt	1 cup	29	tr	0	tr	tr	tr	0	3	3
Del Monte										
Zucchini w/ Italian Tomato Sauce	½ cup (4.2 oz)	30	0	0	0	0	0	0	1	1
TAKE-OUT										
breaded & fried	6 slices (3 oz)	141	11	2	1	5	4	0	1	3
indian pakora	1 serv	46	2	1	tr	–	–	–	2	–
sticks breaded & fried	6 (2 oz)	90	7	2	1	3	2	0	1	2

PART TWO

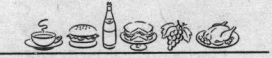

Restaurant Chains

CHOOSE WISELY

Meals eaten away from home make up ⅓ of our daily calories and are usually higher in saturated fat and trans fat and lower in fiber.

FOOD	PORTION	CALS	TOTAL FAT	CHOL	SAT FAT	POLY FAT	MONO FAT	TRANS FAT	FIBER	C
BASKIN-ROBBINS										
BEVERAGES										
Cappuccino Blast w/ Whipped Cream	1 sm (16 oz)	330	14	55	9	–	–	0	0	4
Shake Chocolate Chip	1 sm (16 oz)	660	32	115	20	–	–	1	1	7
Shake Chocolate Chip Cookie Dough	1 sm (16 oz)	750	31	105	20	–	–	1	1	8
Shake Mint Chocolate Chip	1 sm (16 oz)	680	33	110	20	–	–	1	1	7
Shake Vanilla	1 sm (16 oz)	670	33	130	21	–	–	1	0	7
FROZEN YOGURT										
Cherries Jubilee	1 scoop (4 oz)	240	12	45	7	–	–	0	1	2
Vanilla Fat Free	1 scoop (4 oz)	150	0	0	0	0	0	0	0	3
ICE CREAM										
Butter Almond Crunch Reduced Fat No Sugar Added	1 scoop (4 oz)	220	11	25	5	–	–	0	4	
Butter Pecan	1 scoop (4 oz)	280	18	50	9	–	–	0	1	2
Cabana Berry Banana Reduced Fat No Sugar Added	1 scoop (4 oz)	150	6	20	4	–	–	0	3	
Chocolate	1 scoop (4 oz)	260	14	50	9	–	–	0	0	3
Chocolate Chip	1 scoop (4 oz)	270	16	55	10	–	–	0	1	2
Chocolate Chip Cookie Dough	1 scoop (4 oz)	310	15	50	10	–	–	0	0	3
Chocolate Overload Reduced Fat No Sugar Added	1 scoop (4 oz)	190	8	20	5	–	–	0	5	
Gold Medal Ribbon	1 scoop (4 oz)	260	13	45	8	–	–	0	0	33
Mint Chocolate Chip	1 scoop (4 oz)	270	16	55	10	–	–	0	1	2
Nutty Coconut	1 scoop (4 oz)	300	20	45	9	–	–	0	1	2
Oreo Cookies 'N Cream	1 scoop (4 oz)	280	15	50	9	–	–	0	1	2
Peanut Butter 'N Chocolate	1 scoop (4 oz)	320	20	45	9	–	–	0	1	28
Pistachio Almond	1 scoop (4 oz)	290	19	50	9	–	–	0	1	23
Pralines 'N Cream	1 scoop (4 oz)	280	14	45	8	–	–	0	1	31
Reese's Peanut Butter Cup	1 scoop (4 oz)	300	18	50	10	–	–	0	1	2
Rocky Road	1 scoop (4 oz)	290	15	45	8	–	–	0	5	32
Sundae Caramel Soft Serve	1 (10 oz)	580	21	70	13	–	–	1	1	78
Sundae Hot Fudge Soft Serve	1 (10 oz)	610	25	65	18	–	–	1	1	75
Sundae Strawberry Soft Serve	1 (10 oz)	450	18	65	11	–	–	0	1	57

FOOD	PORTION	CALS	TOTAL FAT	CHOL	SAT FAT	POLY FAT	MONO FAT	TRANS FAT	FIBER	SUGAR
Wax Crunch	1 scoop (4 oz)	330	20	45	11	–	–	0	1	28
Vanilla	1 scoop (4 oz)	260	16	65	10	–	–	1	0	26
Vanilla Soft Serve	1 serv (6 oz)	280	11	40	7	–	–	0	0	36
Very Berry Strawberry	1 scoop (4 oz)	320	11	40	7	–	–	0	0	27
ICES										
Sherbet Rainbow	1 scoop (4 oz)	160	2	10	2	–	–	0	0	34
Sorbet Lemon	1 scoop (4 oz)	130	0	0	0	0	0	0	0	33
Sorbet Mango	1 scoop (4 oz)	120	0	0	0	0	0	0	0	30
Sorbet Strawberry	1 scoop (4 oz)	130	0	0	0	0	0	0	0	34

BILLY'S BURGER HUT
BEVERAGES

FOOD	PORTION	CALS	TOTAL FAT	CHOL	SAT FAT	POLY FAT	MONO FAT	TRANS FAT	FIBER	SUGAR
Shake Chocolate	1 (20 oz)	420	10	30	4	–	–	0	0	50
Shake Vanilla	1 (20 oz)	320	10	25	4	–	–	0	0	44
MAIN MENU SELECTIONS										
Big Billy's Roast Beef Sub	1	843	54	151	27	–	–	0	3	12
Billyburger	1	426	22	63	12	–	–	1	3	6
Billyburger w/ Cheese	1	498	35	57	19	–	–	1	4	8
Billy's Best Red Potato Salad	1 serv	190	9	80	2	4	4	0	3	4
Billy's Biggest Burger ½ Pounder w/ Everything	1	852	58	140	–	–	–	2	4	15
Billy's Famous 7 Layer Salad	1 serv	558	49	119	11	25	11	0	2	9
Billy's Seafood Sandwich	1	399	18	42	10	–	–	0	3	9
Caesar Side Salad	1 serv	360	28	70	4	2	20	0	4	1
Chili w/ Cheese & Onion	1 serv	380	12	64	6	–	–	0	7	8
Cowboy Cobb Salad	1 serv	735	45	239	14	9	26	0	9	10
Cowboy Coleslaw	1 serv	180	9	10	2	5	4	0	3	4
French Fries	1 reg	230	12	0	4	–	–	1	1	7
Onion Rings	1 serv	250	10	0	6	–	–	2	1	6
Super Billy Burger w/ Bacon	1	663	41	98	21	–	–	1	4	9

BLIMPIE
DESSERTS

FOOD	PORTION	CALS	TOTAL FAT	CHOL	SAT FAT	POLY FAT	MONO FAT	TRANS FAT	FIBER	SUGAR
Cookie Chocolate Chunk	1 (1.5 oz)	200	10	15	5	–	–	0	0	16
Cookie Oatmeal Raisin	1 (1.5 oz)	180	7	10	3	–	–	0	tr	16
Cookie Peanut Butter	1 (1.5 oz)	210	13	10	5	–	–	0	tr	13
Cookie Sugar	1 (2.5 oz)	320	16	35	6	–	–	0	0	23
Cookie White Chocolate Macadamia Nut	1 (1.5 oz)	200	11	15	5	–	–	0	0	16
SALAD DRESSINGS AND SAUCES										
Dressing Blue Cheese	1 serv 1.5 oz	230	24	25	5	–	–	0	–	2

FOOD	PORTION	CALS	TOTAL FAT	CHOL	SAT FAT	POLY FAT	MONO FAT	TRANS FAT	FIBER	S
Dressing Buttermilk Ranch	1 serv (1.5 oz)	230	24	10	4	–	–	0	–	
Dressing Buttermilk Ranch Light	1 serv (1.5 oz)	70	4	0	1	–	–	0	–	1
Dressing Creamy Caesar	1 serv (1.5 oz)	210	21	10	4	–	–	0	–	
Dressing Creamy Italian	1 serv (1.5 oz)	180	18	0	3	–	–	0	0	
Dressing Dijon Honey Mustard	1 serv (1.5 oz)	180	17	15	3	–	–	0	–	2
Dressing Italian Fat Free	1 serv (1.5 oz)	25	0	0	–	–	–	0	0	3
Dressing Italian Light	1 serv (1.5 oz)	20	1	0	0	–	–	0	–	2
Dressing Peppercorn	1 serv (1.5 oz)	240	26	20	5	–	–	–	0	1
Dressing Thousand Island	1 serv (1.5 oz)	210	20	15	3	–	–	0	0	6
Guacamole	1 serv (1 oz)	45	4	0	1	–	–	0	1	
Mayonnaise	1 serv (1 oz)	200	22	20	3	–	–	0	0	
Sauce Blimpie Special	1 serv (0.5 oz)	40	5	0	0	–	–	0	–	
Sauce Red Hot Original	1 serv (1 oz)	10	0	0	0	0	0	0	0	(
SALADS										
Antipasto	1 serv (11.6 oz)	254	14	60	6	–	–	0	4	
Buffalo Chicken	1 serv (7.7 oz)	220	9	60	5	–	–	0	4	5
Chicken Caesar	1 serv (9.4 oz)	190	8	65	4	–	–	0	3	3
Cole Slaw	1 side (4 oz)	160	9	5	2	–	–	0	2	17
Garden	1 serv (6.5 oz)	30	0	0	0	–	–	–	3	3
Macaroni	1 side (5 oz)	330	22	15	5	–	–	0	2	8
Northwest Potato	1 side (5 oz)	260	17	25	4	–	–	0	3	3
Potato	1 side (4.7 oz)	230	12	10	3	–	–	0	3	8
Tuna	1 serv (9.4 oz)	270	19	55	3	–	–	0	3	3
Ultimate Club	1 serv (10.1 oz)	280	14	65	7	–	–	0	3	5
SANDWICHES										
6 Inch Sub Blimpie Best	1 (10.4 oz)	450	17	50	6	–	–	0	3	10
6 Inch Sub Blimpie Best Super Stacked	1 (12.8 oz)	550	22	90	8	–	–	0	3	12
6 Inch Sub Blimpie Trio Super Stacked	1 (13.5 oz)	510	15	90	5	–	–	0	3	1
6 Inch Sub BLT	1 (7.2 oz)	430	22	25	5	–	–	0	2	6
6 Inch Sub BLT Super Stacked	1 (8.4 oz)	640	41	55	9	–	–	0	2	6
6 Inch Sub Chicken Cheddar Bacon Ranch	1 (12.1 oz)	600	29	85	10	–	–	0	3	8
6 Inch Sub Chicken Teriyaki	1 (8.7 oz)	450	12	65	5	–	–	0	2	13

FOOD	PORTION	CALS	TOTAL FAT	CHOL	SAT FAT	POLY FAT	MONO FAT	TRANS FAT	FIBER	SUGAR
6 Inch Sub Club	1 (10.2 oz)	410	13	45	4	–	–	0	3	9
6 Inch Sub Cuban	1 (8.2 oz)	410	11	65	5	–	–	0	1	6
6 Inch Sub French Dip	1 (13.4 oz)	410	11	65	5	–	–	0	1	3
6 Inch Sub Ham & Swiss	1 (10 oz)	420	14	45	5	–	–	0	3	10
6 Inch Sub Hot Pastrami	1 (7.2 oz)	430	16	65	7	–	–	0	1	5
6 Inch Sub Hot Pastrami Super Stacked	1 (10.1 oz)	570	23	110	10	–	–	0	1	7
6 Inch Sub Meatball	1 (10 oz)	580	31	75	13	–	–	0	4	6
6 Inch Sub Reuben	1 (9.2 oz)	530	20	70	6	–	–	0	3	7
6 Inch Sub Roast Beef & Provolone	1 (10.8 oz)	430	14	55	5	–	–	0	3	7
6 Inch Sub Roast Beef & Provolone On Wheat	1 (11.3 oz)	430	16	60	5	–	–	0	6	6
6 Inch Sub Tuna	1 (8.9 oz)	470	21	55	3	–	–	0	2	5
6 Inch Sub Turkey & Provolone	1 (10.8 oz)	410	13	40	4	–	–	0	3	8
6 Inch Sub Turkey & Provolone On Wheat	1 (11.3 oz)	420	14	45	5	–	–	0	6	8
6 Inch Sub VegiMax	1 (10.2 oz)	520	20	15	6	–	–	0	5	8
Blimpie Burger	1 (6 oz)	460	24	70	10	–	–	1	1	4
Blimpie Dog	1 (6.3 oz)	510	29	55	12	–	–	0	1	7
Ciabatta Buffalo Chicken	1 (11.3 oz)	540	23	65	7	–	–	0	3	5
Ciabatta French Dip	1 (13.8 oz)	430	11	65	5	–	–	0	2	2
Ciabatta Grilled Chicken Caesar	1 (10.1 oz)	580	20	65	5	–	–	0	3	4
Ciabatta Mediterranean	1 (10.1 oz)	450	8	35	3	–	–	0	3	6
Ciabatta Roast Beef Turkey & Cheddar	1 (10 oz)	520	24	65	8	–	–	0	3	6
Ciabatta Sicilian	1 (10 oz)	590	22	60	6	–	–	0	3	9
Ciabatta Spicy Chicken & Pepperoni	1 (10.1 oz)	710	34	80	11	–	–	0	3	4
Ciabatta Tuscan	1 (9.9 oz)	570	20	50	6	–	–	0	3	6
Ciabatta Ultimate Club	1 (7.4 oz)	520	24	65	7	–	–	0	2	5
Wrap Chicken Caesar	1 (9.7 oz)	220	8	60	0	–	–	0	4	5
Wrap Southwestern	1 (10 oz)	530	22	55	6	–	–	0	4	10
SOUPS										
Bean w/ Ham	1 serv (8.6 oz)	140	1	0	0	–	–	0	11	2
Chicken Noodle	1 serv (8.6 oz)	130	4	30	1	–	–	0	2	5
Chicken w/ White & Wild Rice	1 serv (8.6 oz)	250	10	30	3	–	–	0	4	4
Cream Of Broccoli w/ Cheese	1 serv (8.6 oz)	250	19	55	11	–	–	0	tr	2

FOOD	PORTION	CALS	TOTAL FAT	CHOL	SAT FAT	POLY FAT	MONO FAT	TRANS FAT	FIBER	SUG
Cream Of Potato	1 serv (8.6 oz)	190	9	<5	3	–	–	0	3	3
Garden Vegetable	1 serv (8.6 oz)	80	1	0	0	–	–	0	3	5
Grande Chili w/ Bean & Beef	1 serv (8.6 oz)	310	9	20	4	–	–	0	9	9
Tomato Basil w/ Raviolini	1 serv (8.6 oz)	110	1	10	0	–	–	0	0	5
Vegetable Beef	1 serv (8.6 oz)	80	2	5	1	–	–	0	2	3

BURGER KING
BEVERAGES

FOOD	PORTION	CALS	TOTAL FAT	CHOL	SAT FAT	POLY FAT	MONO FAT	TRANS FAT	FIBER	SUG
Apple Juice Minute Maid	1 (6.67 oz)	100	0	0	0	0	0	0	0	21
Barq's Root Beer	1 sm (16 oz)	160	0	0	0	0	0	0	0	46
Cherry Coke	1 sm (16 oz)	150	0	0	0	0	0	0	0	42
Chocolate Milk 1% Low Fat	1 (8 oz)	160	3	15	2	–	–	0	0	25
Coca-Cola Classic	1 sm (16 oz)	140	0	0	0	0	0	0	–	39
Coffee Seattle's Best Decaf Black	1 (16 oz)	0	0	0	0	0	0	0	0	0
Coffee Seattle's Best Regular Black	1 (16 oz)	0	0	0	0	0	0	0	0	0
Coffee Iced Seattle's Best	1 sm	80	2	10	2	–	–	0	0	12
Coffee Iced Seattle's Best Caramel	1 sm	170	4	15	2	–	–	0	0	23
Coffee Iced Seattle's Best Mocha	1 sm	180	3	10	2	–	–	0	1	33
Coffee Iced Seattle's Best Vanilla	1 sm	160	2	10	2	–	–	0	0	32
Diet Coke	1 sm (16 oz)	0	0	0	0	0	0	0	0	0
Dr Pepper	1 sm (16 oz)	140	0	0	0	0	0	0	0	39
Fanta Orange	1 sm (16 oz)	160	0	0	0	0	0	0	0	42
Frappe Caramel	1 (12 oz)	410	19	5	11	–	–	0	0	39
Frappe Mocha	1 (12 oz)	410	19	5	11	–	–	0	0	39
Frozen Coke	1 sm (16 oz)	90	0	0	0	0	0	0	0	25
Hi-C Fruit Punch	1 sm (16 oz)	150	0	0	0	0	0	0	0	42
Iced Tea Southern Style Nestea	1 sm (16 oz)	180	0	0	0	0	0	0	0	50
Iced Tea Sweetened Nestea	1 sm (16 oz)	90	0	0	0	0	0	0	0	24
Iced Tea Unsweetened Nestea	1 sm (16 oz)	0	0	0	0	0	0	0	0	0
Lemonade Light Minute Maid	1 sm (16 oz)	5	0	0	0	0	0	0	0	0
Milk Fat Free	8 oz	90	0	5	0	0	0	0	0	12
Orange Juice Minute Maid	10 oz	140	0	0	0	0	0	0	0	30

FOOD	PORTION	CALS	TOTAL FAT	CHOL	SAT FAT	POLY FAT	MONO FAT	TRANS FAT	FIBER	SUGAR
Shake Chocolate	1 sm (12 oz)	580	17	40	13	–	–	1	0	83
Shake Strawberry	1 sm (12 oz)	500	16	40	12	–	–	1	0	67
Shake Vanilla	1 sm (12 oz)	550	16	40	12	–	–	1	0	81
Smoothie Strawberry Banana	1 (12 oz)	200	0	0	0	0	0	0	2	40
Smoothie Tropical Mango	1 (12 oz)	210	1	0	0	–	–	0	1	41
Sprite	1 sm (16 oz)	140	0	0	0	0	0	0	0	39
Sweet Tea Gold Peak	1 sm (16 oz)	120	0	0	0	0	0	0	0	31
Vault	1 sm (16 oz)	160	0	0	0	0	0	0	0	42
BREAKFAST SELECTIONS										
Biscuit Bacon Egg & Cheese	1 (5.6 oz)	420	25	160	16	–	–	1	1	4
Biscuit Ham Egg & Cheese	1 (6.4 oz)	390	19	165	14	–	–	1	1	4
Biscuit Sausage	1 (4.4 oz)	420	27	35	15	–	–	1	1	3
Biscuit Sausage Egg & Cheese	1 (6.7 oz)	520	34	180	19	–	–	1	1	3
Biscuit Country Ham & Egg	1 (6.4 oz)	420	23	185	15	–	–	0	1	3
BK Breakfast Muffin Bacon Egg & Cheese	1 (4.6 oz)	250	11	165	5	–	–	0	1	2
BK Breakfast Muffin Egg & Cheese	1 (4.4 oz)	220	9	160	4	–	–	0	1	2
BK Breakfast Muffin Ham Egg & Cheese	1 (5.6 oz)	250	9	175	4	–	–	0	1	3
BK Breakfast Muffin Sausage & Cheese	1 (3.9 oz)	330	20	45	7	–	–	0	1	1
BK Breakfast Muffin Sausage Egg & Cheese	1 (5.9 oz)	390	23	195	9	–	–	0	1	2
BK Breakfast Platter Ultimate	1 (17.9 oz)	1450	84	505	30	–	–	1	5	41
Breakfast Burrito Sausage	1 (4.3 oz)	290	17	140	7	–	–	0	1	2
Breakfast Burrito Southwestern	1 (7.8 oz)	580	35	205	13	–	–	0	4	3
Breakfast Syrup	1 serv (1 oz)	120	0	0	0	0	0	0	0	18
Cinnabon Roll	1 (3.4 oz)	300	11	5	5	–	–	0	2	20
Croissan'wich Bacon Egg & Cheese	1 (4.6 oz)	320	18	165	8	–	–	0	1	4
Croissan'wich Double w/ Bacon Egg & Cheese	1 (5.2 oz)	390	24	180	11	–	–	0	1	4
Croissan'wich Double w/ Ham Bacon Egg & Cheese	1 (6.2 oz)	390	22	190	10	–	–	0	1	5
Croissan'wich Double w/ Ham Egg & Cheese	1 (7 oz)	390	19	185	9	–	–	0	1	6

FOOD	PORTION	CALS	TOTAL FAT	CHOL	SAT FAT	POLY FAT	MONO FAT	TRANS FAT	FIBER	SUG
Croissan'wich Double w/ Ham Sausage Egg & Cheese	1 (7.5 oz)	530	34	215	14	–	–	1	1	5
Croissan'wich Double w/ Sausage Bacon Egg & Cheese	1 (6.6 oz)	530	36	210	15	–	–	1	1	4
Croissan'wich Double w/ Sausage Egg & Cheese	1 (8 oz)	660	48	235	18	–	–	1	1	4
Croissan'wich Egg & Cheese	1 (4.4 oz)	280	15	160	7	–	–	0	1	4
Croissan'wich Ham Egg & Cheese	1 (5.9 oz)	450	30	195	11	–	–	0	1	4
Croissan'wich Sausage & Cheese	1 (4 oz)	390	26	45	10	–	–	0	1	3
French Toast Sticks	3 (2.3 oz)	230	11	0	2	–	–	0	1	8
Hash Browns	1 sm (2.9 oz)	250	16	0	4	–	–	4	3	0
Jam Strawberry or Grape	1 pkg (0.4 oz)	30	0	0	0	0	0	0	0	6
Pancakes + Syrup	3 (6.6 oz)	500	19	95	5	–	–	0	1	36
Platter Pancake & Sausage	1 (13.7 oz)	670	34	125	9	–	–	0	1	36
Quaker Oatmeal Maple Brown Sugar	1 serv (6.1 oz)	270	4	5	2	–	–	0	5	29
Quaker Oatmeal Original	1 serv (4.4 oz)	140	4	5	1	–	–	0	3	1
DESSERTS										
Cookies Chocolate Chip	2 (2.7 oz)	330	15	20	8	–	–	0	1	29
Cookies Oatmeal Raisin	2 (2.7 oz)	310	13	20	8	–	–	0	3	26
Cookies White Chocolate Macadamia Nut	2 (2.7 oz)	340	18	20	8	–	–	0	0	28
Dutch Apple Pie	1 (3.8 oz)	320	14	0	6	–	–	0	1	23
Hershey Sundae Pie	1 serv (2.8 oz)	310	19	10	12	–	–	0	1	22
Soft Serve Cone	1 (3.5 oz)	160	4	15	3	–	–	0	0	20
Soft Serve Cup	1 (3.3 oz)	140	4	15	3	–	–	0	0	19
Sundae Brownie	1 (8 oz)	530	17	55	10	–	–	0	2	70
Sundae Caramel	1 (4.9 oz)	280	6	20	4	–	–	0	0	37
Sundae Chocolate Fudge	1 (4.9 oz)	280	7	15	5	–	–	0	1	43
Sundae Mini M&M	1 (7.2 oz)	450	13	30	9	–	–	0	0	62
Sundae Oreo	1 (7.2 oz)	440	12	25	7	–	–	0	1	57
Sundae Strawberry	1 (4.9 oz)	190	4	15	3	–	–	0	0	31
MAIN MENU SELECTIONS										
Apple Slices	1 pkg (2 oz)	30	0	0	0	0	0	0	1	6
BK Stacker Double	1 (5.3 oz)	490	30	90	11	–	–	1	1	7
BK Stacker Quad	1 (8.4 oz)	760	51	170	22	–	–	2	1	8

FOOD	PORTION	CALS	TOTAL FAT	CHOL	SAT FAT	POLY FAT	MONO FAT	TRANS FAT	FIBER	SUGAR
BK Stacker Single	1 (4 oz)	370	21	50	8	–	–	0	1	7
BK Stacker Triple	1 (6.9 oz)	630	41	130	17	–	–	1	1	7
BK Veggie Burger	1 (7.3 oz)	410	16	5	3	–	–	0	7	8
Burger BK Bacon	1 (3.7 oz)	320	17	40	5	–	–	0	1	7
Cheeseburger	1 (4 oz)	280	12	40	6	–	–	0	1	7
Cheeseburger Bacon	1 (4.2 oz)	310	14	45	6	–	–	0	1	7
Cheeseburger Double	1 (5.2 oz)	370	18	70	9	–	–	1	1	7
Cheeseburger Double Bacon	1 (5.6 oz)	440	24	85	10	–	–	1	1	7
Chicken Nuggets	4 (2.2 oz)	190	11	25	2	–	–	0	1	0
Chicken Strips	2 (3.2 oz)	240	13	20	3	–	–	0	0	0
French Fries Salted	1 sm (4.5 oz)	340	15	0	3	–	–	0	4	0
Hamburger	1 (3.5 oz)	240	8	30	4	–	–	0	1	7
Mozzarella Sticks	4 (3.1 oz)	280	15	35	5	–	–	0	2	2
Onion Rings	1 sm (3.2 oz)	320	16	0	3	–	–	0	3	4
Pickles	2 (0.4 oz)	10	0	0	0	0	0	0	0	0
Sandwich Chicken Crispy	1 (9.3 oz)	750	45	70	8	–	–	1	3	8
Sandwich Chicken Crispy Spicy	1 (5.2 oz)	480	27	45	5	–	–	1	2	6
Sandwich Chicken Grilled	1 (8.4 oz)	510	22	80	4	–	–	0	2	6
Sandwich Chicken Original	1 (7.6 oz)	630	39	65	7	–	–	1	3	4
Sandwich Country Pork	1 (10.5 oz)	810	42	75	13	–	–	0	4	10
Sandwich Premium Alaskan Fish	1 (8 oz)	590	31	45	5	–	–	0	3	8
Tacos	2 (6.1 oz)	390	16	30	7	–	–	1	5	4
Whopper	1 (9.7 oz)	630	35	65	10	–	–	1	3	13
Whopper Texas	1 (10.8 oz)	760	48	90	15	–	–	1	3	10
Whopper Texas Double	1 (13.7 oz)	1000	66	155	24	–	–	2	3	11
Whopper w/ Cheese	1 (10.5 oz)	710	42	85	15	–	–	1	3	14
Whopper Double	1 (12.2 oz)	830	50	120	17	–	–	1	3	13
Whopper Double w/ Cheese	1 (14 oz)	990	65	160	24	–	–	2	3	11
Whopper Jr.	1 (5.2 oz)	340	19	40	5	–	–	0	2	6
Whopper Jr. w/ Cheese	1 (5.6 oz)	380	23	55	8	–	–	1	2	6
Whopper Triple	1 (14.6 oz)	1020	65	175	23	–	–	2	3	13
Wrap Chicken Apple & Cranberry Garden Fresh Salad Crispy	1 (7.5 oz)	500	24	40	6	–	–	0	5	19
Wrap Chicken Apple & Cranberry Garden Fresh Salad Grilled	1 (7.3 oz)	430	18	54	5	–	–	0	4	17

FOOD	PORTION	CALS	TOTAL FAT	CHOL	SAT FAT	POLY FAT	MONO FAT	TRANS FAT	FIBER	SUG
Wrap Chicken BLT Garden Fresh Salad Crispy	1 (7.2 oz)	490	27	50	7	–	–	0	4	4
Wrap Chicken BLT Garden Fresh Salad Grilled	1 (7.2 oz)	420	22	55	6	–	–	0	4	3
Wrap Chicken Caesar Garden Fresh Salad Crispy	1 (8.2 oz)	460	23	35	5	–	–	0	5	4
Wrap Chicken Caesar Garden Fresh Salad Grilled	1 (8 oz)	380	18	40	4	–	–	0	5	3
Wrap Honey Mustard Crispy Chicken	1 (5 oz)	390	23	35	6	–	–	0	2	6
Wrap Honey Mustard Grilled Chicken	1 (5.2 oz)	370	19	55	5	–	–	0	1	6
Wrap Ranch Crispy Chicken	1 (5 oz)	370	23	35	6	–	–	1	2	1
Wrap Ranch Grilled Chicken	1 (5.2 oz)	350	18	55	5	–	–	0	1	1
SALAD DRESSINGS AND SAUCES										
Dipping Sauce Barbecue	1 serv (1 oz)	40	0	0	0	0	0	0	0	10
Dipping Sauce BBQ Roasted Jalapeno	1 serv (1 oz)	50	0	0	0	0	0	0	0	11
Dipping Sauce Honey Mustard	1 serv (1 oz)	90	6	10	1	–	–	0	0	7
Dipping Sauce King Kung Pao	1 serv (1 oz)	60	0	0	0	0	0	0	0	12
Dipping Sauce Ranch	1 serv (1 oz)	140	15	5	3	–	–	0	0	1
Dipping Sauce Sweet And Sour	1 serv (1 oz)	45	0	0	0	0	0	0	0	10
Dipping Sauce Zesty Onion Ring	1 serv (1 oz)	150	15	15	3	–	–	0	1	2
Dressing Ken's Apple Cider Vinaigrette	1 pkg (1.75 oz)	210	18	10	3	–	–	0	0	7
Dressing Ken's Avocado Ranch	1 pkg (1.8 oz)	170	17	15	3	–	–	0	0	3
Dressing Ken's Citrus Caesar	1 pkg (1.8 oz)	180	18	5	4	–	–	0	0	2
Dressing Ken's Honey Mustard	1 pkg (1.8 oz)	220	23	15	3	–	–	0	1	12
Dressing Ken's Lite Honey Balsamic	1 pkg (1.75 oz)	120	7	0	1	–	–	0	0	11
Ketchup	1 pkg (0.4 oz)	10	0	0	0	0	0	0	0	2
Mayonnaise	1 pkg (0.4 oz)	80	9	10	1	–	–	0	0	0
Sauce French Fry	1 serv (1 oz)	90	7	5	1	–	–	0	0	3

FOOD	PORTION	CALS	TOTAL FAT	CHOL.	SAT FAT	POLY FAT	MONO FAT	TRANS FAT	FIBER	SUGAR
Sauce Marinara	1 serv (1 oz)	15	0	0	0	0	0	0	1	3
Sauce Picante/Taco	1 serv (1 oz)	10	0	0	0	0	0	0	0	1
SALADS										
Chicken Apple & Cranberry Garden Fresh w/ Tendercrisp & Dressing	1 (14 oz)	700	41	80	9	–	–	0	5	37
Chicken Apple & Cranberry Garden Fresh w/ Tendergrill & Dressing	1 (13.6 oz)	560	30	90	7	–	–	0	4	34
Chicken BLT Garden Fresh w/ Tendercrisp & Dressing	1 (14 oz)	690	48	100	12	–	–	1	4	8
Chicken BLT Garden Fresh w/ Tendergrill & Dressing	1 (13.6 oz)	550	37	115	10	–	–	0	3	5
Chicken Caesar Garden Fresh w/ Tendercrisp & Dressing	1 (13.5 oz)	670	43	80	7	–	–	0	5	8
Chicken Caesar Garden Fresh w/ Tendergrill & Dressing	1 (13.1 oz)	530	32	95	5	–	–	0	3	6
Croutons Homestyle Caesar	1 pkg (0.5 oz)	60	2	10	0	–	–	0	0	1
Side Caesar w/ Dressing	1 (5 oz)	220	20	10	4	–	–	0	2	3
Side Garden w/ Avocado Ranch Dressing	1 (5.2 oz)	230	21	30	5	–	–	0	2	3

CARIBOU COFFEE

BEVERAGES

FOOD	PORTION	CALS	TOTAL FAT	CHOL.	SAT FAT	POLY FAT	MONO FAT	TRANS FAT	FIBER	SUGAR
Americano No Whip	1 sm (11 oz)	0	0	0	0	0	0	0	0	0
Apple Blast Cooler No Whip	1 sm (17 oz)	300	11	40	7	–	–	0	0	48
Apple Blast w/ Whip	1 med (17 oz)	400	11	40	7	–	–	0	0	71
Berry Black Tea Growlers	1 sm (9 oz)	110	0	0	0	0	0	0	0	26
Berry Mocha 2% Milk w/ Whip	1 sm (14 oz)	570	31	65	20	–	–	0	1	63
Berry Mocha Cooler Northern Lite No Whip	1 sm (17 oz)	170	3	0	3	–	–	0	8	27
Berry Mocha Cooler w/ Whip	1 sm (18 oz)	560	20	55	13	–	–	0	0	83
Berry Mocha Northern Lite Skim Milk No Whip	1 sm (11 oz)	185	6	5	4	–	–	0	0	22
Black Forest Caribou Cooler w/ Whip	1 sm (19 oz)	650	28	85	18	–	–	0	4	85
Black Tea	1 sm (12 oz)	0	0	0	0	0	0	0	0	0

FOOD	PORTION	CALS	TOTAL FAT	CHOL	SAT FAT	POLY FAT	MONO FAT	TRANS FAT	FIBER	SUG
Black Tea Peach Growlers	1 sm (9 oz)	90	0	0	0	0	0	0	0	22
Black Tea Peach No Whip	1 med (24 oz)	104	0	0	0	0	0	0	0	33
Breve No Whip	1 sm (12 oz)	350	31	100	19	–	–	0	0	0
Campfire Mocha 2% Milk w/ Whip	1 med (14 oz)	560	31	65	20	–	–	0	1	62
Campfire Mocha Cooler w/ Whip	1 sm (18 oz)	510	20	55	13	–	–	0	0	81
Cappuccino 2% Milk No Whip	1 sm (6 oz)	45	2	5	1	–	–	0	0	4
Caramel Caribou Cooler Northern Lite No Whip	1 sm (16 oz)	90	2	0	2	–	–	0	6	11
Caramel Caribou Cooler w/ Whip	1 sm (17 oz)	420	16	40	11	–	–	0	0	63
Caramel High Rise 2% Milk w/ Whip	1 med (17 oz)	360	18	65	12	–	–	0	0	40
Caramel High Rise Northern Lite Skim Milk Nonfat Whip	1 sm (12 oz)	115	1	5	0	–	–	0	0	15
Chai 2% Milk No Whip	1 sm (13 oz)	250	6	25	4	–	–	0	0	38
Chai Blended 2% Milk No Whip	1 sm (16 oz)	210	4	10	2	–	–	0	0	39
Chai Iced 2% Milk No Whip	1 sm (13 oz)	210	4	10	2	–	–	0	0	39
Coffee Caribou Cooler Northern Lite No Whip	1 sm (16 oz)	100	2	0	2	–	–	0	7	13
Coffee Of The Day w/o Milk & Whip	1 sm (12 oz)	5	0	0	0	0	0	0	0	0
Cold Press Growlers	1 sm (8 oz)	0	0	0	0	0	0	0	0	0
Cold Press Iced Coffee No Whip	1 sm (14 oz)	5	0	0	0	0	0	0	0	0
Cookies & Cream Snowdrift 2% Milk w/ Whip	1 sm (19 oz)	590	25	70	13	–	–	0	1	71
Depth Charge	1 sm (12 oz)	5	0	0	0	0	0	0	0	0
Espresso	1 sm (3 oz)	0	0	0	0	0	0	0	0	0
Espresso Caribou Cooler No Whip	1 sm (16 oz)	210	35	0	4	–	–	0	0	36
Espresso Caribou Cooler Northern Lite No Whip	1 sm (16 oz)	80	2	0	2	–	–	0	6	11
Green Tea	1 sm (12 oz)	0	0	0	0	0	0	0	0	0
Green Tea Lemonade Growlers	1 sm (9 oz)	140	0	0	0	0	0	0	0	35

FOOD	PORTION	CALS	TOTAL FAT	CHOL	SAT FAT	POLY FAT	MONO FAT	TRANS FAT	FIBER	SUGAR
Green Tea Lemonade No Whip	1 med (24 oz)	210	0	0	0	0	0	0	0	52
Herbal Tea	1 sm (12 oz)	0	0	0	0	0	0	0	0	0
Hot Chocolate 2% Milk w/ Whip	1 sm (10 oz)	410	26	65	17	–	–	0	1	33
Hot Chocolate Lite Skim Milk Nonfat Whip	1 sm (11 oz)	215	6	10	4	–	–	0	0	27
Juice Lemon Ginger Pomegranate	1 med (24 oz)	260	0	0	0	0	0	0	0	57
Juice Lemon Ginger Pomegranate Growlers	1 sm (9 oz)	170	0	0	0	0	0	0	0	38
Juice Very Berry	1 med (24 oz)	160	0	0	0	0	0	0	0	34
Juice Very Berry Growlers	1 sm (9 oz)	110	0	0	0	0	0	0	0	23
Latte 2% Milk No Whip	1 sm (12 oz)	140	6	22	4	–	–	0	0	13
Latte Iced 2% Milk No Whip	1 sm (12 oz)	80	3	10	2	–	–	0	0	7
Latte Iced Northern Lite Skim Milk No Whip	1 sm (12 oz)	45	0	0	0	0	0	0	0	6
Latte Northern Lite Skim Milk No Whip	1 sm (12 oz)	90	5	5	0	–	–	0	0	12
Macchiato 2% Milk No Whip	1 sm (4 oz)	15	1	0	0	–	–	0	0	1
Mint Condition 2% Milk w/ Whip	1 sm (14 oz)	520	31	65	20	–	–	0	1	65
Mint Condition Cooler w/ Whip	1 sm (18 oz)	570	20	55	13	–	–	0	0	84
Mint Snowdrift 2% Milk w/ Whip	1 sm (18 oz)	490	21	70	12	–	–	0	0	64
Mocha 2% Milk w/ Whip	1 sm (10 oz)	360	24	55	15	–	–	0	1	28
Mocha Cooler Northern Lite No Whip	1 sm (17 oz)	190	3	0	3	–	–	0	9	29
Mocha Cooler w/ Whip	1 sm (18 oz)	530	21	60	13	–	–	0	0	70
Mocha Iced 2% Milk No Whip	1 sm (13 oz)	250	8	25	4	–	–	0	0	35
Mocha Iced Northern Lite Skim Milk No Whip	1 sm (12 oz)	140	3	10	2	–	–	0	0	20
Mocha Northern Lite Skim Milk Nonfat Whip	1 sm (10 oz)	185	6	5	4	–	–	0	0	22
Oolong Tea Iced Pomegranate 2% Milk No Whip	1 sm (13 oz)	140	3	10	2	–	–	0	0	26

FOOD	PORTION	CALS	TOTAL FAT	CHOL	SAT FAT	POLY FAT	MONO FAT	TRANS FAT	FIBER	SUG
Oolong Tea Pomegranate 2% Milk No Whip	1 sm (13 oz)	200	6	25	4	–	–	0	0	29
Rooibos Tea Iced Vanilla	1 sm (13 oz)	140	3	10	2	–	–	0	0	26
Rooibos Tea Vanilla 2% Milk No Whip	1 sm (13 oz)	200	6	25	4	–	–	0	0	28
Smoothie Mango Orange Key Lime No Whip	1 sm (19 oz)	360	0	0	0	0	0	0	0	82
Smoothie Strawberry Banana No Whip	1 sm (18 oz)	300	0	0	0	0	0	0	0	66
Smoothie White Peach Berry No Whip	1 sm (19 oz)	260	0	0	0	0	0	0	0	56
Tea Berry Black No Whip	1 med (24 oz)	170	0	0	0	0	0	0	0	39
Turtle Mocha 2% Milk w/ Whip	1 med (14 oz)	580	31	65	20	–	–	0	1	66
Turtle Mocha Cooler Northern Lite No Whip	1 sm (17 oz)	488	3	0	3	–	–	0	8	27
Turtle Mocha Cooler w/ Whip	1 sm (18 oz)	570	20	55	13	–	–	0	0	85
Turtle Mocha Northen Lite Skim Milk Nonfat Whip	1 sm (11 oz)	185	6	5	4	–	–	0	0	22
Vanilla Caribou Cooler	1 sm (17 oz)	410	16	40	11	–	–	0	0	60
Vanilla Caribou Cooler Northern Lite No Whip	1 sm (16 oz)	90	2	0	2	–	–	0	6	11
Vanilla White Chocolate Mocha 2% Milk w/ Whip	1 sm (14 oz)	570	31	65	20	–	–	0	1	63
Vanilla White Chocolate Mocha Cooler Northern Lite No Whip	1 sm (17 oz)	170	3	0	3	–	–	0	8	27
Vanilla White Chocolate Mocha Cooler w/ Whip	1 sm (18 oz)	560	20	55	13	–	–	0	0	82
Vanilla White Chocolate Mocha Northern Lite Skim Milk Nonfat Whip	1 sm (11 oz)	185	6	5	4	–	–	0	0	22
White Tea Mint Lime Growlers	1 sm (9 oz)	160	0	0	0	0	0	0	0	39
White Tea Mint Lime No Whip	1 med (24 oz)	240	0	0	0	0	0	0	0	58
FOOD										
Croissant Butter	1 (2.5 oz)	280	13	30	8	–	–	0	1	5
Daybreaker Chicken Apple Sausage	1 (6.4 oz)	410	20	235	10	–	–	1	1	9

FOOD	PORTION	CALS	TOTAL FAT	CHOL	SAT FAT	POLY FAT	MONO FAT	TRANS FAT	FIBER	SUGAR
Daybreaker Egg White & Turkey Bacon	1 (5 oz)	320	13	40	7	–	–	1	3	7
Daybreaker Veggie	1 (5.5 oz)	370	16	180	8	–	–	1	4	7
Mini Turkey Bacon	1 (2.4 oz)	190	10	85	3	–	–	0	1	1
Mini Turkey Sausage	1 (4 oz)	310	16	115	8	–	–	0	1	4
Muffin Carrot Cake	1 (5 oz)	510	24	70	7	–	–	0	2	47
Muffin Maine Blueberry	1 (5 oz)	620	38	100	12	–	–	1	1	33
Muffin Triple Berry	1 (5 oz)	600	34	100	10	–	–	1	1	42
Oatmeal Apple Cinnamon	1 serv (8 oz)	330	3	0	1	–	–	0	8	22
Oatmeal Blueberry Almond	1 serv (8 oz)	370	8	0	1	–	–	0	9	17
Oatmeal Classic	1 serv (6.6 oz)	260	3	0	1	–	–	0	7	8
Oatmeal Maple Brown Sugar Crunch	1 serv (7.2 oz)	206	4	5	1	–	–	0	7	16
Oatmeal Very Berry	1 serv (9 oz)	400	8	0	1	–	–	0	10	34
Sandwich Aged Cheddar Roast	1 (6.5 oz)	480	22	65	10	–	–	1	2	8
Sandwich Gouda Turkey Pesto	1 (7.2 oz)	510	24	80	13	–	–	1	2	7
Sandwich Italian Chicken Melt	1 (7 oz)	470	21	75	11	–	–	0	7	6
Sandwich Three Cheese	1 (5.2 oz)	500	25	60	14	–	–	1	1	9

CHICK-FIL-A
BEVERAGES

FOOD	PORTION	CALS	TOTAL FAT	CHOL	SAT FAT	POLY FAT	MONO FAT	TRANS FAT	FIBER	SUGAR
Coca-Cola	1 med	170	0	0	0	0	0	0	0	47
Coffee 100% Colombian	1 med	5	0	0	0	0	0	0	0	0
Diet Coke	1 med	0	0	0	0	0	0	0	0	0
Dr Pepper	1 med	180	0	0	0	0	0	0	0	48
Iced Tea Sweetened	1 med	130	0	0	0	0	0	0	0	32
Iced Tea Unsweetened	1 med	0	0	0	0	0	0	0	0	0
Lemonade	1 med	240	0	0	0	0	0	0	0	58
Lemonade Diet	1 med	20	0	0	0	0	0	0	0	2
Milkshake Chocolate	1 sm	600	23	75	14	–	–	0	1	86
Milkshake Peach	1 sm	780	19	65	11	–	–	0	1	118
Milkshake Strawberry	1 sm	610	23	75	13	–	–	0	1	85

BREAKFAST SELECTIONS

FOOD	PORTION	CALS	TOTAL FAT	CHOL	SAT FAT	POLY FAT	MONO FAT	TRANS FAT	FIBER	SUGAR
Bagel Multigrain Chicken Egg & Cheese	1	490	20	240	6	–	–	0	3	8
Biscuit Bacon Egg & Cheese	1	500	27	230	12	–	–	0	2	6
Biscuit Chicken	1	440	20	25	8	–	–	0	3	6

FOOD	PORTION	CALS	TOTAL FAT	CHOL	SAT FAT	POLY FAT	MONO FAT	TRANS FAT	FIBER	SUGAR
Biscuit Plain	1	310	14	0	7	–	–	0	2	5
Biscuit Sausage	1	590	39	45	15	–	–	0	2	5
Biscuit Spicy Chicken	1	450	20	30	8	–	–	0	2	5
Breakfast Burrito Chicken	1	450	20	260	8	–	–	0	2	3
Breakfast Burrito Sausage	1	510	28	270	12	–	–	0	2	3
Chick-N-Minis	3	280	10	40	3	–	–	0	1	5
Cinnamon Cluster	1 serv	430	17	30	7	–	–	0	2	29
Hashbrowns	1 serv	270	18	0	4	–	–	0	2	0
Yogurt Parfait	1	230	3	10	2	–	–	0	0	35
Yogurt Parfait w/ Chocolate Cookie Crumbs	1	240	5	10	2	–	–	0	0	36
Yogurt Parfait w/ Granola	1	290	6	10	2	–	–	0	1	39
DESSERTS										
Cheesecake	1 slice	310	23	115	13	–	–	1	1	14
Fudge Nut Brownie	1	370	19	25	6	–	–	0	3	28
Icedream	1 cup	290	7	25	5	–	–	0	0	49
Icedream Cone	1	170	4	15	2	–	–	0	0	25
Lemon Pie	1 slice	360	13	30	6	–	–	0	1	21
MAIN MENU SELECTIONS										
Chick-N-Strips	3	360	17	80	4	–	–	0	1	2
Cool Wrap Chargrilled Chicken	1	410	12	55	4	–	–	0	9	8
Cool Wrap Chicken Caesar	1	460	15	65	6	–	–	0	8	6
Cool Wrap Spicy Chicken	1	410	12	60	4	–	–	0	8	5
Hearty Breast of Chicken Soup	1 med	140	4	25	1	–	–	0	2	3
Nuggets	8	260	12	70	3	–	–	0	1	1
Sandwich Chargrilled Chicken	1	290	5	55	1	–	–	0	3	9
Sandwich Chargrilled Chicken Club	1	410	12	80	5	–	–	0	3	10
Sandwich Chicken	1	430	17	60	4	–	–	0	3	6
Sandwich Chicken Deluxe	1	490	22	70	6	–	–	0	3	8
Sandwich Chicken Salad On Wheat Bread	1	490	19	80	3	–	–	0	5	12
Sandwich Spicy Chicken	1	480	20	65	5	–	–	0	3	6
Sandwich Spicy Chicken Deluxe	1	570	27	80	8	–	–	0	4	8
Waffle Potato Fries	1 med	360	19	0	3	–	–	0	5	0

FOOD	PORTION	CALS	TOTAL FAT	CHOL	SAT FAT	POLY FAT	MONO FAT	TRANS FAT	FIBER	SUGAR
SALAD DRESSINGS AND SAUCES										
Dressing Berry Balsamic Vinaigrette Reduced Fat	½ pkg (1.25 oz)	70	2	0	0	–	–	0	0	9
Dressing Blue Cheese	½ pkg (1.25 oz)	160	16	20	3	–	–	0	0	1
Dressing Buttermilk Ranch	½ pkg (1.25 oz)	160	17	5	3	–	–	0	0	1
Dressing Caesar	½ pkg (1.25 oz)	160	17	30	3	–	–	0	0	0
Dressing Honey Mustard Fat Free	½ pkg (1.25 oz)	60	0	0	0	0	0	0	0	12
Dressing Italian Light	½ pkg (1.25 oz)	15	1	0	0	–	–	0	0	2
Dressing Spicy	½ pkg (1.25 oz)	140	14	5	2	–	–	0	0	1
Dressing Thousand Island	½ pkg (1.25 oz)	150	14	10	2	–	–	0	0	4
Sauce Barbecue	½ pkg (0.5 oz)	45	0	0	0	0	0	0	0	9
Sauce Buffalo	½ pkg (0.4 oz)	10	0	0	0	0	0	0	0	0
Sauce Buttermilk Ranch	½ pkg (0.4 oz)	110	12	5	2	–	–	0	0	1
Sauce Chick-fil-A	½ pkg (0.5 oz)	140	13	10	2	–	–	0	0	6
Sauce Honey Mustard	½ pkg (1.25 oz)	45	0	0	0	0	0	0	0	10
Sauce Honey Roasted BBQ	½ pkg	60	5	5	1	–	–	0	0	2
Sauce Polynesian	½ pkg (0.5 oz)	110	6	0	1	–	–	0	0	5
SALADS										
Carrot & Raisin Salad	1 med	260	12	5	2	–	–	0	4	32
Chargrilled & Fruit	1 serv	220	6	55	4	–	–	0	4	17
Chargrilled Chicken Garden Salad	1 serv	180	6	65	4	–	–	0	4	6
Chicken Salad Bacon & Egg	1 cup	350	22	120	4	–	–	0	1	6
Chick-N-Strips Salad	1 serv	460	22	90	6	–	–	0	5	6
Cole Slaw	1 med	360	31	20	5	–	–	0	3	16
Croutons Garlic & Butter	1 pkg	60	2	0	0	–	–	0	0	1
Fruit Cup	1 serv	70	0	0	0	0	0	0	2	14
Harvest Nut Granola	1 pkg	60	3	0	0	–	–	0	1	3
Honey Roasted Sunflower Kernels	1 pkg	90	7	0	1	–	–	0	1	1
Side Salad	1 serv	70	5	15	3	–	–	0	2	2
Southwest Chargrilled Salad	1 serv	240	9	60	4	–	–	0	5	6
Tortilla Strips	1 pkg	80	4	0	0	–	–	0	1	1

FOOD	PORTION	CALS	TOTAL FAT	CHOL	SAT FAT	POLY FAT	MONO FAT	TRANS FAT	FIBER	SUC
DAIRY QUEEN										
BEVERAGES										
Arctic Rush All Flavors	1 sm (13.6 oz)	210	0	0	0	0	0	0	0	41
Arctic Rush Float All Flavors	1 sm (13.2 oz)	330	6	20	4	–	–	0	0	61
Arctic Rush Freeze All Flavors	1 sm (11.8 oz)	380	10	35	6	–	–	1	0	58
Barq's	1 sm (17 oz)	180	0	0	0	0	0	0	0	48
Coca-Cola	1 sm (16.8 oz)	160	0	0	0	0	0	0	0	43
Coffee Black	1 (12 oz)	0	0	0	0	0	0	0	0	0
Diet Coca-Cola	1 sm (16.5 oz)	0	0	0	0	0	0	0	0	0
Diet Pepsi	1 sm (17 oz)	0	0	0	0	0	0	0	0	0
Dr Pepper	1 sm (16.8 oz)	160	0	0	0	0	0	0	0	43
Lemonade Chiller Classic	1 sm (12.4 oz)	250	0	0	0	0	0	0	0	54
Lemonade Chiller Strawberry	1 sm (13.8 oz)	280	0	0	0	0	0	0	0	61
Malt Banana	1 sm (13 oz)	540	19	45	14	–	–	1	1	65
Malt Caramel	1 sm (13.3 oz)	610	20	50	15	–	–	1	0	72
Malt Cherry	1 sm (13.3 oz)	560	19	54	14	–	–	1	0	71
Malt Chocolate	1 sm (13.3 oz)	590	21	45	14	–	–	1	1	79
Malt Hot Fudge	1 sm (13.3 oz)	620	22	45	18	–	–	1	1	73
Malt Peanut Butter	1 sm (13.3 oz)	700	34	45	16	–	–	1	1	65
Malt Strawberry	1 sm (13.3 oz)	550	19	45	14	–	–	1	0	68
Malt Vanilla	1 sm (13.3 oz)	580	19	50	14	–	–	1	0	73
Milk 2%	8 oz	110	5	15	3	–	–	0	0	11
MooLatte Cappuccino	1 sm (13 oz)	450	16	30	12	–	–	1	0	58
MooLatte Caramel	1 sm (13.5 oz)	520	16	35	13	–	–	1	0	64
MooLatte French Vanilla	1 sm (13.6 oz)	500	15	30	12	–	–	1	0	67
MooLatte Mocha	1 sm (13.2 oz)	500	19	30	13	–	–	1	0	65
Mountan Dew	1 sm (17 oz)	190	0	0	0	0	0	0	0	51
Mug	1 sm (17 oz)	160	0	0	0	0	0	0	0	47
Pepsi	1 sm (16.5 oz)	160	0	0	0	0	0	0	0	44
Shake Banana	1 sm (12.6 oz)	480	18	45	14	–	–	1	1	56
Shake Caramel	1 sm (12.8 oz)	560	20	50	15	–	–	1	0	63
Shake Cherry	1 sm (12.8 oz)	500	18	45	14	–	–	1	0	61
Shake Chocolate	1 sm (12.8 oz)	540	20	45	14	–	–	1	1	69
Shake Hot Fudge	1 sm (12.8 oz)	560	22	45	17	–	–	1	1	64
Shake Peanut Butter	1 sm (12.8 oz)	640	33	45	16	–	–	1	1	56
Shake Strawberry	1 sm (12.8 oz)	490	18	45	14	–	–	1	0	59
Shake Vanilla	1 sm (12.8 oz)	520	19	45	14	–	–	1	0	63
Sierra Mist	1 sm (17 oz)	170	0	0	0	0	0	0	0	43
Sprite	1 sm (17 oz)	150	0	0	0	0	0	0	0	42

FOOD	PORTION	CALS	TOTAL FAT	CHOL	SAT FAT	POLY FAT	MONO FAT	TRANS FAT	FIBER	SUGAR
BREAKFAST SELECTIONS										
Biscuit Sandwich Bacon	1 (4.8 oz)	380	24	185	9	–	–	1	1	1
Biscuit Sandwich Ham	1 (5.4 oz)	360	21	185	8	–	–	1	1	2
Biscuit Sandwich Sausage	1 (5.4 oz)	440	30	195	10	–	–	1	1	1
Biscuit Twin Pack Sausage	1 (6.3 oz)	600	36	50	15	–	–	0	2	2
Biscuits & Gravy	1 serv (12.8 oz)	730	47	15	17	–	–	2	2	4
Hashbrowns	1 serv (2.5 oz)	190	12	0	3	–	–	1	2	0
Platter Country	1 (11 oz)	780	46	340	16	–	–	2	4	3
Platter Pancake	1 (5.6 oz)	310	6	0	1	–	–	0	3	9
Platter Ultimate Hashbrown	1 (12.4 oz)	660	43	370	14	–	–	3	5	1
Ultimate Breakfast Burrito Ultimate	1 (10 oz)	640	37	210	12	–	–	2	4	2
CHILDREN'S MENU SELECTIONS										
Applesauce	1 serv (4 oz)	90	0	0	0	0	0	0	1	22
Banana	1 (4.4 oz)	110	0	0	0	0	0	0	3	15
Cheeseburger	1 (5.5 oz)	400	18	65	9	–	–	1	1	8
Chicken Strips	2 (2.8 oz)	220	12	40	2	–	–	0	2	0
Fries	1 serv (2.5 oz)	190	8	0	1	–	–	0	2	0
Grilled Cheese	1 (3.6 oz)	320	13	35	8	–	–	0	1	2
Hot Dog	1 (3.9 oz)	290	17	35	7	–	–	1	1	4
ICE CREAM										
Banana Split	1 (13 oz)	520	14	30	10	–	–	1	4	73
Blizzard Banana Cream Pie	1 sm (10.8 oz)	570	21	50	14	–	–	1	1	64
Blizzard Banana Split	1 sm (10.4 oz)	440	14	45	9	–	–	1	1	58
Blizzard Butterfinger	1 sm (9.2 oz)	460	17	45	12	–	–	1	1	58
Blizzard Chocolate Xtreme	1 sm (10 oz)	650	29	50	16	–	–	1	2	69
Blizzard Cookie Dough	1 sm (11.2 oz)	710	28	55	16	–	–	1	1	75
Blizzard Double Fudge Cookie Dough	1 sm (11.3 oz)	750	32	55	16	–	–	1	2	77
Blizzard French Silk Pie	1 sm (10.1 oz)	670	30	50	19	–	–	1	1	69
Blizzard Georgia Mud Fudge	1 sm (10 oz)	680	35	50	13	–	–	1	3	63
Blizzard Hawaiian	1 sm (9.9 oz)	440	15	40	10	–	–	1	1	55
Blizzard Heath	1 sm (10 oz)	600	26	50	16	–	–	1	1	73
Blizzard Midnight Truffle	1 sm (12 oz)	750	37	55	21	–	–	1	3	80
Blizzard Mint Oreo	1 sm (10 oz)	560	18	40	10	–	–	1	1	69
Blizzard Oreo CheeseQuake	1 sm (9.7 oz)	580	25	75	14	–	–	1	1	58
Blizzard Oreo Cookies	1 sm (9.9 oz)	550	20	40	10	–	–	1	1	61
Blizzard Reese's Peanut Butter Cups	1 sm (10 oz)	530	21	45	11	–	–	1	1	62

FOOD	PORTION	CALS	TOTAL FAT	CHOL	SAT FAT	POLY FAT	MONO FAT	TRANS FAT	FIBER	SUG
Blizzard Snickers	1 sm (11.4 oz)	670	26	50	13	–	–	1	1	83
Blizzard Strawberry CheeseQuake	1 sm (9.8 oz)	510	20	75	13	–	–	1	0	54
Buster Bar Treat	1 (5.2 oz)	460	28	15	16	–	–	0	2	36
Cake 8 Inch Round	1/8 (7.3 oz)	410	15	30	11	–	–	1	1	46
Cake Blizzard Chocolate Xtreme 8 Inch	1/8 cake (8.7 oz)	620	29	35	20	–	–	1	2	64
Cake Blizzard Oreo 8 Inch	1/8 (8 oz)	550	24	30	17	–	–	0	1	58
Cake Blizzard Reese's Peanut Butter Cups 8 Inch	1/8 (8.4 oz)	580	27	30	19	–	–	0	2	62
Cone Chocolate	1 sm (5 oz)	240	7	20	5	–	–	0	0	25
Cone Vanilla	1 sm (5 oz)	230	7	25	5	–	–	0	0	26
Cone Dipped Chocolate	1 sm (5.5 oz)	330	15	25	12	–	–	0	0	31
Cone Kids' Chocolate	1 (3.5 oz)	180	5	15	4	–	–	0	0	17
Cone Kids' Dipped Chocolate	1 (3.7 oz)	220	9	15	7	–	–	0	0	30
Cone Kids' Vanilla	1 (3.5 oz)	170	5	15	3	–	–	0	0	18
Dilly Bar Butterscotch	1 (3 oz)	210	11	15	9	–	–	0	0	20
Dilly Bar Cherry	1 (3 oz)	210	12	15	8	–	–	0	0	20
Dilly Bar Chocolate	1 (3 oz)	240	15	15	9	–	–	0	1	20
Dilly Bar Chocolate Mint	1 (3 oz)	240	15	15	9	–	–	0	1	20
Dilly Bar Heath	1 (3 oz)	220	13	15	10	–	–	0	0	22
Dilly Bar No Sugar Added	1 (3 oz)	190	13	15	10	–	–	0	5	5
DQ Heart Cake	1/10 cake (5 oz)	290	11	20	8	–	–	1	1	32
DQ Log Cake	1/8 cake (5 oz)	310	12	15	8	–	–	1	1	33
DQ Sandwich	1 (3 oz)	190	5	10	3	–	–	0	1	18
DQ Sheet Cake	1/24 cake (5.4 oz)	320	13	20	9	–	–	1	1	35
Fudge Bar	1 (2.3 oz)	50	0	0	0	0	0	0	6	4
Oreo Brownie Earthquake Treat	1 (10.7 oz)	740	27	65	15	–	–	1	2	86
Parfait Peanut Buster	1 (10.6 oz)	710	31	35	18	–	–	1	3	71
Peanut Butter Bash	1 (9 oz)	580	27	35	15	–	–	1	2	55
Pecan Mudslide Treat	1 (9.6 oz)	640	30	35	12	–	–	1	2	58
Starkiss Bar Cherry	1 (3 oz)	80	0	0	0	0	0	0	0	17
Starkiss Bar Stars & Stripes	1 (3 oz)	80	0	0	0	0	0	0	0	17
Strawberry Shortcake	1 (8.9 oz)	480	17	70	13	–	–	1	1	62
Sundae Banana	1 sm (5.7 oz)	230	7	25	5	–	–	0	1	29
Sundae Caramel	1 sm (5.7 oz)	300	8	25	5	–	–	0	0	35
Sundae Cherry	1 sm (5.7 oz)	240	7	25	5	–	–	0	0	33
Sundae Chocolate	1 sm (5.7 oz)	280	8	25	5	–	–	0	1	41

FOOD	PORTION	CALS	TOTAL FAT	CHOL	SAT FAT	POLY FAT	MONO FAT	TRANS FAT	FIBER	SUGAR
Sundae Hot Fudge	1 sm (5.7 oz)	300	10	25	8	–	–	0	0	36
Sundae Marshmallow	1 sm (5.7 oz)	290	7	25	5	–	–	0	0	42
Sundae Peanut Butter	1 sm (5.7 oz)	390	22	25	7	–	–	0	1	28
Sundae Pineapple	1 sm (5.7 oz)	230	7	25	5	–	–	0	0	32
Sundae Strawberry	1 sm (6.7 oz)	260	7	25	5	–	–	0	0	36
Sundae Waffle Bowl Chocolate Covered Strawberry	1 (11.2 oz)	760	38	30	30	–	–	1	2	74
Sundae Waffle Bowl Fudge Brownie Temptation	1 (11.2 oz)	940	48	40	22	–	–	1	2	89
Sundae Waffle Bowl Turtle	1 (10.7 oz)	810	35	35	18	–	–	1	2	72
Vanilla Orange Bar	1 (2.3 oz)	60	0	0	0	0	0	0	6	4
Waffle Cone Chocolate Coated w/ Soft Serve	1 (8.6 oz)	540	21	35	13	–	–	1	1	57
Waffle Cone w/ Soft Serve	1 (7.9 oz)	420	13	35	7	–	–	1	0	47
MAIN MENU SELECTIONS										
Breaded Mushrooms	1 serv (4 oz)	250	9	0	–	–	–	0	2	1
Burger DQ Ultimate	1 (9 oz)	780	48	150	22	–	–	2	1	7
Cheese Curds	1 serv (4.9 oz)	550	45	150	25	–	–	0	0	0
Cheeseburger Deluxe	1 (6.2 oz)	400	19	65	9	–	–	1	1	9
Cheeseburger Deluxe Double	1 (8.7 oz)	640	34	125	18	–	–	2	1	9
Cheeseburger Original	1 (5.5 oz)	400	18	65	9	–	–	1	1	8
Cheeseburger Original Double	1 (7.9 oz)	630	34	125	18	–	–	2	1	9
Chick Strip Basket w/ Country Gravy	4 pieces (15.2 oz)	1030	53	80	9	–	–	1	9	4
Chili	1 cup (8 oz)	470	16	55	7	–	–	0	2	2
Chili Cheese Dog	1 (4.8 oz)	380	24	55	11	–	–	1	1	3
Chili Cheese Dog Foot-Long	1 (8.2 oz)	670	43	95	19	–	–	2	2	5
Chili Dog	1 (4.8 oz)	330	20	40	8	–	–	1	1	5
Corn Dog	1 (2.6 oz)	260	15	20	4	–	–	0	1	7
French Fries	1 reg (4 oz)	310	13	0	2	–	–	0	3	0
Fries Chili Cheese	1 serv (15 oz)	1020	51	55	15	–	–	1	10	4
GrillBurger ½ Lb FlameThrower	1 (11.3 oz)	1000	74	170	26	–	–	2	2	9
GrillBurger ½ Lb w/ Cheese	1 (11.3 oz)	800	51	135	20	–	–	2	3	13
GrillBurger ¼ Lb Bacon Cheese	1 (8.5 oz)	630	37	95	13	–	–	1	2	13

FOOD	PORTION	CALS	TOTAL FAT	CHOL	SAT FAT	POLY FAT	MONO FAT	TRANS FAT	FIBER	SUGAR
GrillBurger ¼ Lb Mushroom Swiss	1 (6.9 oz)	570	35	75	11	–	–	1	5	8
GrillBurger ¼ Lb w/ Cheese	1 (8.1 oz)	540	30	70	11	–	–	1	3	13
Hamburger Deluxe	1 (5.7 oz)	350	14	50	7	–	–	1	1	9
Hamburger Deluxe Double	1 (7.7 oz)	540	26	100	13	–	–	1	1	9
Hot Dog	1 (4 oz)	290	17	35	7	–	–	1	1	4
Hot Dog Foot-Long	1 (7 oz)	560	35	65	14	–	–	1	2	6
Onion Rings	1 serv (4 oz)	360	16	0	2	–	–	0	2	3
Popcorn Shrimp Basket	1 (15 oz)	1000	49	125	22	–	–	0	7	3
Quesadilla Basket Chicken	1 (18 oz)	1160	60	115	25	–	–	2	6	7
Quesadilla Basket Veggie	1 (16.2 oz)	1100	59	90	25	–	–	2	7	6
Sandwich Barbecue Beef	1 (5 oz)	350	14	40	4	–	–	1	2	8
Sandwich Barbecue Pork	1 (5 oz)	310	9	50	3	–	–	0	2	9
Sandwich Crispy Chicken	1 (7.4 oz)	600	30	55	5	–	–	0	7	8
Sandwich Crispy Fish	1 (6.5 oz)	470	22	20	3	–	–	0	2	7
Sandwich Crispy Flame Thrower Chicken	1 (9.4 oz)	830	51	95	11	–	–	0	8	9
Sandwich Grilled Chicken	1 (6.3 oz)	360	15	50	3	–	–	0	1	5
Sandwich Iron Grilled Cheese	1 (5 oz)	420	14	35	8	–	–	0	2	3
Sandwich Iron Grilled Classic Club	1 (9.4 oz)	600	24	85	8	–	–	0	3	4
Sandwich Iron Grilled Supreme BLT	1 (6 oz)	600	34	75	9	–	–	0	2	2
Sandwich Iron Grilled Turkey	1 (8.2 oz)	550	23	85	7	–	–	0	2	2
Wrap Crispy Chicken	1 (4 oz)	350	21	35	5	–	–	0	2	1
Wrap Crispy Flame Thrower Chicken	1 (4 oz)	360	22	35	5	–	–	0	2	1
Wrap Grilled Chicken	1 (4 oz)	280	15	30	4	–	–	0	1	1
SALAD DRESSINGS AND SAUCES										
Country Gravy	1 serv (4 oz)	90	6	0	2	–	–	0	0	1
Dipping Sauce Bleu Cheese	1 serv (2 oz)	210	21	5	4	–	–	0	0	4
Dipping Sauce Honey Mustard	1 serv (2 oz)	250	21	20	3	–	–	0	0	9
Dipping Sauce Ranch	1 serv (2 oz)	320	35	20	5	–	–	1	0	2
Dipping Sauce Sweet & Sour	1 serv (2 oz)	90	0	0	0	0	0	0	0	22
Dipping Sauce Wild Buffalo	1 serv (1.3 oz)	110	12	0	2	–	–	0	0	0
Dressing Italian Fat Free	1 serv (1.5 oz)	15	0	0	0	0	0	0	0	2
Dressing Ranch Fat Free	1 serv (1.5 oz)	35	0	0	0	0	0	0	0	4
Dressing Red French Fat Free	1 serv (1.5 oz)	40	0	0	0	0	0	0	0	7

FOOD	PORTION	CALS	TOTAL FAT	CHOL	SAT FAT	POLY FAT	MONO FAT	TRANS FAT	FIBER	SUGAR
Dressing Thousand Island Fat Free	1 serv (1.5 oz)	60	0	0	0	0	0	0	0	10
SALADS										
Crispy Chicken	1 (14.9 oz)	470	26	85	9	–	–	0	7	8
Grilled Chicken	1 (14.9 oz)	330	15	80	8	–	–	0	4	8
Side Salad	1 (4 oz)	20	0	0	0	0	0	0	2	3

DENNY'S

BEVERAGES

FOOD	PORTION	CALS	TOTAL FAT	CHOL	SAT FAT	POLY FAT	MONO FAT	TRANS FAT	FIBER	SUGAR
Apple Juice	1 sm (10 oz)	141	0	0	0	0	0	0	0	11
Cappuccino	1 (8 oz)	100	2	0	2	–	–	0	1	24
Chocolate Milk	1 sm (10 oz)	160	3	10	2	–	–	0	1	25
Hot Chocolate	1 (8 oz)	100	2	0	2	–	–	0	1	24
Iced Tea Raspberry	1 serv (16 oz)	78	0	0	0	0	0	0	0	–
Lemonade	1 serv (15 oz)	150	0	0	0	0	0	0	0	31
Milk	1 sm (10 oz)	130	5	20	3	–	–	0	0	12
Orange Juice	1 sm (10 oz)	140	0	0	0	0	0	0	0	30
Ruby Red Grapefruit	1 sm (10 oz)	164	0	0	0	0	0	0	0	36
Tomato Juice	1 sm (10 oz)	56	0	0	0	0	0	0	2	–

BREAKFAST SELECTIONS

FOOD	PORTION	CALS	TOTAL FAT	CHOL	SAT FAT	POLY FAT	MONO FAT	TRANS FAT	FIBER	SUGAR
All American Slam w/o Choices	1 serv (10 oz)	800	68	775	25	–	–	0	1	1
Bacon Strips	4	140	11	30	4	–	–	0	0	1
Bacon Turkey	4 slices	150	8	65	2	–	–	0	0	0
Banana	1	110	0	0	0	0	0	0	4	14
Egg	1 (2 oz)	120	11	210	3	–	–	0	0	0
Eggs White	1 serv (4 oz)	50	1	0	0	–	–	0	0	0
English Muffin w/o Margarine	1	130	1	0	0	–	–	0	1	1
Grand Slam Slugger w/o Choices	1 serv (13 oz)	780	42	475	13	–	–	0	3	13
Grapes	1 serv (3 oz)	55	0	0	0	0	0	0	4	13
Grits w/ Margarine	1 serv (12 oz)	220	3	0	1	–	–	0	3	0
Ham Slice Grilled Honey	1 (3 oz)	120	5	45	4	–	–	1	0	6
Hash Browns	1 serv	210	12	0	3	–	–	0	2	1
Hash Browns Cheddar Cheese	1 serv (5 oz)	300	19	20	7	–	–	0	2	2
Hash Browns Everything	1 serv (8 oz)	340	21	20	8	–	–	0	2	3
Lumberjack Slam w/o Choices	1 serv (15 oz)	940	47	555	17	–	–	1	4	19

FOOD	PORTION	CALS	TOTAL FAT	CHOL	SAT FAT	POLY FAT	MONO FAT	TRANS FAT	FIBER	SUGAR
Moon Over My Hammy Omelette w/ Hash Browns w/o Choices	1 serv (16 oz)	770	53	790	18	–	–	0	2	5
Oatmeal w/ Milk	1 serv (16 oz)	290	8	20	4	–	–	0	4	20
Omelette Southern w/ Hash Browns w/o Bread	1 serv (18 oz)	1070	80	795	30	–	–	0	4	3
Omelette Veggie Cheese w/o Choices	1 serv (13 oz)	460	33	740	12	–	–	0	2	4
Omelette w/ Hash Browns w/o Choices	1 serv (16 oz)	700	46	770	13	–	–	0	2	5
Pancakes Buttermilk	2	330	4	0	1	–	–	0	2	12
Platter Chocolate Chip Pancakes w/o Meat	1 serv (13 oz)	640	22	480	9	–	–	0	4	28
Sausage Links	4 (3 oz)	370	34	70	13	–	–	0	3	0
Senior Omelette w/o Choices	1 serv (9 oz)	470	37	510	15	–	–	0	1	3
Senior Scrambled Eggs & Cheddar	1 serv (13 oz)	870	48	525	18	–	–	0	4	12
Senior Slam Belgian Waffle w/ Egg w/o Choices	1 serv (8 oz)	450	31	455	16	–	–	0	0	1
Skillet Bananas Foster French Toast w/o Meat	1 serv (15 oz)	860	33	720	9	–	–	0	3	44
Slam Belgian Waffle w/ Margarine w/o Syrup	1 serv (13 oz)	1030	77	715	27	–	–	0	2	2
Slam Everyday Value w/ Bacon	1 serv (12 oz)	650	30	440	8	–	–	0	2	13
Slam Everyday Value w/ Sausage	1 serv (13 oz)	760	42	460	12	–	–	0	3	12
Slam French Toast	1 serv (15 oz)	940	55	850	17	–	–	0	3	13
Ultimate Omelette w/o Choices	1 serv (12 oz)	620	48	740	11	–	–	0	2	3
CHILDREN'S MENU SELECTIONS										
Jr Grand Slam	1 serv (5 oz)	380	19	235	6	–	–	0	2	7
Oreo Blender Blaster	1 serv (12 oz)	680	33	90	17	–	–	0	3	65
Pancake Softball w/ Meat	1 serv (4 oz)	250	11	20	4	–	–	0	1	5
Pancakes Chocolate Chip-In	1 serv (7 oz)	450	18	25	7	–	–	0	3	17
Pit Stop Pizza w/o Side	1 serv (8 oz)	590	26	35	6	–	–	0	5	4
Slam Dribblers	1 serv (6 oz)	410	11	10	3	–	–	0	2	41
Slap Shot Slider w/o Side	1 (4 oz)	310	15	60	6	–	–	1	1	3
Spaghetti Set Go w/o Side	1 serv (6 oz)	260	7	0	2	–	–	0	7	4
Track & Cheese w/o Side	1 serv (7 oz)	340	11	25	3	–	–	0	2	11

DESSERTS

FOOD	PORTION	CALS	TOTAL FAT	CHOL	SAT FAT	POLY FAT	MONO FAT	TRANS FAT	FIBER	SUGAR
Apple Crisp A La Mode	1 serv (13 oz)	740	21	35	9	–	–	0	5	89
Blender Blaster Oreo	1 serv (14 oz)	890	44	105	20	–	–	0	3	77
Cake Carrot	1 serv (8 oz)	820	45	125	16	–	–	0	2	77
Cake Hershey's Chocolate	1 serv (5 oz)	580	28	40	15	–	–	0	2	55
Cheesecake New York Style	1 serv (7 oz)	640	41	195	26	–	–	0	0	44
Float Rootbeer or Cola	1 (16 oz)	430	17	65	9	–	–	0	0	63
Hot Fudge Brownie A La Mode	1 serv (9 oz)	830	37	65	18	–	–	0	4	95
Milkshake	1 (12 oz)	560	26	100	16	–	–	0	tr	65
Pie Apple	1 serv (7 oz)	480	22	0	9	–	–	0	3	35
Pie Chocolate Peanut Butter Silk	1 serv (6 oz)	680	47	70	24	–	–	0	4	39
Pie Coconut Cream	1 serv (7 oz)	630	39	0	24	–	–	0	1	43
Pie Cookies & Cream	1 serv (7 oz)	630	39	5	29	–	–	0	3	44
Pie French Silk	1 serv (5 oz)	770	57	105	30	–	–	2	2	38
Pie Key Lime	1 serv (7 oz)	560	20	25	8	–	–	4	0	68
Pie Lemon Meringue	1 serv (7 oz)	500	19	0	11	–	–	0	1	56
Pie Pecan	1 serv (7 oz)	730	36	110	12	–	–	0	2	36
Pie Pumpkin	1 serv (7 oz)	500	18	80	8	–	–	0	3	34
Sundae Oreo	1 (9 oz)	760	37	60	21	–	–	0	3	76
Sundae Single Scoop	1 (4 oz)	300	16	40	11	–	–	0	1	16
Topping Cherry	1 serv (2 oz)	57	0	0	0	0	0	0	0	12
Topping Chocolate	1 serv (2 oz)	133	1	0	0	–	–	0	1	32
Topping Fudge	1 serv (2 oz)	201	10	3	7	–	–	0	1	29
Topping Strawberry	1 serv (2 oz)	77	1	0	0	–	–	0	1	–

MAIN MENU SELECTIONS

FOOD	PORTION	CALS	TOTAL FAT	CHOL	SAT FAT	POLY FAT	MONO FAT	TRANS FAT	FIBER	SUGAR
Basket Of Puppies w/o Syrup	10 pieces	520	11	0	2	–	–	0	3	16
Burger Bacon Cheddar w/o Choices	1 (15 oz)	900	50	160	22	–	–	0	3	10
Burger Classic & Fries	1 serv (19 oz)	1190	62	110	21	–	–	0	8	11
Burger Mushroom Swiss w/o Choices	1 (18 oz)	880	49	130	22	–	–	0	4	13
Burger Veggie w/ Dressing w/o Choices	1 (11 oz)	520	12	20	5	–	–	0	9	23
Cheeseburger Double w/o Choices	1 serv (23 oz)	1420	87	260	41	–	–	5	4	12
Chicken Strips Sweet & Tangy BBQ w/o Dipping Sauce	1 serv (13 oz)	820	30	115	0	–	–	0	58	29

FOOD	PORTION	CALS	TOTAL FAT	CHOL	SAT FAT	POLY FAT	MONO FAT	TRANS FAT	FIBER	SUGAR
Chicken Wings Sweet & Tangy BBQ	1 serv (8 oz)	450	18	185	5	–	–	0	1	38
Chicken Wings w/ Buffalo Sauce	1 serv (8 oz)	330	20	185	5	–	–	0	1	2
Chopped Steak Mushroom Swiss w/o Choices	1 serv (13 oz)	900	66	165	28	–	–	1	1	4
Chopped Steak Spicy Cowboy w/o Choices	1 serv (15 oz)	1050	63	170	27	–	–	0	3	41
Club Sandwich w/o Choices	1 (10 oz)	550	32	50	5	–	–	0	3	7
Coleslaw	1 serv (5 oz)	260	22	35	4	–	–	0	3	12
Corn	1 serv (4 oz)	130	3	0	0	–	–	0	1	3
Cottage Cheese	1 serv (3 oz)	70	2	10	1	–	–	0	0	3
Country Fried Steak w/ Gravy	1 serv (13 oz)	990	65	75	23	–	–	0	6	0
Dippable Veggies w/o Dressing	1 serv (2.5 oz)	30	0	0	0	0	0	0	1	3
Fiesta Corn	1 serv (4 oz)	100	0	0	0	0	0	0	3	4
Fit Fare Grilled Tilapia	1 serv (17 oz)	600	11	110	3	–	–	0	3	7
Fit Fare Sweet & Tangy BBQ Chicken w/ Vegetables & Tomatoes	1 serv (13 oz)	640	14	180	4	–	–	0	2	32
French Fries Salted	1 serv (5 oz)	430	23	0	5	–	–	0	5	0
Fried Shrimp Platter w/ Fries	1 serv (18 oz)	1050	59	150	11	–	–	0	13	24
Garlic Dinner Bread	2 pieces	170	9	0	2	–	–	0	1	0
Green Beans	1 serv (3 oz)	25	0	0	0	0	0	0	2	2
Haddock Fillet w/o Bread	1 serv (20 oz)	1330	81	130	14	–	–	1	8	18
Homestyle Meatloaf w/ Gravy	1 serv (7 oz)	600	46	200	17	–	–	3	0	33
Lemon Pepper Tilapia w/o Choices	1 serv (13 oz)	640	27	160	14	–	–	0	2	3
Mashed Potatoes Plain	1 serv (5 oz)	170	7	20	1	–	–	0	1	1
Mashed Potatoes Smoked Cheddar	1 serv (4 oz)	120	5	10	3	–	–	0	1	1
Mozzarella Sticks w/o Sauce	1 serv (8 oz)	560	20	185	17	–	–	0	2	4
Onion Rings	1 serv (5 oz)	520	36	0	2	–	–	0	3	6
Quesadilla Cheese	1 (8 oz)	690	42	75	21	–	–	1	6	5
Ranchero Tilapia w/o Bread	1 serv (19 oz)	450	15	120	5	–	–	0	4	4
Sampler w/o Sauce	1 serv (17 oz)	1380	71	80	6	–	–	0	6	11
Sandwich Bacon Lettuce & Tomato w/o Choices	1 (7 oz)	520	35	35	8	–	–	0	2	7

FOOD	PORTION	CALS	TOTAL FAT	CHOL	SAT FAT	POLY FAT	MONO FAT	TRANS FAT	FIBER	SUGAR
Sandwich Chicken Ranch Melt w/o Choices	1 serv (12 oz)	790	38	85	11	–	–	0	3	3
Sandwich Fried Cheese Melt w/ Marinara Sauce w/o Choices	1 (12 oz)	830	40	75	17	–	–	0	3	8
Sandwich Hickory Grilled Chicken w/o Choices	1 (15 oz)	1020	60	115	14	–	–	0	4	15
Sandwich Patty Melt w/o Choices	1 (13 oz)	1040	73	160	29	–	–	0	4	10
Sandwich Philly Melt Prime Rib w/o Choices	1 serv (13 oz)	670	36	75	11	–	–	0	3	5
Sandwich Pulled BBQ Chicken w/ Coleslaw	1 serv (14 oz)	670	23	60	24	–	–	0	4	53
Sandwich Smoked Chicken Melt w/o Choices	1 (12 oz)	840	45	105	14	–	–	0	3	11
Sandwich Spicy Buffalo Chicken Melt w/o Choices	1 (15 oz)	860	48	70	12	–	–	0	3	3
Sandwich The Super Bird w/o Choices	1 (11 oz)	620	31	65	10	–	–	0	4	6
Seasoned Fries	1 serv (5 oz)	510	33	0	6	–	–	0	5	0
Senior Country Fried Steak w/o Choices	1 serv (8 oz)	520	34	40	12	–	–	3	3	0
Senior Grilled Chicken w/o Choices	1 serv (5 oz)	200	6	90	2	–	–	0	0	0
Senior Grilled Shrimp Skewer w/o Choices	1 serv (8 oz)	280	6	135	2	–	–	0	2	2
Senior Homestyle Meatloaf w/o Choices	1 serv (4 oz)	290	23	100	9	–	–	1	0	2
Senior Mini Burgers Bacon Cheddar w/o Choices	1 (11 oz)	720	39	115	19	–	–	0	2	7
Senior Sandwich Club w/o Choices	1 (10 oz)	570	34	60	7	–	–	0	4	7
Senior Sandwich Grilled Cheese Deluxe w/o Choices	1 (7 oz)	520	28	40	11	–	–	0	2	5
Senior Slam French Toast w/ Egg	1 serv (5 oz)	300	14	280	4	–	–	0	1	5
Senior Starter w/o Choice	1 serv (3 oz)	210	19	230	6	–	–	0	1	0
Shrimp Breaded	6	190	8	70	2	–	–	0	2	5
Shrimp Grilled Skewer	1	90	4	135	1	–	–	0	0	0

FOOD	PORTION	CALS	TOTAL FAT	CHOL	SAT FAT	POLY FAT	MONO FAT	TRANS FAT	FIBER	SUGAR
Skillet Bacon Chipotle Chicken w/o Sides	1 serv (7 oz)	360	18	125	7	–	–	0	0	3
Skillet Prime Rib Premium	1 serv (21 oz)	850	46	540	15	–	–	0	7	9
Skillet Santa Fe	1 serv (14 oz)	710	52	485	15	–	–	0	5	5
Skillet Ultimate	1 serv (15 oz)	740	56	475	17	–	–	0	6	5
Slamburger Bacon w/ Fries	1 serv (15 oz)	1030	59	350	24	–	–	0	2	9
Smothered Cheese Fries	1 serv (10 oz)	860	53	65	17	–	–	1	7	3
Spinach Sauteed	1 serv (2 oz)	70	6	0	1	–	–	0	2	0
Spinach w/ Pico De Gallo	1 serv (3 oz)	110	8	5	2	–	–	0	2	1
T-Bone Steak w/o Choices	1 serv (12 oz)	640	42	135	14	–	–	1	0	0
T-Bone Steak & Breaded Shrimp	1 serv (13 oz)	830	50	204	15	–	–	1	2	5
T-Bone Steak & Shrimp Skewer	1 serv (12 oz)	730	46	270	15	–	–	1	0	0
The Big Dipper w/ Salsa w/o Dipping Sauce	10 pieces	1230	50	85	23	–	–	0	14	13
Three Dip & Chips	1 serv (12 oz)	560	25	70	11	–	–	0	7	5
Tomatoes Slices	2	10	0	0	0	0	0	0	1	2
Tsing Tsing Chicken	1 serv (14 oz)	900	26	130	5	–	–	0	4	28
Vegetable Rice Pilaf	1 serv (5 oz)	190	3	0	0	–	–	0	2	2
Wrap Buffalo Chicken	1 (14 oz)	830	28	65	7	–	–	0	8	5
Zesty Nachos	1 serv (22 oz)	1340	61	210	29	–	–	0	12	10
SALAD DRESSINGS AND TOPPINGS										
BBQ Sweet & Spicy	1 serv (1.5 oz)	110	0	0	0	0	0	0	1	0
Cherry Topping	1 serv (3 oz)	86	0	0	0	0	0	0	0	12
Croutons	1 serv (0.25 oz)	90	3	0	0	–	–	0	0	0
Dressing Bleu Cheese	1 serv (1 oz)	110	11	20	3	–	–	0	0	1
Dressing Caesar	1 serv (1 oz)	100	10	5	0	–	–	2	0	0
Dressing French	1 serv (1 oz)	74	5	7	0	–	–	0	0	4
Dressing Honey Mustard	1 serv (1 oz)	160	15	10	0	–	–	3	0	4
Dressing Italian Fat Free	1 serv (1 oz)	9	0	0	0	0	0	0	0	2
Dressing Ranch	1 serv (1 oz)	130	14	5	3	–	–	0	0	0
Dressing Ranch Fat Free	1 serv (1 oz)	25	0	0	0	0	0	0	1	1
Dressing Thousand Island	1 serv (1 oz)	107	10	14	0	–	–	2	0	4
Pico De Gallo	1 serv (3 oz)	21	0	0	0	0	0	0	1	3
Sour Cream	1 serv (1.5 oz)	91	9	19	–	–	–	–	0	0
Syrup Maple Flavored	3 tbsp (1.5 oz)	143	0	0	0	0	0	0	0	28
Syrup Sugar Free Maple	1 serv (1.5 oz)	23	0	0	0	0	0	0	0	1
Whipped Margarine	1 tbsp	50	6	0	2	–	–	0	0	0

FOOD	PORTION	CALS	TOTAL FAT	CHOL	SAT FAT	POLY FAT	MONO FAT	TRANS FAT	FIBER	SUGAR
SALADS										
Cranberry Apple w/ Chicken w/o Dressing	1 serv (11 oz)	320	10	90	2	–	–	0	3	17
Deluxe Salad w/ Chicken Strips w/o Choices	1 serv (18 oz)	590	29	90	5	–	–	0	4	7
Deluxe Salad w/ Grilled Chicken Breast w/o Choices	1 serv (17 oz)	340	13	110	6	–	–	0	4	7
Nacho	1 serv (20 oz)	850	52	165	27	–	–	1	9	19
SOUPS										
Broccoli & Cheddar	1 serv (12 oz)	370	16	40	10	–	–	0	7	14
Chicken Noodle	1 serv (12 oz)	140	4	110	2	–	–	0	2	6
Clam Chowder	1 serv (12 oz)	270	17	35	12	–	–	0	1	12
Loaded Baked Potato	1 serv (12 oz)	310	23	45	11	–	–	0	2	5
Vegetable Beef	1 serv (12 oz)	140	5	10	0	–	–	0	3	3
DUNKIN' DONUTS										
BAKED SELECTIONS										
Coffee Roll	1	370	18	0	7	–	–	0	2	17
Donut Double Chocolate Cake	1	290	16	0	7	–	–	0	1	17
Donut Glazed	1	220	9	0	4	–	–	0	1	12
Donut Glazed Cake	1	320	18	25	8	–	–	0	1	18
Donut Triple Chocolate	1	420	27	0	12	–	–	0	2	22
French Cruller	1	250	20	35	9	–	–	0	0	10
Munchkin Glazed Cake	1	60	3	5	2	–	–	0	0	4
BEVERAGES										
Cappuccino	1 sm (10 oz)	80	4	15	3	–	–	0	0	7
Cappuccino Frozen w/ Skim Milk	1 sm (16 oz)	280	0	0	0	0	0	0	0	53
Cappuccino Frozen w/ Whole Milk w/ Sugar	1 sm (16 oz)	300	4	15	3	–	–	0	0	53
Cappuccino	1 sm (10 oz)	140	4	15	3	–	–	0	0	24
Coffee French Vanilla	1 sm (10 oz)	10	0	0	0	0	0	0	0	0
Coffee Hazelnut	1 sm (10 oz)	10	0	0	0	0	0	0	0	0
Coffee Mocha	1 sm (10 oz)	110	0	0	0	0	0	0	1	23
Coffee Mocha w/ Cream	1 sm (10 oz)	170	6	20	4	–	–	0	1	23
Coffee Raspberry	1 sm (10 oz)	15	0	0	0	0	0	0	0	0
Coffee White Chocolate w/ Cream	1 sm (10 oz)	160	6	20	4	–	–	0	0	19
Coffee w/ Milk	1 sm (10 oz)	25	1	5	1	–	–	0	0	1

FOOD	PORTION	CALS	TOTAL FAT	CHOL	SAT FAT	POLY FAT	MONO FAT	TRANS FAT	FIBER	SUGAR
Coffee w/ Skim Milk & Splenda	1 sm (10 oz)	25	0	0	0	0	0	0	0	2
Coffee w/ Splenda	1 sm (10 oz)	15	0	0	0	0	0	0	0	0
Coolatta Coffee w/ Cream	1 sm (16 oz)	400	23	80	14	–	–	1	0	43
Coolatta Coffee w/ Milk	1 sm (16 oz)	240	4	15	3	–	–	0	0	49
Coolatta Coffee w/ Skim Milk	1 sm (16 oz)	210	0	0	0	0	0	0	0	49
Coolatta Strawberry Fruit	1 sm (16 oz)	300	0	0	0	0	0	0	0	65
Coolatta Vanilla Bean	1 sm (16 oz)	430	6	20	4	–	–	0	0	86
Iced Coffee Mocha w/ Cream	1 sm (16 oz)	180	6	20	4	–	–	0	1	23
Iced Coffee White Chocolate w/ Cream	1 sm (16 oz)	170	6	20	4	–	–	0	1	19
Latte Caramel Swirl	1 sm (10 oz)	220	6	25	4	–	–	0	0	34
Latte Lite	1 sm (10 oz)	80	0	0	0	0	0	0	0	10
Latte Lite Vanilla	1 sm (10 oz)	90	0	0	0	0	0	0	0	10
Latte Mocha Raspberry	1 med (16 oz)	340	9	35	6	–	–	0	2	48
Latte Mocha Spice	1 med (16 oz)	330	9	35	6	–	–	0	2	48
Latte Mocha Swirl	1 sm (10 oz)	220	6	25	4	–	–	0	1	32
Latte w/ Sugar	1 sm (10 oz)	170	6	25	4	–	–	0	0	27
Latte White Chocolate	1 med (16 oz)	320	9	40	6	–	–	0	0	43
SANDWICHES										
Bagel Bacon Egg Cheese	1	510	17	195	6	–	–	0	5	7
English Muffin Egg White & Cheese	1	270	5	10	3	–	–	0	2	3
English Muffin Ham Egg White & Cheese	1	310	7	30	4	–	–	0	2	3
English Muffin Wheat Egg White & Cheese	1	260	6	10	3	–	–	0	2	3
English Muffin Wheat Ham Egg White & Cheese	1	300	8	30	4	–	–	0	2	3
Flatbread Grilled Cheese	1	380	18	45	9	–	–	1	1	2
Flatbread Ham & Cheese	1	320	11	40	5	–	–	0	1	2
Flatbread Turkey Cheddar & Bacon	1	410	20	50	7	–	–	0	1	2
Pressed Cuban	1	680	33	120	13	–	–	0	2	6
SOUPS										
Broccoli Cheddar	1 serv (8 oz)	190	11	35	6	–	–	0	2	5
Chicken Noodle	1 serv (8 oz)	130	3	45	1	–	–	0	1	1

FOOD	PORTION	CALS	TOTAL FAT	CHOL	SAT FAT	POLY FAT	MONO FAT	TRANS FAT	FIBER	SUGAR
EINSTEIN BROS BAGELS										
BAGELS AND BREADS										
Bagel Asiago Cheese	1 (4 oz)	310	5	15	3	–	–	0	2	5
Bagel Black Russian	1 (3.9 oz)	280	4	0	0	–	–	0	3	4
Bagel Blueberry	1 (3.8 oz)	300	1	0	0	–	–	0	3	11
Bagel Chocolate Chip	1 (3.8 oz)	290	3	0	1	–	–	0	3	10
Bagel Cinnamon Raisin	1 (3.8 oz)	290	1	0	0	–	–	0	3	13
Bagel Cinnamon Sugar	1 (3.9 oz)	290	3	0	1	–	–	1	2	12
Bagel Cranberry	1 (3.8 oz)	270	1	0	0	–	–	0	2	12
Bagel Croutons	1 serv (1 oz)	90	5	0	1	–	–	0	0	1
Bagel Egg	1 (3.5 oz)	300	5	120	2	–	–	0	2	6
Bagel Everything	1 (3.7 oz)	270	2	0	0	–	–	0	2	5
Bagel Garlic	1 (3.7 oz)	270	3	0	0	–	–	0	2	5
Bagel Green Chili	1 (5.4 oz)	350	8	25	5	–	–	0	2	6
Bagel Honey Whole Wheat	1 (3.6 oz)	260	1	0	0	–	–	0	3	8
Bagel Onion	1 (3.7 oz)	270	1	0	0	–	–	0	2	5
Bagel Plain	1 (3.5 oz)	260	1	0	0	–	–	0	2	5
Bagel Poppy	1 (3.7 oz)	280	3	0	0	–	–	0	2	5
Bagel Potato	1 (3.5 oz)	270	4	0	1	–	–	0	2	5
Bagel Power	1 (4 oz)	310	5	0	1	–	–	0	4	16
Bagel Pumpernickel	1 (3.5 oz)	240	2	0	0	–	–	0	3	4
Bagel Salt	1 (3.7 oz)	260	1	0	0	–	–	0	2	5
Bagel Sesame	1 (3.7 oz)	280	3	0	0	–	–	0	2	5
Bagel Six Cheese	1 (4.3 oz)	330	6	15	4	–	–	0	2	5
Bagel Spinach Florentine	1 (4.7 oz)	340	8	20	4	–	–	0	2	5
Bagel Poppers Cinnamon Sugar	1 (5 oz)	450	9	0	2	–	–	0	4	29
Bagel Poppers Pretzel w/ Nacho Cheese	1 (5 oz)	320	8	5	2	–	–	1	2	6
Bagel Poppers Sweet Cream Cheese	1 (6 oz)	440	7	5	2	–	–	0	3	30
Bagel Thin Singles Everything	1 (2 oz)	150	2	0	0	–	–	0	1	2
Bagel Thin Singles Honey Whole Wheat	1 (2 oz)	140	2	0	0	–	–	0	4	4
Bagel Thin Singles Plain	1 (2 oz)	140	1	0	0	–	–	0	1	2
Bread Ciabatta	1 serv (4.25 oz)	300	4	0	0	–	–	0	2	1
Pizza Bagel Pepperoni	1 (6 oz)	450	15	45	9	–	–	0	3	7
Roll Challah	1 (2.75 oz)	210	3	10	1	–	–	0	1	5

FOOD	PORTION	CALS	TOTAL FAT	CHOL	SAT FAT	POLY FAT	MONO FAT	TRANS FAT	FIBER	SUG
BEVERAGES										
Americano	1 reg (12 oz)	0	0	0	0	0	0	0	0	0
Barq's Root Beer	1 reg (20 oz)	260	0	0	0	0	0	0	0	75
Cafe Latte Nonfat Milk	1 reg (12 oz)	100	0	0	0	0	0	0	0	15
Cafe Latte Reduced Fat Milk	1 reg (12 oz)	150	7	25	4	–	–	0	0	15
Cappuccino	1 reg (12 oz)	140	8	25	5	–	–	0	0	11
Cappuccino Nonfat Milk	1 reg (12 oz)	70	0	5	0	0	0	0	0	11
Cappuccino Reduced Fat Milk	1 reg (12 oz)	90	4	15	2	–	–	0	0	8
Chai Tea Latte	1 reg (12 oz)	230	3	10	2	–	–	0	0	45
Chai Tea Latte Nonfat Milk	1 reg (12 oz)	210	0	0	0	0	0	0	0	45
Chai Tea Latte Reduced Fat Milk	1 reg (12 oz)	220	2	5	1	–	–	0	0	45
Coca-Cola	1 reg (20 oz)	230	0	0	0	0	0	0	0	65
Coca-Cola Cherry	1 reg (20 oz)	250	0	0	0	0	0	0	0	70
Coffee Black All Sizes	1	0	0	0	0	0	0	0	0	0
Diet Coke	1 reg (20 oz)	0	0	0	0	0	0	0	0	0
Espresso Single	1 (2 oz)	0	0	0	0	0	0	0	0	0
Fanta Orange	1 (20 oz)	270	0	0	0	0	0	0	0	73
Frozen Blended Cafe Caramel	1 (18 oz)	520	9	45	3	–	–	0	0	66
Frozen Blended Cafe Mocha	1 (18 oz)	510	8	40	3	–	–	0	0	64
Frozen Blended Strawberry	1 (18 oz)	450	19	65	14	–	–	0	3	64
Frozen Blended Wild Berry	1 (18 oz)	350	3	5	2	–	–	0	5	62
Half & Half	1 oz	40	3	15	2	–	–	0	0	1
Hi-C Fruit Punch	1 (20 oz)	270	0	0	0	0	0	0	0	74
Hot Chocolate	1 reg (12 oz)	270	8	25	5	–	–	0	1	36
Hot Chocolate Nonfat Milk	1 reg (12 oz)	220	2	5	1	–	–	0	1	36
Iced Americano	1 med	0	0	0	0	0	0	0	0	0
Iced Coffee	1 med	0	0	0	0	0	0	0	0	0
Iced Latte	1 med (12 oz)	110	6	20	4	–	–	0	0	9
Iced Latte Nonfat Milk	1 med (16 oz)	60	0	0	0	0	0	0	0	9
Iced Latte Reduced Fat Milk	1 med (16 oz)	90	4	15	3	–	–	0	0	9
Iced Mocha	1 med (16 oz)	220	6	15	4	–	–	0	0	32
Iced Mocha Nonfat Milk	1 med (16 oz)	180	0	0	0	0	0	0	0	33
Iced Mocha Reduced Fat Milk	1 med (16 oz)	200	4	15	2	–	–	0	0	33
Macchiato Caramel	1 reg (12 oz)	300	8	25	5	–	–	0	0	43
Macchiato Caramel Nonfat Milk	1 reg (12 oz)	260	0	5	0	0	0	0	0	50

FOOD	PORTION	CALS	TOTAL FAT	CHOL	SAT FAT	POLY FAT	MONO FAT	TRANS FAT	FIBER	SUGAR
Macchiato Caramel Reduced Fat Milk	1 reg (12 oz)	290	5	20	3	–	–	0	0	50
Minute Maid Lemonade Lite	1 reg (20 oz)	40	0	0	0	0	0	0	0	5
Mocha	1 reg (12 oz)	260	9	25	5	–	–	0	0	32
Mocha Nonfat Milk	1 reg (12 oz)	180	0	5	0	0	0	0	0	32
Mocha Reduced Fat Milk	1 reg (12 oz)	220	5	20	3	–	–	0	0	32
Nestea Iced Tea Unsweetened	1 reg (20 oz)	0	0	0	0	0	0	0	0	0
Pibb Xtra	1 reg (20 oz)	250	0	0	0	0	0	0	0	65
Skim Milk	8 oz	80	0	5	0	0	0	0	0	13
Sprite	1 reg (20 oz)	230	0	0	0	0	0	0	0	63
Whole Milk	8 oz	150	8	25	5	–	–	0	0	11
DESSERTS										
Cinnamon Twist	1 (4 oz)	370	18	0	7	–	–	0	2	19
Coffee Cake Apple Cinnamon	1 serv (7 oz)	700	28	5	10	–	–	0	1	57
Coffee Cake Chocolate Chip	1 serv (6.4 oz)	800	36	5	14	–	–	0	3	62
Coffee Cake Mixed Berry	1 serv (7 oz)	710	29	5	10	–	–	0	2	59
Cookie Chocolate Chip	1 (2.75 oz)	360	18	15	9	–	–	0	2	29
Cookie Chocolate Mudslide	1 (2.8 oz)	320	17	60	9	–	–	0	1	38
Cookie Iced Sugar	1 (3.7 oz)	480	15	25	7	–	–	0	1	51
Cookie Oatmeal Raisin	1 (3 oz)	320	11	25	5	–	–	0	2	31
Marshmallow Crispy Treat	1 (4 oz)	410	7	0	2	–	–	0	0	37
Muffin Blueberry	1 (5 oz)	480	23	100	3	–	–	0	1	35
Muffin Double Chocolate	1 (5 oz)	440	24	90	3	–	–	0	2	32
Muffin Strawberry White Chocolate	1 (6 oz)	500	22	85	5	–	–	0	1	44
Strudel Cinnamon Walnut	1 piece (6 oz)	640	35	70	15	–	–	0	4	26
SALAD DRESSINGS										
Caesar	1 serv (3 oz)	410	44	25	7	–	–	0	0	3
Vinaigrette Chipotle	1 serv (3 oz)	290	26	0	4	–	–	1	1	11
Vinaigrette Raspberry	1 serv (3 oz)	410	44	25	7	–	–	0	0	3
SALADS										
Bros Bistro	1 (10.5 oz)	820	68	25	11	–	–	1	7	29
Bros Bistro Half	1 serv (5.3 oz)	410	34	15	5	–	–	1	3	15
Bros Bistro w/ Chicken	1 (14.5 oz)	950	71	115	12	–	–	1	7	29
Bros Bistro w/ Chicken Half	1 serv (7.3 oz)	470	36	55	6	–	–	1	4	14
Caesar	1 (9.5 oz)	600	53	40	11	–	–	0	4	5
Caesar Half	1 serv (4.5 oz)	280	25	20	5	–	–	0	2	2
Caesar w/ Chicken	1 (14 oz)	730	56	130	12	–	–	0	4	5

FOOD	PORTION	CALS	TOTAL FAT	CHOL	SAT FAT	POLY FAT	MONO FAT	TRANS FAT	FIBER	S
Caesar w/ Chicken Half	1 (6.5 oz)	340	27	65	6	–	–	0	2	2
Chipotle	1 (11.7 oz)	590	37	20	8	–	–	1	11	14
Chipotle Half	1 serv (5.8 oz)	290	19	10	4	–	–	0	5	7
Chipotle w/ Chicken	1 (15.7 oz)	720	41	110	9	–	–	1	11	15
Chipotle w/ Chicken Half	1 serv (7.8 oz)	360	20	55	5	–	–	0	5	7
Fruit	1 (11 oz)	140	0	0	0	0	0	0	3	30
Fruit Cup	1 (5 oz)	60	0	0	0	0	0	0	2	14
Potato	1 serv (3 oz)	160	12	10	3	–	–	0	1	1
SANDWICHES										
Bagel Asiago Tasty Turkey	1 (13 oz)	540	18	90	10	–	–	0	4	9
Bagel Dogs Asiago	1 (7 oz)	550	28	55	12	–	–	1	2	5
Bagel Dogs Chicken Apple	1 (5 oz)	290	13	0	4	–	–	0	1	6
Bagel Dogs Original	1 (7 oz)	540	27	50	11	–	–	1	2	5
Bagel Thin Asparagus Mushroom & Swiss	1 (6 oz)	290	13	25	5	–	–	0	5	5
Bagel Thin BLT w/ Avocado	1 (7 oz)	400	25	30	5	–	–	0	7	7
Bagel Thin Panini Bacon & Cheese	1 (6 oz)	400	20	60	11	–	–	0	4	4
Bagel Thin Tuna	1 (8 oz)	320	16	30	3	–	–	0	5	7
Bagel Thin Turkey	1 (8 oz)	270	6	50	3	–	–	0	2	5
Bagel Thin Turkey Sausage w/ Salsa	1 (6 oz)	240	6	30	1	–	–	0	4	6
Breakfast Wrap Sante Fe	1 (12 oz)	720	37	445	15	–	–	0	6	8
Breakfast Wrap Spicy Elmo	1 (11 oz)	720	40	435	17	–	–	0	6	6
Challah Club Mex	1 (11 oz)	740	48	105	11	–	–	1	2	8
Deli Albacore Tuna Salad	1 (9 oz)	390	12	25	2	–	–	0	4	7
Deli Chicken Salad	1 (10 oz)	480	17	75	3	–	–	0	6	12
Deli Ham	1 (11 oz)	610	31	75	8	–	–	1	4	9
Deli Open Face Melts Ham & Swiss	1 (9 oz)	480	15	80	8	–	–	0	3	8
Deli Open Face Melts Turkey & Cheddar	1 (9 oz)	490	15	75	8	–	–	0	3	6
Deli Turkey Breast	1 (11 oz)	590	29	70	7	–	–	1	4	7
Egg Bacon & Cheddar	1 (9 oz)	590	25	410	11	–	–	0	2	8
Egg Cheese Only	1 (8 oz)	510	20	395	9	–	–	0	2	7
Egg Ham & Swiss	1 (10 oz)	550	20	415	9	–	–	0	2	8
Egg Spinach Mushroom & Swiss	1 (10 oz)	560	24	395	10	–	–	0	3	8
Egg Turkey Sausage & Cheddar	1 (10 oz)	580	24	425	10	–	–	0	2	8

FOOD	PORTION	CALS	TOTAL FAT	CHOL	SAT FAT	POLY FAT	MONO FAT	TRANS FAT	FIBER	SUGAR
Egg Paninis Southwest Turkey Sausage	1 (12 oz)	680	29	435	12	–	–	0	4	5
Egg Paninis Spinach & Bacon	1 (12 oz)	830	47	435	16	–	–	1	5	4
Nova Lox & Bagel	1 (9 oz)	480	18	45	9	–	–	0	3	10
Panini Italian Chicken	1 (13 oz)	820	41	135	13	–	–	1	5	3
Panini Turkey Club	1 (13 oz)	790	41	100	11	–	–	1	6	5
Wrap California Chicken	1 (16 oz)	720	35	130	11	–	–	0	9	7
Wrap Chipotle Turkey	1 (13 oz)	750	38	85	13	–	–	0	9	12
Wrap Turkey Tornado	1 (7 oz)	270	4	35	0	–	–	0	5	4
SOUPS										
Broccoli Cheese	1 cup (8.75 oz)	290	21	55	12	–	–	0	2	5
Chicken Noodle	1 cup (87.5 oz)	120	4	15	0	–	–	0	2	1
Turkey Chili	1 cup (8.75 oz)	170	5	25	0	–	–	0	5	5
SPREADS										
Butter Blend	1 serv (1 oz)	170	18	0	5	–	–	0	0	0
Cream Cheese Light Whipped Plain	1 serv (1.25 oz)	80	6	20	4	–	–	0	2	3
Cream Cheese Onion & Chive	1 serv (1.25 oz)	120	11	35	7	–	–	0	0	2
Cream Cheese Plain	1 serv (1.25 oz)	120	12	35	8	–	–	0	0	2
Cream Cheese Reduced Fat Blueberry	1 serv (1.25 oz)	120	9	25	6	–	–	0	0	9
Cream Cheese Reduced Fat Garden Vegetable	1 serv (1.25 oz)	110	9	25	6	–	–	0	0	2
Cream Cheese Reduced Fat Garlic Herb	1 serv (1.25 oz)	110	9	25	6	–	–	0	0	2
Cream Cheese Reduced Fat Honey Almond	1 serv (1.25 oz)	120	9	25	5	–	–	0	0	7
Cream Cheese Reduced Fat Jalapeno Salsa	1 serv (1.25 oz)	110	9	25	6	–	–	0	0	2
Cream Cheese Reduced Fat Plain	1 serv (1.25 oz)	110	9	25	6	–	–	0	0	2
Cream Cheese Reduced Fat Strawberry	1 serv (1.25 oz)	120	9	25	6	–	–	0	0	7
Cream Cheese Reduced Fat Sundried Tomato Basil	1 serv (1.25 oz)	110	9	0	6	–	–	0	0	2
Cream Cheese Smoked Salmon	1 serv (1.25 oz)	110	11	35	6	–	–	0	0	2
Honey Butter	1 serv (1 oz)	140	12	0	4	–	–	0	0	7
Hummus	1 serv (1 oz)	70	3	0	0	–	–	0	4	0

FOOD	PORTION	CALS	TOTAL FAT	CHOL	SAT FAT	POLY FAT	MONO FAT	TRANS FAT	FIBER	SUG
Mayo Ancho	1 serv (1.5 oz)	310	33	25	5	–	–	0	0	1
Mustard Creamy	1 serv (1.5 oz)	270	29	20	5	–	–	0	0	1
Mustard Deli	1 tsp (5 g)	5	0	0	0	0	0	0	0	0
Mustard Yellow	1 tbsp (5 g)	0	0	0	0	0	0	0	0	0
Peanut Butter Creamy	1 serv (2 oz)	330	28	5	6	–	–	1	4	5
Salsa Ancho Lime	1 serv (1.5 oz)	20	1	0	0	–	–	0	0	2
Spicy Roasted Tomato	1 serv (1.5 oz)	210	22	20	4	–	–	0	1	1

ELEVATION BURGER
DESSERTS

FOOD	PORTION	CALS	TOTAL FAT	CHOL	SAT FAT	POLY FAT	MONO FAT	TRANS FAT	FIBER	SUG
Cone 1 Scoop Chocolate	1 (5 oz)	310	13	55	9	–	–	0	0	31
Cone 1 Scoop Coffee	1 (5 oz)	310	13	55	10	–	–	0	0	28
Cone 1 Scoop Vanilla	1 (5 oz)	310	15	55	9	–	–	0	0	22
Cookie	1 lg	380	22	45	11	–	–	0	4	23
Cookies	3 sm	270	15	30	9	–	–	0	3	18

MAIN MENU SELECTIONS

FOOD	PORTION	CALS	TOTAL FAT	CHOL	SAT FAT	POLY FAT	MONO FAT	TRANS FAT	FIBER	SUG
Cheeseburger	1	420	21	65	11	–	–	0	1	4
Cheeseburger Wrapped In Lettuce	1	280	19	65	11	–	–	0	1	1
Elevation Salad w/o Dressing	1 (7.8 oz)	230	17	0	2	–	–	0	5	15
Fresh Fries	1 boat	520	26	0	5	–	–	0	5	3
Grilled Cheese	1	330	17	50	10	–	–	0	1	4
Half-The-Guilt Burger #1	1	480	19	50	8	–	–	0	4	4
Half-The-Guilt Burger #1 Wrapped In Lettuce	1	340	17	50	8	–	–	0	4	1
Half-The-Guilt Burger #2	1	500	22	40	7	–	–	0	5	6
Hamburger	1	330	14	40	6	–	–	0	1	4
Hamburger Wrapped In Lettuce	1	190	12	40	6	–	–	0	1	1
Mandarin Oranges	1 serv (4 oz)	70	0	0	0	0	0	0	1	18
Side Salad w/o Dressing	1 (3.2 oz)	20	0	0	0	0	0	0	2	2
The Elevation Burger Double Meat	1	510	26	80	12	–	–	0	1	4
The Elevation Burger Double Meat Double Cheese	1	690	41	130	22	–	–	0	1	4
The Elevation Burger Double Meat Double Cheese Wrapped In Lettuce	1	550	39	130	22	–	–	0	0	1

FOOD	PORTION	CALS	TOTAL FAT	CHOL	SAT FAT	POLY FAT	MONO FAT	TRANS FAT	FIBER	SUGAR
The Elevation Burger Double Meat Wrapped In Lettuce	1	370	24	80	12	–	–	0	1	1
Veggie Burger #1	1	300	7	10	2	–	–	0	4	4
Veggie Burger #1 Wrapped In Lettuce	1	160	5	10	2	–	–	0	4	1
Veggie Burger #2	1	320	10	0	1	–	–	0	5	6
Veggie Burger #2 Wrapped In Lettuce	1	180	8	0	1	–	–	0	5	3
Vertigo Burger 3 Patties	1	690	38	120	18	–	–	0	1	4
Vertigo Burger Wrapped In Lettuce	1	550	36	120	18	–	–	0	1	1
SALAD DRESSINGS AND SAUCES										
Balsamic Mustard	1 serv (0.2 oz)	5	0	0	0	0	0	0	0	1
Dressing Blue Cheese	1 serv (1 oz)	130	14	15	3	–	–	0	0	0
Dressing Ranch	1 serv (1 oz)	160	17	10	3	–	–	0	0	1
Elevation Sauce	1 serv (0.2 oz)	5	0	0	0	0	0	0	0	1
Hot Pepper Relish	1 serv (0.7 oz)	0	0	0	0	0	0	0	0	0
SHAKES AND TOPPINGS										
Bananas	1 serv (1.4 oz)	35	0	0	0	0	0	0	1	5
Blueberries	1 serv (1.5 oz)	25	0	0	0	0	0	0	2	5
Malt Powder	1 serv (1 oz)	110	1	0	1	–	–	0	0	18
Mangoes	1 serv (1.5 oz)	25	0	0	0	0	0	0	1	6
Oreo Cookies	1 serv (0.6 oz)	80	4	0	1	–	–	0	1	7
Organic Cheesecake Powder	1 tbsp	45	0	0	0	0	0	0	0	12
Shake Chocoate	1 (15.5 oz)	710	32	135	21	–	–	0	0	75
Shake Coffee	1 (15.5 oz)	710	32	135	24	–	–	0	0	70
Shake Vanilla	1 (15.5 oz)	710	37	135	21	–	–	0	0	55
Strawberries	1 serv (4.1 oz)	35	0	0	0	0	0	0	2	6
Syrup Black Cherry	1 serv (0.9 oz)	70	0	0	0	0	0	0	0	18
Syrup Chocolate	1 serv (3.6 oz)	260	0	0	0	0	0	0	3	52
Syrup Guava	1 serv (0.9 oz)	70	0	0	0	0	0	0	0	16
Syrup Key Lime Pie	1 serv (0.9 oz)	60	0	0	0	0	0	0	0	15
Syrup Mango	1 serv (0.9 oz)	90	0	0	0	0	0	0	0	21
Syrup Orange	1 serv (0.9 oz)	60	0	0	0	0	0	0	0	15
Syrup Pineapple	1 serv (0.9 oz)	70	0	0	0	0	0	0	0	15

FRESHENS
CREPES

FOOD	PORTION	CALS	TOTAL FAT	CHOL	SAT FAT	POLY FAT	MONO FAT	TRANS FAT	FIBER	SUGAR
Breakfast Denver	1 serv	460	24	480	11	–	–	0	1	7

FOOD	PORTION	CALS	TOTAL FAT	CHOL	SAT FAT	POLY FAT	MONO FAT	TRANS FAT	FIBER	SUG
Breakfast Egg White Florentine	1 serv	270	8	45	5	–	–	0	2	5
Breakfast Steak & Egg	1 serv	480	26	485	12	–	–	0	1	6
Breakfast Wake Up	1 serv	420	22	470	11	–	–	0	1	5
Dessert Cheesecake Cherry	1 serv	590	19	115	10	–	–	1	2	23
Dessert Cheesecake Supreme	1 serv	510	20	80	9	–	–	0	3	35
Dessert Nutella Supreme	1 serv	600	22	50	8	–	–	0	5	50
Dessert The Guilty Pleasure	1 serv	540	13	35	3	–	–	0	5	46
Honey Mustard Chicken	1 serv	470	14	105	6	–	–	0	3	16
Savory Buffalo Chicken	1 serv	480	14	105	8	–	–	0	5	12
Savory Caesar Salad	1 serv	500	19	105	8	–	–	0	5	14
Savory Fajita Chicken	1 serv	500	13	110	7	–	–	0	6	17
Savory Fajita Steak	1 serv	530	19	110	9	–	–	0	5	16
Savory Greek Salad	1 serv	370	9	50	4	–	–	0	5	15
Savory Harvest Salad	1 serv	520	12	90	4	–	–	0	6	29
Savory Havana Chicken	1 serv	470	15	115	6	–	–	0	3	11
Savory Pesto Chicken	1 serv	440	13	95	5	–	–	0	5	11
Savory Philly Cheese Chicken	1 serv	610	25	120	10	–	–	0	7	13
Savory Philly Cheese Steak	1 serv	650	30	120	12	–	–	0	6	12
Savory Pizza Cali	1 serv	270	30	115	16	–	–	0	5	12
Savory Southwest Chicken	1 serv	610	27	105	8	–	–	0	5	16
Savory Southwest Steak	1 serv	650	32	100	10	–	–	0	4	15
Savory Tomato Cheese & Basil	1 serv	460	18	80	11	–	–	0	5	11
SMOOTHIES										
Blended Fruit Berry Breeze	1	290	0	0	0	0	0	0	2	66
Blended Fruit Caribbean Craze	1	260	0	0	0	0	0	0	2	58
Blended Fruit Citrus Mango	1	390	7	10	5	–	–	0	1	67
Blended Fruit Jamaican Jammer	1	290	0	0	0	0	0	0	2	56
Blended Fruit Orange Sunrise	1	260	3	10	2	–	–	0	2	44
Blended Fruit Peach Sunset	1	230	0	0	0	0	0	0	2	53
Blended Fruit Strawberry Kiwi	1	290	0	0	0	0	0	0	1	67
Blended Fruit Strawberry Shooter	1	250	0	0	0	0	0	0	1	59

FOOD	PORTION	CALS	TOTAL FAT	CHOL	SAT FAT	POLY FAT	MONO FAT	TRANS FAT	FIBER	SUGAR
Blended Fruit Strawberry Squeeze	1	250	0	0	0	0	0	0	1	48
Blended Fruit Tropical Pineapple	1	380	4	0	3	–	–	0	1	82
Fro-Yo Blasts Reese's Pieces & Peanut Butter	1	600	19	5	7	–	–	0	3	84
Fro-Yo Cookie Dough	1	490	6	5	3	–	–	0	1	82
Fro-Yo M&M's	1	490	10	10	–	–	–	0	2	83
Fro-Yo Oreo Overload	1	370	4	5	1	–	–	0	1	62
High Protein Peanut Butter	1	460	12	25	3	–	–	0	2	61
High Protein Strawberries 'N Cream	1	370	1	20	0	–	–	0	1	56
Indulgent Shake Chocolate	1	440	3	10	2	–	–	0	1	83
Indulgent Shake Oreo Cream	1	530	6	10	2	–	–	0	1	91
Indulgent Shake Strawberry	1	400	2	10	1	–	–	0	1	79
Indulgent Shake Vanilla	1	410	2	10	1	–	–	0	1	84
Low-Cal Mango Beach No Sugar Added	1	70	0	0	0	0	0	0	1	5
Low-Cal Peach Breeze No Sugar Added	1	80	0	0	0	0	0	0	1	9
Low-Cal Strawberry Oasis No Sugar Added	1	70	0	0	0	0	0	0	1	9
Rainforest Energy Acai	1	280	3	0	0	–	–	0	3	57
Rainforest Energy Brazilian	1	290	3	0	–	–	–	0	3	59
Rainforest Energy Mangosteen	1	320	0	0	0	0	0	0	2	73
YOGURT										
Chocolate Cake Cone	1	150	0	0	0	0	0	0	1	26
Chocolate Cup	11 oz	280	1	5	0	–	–	0	2	56
Chocolate Waffle Cone	1	250	2	5	0	–	–	0	2	38
Granola Parfait w/ 2 Fruits	1 serv	400	8	5	0	–	–	0	6	45
Tart Cup	11 oz	300	0	0	0	0	0	0	0	55
Tart Cup	7 oz	190	0	0	0	0	0	0	0	35
Vanilla Cake Cone	1	160	0	0	0	0	0	0	0	28
Vanilla Cup	7 oz	180	0	0	0	0	0	0	0	38
Vanilla Cup	11 oz	290	0	0	0	0	0	0	1	60
Vanilla Waffle Cone	1	250	1	5	0	–	–	0	1	40

FOOD	PORTION	CALS	TOTAL FAT	CHOL	SAT FAT	POLY FAT	MONO FAT	TRANS FAT	FIBER	SUG
FRUITFULL										
BREADS										
Almond Cherry	½ slice (2 oz)	226	11	23	2	–	–	–	1	17
Apple Spice	½ slice (2 oz)	186	7	19	1	–	–	–	1	18
Banana	½ slice (2 oz)	165	6	22	1	–	–	–	1	11
Cappuccino Chocolate Chip	½ slice (2 oz)	229	13	35	3	–	–	–	1	16
Carrot	½ slice (2 oz)	190	9	24	1	–	–	–	0	12
Chocolate	½ slice (2 oz)	120	0	0	0	0	0	0	2	16
Old Fashion Pound Cake	½ slice (2 oz)	227	13	51	3	–	–	–	0	14
Orange Cranberry	½ slice (2 oz)	130	0	0	0	0	0	0	0	12
Pumpkin	½ slice (2 oz)	130	0	0	0	0	0	0	1	19
Sweet Potato	½ slice (2 oz)	176	6	19	1	–	–	–	1	17
Zucchini	½ slice (2 oz)	190	9	22	1	–	–	–	1	13
FROZEN BARS										
Cream Banana	1 (4 oz)	110	3	20	2	–	–	0	0	13
Cream Coconut	1 (4 oz)	130	5	15	4	–	–	0	0	13
Cream Horchata	1 (4 oz)	240	14	45	10	–	–	0	tr	21
Cream Mango Cream	1 (4 oz)	170	7	20	5	–	–	0	tr	20
Cream Peaches 'N' Cream	1 (4 oz)	150	5	25	4	–	–	0	2	21
Cream Pina Colada	1 (4 oz)	90	3	10	2	–	–	0	tr	15
Cream Raspberry Cream	1 (4 oz)	110	3	10	2	–	–	0	0	12
Cream Sapote Lucuma	1 (4 oz)	180	8	22	5	–	–	0	<2	29
Cream Strawberry Cream	1 (4 oz)	110	3	15	1	–	–	0	0	17
Juice Fuzzy Navel	1 (4 oz)	70	0	0	0	0	0	0	0	15
Juice Green Tea Melon	1 (4 oz)	90	0	0	0	0	0	0	–	16
Juice Guava	1 (4 oz)	70	0	0	0	0	0	0	–	11
Juice Lemon	1 (4 oz)	90	0	0	0	0	0	0	–	22
Juice Lime	1 (4 oz)	80	0	0	0	0	0	0	0	19
Juice Passionate Cherry	1 (4 oz)	80	0	0	0	0	0	0	–	16
Juice Pineapple	1 (4 oz)	80	0	0	0	0	0	0	0	0
Juice Raspberry	1 (4 oz)	70	0	0	0	0	0	0	0	18
Juice Strawberry	1 (4 oz)	70	0	0	0	0	0	0	0	13
Juice Tamarind	1 (4 oz)	90	0	0	0	0	0	0	–	21
Juice Tropical Splash	1 (4 oz)	80	0	0	0	0	0	0	0	17
Juice Watermelon	1 (4 oz)	60	0	0	0	0	0	0	–	13
Mamey Sapote Lucuma	1 (4 oz)	180	8	22	5	–	–	0	<2	–
SNACKS										
All About Almonds	1 pkg (1 oz)	170	15	0	1	–	–	0	4	0
Blueberry Thrill	1 pkg (1 oz)	150	8	0	1	–	–	0	3	9
Buzzworthy Banana	1 pkg (1.1 oz)	140	8	0	3	–	–	0	2	11

FOOD	PORTION	CALS	TOTAL FAT	CHOL	SAT FAT	POLY FAT	MONO FAT	TRANS FAT	FIBER	SUGAR
Calypso Cashews	1 pkg (1.1 oz)	170	13	1	2	–	–	0	1	2
Chocolate Covered Nuts	1 pkg (1.5 oz)	230	16	5	7	–	–	0	1	18
Chocolate Twisted Bliss	1 pkg (1.4 oz)	190	8	6	6	–	–	0	1	16
Cin-sational Apple Crunch	1 pkg (1 oz)	160	10	0	2	–	–	0	1	8
Dark Chocolate Covered Almonds	1 pkg (1.4 oz)	210	16	2	6	–	–	0	3	14
Dark Chocolate Covered Cashews	1 pkg (1.4 oz)	220	16	2	6	–	–	0	3	14
Dark Chocolate Covered Cranberries	1 pkg (1.4 oz)	180	9	2	5	–	–	0	2	24
Debbie Loves Fruit	1 pkg (1 oz)	110	2	0	2	–	–	0	1	16
Eat Your Veggies	1 pkg (1.5 oz)	180	8	0	1	–	–	0	3	7
Got Nuts?	1 pkg (1.1 oz)	180	13	1	1	–	–	0	2	1
Hit The Road Jack	1 pkg (1.1 oz)	130	6	0	1	–	–	0	1	16
Honey I Ate The Peanuts	1 pkg (1 oz)	160	12	0	2	–	–	0	2	6
Just Peachy	1 pkg (1.4 oz)	140	0	0	0	0	0	0	0	22
Mammoth Malts	1 pkg (1 oz)	150	7	3	4	–	–	0	0	18
Nice Catch Swedish Fish	1 pkg (1.4 oz)	140	0	0	0	0	0	0	0	22
Off The Hook Gummy Worms	1 pkg (1.5 oz)	130	0	0	0	0	0	0	0	21
PB Pretzel Poppers	1 pkg (1 oz)	140	7	0	2	–	–	0	2	2
Power Pistachios	1 pkg (1.5 oz)	260	23	0	4	–	–	0	4	3
Pumpkin Seeds	1 pkg (1 oz)	180	15	0	2	–	–	0	1	0
Reggae Rice Crackers	1 pkg (1.1 oz)	110	0	0	0	0	0	0	0	1
Rockin' Raisins	1 pkg (1.4 oz)	170	7	4	4	–	–	0	1	19
Rocky Mountain Munch	1 pkg (1.1 oz)	120	4	0	2	–	–	0	1	14
Smokin' Nuts	1 pkg (1.3 oz)	170	15	0	1	–	–	0	3	2
Soft Twisters Green Apple	1 pkg (1 oz)	120	0	0	0	0	0	0	0	14
Soft Twisters Watermelon	1 pkg (1.3 oz)	120	0	0	0	0	0	0	0	14
Sour Wiggle Giggle	1 pkg (1.5 oz)	150	0	0	0	0	0	0	0	22
Strawberry Fields	1 pkg (1 oz)	140	7	0	3	–	–	0	1	9
Sunflower Seeds Tummy	1 pkg (1.1 oz)	190	14	0	2	–	–	0	2	1
Swinging Sesame Stix	1 pkg (1.1 oz)	180	13	0	2	–	–	0	2	0
Whassup Wasabi	1 pkg (1.1 oz)	150	7	0	1	–	–	0	2	1

HARDEE'S
BEVERAGES

FOOD	PORTION	CALS	TOTAL FAT	CHOL	SAT FAT	POLY FAT	MONO FAT	TRANS FAT	FIBER	SUGAR
Ice Cream Malt	1 (14.5 oz)	780	35	105	24	–	–	–	0	76
Ice Cream Shake	1 (14 oz)	710	33	100	23	–	–	–	0	68

FOOD	PORTION	CALS	TOTAL FAT	CHOL	SAT FAT	POLY FAT	MONO FAT	TRANS FAT	FIBER	SUG
BREAKFAST SELECTIONS										
Big Country Breakfast Platter Bacon w/o Syrup Jam & Butter	1 (11.6 oz)	870	44	390	11	–	–	–	6	12
Biscuit Bacon Egg Cheese	1 (5.2 oz)	450	26	195	9	–	–	–	3	2
Biscuit Chicken Fillet	1 (6 oz)	550	32	45	7	–	–	–	4	3
Biscuit Cinnamon 'N' Raisin	1 (2.8 oz)	300	15	0	4	–	–	–	1	17
Biscuit Country Ham	1 (4.2 oz)	370	19	35	6	–	–	–	3	2
Biscuit Country Steak	1 (5 oz)	510	31	25	9	–	–	–	4	3
Biscuit Ham Egg Cheese	1 (6.1 oz)	440	24	205	8	–	–	–	3	2
Biscuit Jelly	1 (4 oz)	430	26	0	6	–	–	–	3	9
Biscuit Loaded Omelet	1 (6 oz)	520	33	215	12	–	–	–	3	2
Biscuit Made From Scratch	1 (3 oz)	300	15	0	4	–	–	–	3	2
Biscuit Monster	1 (8.3 oz)	720	49	250	18	–	–	–	3	3
Biscuit 'N' Gravy	1 (8 oz)	460	26	10	7	–	–	–	3	2
Biscuit Sausage	1 (4.4 oz)	490	33	30	10	–	–	–	3	3
Biscuit Sausage & Egg	1 (6 oz)	550	37	210	12	–	–	–	3	3
Breakfast Bowl Low Carb	1 (8.6 oz)	690	58	630	23	–	–	–	1	1
Breakfast Burrito Loaded	1 (8.9 oz)	710	45	430	19	–	–	–	2	1
Breakfast Sandwich Frisco	1 (6.8 oz)	440	19	215	8	–	–	–	2	5
Grits	1 serv (5 oz)	110	5	0	1	–	–	–	1	0
Hash Rounds	1 sm (3 oz)	260	17	0	4	–	–	–	3	1
Pancakes w/o Syrup Jam & Butter	3 (4.8 oz)	310	5	30	1	–	–	–	2	14
Sunrise Croissant w/ Ham	1 (5.7 oz)	440	27	220	12	–	–	–	1	4
CHILDREN'S MENU SELECTIONS										
French Fries	1 serv (2.8 oz)	330	11	0	2	–	–	–	3	0
Kids Meal Cheeseburger	1 (7.1 oz)	540	26	40	6	–	–	–	4	6
Kids Meal Chicken Tenders	1 serv (5.7 oz)	400	19	45	4	–	–	–	4	0
Kids Meal Hamburger	1 (6.7 oz)	490	23	30	5	–	–	–	4	6
DESSERTS										
Apple Turnover w/o Cinnamon Sugar Topping	1 (3 oz)	270	13	5	4	–	–	–	1	11
Cookie Chocolate Chip	1 (2.4 oz)	290	11	20	5	–	–	–	0	26
Ice Cream Bowl Single Scoop	1 (4 oz)	240	13	45	8	–	–	–	0	22
Ice Cream Cone Single Scoop	1 (4.4 oz)	290	13	45	8	–	–	–	0	26
Peach Cobbler	1 sm (6.3 oz)	290	7	0	1	–	–	–	1	45
MAIN MENU SELECTIONS										
Burger Original Turkey	1 (8.2 oz)	390	17	75	4	–	–	–	3	7

FOOD	PORTION	CALS	TOTAL FAT	CHOL	SAT FAT	POLY FAT	MONO FAT	TRANS FAT	FIBER	SUGAR
Cheeseburger	1 sm (4.4 oz)	310	15	40	6	–	–	–	1	6
Cheeseburger Double	1 (5.8 oz)	410	21	70	9	–	–	–	2	7
Cheeseburger Little Thick	1 (5.8 oz)	420	23	65	9	–	–	–	3	8
Chicken Tenders Hand Breaded	3 (4.5 oz)	260	13	70	3	–	–	–	2	0
Cole Slaw	1 sm (4 oz)	170	10	10	2	–	–	–	2	16
Crispy Curls	1 sm (4 oz)	360	18	0	4	–	–	–	4	0
French Fries	1 sm (4 oz)	340	16	0	3	–	–	–	4	0
Fried Chicken Breast	1 (5.2 oz)	370	15	75	4	–	–	–	0	0
Fried Chicken Leg	1 (2.4 oz)	170	7	45	2	–	–	–	0	0
Fried Chicken Thigh	1 (4.2 oz)	330	15	60	4	–	–	–	0	0
Fried Chicken Wing	1 (2.3 oz)	200	8	30	2	–	–	–	0	0
Hamburger	1 sm (4 oz)	270	11	30	4	–	–	–	1	6
Hot Ham 'N' Cheese	1 (4.6 oz)	280	11	35	5	–	–	–	1	4
Hot Ham 'N' Cheese Big	1 (8.4 oz)	480	19	75	8	–	–	–	3	6
Jumbo Chili Dog	1 (5 oz)	370	25	50	8	–	–	–	2	6
Mashed Potatoes	1 sm (5 oz)	90	2	0	0	–	–	–	0	1
Onion Rings Beer Battered	1 serv (4.3 oz)	410	24	0	5	–	–	–	3	5
Roast Beef Big	1 (7.2 oz)	460	20	70	7	–	–	–	4	5
Sandwich Charbroiled BBQ Chicken	1 (7.5 oz)	310	6	45	1	–	–	–	3	15
Sandwich Charbroiled Chicken Club	1 (8.6 oz)	540	31	80	8	–	–	–	3	10
Sandwich Fish Supreme	1 (7 oz)	530	34	40	6	–	–	–	3	9
Sandwich Hand Breaded Chicken Fillet	1 (10.9 oz)	680	38	90	7	–	–	–	4	7
Sandwich Low Carb Charbroiled Chicken Club	1 (8 oz)	340	22	75	7	–	–	–	1	8
Sandwich Roast Beef Regular	1 (4.5 oz)	290	14	40	5	–	–	–	2	4
Sandwich Spicy Chicken	1 (5.5 oz)	430	24	30	5	–	–	–	3	3
Side Salad w/o Dressing	1 (6.7 oz)	120	7	20	5	–	–	–	2	4
Thickburger 1/3 Lb Cheeseburger	1 (8.8 oz)	630	33	80	13	–	–	–	3	10
Thickburger 1/3 Lb Bacon Cheese	1 (11.7 oz)	850	56	105	18	–	–	–	4	7
Thickburger 1/3 Lb Frisco	1 (10.5 oz)	880	59	115	20	–	–	–	2	6
Thickburger 1/3 Lb Low Carb	1 (9.7 oz)	480	36	90	13	–	–	–	1	6
Thickburger 1/3 Lb Mushroom & Swiss	1 (9.2 oz)	670	38	95	16	–	–	–	3	5
Thickburger 1/3 Lb Original	1 (12.4 oz)	810	52	95	16	–	–	–	4	10

FOOD	PORTION	CALS	TOTAL FAT	CHOL	SAT FAT	POLY FAT	MONO FAT	TRANS FAT	FIBER	SUG
Thickburger ⅔ Lb Double	1 (16.5 oz)	1160	78	180	28	–	–	–	4	10
Thickburger ⅔ Lb Monster	1 (13.4 oz)	1300	93	210	35	–	–	–	3	5
Thickburger Little	1 (8 oz)	570	39	80	12	–	–	–	3	7
Thickburger The Six Dollar	1 (14 oz)	940	63	125	23	–	–	–	4	16

IHOP

FOOD	PORTION	CALS	TOTAL FAT	CHOL	SAT FAT	POLY FAT	MONO FAT	TRANS FAT	FIBER	SUG
Pancake Buttermilk	5	770	25	115	9	–	–	1	7	22
Pancake Buttermilk Short Stack	3	490	18	80	8	–	–	1	4	13
Pancake Chocolate Chip	4	720	24	80	10	–	–	1	8	32
Pancake Double Blueberry	4	800	17	80	5	–	–	1	11	57
Pancake Harvest Grain 'N Nut	4	920	49	125	11	–	–	0	10	22
Pancake New York Cheesecake	4	1100	44	190	21	–	–	2	8	53
Pancake Strawberry Banana	4	760	17	80	5	–	–	1	10	41

JERSEY MIKE'S
SANDWICHES

FOOD	PORTION	CALS	TOTAL FAT	CHOL	SAT FAT	POLY FAT	MONO FAT	TRANS FAT	FIBER	SUG
#05 Super Sub	1 (11.9 oz)	290	14	85	7	–	–	0	2	5
#05 Super Sub Wheat	1 (16 oz)	280	19	85	8	–	–	0	5	11
#05 Super Sub White	1 (16 oz)	580	19	85	9	–	–	0	4	9
#06 Roast Beef & Provolone In A Tub	1 (12.2 oz)	430	20	125	9	–	–	1	2	5
#06 Roast Beef & Provolone Wheat	1 reg (16.2 oz)	720	25	125	10	–	–	1	5	11
#06 Roast Beef & Provolone White	1 reg (16.2 oz)	730	25	125	11	–	–	1	4	8
#07 Turkey Breast & Provolone In A Tub	1 (11.4 oz)	250	11	65	6	–	–	0	2	5
#07 Turkey Breast & Provolone Wheat	1 reg (15.4 oz)	540	16	65	6	–	–	0	5	11
#07 Turkey Breast & Provolone White	1 (15.4 oz)	550	15	65	7	–	–	0	4	8
#08 Club Sub w/ Mayonnaise In A Tub	1 (13.2 oz)	600	47	100	14	–	–	0	2	5
#08 Club Sub w/ Mayonnaise Wheat	1 (17.2 oz)	890	52	100	15	–	–	0	5	11
#08 Club Sub w/ Mayonnaise White	1 (17.2 oz)	890	52	100	16	–	–	1	4	9

FOOD	PORTION	CALS	TOTAL FAT	CHOL	SAT FAT	POLY FAT	MONO FAT	TRANS FAT	FIBER	SUGAR
#09 Club Sub Supreme w/ Mayonnaise In A Tub	1 (13.2 oz)	650	47	120	13	–	–	1	2	5
#09 Club Supreme w/ Mayonnaise Wheat	1 reg (17.2 oz)	940	52	120	14	–	–	1	5	11
#09 Club Supreme w/ Mayonnaise White	1 (17.2 oz)	940	52	120	15	–	–	1	4	9
#10 Albacore Tuna In A Tub	1 (12.2 oz)	620	55	55	8	–	–	0	3	5
#10 Albacore Tuna Wheat	1 (16.2 oz)	910	59	55	9	–	–	0	6	11
#10 Albacore Tuna White	1 (16.2 oz)	910	59	55	10	–	–	0	4	9
#13 Original Italian In A Tub	1 (12.9 oz)	390	22	95	10	–	–	0	2	5
#13 Original Italian Wheat	1 reg (16.9 oz)	680	27	95	11	–	–	0	5	11
#13 Original Italian White	1 reg (16.9 oz)	680	27	96	11	–	–	0	4	9
#14 Veggie White	1 reg (15.7 oz)	750	36	100	21	–	–	1	5	10
American Classic In A Tub	1 (11.4 oz)	270	14	80	7	–	–	0	2	5
American Classic Wheat	1 reg (15.4 oz)	560	18	80	8	–	–	0	5	11
American Classic White	1 reg (15.4 oz)	560	18	80	9	–	–	0	4	8
BLT In A Tub	1 (8.2 oz)	280	21	45	9	–	–	0	2	5
BLT Wheat	1 reg (12.2 oz)	570	26	45	10	–	–	1	5	10
BLT White	1 reg (12.2 oz)	570	26	45	11	–	–	0	4	8
Hot Sub #15 Meatball & Cheese Wheat	1 reg (13.5 oz)	890	52	95	21	–	–	2	6	12
Hot Sub #15 Meatball & Cheese White	1 reg (13.5 oz)	890	51	95	–	–	–	2	5	10
Hot Sub #17 Chicken Philly Wheat	1 reg (13 oz)	630	25	175	13	–	–	0	4	12
Hot Sub BBQ Beef Wheat	1 reg (11.2 oz)	710	16	110	5	–	–	0	4	23
Hot Sub BBQ Beef White	1 reg (11.2 oz)	720	16	110	6	–	–	1	3	20
Hot Sub Big Kahuna Chicken Wheat	1 reg (14.2 oz)	680	29	190	16	–	–	1	5	13
Hot Sub Big Kahuna Chicken White	1 reg (14.2 oz)	690	29	190	17	–	–	1	3	11
Hot Sub Big Kahuna Wheat	1 reg (14.2 oz)	670	28	140	14	–	–	1	5	12
Hot Sub Big Kahuna White	1 reg (14.2 oz)	680	28	140	15	–	–	1	3	10
Hot Sub Cheese Steak Buffalo Chicken Wheat	1 reg (20.2 oz)	940	55	185	19	–	–	0	5	17
Hot Sub Cheese Steak Buffalo Chicken White	1 reg (20.2 oz)	940	55	185	20	–	–	0	4	14
Hot Sub Cheese Steak California Chicken Wheat	1 reg (17.4 oz)	890	53	190	18	–	–	0	5	14

FOOD	PORTION	CALS	TOTAL FAT	CHOL	SAT FAT	POLY FAT	MONO FAT	TRANS FAT	FIBER	SUGAR
Hot Sub Cheese Steak California Chicken White	1 reg (17.4 oz)	890	52	190	18	–	–	1	4	12
Hot Sub Cheese Steak California Wheat	1 reg (17.4 oz)	870	51	140	15	–	–	1	5	12
Hot Sub Cheese Steak California White	1 reg (17.4 oz)	880	51	140	16	–	–	1	4	10
Hot Sub Cheese Steak Teriyaki Chicken Wheat	1 reg (14.9 oz)	680	25	175	13	–	–	0	4	20
Hot Sub Cheese Steak Teriyaki Chicken White	1 reg (14.9 oz)	680	25	175	14	–	–	0	3	18
Hot Sub Chicka Phila Roni Wheat	1 reg (12.5 oz)	620	19	90	12	–	–	1	3	7
Hot Sub Chicka Phila Roni White	1 reg (12.5 oz)	605	12	90	12	–	–	1	1	5
Hot Sub Chicken Parmesan Wheat	1 reg (11 oz)	650	22	60	7	–	–	0	5	7
Hot Sub Chicken Philly White	1 reg (13 oz)	630	25	175	14	–	–	0	3	10
Hot Sub Chipotle Chicken Wheat	1 reg (14.4 oz)	910	56	195	19	–	–	0	4	12
Hot Sub Chipotle Chicken White	1 reg (14.4 oz)	920	56	195	19	–	–	1	3	10
Hot Sub Chipotle Steak Wheat	1 reg (14.4 oz)	900	55	145	16	–	–	1	4	11
Hot Sub Chipotle Steak White	1 reg (14.4 oz)	910	55	145	17	–	–	1	3	9
Hot Sub Chipotle Turkey Wheat	1 reg (17.4 oz)	865	50	95	14	–	–	1	6	10
Hot Sub Chipotle Turkey White	1 reg (17.4 oz)	870	50	95	15	–	–	1	4	8
Hot Sub Grilled Chicken Wheat	1 reg (12.7 oz)	670	33	65	5	–	–	0	4	8
Hot Sub Grilled Chicken White	1 reg (12.7 oz)	670	33	65	6	–	–	0	3	6
Hot Sub Pastrami & Swiss Wheat	1 reg (10.7 oz)	580	18	95	87	–	–	1	3	8
Hot Sub Pastrami & Swiss White	1 reg (10.7 oz)	590	17	95	9	–	–	1	2	6
Hot Sub Reuben Wheat	1 reg (12.2 oz)	700	27	95	9	–	–	0	5	14
Hot Sub Reuben White	1 reg (12.2 oz)	710	27	95	10	–	–	1	3	11
Hot Sub Sausage Wheat	1 reg (11.5 oz)	600	27	65	8	–	–	0	5	12

FOOD	PORTION	CALS	TOTAL FAT	CHOL	SAT FAT	POLY FAT	MONO FAT	TRANS FAT	FIBER	SUGAR
Hot Sub Sausage White	1 reg (11.4 oz)	600	26	65	8	–	–	0	4	10
Hot Sub Steak Philly Wheat	1 reg (13 oz)	620	24	125	11	–	–	1	4	11
Hot Sub Steak Philly White	1 reg (13 oz)	620	23	125	12	–	–	1	3	9
Jersey Shore Favorite In A Tub	1 (11.4 oz)	270	14	80	7	–	–	0	2	5
Jersey Shore Favorite Wheat	1 reg (15.4 oz)	560	18	80	8	–	–	0	5	11
Jersey Shore Favorite White	1 reg (15.4 oz)	570	18	80	9	–	–	0	4	9
Veggie In A Tub	1 (11.7 oz)	460	32	100	19	–	–	1	3	7
Veggie Wheat	1 reg (15.72 oz)	720	33	75	18	–	–	1	6	11
Wrap Baja Chicken	1 (15.6 oz)	610	23	90	11	–	–	0	8	7
Wrap Buffalo Chicken	1 (14.6 oz)	740	37	95	14	–	–	0	6	6
Wrap Chicken Caesar	1 (12 oz)	580	23	65	5	–	–	0	6	4
Wrap Grilled Ham & Cheese	1 (14 oz)	740	41	80	13	–	–	0	5	11
Wrap Grilled Roast Beef & Cheese	1 (15 oz)	830	45	100	14	–	–	1	5	12
Wrap Grilled Veggie	1 (17 oz)	910	57	105	22	–	–	1	8	10
Wrap Turkey w/ Honey Mustard Sauce	1 (13 oz)	540	20	50	4	–	–	0	7	10
SOUPS										
Beef Steak & Black Bean	1 cup (8.7 oz)	140	2	10	0	–	–	0	9	3
Boston Clam Chowder	1 cup (8.5 oz)	130	6	15	2	–	–	0	0	0
Broccoli Cheese	1 cup (8.7 oz)	140	9	25	5	–	–	0	0	2
Cape Cod Clam Chowder	1 cup (8.7 oz)	140	6	10	2	–	–	1	0	1
Chicken & Dumplings	1 cup (8.7 oz)	250	18	45	7	–	–	3	0	4
Chicken Gumbo	1 cup (9 oz)	100	5	20	2	–	–	0	1	2
Chicken Noodle	1 cup (8.7 oz)	90	4	15	1	–	–	0	0	0
Chicken Pot Pie	1 cup (8.7 oz)	230	14	45	5	–	–	3	1	3
Chicken Tortilla	1 cup (8.7 oz)	140	3	20	1	–	–	0	5	2
Cream Of Broccoli	1 cup (8.7 oz)	90	6	15	3	–	–	0	1	3
Cream Of Potato	1 cup (8.7 oz)	180	8	25	5	–	–	0	1	0
Creamy Tomato Bisque	1 cup (8.5 oz)	90	4	0	1	–	–	0	1	5
French Onion	1 cup (8.7 oz)	80	1	0	0	–	–	0	3	3
Italian Wedding	1 cup (8.5 oz)	120	5	10	3	–	–	0	1	1
Lumberjack Vegetable	1 cup (8.5 oz)	120	5	5	2	–	–	0	5	4
Maryland Crab	1 cup (8.7 oz)	70	1	10	0	–	–	0	2	4
Minestrone	1 cup (8.7 oz)	70	3	0	1	–	–	1	0	6
Potato w/ Bacon	1 cup (8.5 oz)	130	5	5	2	–	–	0	1	2
Spicy Chili w/ Beans	1 cup (9.6 oz)	240	8	40	4	–	–	1	7	5
Split Pea w/ Ham	1 cup (8.5 oz)	150	2	5	1	–	–	0	3	4

FOOD	PORTION	CALS	TOTAL FAT	CHOL	SAT FAT	POLY FAT	MONO FAT	TRANS FAT	FIBER	SUGAR
Timberline Chili w/ Beans	1 cup (8.7 oz)	280	9	30	4	–	–	1	7	9
Tomato Florentine	1 cup (8.7 oz)	90	1	0	0	–	–	0	1	6
Vegetable Beef & Barley	1 cup (8.7 oz)	90	3	10	1	–	–	0	2	1
Vegetarian Vegetable	1 cup (8.7 oz)	80	1	0	0	–	–	0	4	4
Wild & Brown Rice w/ Chicken	1 cup (8.7 oz)	310	15	75	5	–	–	1	1	1
Wisconsin Cheese	1 cup (8.5 oz)	220	16	20	5	–	–	0	0	8

JOE'S CRAB SHACK
DESSERTS

FOOD	PORTION	CALS	TOTAL FAT	CHOL	SAT FAT	POLY FAT	MONO FAT	TRANS FAT	FIBER	SUGAR
Big Cheese Cheesecake	1 serv	980	64	325	37	–	–	0	3	70
Chocolate Shack Attack	1 serv	1530	63	120	29	–	–	0	10	155
Crabby Apple Crumble	1 serv	1400	51	115	0	–	–	0	4	161
Key Lime Wave	1 serv	1230	55	525	38	–	–	0	2	135
Sea Turtle Sundae	1	1240	57	105	25	–	–	0	6	125

MAIN MENU SELECTIONS

FOOD	PORTION	CALS	TOTAL FAT	CHOL	SAT FAT	POLY FAT	MONO FAT	TRANS FAT	FIBER	SUGAR
Blackened Tilapia	1 serv	1190	64	240	16	–	–	14	6	4
Broccoli Flowers	1 serv	80	6	0	1	–	–	0	3	2
Bucket of Shrimp	12	190	3	285	0	–	–	0	1	5
Buckets of Crab Dungeness w/o Butter	1	480	3	120	0	–	–	0	7	6
Buckets of Crab King w/o Butter	1	430	3	65	0	–	–	0	7	6
Buckets Of Crab Snow w/o Butter	1	470	4	100	0	–	–	0	7	6
Burger Surf 'N Turf	1	1260	85	205	23	–	–	9	4	8
Calamari Fried	1 serv	900	58	265	11	–	–	0	5	2
Cheeseburger Chipotle Bacon	1	1010	68	165	26	–	–	9	3	13
Cheesy New Potatoes	1 serv	250	15	35	9	–	–	1	2	1
Classic Sampler	1 serv	1460	103	295	32	–	–	1	8	5
Coleslaw	1 serv	110	7	0	2	–	–	0	2	10
Crab Cake Dinner	1	1470	109	260	21	–	–	14	9	14
Crab Daddy Feast w/o Butter	1	510	4	125	0	–	–	0	7	6
Crab Nachos	1 serv	2000	145	295	53	–	–	2	14	8
Crab Stuffed Mushrooms	1 serv	800	40	135	17	–	–	2	5	4
Crawfish Half & Half	1 serv	860	47	180	16	–	–	0	4	11
Crazy Good Crab Dip	1 serv	1270	87	245	34	–	–	2	7	4
Crunchy Catfish	1 serv	1440	94	65	18	–	–	0	10	10
Diablo Mussels	1 serv	1060	54	105	12	–	–	7	5	5

FOOD	PORTION	CALS	TOTAL FAT	CHOL	SAT FAT	POLY FAT	MONO FAT	TRANS FAT	FIBER	SUGAR
Dipping Butter	1 serv	400	44	360	10	–	–	14	0	0
Dirty Rice	1 serv	170	3	20	1	–	–	0	1	1
Double Dip	1 serv	1260	81	170	32	–	–	2	8	3
Ear Of Corn	1	60	1	0	0	–	–	0	2	2
Fish & Chips	1 serv	1430	92	110	17	–	–	0	10	12
Fish & Shrimp	1 serv	1540	92	170	18	–	–	0	7	18
French Fries	1 serv	370	19	0	4	–	–	0	5	0
Fried Oysters	1 serv	1060	64	40	12	–	–	0	9	1
Garlicky Mussels	1 serv	880	42	75	9	–	–	7	4	1
Get Stuffed Snapper	1 serv	830	43	200	14	–	–	3	4	6
Great Balls Of Fire	1 serv	970	66	70	19	–	–	0	8	4
Grilled Sunset Salmon	1 serv	890	45	135	10	–	–	4	8	25
Homestyle Chicken Tenders	1 serv	1450	81	155	16	–	–	0	6	15
Hush Puppies	1 serv	700	34	0	6	–	–	0	8	2
Joe's Steak Deal	1 serv	710	32	120	8	–	–	0	8	2
Lobster Daddy Feast w/o Butter	1	580	4	320	1	–	–	0	7	6
Maui Mahi	1 serv	680	28	200	7	–	–	4	8	9
Mozzarella Sticks	1 serv	710	36	50	14	–	–	1	6	4
New England Clam Chowder	1 cup	250	13	55	8	–	–	0	2	1
Onion Strings	1 serv	470	23	0	5	–	–	0	6	4
Pan Fried Cheesy Chicken	1 serv	1590	100	235	34	–	–	18	7	8
Pasta-laya	1 serv	1820	94	335	24	–	–	14	12	10
Platter Caribbean Feast	1	1280	59	385	16	–	–	7	16	29
Platter East Coast	1	2110	144	335	27	–	–	9	13	9
Platter Fisherman's	1	1970	129	280	27	–	–	0	11	21
Platter Seaside	1	1540	92	160	18	–	–	0	8	19
Platter Shrimp	1	1490	84	205	20	–	–	0	18	33
Platter Shrimp Trio	1	1050	53	350	14	–	–	2	19	21
Platter The Big Hook	1	2750	168	330	37	–	–	2	26	27
Ribeye	1 serv	1150	82	205	34	–	–	5	5	4
Salmon Orleans	1 serv	1000	65	285	20	–	–	7	1	2
Sandwich Chicken Club Blackened	1	990	71	135	22	–	–	14	2	5
Sandwich Chicken Club Grilled	1	790	49	135	17	–	–	7	2	5
Sandwich Crab Cake	1	810	61	135	12	–	–	10	3	4
Sandwich Mahi Blackened	1	850	53	205	12	–	–	8	2	7
Seafood Fun-Do	1 serv	1310	69	180	24	–	–	6	7	2
Shrimp Coconut	1 serv	1230	72	90	20	–	–	0	25	24

FOOD	PORTION	CALS	TOTAL FAT	CHOL	SAT FAT	POLY FAT	MONO FAT	TRANS FAT	FIBER	SUGAR
Shrimp Crab Stuffed	1 serv	710	37	335	8	–	–	4	5	4
Shrimp Crispy	1 serv	1060	58	180	12	–	–	0	7	16
Shrimp Grilled Malibu	1 serv	540	19	290	4	–	–	0	5	9
Shrimp Pasta Alfredo	1 serv	1650	85	400	36	–	–	1	8	3
Shrimp Popcorn	1 serv	990	54	120	10	–	–	0	9	16
Skillet Paella	1 serv	1990	84	390	18	–	–	7	12	17
Snapper Pontchartrain	1 serv	1090	74	180	21	–	–	16	6	5
Steak & Malibu Shrimp	1 serv	660	22	265	6	–	–	0	5	6
Steampots Bean Town	1	1470	78	705	20	–	–	14	7	6
Steampots Joe's Classic	1	1210	75	285	19	–	–	14	7	6
Steampots Old Bay	1	1200	74	170	19	–	–	14	7	6
Steampots Ragin' Cajun	1	1590	107	250	26	–	–	28	10	9
Steampots Samuel Adams	1	1180	74	175	19	–	–	14	7	6
Steampots Sunset Fire Grilled	1	1260	75	285	19	–	–	14	9	7
Steampots The Diablo	1	1420	84	175	19	–	–	21	9	11
Steampots The KJ	1	1330	85	120	19	–	–	25	7	7
Steampots The Orleans	1	1310	65	730	16	–	–	14	8	7
SALADS										
Aruba Chicken	1	780	49	130	14	–	–	0	7	22
Aruba Shrimp	1	860	61	75	18	–	–	0	15	23
Caesar	1	450	37	35	9	–	–	0	5	5
Caesar Chicken	1	670	46	130	11	–	–	0	5	5
Caesar Chicken Chipotle	1	760	46	110	9	–	–	0	10	9
Caesar Crab Cake Chipotle	1	970	72	140	14	–	–	7	11	11
Caesar Shrimp	1	530	38	180	10	–	–	0	5	5
Caesar Side	1	220	18	15	5	–	–	0	2	2
Classic Cobb Chicken	1	790	46	325	15	–	–	0	10	11
Classic Cobb Shrimp	1	650	39	370	14	–	–	0	10	11
Classic Cobb Snow	1	630	38	270	14	–	–	0	10	11
House Side w/o Dressing	1	120	7	15	3	–	–	0	2	3

LONG JOHN SILVER'S
BEVERAGES

FOOD	PORTION	CALS	TOTAL FAT	CHOL	SAT FAT	POLY FAT	MONO FAT	TRANS FAT	FIBER	SUGAR
Diet Mountain Dew	1 med (32 oz)	0	0	0	0	0	0	0	0	0
Diet Pepsi	1 med (32 oz)	0	0	0	0	0	0	0	0	0
Dr Pepper	1 med (32 oz)	400	0	0	0	0	0	0	0	108
Iced Tea Unsweetened	1 med (32 oz)	0	0	0	0	0	0	0	0	0
Iceflow Lemonade	1 sm (16 oz)	190	0	0	0	0	0	0	0	40

FOOD	PORTION	CALS	TOTAL FAT	CHOL	SAT FAT	POLY FAT	MONO FAT	TRANS FAT	FIBER	SUGAR
Iceflow Strawberry Lemonade	1 sm (16 oz)	240	0	0	0	0	0	0	0	48
Lipton Raspberry Tea	1 med (32 oz)	320	0	0	0	0	0	0	0	84
Mountain Dew	1 med (32 oz)	440	0	0	0	0	0	0	0	116
Pepsi	1 med (32 oz)	400	0	0	0	0	0	0	0	108
Pepsi Wild Cherry	1 med (32 oz)	400	0	0	0	0	0	0	0	112
Sierra Mist	1 med (32 oz)	400	0	0	0	0	0	0	0	108
Tropicana Fruit Punch	1 med (32 oz)	440	0	0	0	0	0	0	0	120
Tropicana Lemonade	1 med (32 oz)	400	0	0	0	0	0	0	0	108
DESSERTS										
Pie Chocolate Cream	1 slice (2.6 oz)	280	17	10	10	–	–	0	1	19
Pie Pineapple Cream	1 slice (3.1 oz)	300	17	10	11	–	–	0	0	25
MAIN MENU SELECTIONS										
Battered Alaskan Pollock	1 piece (3.2 oz)	140	16	35	4	–	–	5	0	0
Battered Shrimp	3 (1.5 oz)	130	9	45	3	–	–	3	0	0
Bites Broccoli Cheddar	5 (3.3 oz)	230	12	15	5	–	–	3	2	2
Bites Jalapeno Cheddar	5 (2.9 oz)	240	14	15	5	–	–	4	2	2
Breaded Clam Strips	1 box (3 oz)	320	19	35	5	–	–	7	2	1
Breaded Mozzarella Sticks	3 (1.8 oz)	150	9	10	4	–	–	0	1	0
Breadstick	1 (2 oz)	170	4	0	1	–	–	1	1	2
Buttered Langostino Lobster Bites	1 box (3.2 oz)	230	9	60	3	–	–	3	2	0
Chicken Strip	1 (1.8 oz)	140	8	20	2	–	–	3	0	0
Cole Slaw	1 serv (4 oz)	200	15	20	3	–	–	0	3	10
Corn Cobbette w/ Butter	1 (3.6 oz)	150	10	0	2	–	–	0	3	6
Corn Cobbette w/o Butter	1 (3.3 oz)	90	3	0	1	–	–	0	3	6
Crumblies	1 serv (1 oz)	170	12	0	3	–	–	4	1	0
Freshside Grille Salmon Entree	1 serv (10.7 oz)	280	7	50	2	–	–	0	3	5
Freshside Grille Shrimp Scampi Entree	1 serv (10.7 oz)	330	15	135	4	–	–	0	3	5
Freshside Grille Tilapia Entree	1 serv (10.2 oz)	250	5	60	2	–	–	0	3	4
Fries Basket Portion	1 serv (4 oz)	310	14	0	4	–	–	4	4	0
Fries Platter Portion	1 serv (3 oz)	230	10	0	3	–	–	3	3	0
Grilled Pacific Salmon Filets	2 (4.5 oz)	150	5	50	1	–	–	0	0	1
Grilled Tilapia Filet	1 (4 oz)	110	3	55	1	–	–	0	0	1
Hushpuppy	1 (0.8 oz)	60	3	0	1	–	–	1	1	1
Jalapeno Peppers	1 (1.3 oz)	15	0	0	0	0	0	0	0	1

FOOD	PORTION	CALS	TOTAL FAT	CHOL	SAT FAT	POLY FAT	MONO FAT	TRANS FAT	FIBER	SUGAR
Longostino Lobster Stuffed Crab Cake	1 (2.2 oz)	170	9	30	2	–	–	0	1	0
Popcorn Shrimp	1 box (2.9 oz)	270	16	75	4	–	–	5	1	1
Rice	1 serv (5 oz)	180	1	0	1	–	–	0	2	1
Sandwich Alaskan Pollock	1 (6.6 oz)	470	23	40	5	–	–	5	3	4
Sandwich Chicken Strip	1 (6.6 oz)	440	30	50	6	–	–	5	4	2
Sandwich Ultimate Alaskan Pollock	1 (7.2 oz)	240	27	55	8	–	–	5	3	4
Sandwich Zesty Chicken Strip	1 (4.5 oz)	380	19	25	4	–	–	3	3	2
Shrimp Scampi	8 pieces	200	13	135	3	–	–	0	0	1
Soup Broccoli Cheese	1 bowl (7.4 oz)	220	18	30	8	–	–	0	1	2
Taco Baja Chicken Strip	1 (4.3 oz)	370	23	25	5	–	–	4	3	2
Taco Baja Fish	1 (4 oz)	360	23	25	5	–	–	4	3	2
Vegetable Medley	1 serv (4 oz)	50	2	0	1	–	–	0	3	3
SAUCES										
BBQ	1 serv (1 oz)	40	0	0	0	0	0	0	0	6
Cocktail	1 serv (1 oz)	25	0	0	0	0	0	0	0	5
Honey Mustard	1 serv (1 oz)	100	6	0	2	–	–	0	0	6
Ketchup	1 pkg (0.3 oz)	10	0	0	0	0	0	0	0	2
Lemon Juice	1 serv (4 g)	0	0	0	0	0	0	0	0	0
Louisiana Hot Sauce	1 tsp (5 g)	0	0	0	0	0	0	0	0	0
Malt Vinegar	1 serv (0.5 oz)	0	0	0	0	0	0	0	0	0
Marinara	1 serv (1 oz)	15	0	0	0	0	0	0	1	2
Ranch	1 serv (1 oz)	160	17	15	3	–	–	0	0	1
Sweet & Sour	1 serv (1 oz)	45	0	0	0	0	0	0	0	7
Tartar	1 serv (1 oz)	100	9	15	2	–	–	0	3	
MAGGIE MOO'S										
BEVERAGES										
Shake Caramel Cowpuccino	1 (15 oz)	740	43	170	31	–	–	0	0	70
Shake Cinnamoo Swirl	1 (16 oz)	780	44	165	32	–	–	0	1	73
Shake Cookies 'N' Cream	1 (15 oz)	740	44	165	30	–	–	0	0	65
Shake Moocha Cowpuccino	1 (15 oz)	710	41	165	30	–	–	0	0	69
Shake Peanut Butter S'Moo	1 (16 oz)	780	46	155	30	–	–	0	4	69
Shake Strawberries 'N' Cream	1 (15 oz)	620	37	150	27	–	–	0	1	58
Zoomer Caramel Coffee	1 (15 oz)	380	13	0	9	–	–	0	0	53
Zoomer Creamy Mango	1 (17 oz)	400	3	0	2	–	–	0	1	88
Zoomer Mocha Coffee	1 (17 oz)	460	11	0	7	–	–	0	0	74

FOOD	PORTION	CALS	TOTAL FAT	CHOL	SAT FAT	POLY FAT	MONO FAT	TRANS FAT	FIBER	SUGAR
Zoomer Raspberry Pomegranate	1 (17 oz)	460	0	0	0	0	0	0	3	104
Zoomer Strawberry Banana	1 (18 oz)	350	10	0	6	–	–	0	3	51
Zoomer Triple Berry Pomegranate	1 (17 oz)	460	1	0	0	–	–	0	3	106
CONES										
Dark Chocolate	1 (1.5 oz)	200	7	5	5	–	–	0	1	18
Dark Chocolate w/ Butterfinger	1 (2 oz)	260	10	5	6	–	–	0	1	24
Dark Chocolate w/ Heath Bar	1 (2 oz)	280	12	10	6	–	–	0	1	26
Dark Chocolate w/ Peanuts	1 (2 oz)	280	15	5	6	–	–	0	2	18
Plain	1 (1 oz)	120	3	5	–	–	–	0	0	10
White Chocolate	1 (1.5 oz)	200	7	10	5	–	–	0	0	19
White Chocolate w/ Sprinkles	1 (2 oz)	210	7	10	5	–	–	0	0	22
ICE CREAM										
Amooretto Cream	1 serv (6 oz)	380	23	95	17	–	–	0	0	34
Apple Strudel	1 serv (6 oz)	380	21	85	15	–	–	0	0	39
Banana Pudding	1 serv (6 oz)	330	18	75	13	–	–	0	1	32
Black Cherry	1 serv (6 oz)	380	23	95	17	–	–	0	0	35
Blueberry Muffin	1 serv (6 oz)	390	20	75	14	–	–	0	1	37
Brownie Batter	1 serv (6 oz)	420	21	85	15	–	–	0	1	42
Butter Pecan	1 serv (6 oz)	380	21	85	15	–	–	0	0	40
Cake 6 inch Better Batter	⅛ cake (5.7 oz)	480	24	55	16	–	–	0	1	45
Cake 6 inch Chocolate Cream	⅛ cake (6.4 oz)	580	33	80	22	–	–	0	3	53
Cake 8 inch Caramel Drizzle	1/14 cake (6 oz)	530	33	65	18	–	–	0	11	45
Cake 8 inch Chocolate Espresso	1/14 cake (5.6 oz)	460	25	150	17	–	–	0	1	48
Cake 8 inch Chocolate Heaven	1/14 cake (5 oz)	400	22	60	16	–	–	0	2	38
Cake 8 inch Cookie Dreams	1/14 cake (5.3 oz)	440	22	55	15	–	–	2	1	41
Cake 8 inch Cookies 'N' Cream	1/14 cake (5.3 oz)	430	24	65	15	–	–	0	1	38
Cake 8 inch Cotton Candy Carnival	1/14 cake (5.9 oz)	490	25	65	18	–	–	0	1	50
Cake 8 inch Fudge Fantasy	1/14 cake (5.4 oz)	410	22	60	17	–	–	0	0	40
Cake 8 inch Maggie S'Mores	1/14 cake (7 oz)	610	23	55	15	–	–	0	2	61

FOOD	PORTION	CALS	TOTAL FAT	CHOL	SAT FAT	POLY FAT	MONO FAT	TRANS FAT	FIBER	SUGAR
Cake 8 inch Maggie's Mud	1/14 cake (5.3 oz)	440	25	60	16	–	–	0	2	41
Cake 8 inch Pecan Perfection	1/14 cake (5.6 oz)	500	33	60	16	–	–	0	3	39
Cake 8 inch Sprinkle	1/14 cake (5.7 oz)	370	19	55	14	–	–	0	0	38
Cake 8 inch Strawberry Cheesecream	1/14 cake (6.3 oz)	530	23	55	15	–	–	0	1	46
Cake 8 inch Truffle Dream	1/14 cake (5.8 oz)	500	28	75	19	–	–	0	2	46
Cake 8 inch Turtle	1/14 cake (6.3 oz)	590	40	65	18	–	–	0	2	42
Cappuccino	1 serv (6 oz)	380	22	90	16	–	–	0	0	36
Caramel Apple	1 serv (6 oz)	400	21	85	15	–	–	0	0	41
Carrot Cake	1 serv (6 oz)	420	21	80	15	–	–	0	0	39
Cheesecake	1 serv (6 oz)	380	21	85	16	–	–	0	0	36
Choco Mallo	1 serv (6 oz)	360	19	75	14	–	–	0	1	36
Chocolate	1 serv (6 oz)	390	22	80	16	–	–	0	2	37
Chocolate Banana	1 serv (6 oz)	370	20	80	15	–	–	0	2	35
Chocolate Better Batter	1 serv (6 oz)	420	21	50	15	–	–	0	1	41
Chocolate Peanut Butter	1 serv (6 oz)	450	28	80	16	–	–	0	2	35
Chocolate Raspberry	1 serv (6 oz)	380	20	80	15	–	–	0	2	39
Cinnamoo	1 serv (6 oz)	380	23	95	17	–	–	0	0	33
Cinnamoo Bun	1 serv (6 oz)	530	23	60	14	–	–	0	1	40
Cocoa Amooretto	1 serv (6 oz)	390	23	90	16	–	–	0	1	36
Cool Mint	1 serv (6 oz)	380	23	95	17	–	–	0	0	34
Cotton Candy	1 serv (6 oz)	380	23	95	17	–	–	0	0	34
Creamy Coconut	1 serv (6 oz)	380	23	95	17	–	–	0	0	33
Cupcake Better Batter	1	430	21	45	15	–	–	0	1	45
Cupcake Caramel Pumpkin Pie	1	500	26	50	19	–	–	0	1	46
Cupcake Cherry Chocolate	1	280	13	50	8	–	–	0	1	22
Cupcake Chocolate	1	400	22	65	13	–	–	0	2	37
Cupcake Chocolate Heaven	1	340	18	45	13	–	–	0	1	31
Cupcake Cool Swirl	1	370	19	45	14	–	–	1	0	36
Cupcake Cotton Candy Carnival	1	330	18	50	13	–	–	0	0	32
Cupcake Maggie O	1	360	18	55	10	–	–	0	1	29
Cupcake Pecan Pie	1	440	28	45	17	–	–	0	1	31
Cupcake Snowcap Blush	1	360	18	45	13	–	–	0	1	36

FOOD	PORTION	CALS	TOTAL FAT	CHOL	SAT FAT	POLY FAT	MONO FAT	TRANS FAT	FIBER	SUGAR
Cupcake Sprinkle	1	340	18	50	13	–	–	0	0	34
Dark Chocolate	1 serv	390	23	90	16	–	–	0	2	35
Egg Nog	1 serv (6 oz)	390	22	90	16	–	–	0	0	38
Espresso Bean	1 serv (6 oz)	380	22	90	16	–	–	0	0	36
French Vanilla	1 serv	390	22	90	16	–	–	0	0	38
Fresh Banana	1 serv (6 oz)	340	19	80	14	–	–	0	1	32
Key Lime	1 serv	380	18	70	13	–	–	0	0	48
Maggie's Fudge	1 serv	630	34	120	26	–	–	0	0	62
Mint Chocolate	1 serv (6 oz)	390	23	80	16	–	–	0	1	37
Mocha	1 serv (6 oz)	390	23	850	14	–	–	0	1	29
Peanut Butter	1 serv (6 oz)	480	33	80	17	–	–	0	1	31
Pina Cowlada	1 serv (6 oz)	360	21	85	15	–	–	0	0	33
Pink Bubblegum	1 serv (6 oz)	380	23	85	17	–	–	0	0	34
Pink Peppermint Stick	1 serv (6 oz)	420	21	85	15	–	–	0	0	47
Pistachio	1 serv (6 oz)	380	23	95	17	–	–	0	0	34
Pizza 10 inch Cheese	1/10 pie (5.4 oz)	340	18	65	12	–	–	0	0	31
Pizza 10 inch Chocolate Lover's	1/10 pie	390	20	70	13	–	–	0	1	35
Pizza 10 inch Supreme	1/10 pie (6.1 oz)	450	24	70	15	–	–	0	1	43
Pumpkin Pie	1 serv (6 oz)	370	21	850	15	–	–	0	0	36
Raspberry	1 serv (6 oz)	370	21	85	15	–	–	0	0	37
Red Velvet Cake	1 serv (6 oz)	420	21	75	14	–	–	0	1	41
Rum Raisin	1 serv (6 oz)	380	23	95	17	–	–	0	0	35
Southern Peaches	1 serv (6 oz)	330	16	65	12	–	–	0	0	36
Strawberry	1 serv	350	21	85	15	–	–	0	0	33
Strawberry Banana No Sugar Added	1 serv (6 oz)	170	6	0	5	–	–	0	0	0
Udderly Cream	1 serv (6 oz)	380	23	95	17	–	–	0	0	34
Vanilla	1 serv (6 oz)	380	23	95	17	–	–	0	0	35
Vanilla Low Fat Lactose Free	1 serv (6 oz)	130	5	0	3	–	–	0	0	18
Very Yellow Marshmallow	1 serv (6 oz)	350	20	80	14	–	–	0	0	34

MANHATTAN BAGEL
BAGELS AND BAKED GOODS

FOOD	PORTION	CALS	TOTAL FAT	CHOL	SAT FAT	POLY FAT	MONO FAT	TRANS FAT	FIBER	SUGAR
Bagel Blueberry	1 (3.8 oz)	300	1	0	0	–	–	0	3	11
Bagel Blueberry Glaze	1 (4.5 oz)	360	0	0	0	0	0	0	3	25
Bagel Cheddar	1 (4 oz)	320	2	0	0	–	–	0	3	3
Bagel Chocolate Chip	1 (3.8 oz)	290	3	0	1	–	–	0	3	10
Bagel Cinnamon Raisin	1 (4 oz)	330	1	0	0	–	–	0	3	10
Bagel Egg	1 (4 oz)	320	2	120	0	–	–	0	3	3

FOOD	PORTION	CALS	TOTAL FAT	CHOL	SAT FAT	POLY FAT	MONO FAT	TRANS FAT	FIBER	SUGAR
Bagel Everything	1 (4.3 oz)	350	3	0	0	–	–	0	3	3
Bagel French Toast	1 (3.5 oz)	300	6	55	2	–	–	0	2	9
Bagel Garlic	1 (4.3 oz)	340	1	0	0	–	–	0	3	3
Bagel Honey Whole Wheat	1 (3.5 oz)	250	1	0	0	–	–	0	3	8
Bagel Honey Whole Wheat Everything	1 (3.8 oz)	280	3	0	0	–	–	0	3	8
Bagel Jalapeno Cheddar	1 (4 oz)	320	2	0	0	–	–	0	3	3
Bagel Onion	1 (4.3 oz)	340	1	0	0	–	–	0	3	3
Bagel Plain	1 (4 oz)	320	1	0	0	–	–	0	3	3
Bagel Poppy	1 (4.3 oz)	360	5	0	0	–	–	0	3	3
Bagel Pumpernickel	1 (3.5 oz)	240	2	0	0	–	–	0	3	4
Bagel Rye	1 (4 oz)	310	2	0	0	–	–	0	3	3
Bagel Salt	1 (4.3 oz)	320	1	0	0	–	–	0	3	3
Bagel Sesame Seed	1 (4.5 oz)	360	5	0	0	–	–	0	3	3
Bagel Mini Plain	1 (1.8 oz)	130	1	0	0	–	–	0	1	1
Bagel Thin Honey Whole Wheat	1 (2 oz)	120	2	0	0	–	–	0	4	3
Bagel Thin Plain	1 (2 oz)	120	1	0	0	–	–	0	1	2

MCDONALD'S
BEVERAGES

FOOD	PORTION	CALS	TOTAL FAT	CHOL	SAT FAT	POLY FAT	MONO FAT	TRANS FAT	FIBER	SUGAR
Apple Juice Minute Maid Juice Box	1 box (6.8 oz)	100	0	0	0	0	0	0	0	22
Coca-Cola Classic	1 sm (16 oz)	150	0	0	0	0	0	0	0	40
Coffee Black	1 sm (12 oz)	0	0	0	0	0	0	0	0	0
Coffee Cream	1 pkg (0.4 oz)	20	2	10	2	–	–	0	0	0
Diet Coke	1 sm (16 oz)	0	0	0	0	0	0	0	0	0
Dr Pepper	1 sm (16 oz)	150	0	0	0	0	0	0	0	39
Dr Pepper Diet	1 sm (16 oz)	0	0	0	0	0	0	0	0	0
Frappe Caramel	1 sm (12 oz)	450	20	55	13	–	–	1	0	56
Frappe Mocha	1 sm (12 oz)	450	20	55	13	–	–	1	1	56
Hi-C Orange Lavaburst	1 sm (16 oz)	160	0	0	0	0	0	0	0	44
Hot Chocolate Peppermint w/ Nonfat Milk	1 (12 oz)	220	4	5	3	–	–	0	0	34
Iced Coffee Caramel	1 sm (16 oz)	130	5	20	4	–	–	0	1	20
Iced Coffee Hazelnut	1 sm (16 oz)	130	5	20	4	–	–	0	0	21
Iced Coffee Regular	1 sm (16 oz)	140	5	20	4	–	–	0	0	22
Iced Coffee Vanilla	1 sm (16 oz)	130	5	20	4	–	–	0	0	21
Iced Coffee w/ Sugar Free Vanilla Syrup	1 sm (16 oz)	60	5	20	4	–	–	0	0	1

FOOD	PORTION	CALS	TOTAL FAT	CHOL	SAT FAT	POLY FAT	MONO FAT	TRANS FAT	FIBER	SUGAR
Iced Mocha w/ Nonfat Milk	1 sm (12 oz)	230	7	10	5	–	–	0	0	29
Iced Tea	1 sm (16 oz)	0	0	0	0	0	0	0	0	0
McCafe Shake Chocolate	1 (12 oz)	570	17	50	11	–	–	1	1	76
McCafe Shake Strawberry	1 (12 oz)	560	18	50	1	–	–	1	0	79
McCafe Shake Vanilla	1 (12 oz)	530	17	50	11	–	–	1	0	63
Milk Lowfat 1%	1 jug (8.3 oz)	100	3	10	2	–	–	0	0	12
Orange Juice Minute Maid	1 sm (12 oz)	150	0	0	0	0	0	0	0	30
Peppermint Mocha w/ Nonfat Milk	1 sm (12 oz)	220	4	5	3	–	–	0	0	33
Powerade Mountain Blast	1 sm (16 oz)	100	0	0	0	0	0	0	0	21
Smoothie Strawberry Banana	1 (12 oz)	210	1	5	0	–	–	0	2	44
Smoothie Wild Berry	1 (12 oz)	210	1	5	0	–	–	0	3	4
Sprite	1 sm (16 oz)	150	0	0	0	0	0	0	0	39
Sweet Tea	1 sm (16 oz)	150	0	0	0	0	0	0	0	36
BREAKFAST SELECTIONS										
Big Breakfast Regular Biscuit	1 (9.5 oz)	740	48	555	17	–	–	0	3	3
Big Breakfast w/ Hotcakes Regular Biscuit	1 (14.8 oz)	1090	56	575	19	–	–	0	6	17
Biscuit Regular Bacon Egg Cheese	1 (4.9 oz)	420	23	240	12	–	–	0	2	3
Biscuit Regular Sausage	1 (4.1 oz)	430	27	30	12	–	–	0	2	2
Biscuit Regular Sausage w/ Egg	1 (5.7 oz)	510	33	250	14	–	–	0	2	2
Chicken Biscuit Southern Style Regular	1 (5 oz)	410	20	30	8	–	–	0	2	3
Cinnamon Melts	1 serv (4 oz)	460	19	15	9	–	–	0	3	32
Fruit 'n Yogurt Parfait	1 (5.2 oz)	150	2	5	1	–	–	0	1	23
Hash Brown	1 (2 oz)	150	9	0	2	–	–	0	2	0
Hotcake Syrup	1 pkg (2 oz)	180	0	0	0	0	0	0	0	32
Hotcakes	1 serv (5.3 oz)	350	9	20	2	–	–	0	3	14
Hotcakes w/ Sausage	1 serv (6.8 oz)	520	24	50	7	–	–	0	3	14
McGriddles Bacon Egg Cheese	1 (5.8 oz)	410	18	240	8	–	–	0	2	15
McGriddles Sausage	1 serv (5 oz)	420	22	35	8	–	–	0	2	15
McGriddles Sausage Egg & Cheese	1 serv (7.1 oz)	550	31	265	12	–	–	0	2	15
McMuffin Egg	1 (4 oz)	300	12	260	5	–	–	0	2	3
McMuffin Sausage	1 (4 oz)	370	22	45	8	–	–	0	2	2
McMuffin Sausage w/ Egg	1 (5.8 oz)	450	27	285	10	–	–	0	2	2

FOOD	PORTION	CALS	TOTAL FAT	CHOL	SAT FAT	POLY FAT	MONO FAT	TRANS FAT	FIBER	SUGAR
Oatmeal Fruit & Maple	1 serv (9.2 oz)	290	5	10	2	–	–	0	5	32
Oatmeal Fruit & Maple w/o Brown Sugar	1 serv (9.2 oz)	260	5	5	2	–	–	0	5	18
DESSERTS										
Baked Hot Apple Pie	1 (2.7 oz)	250	13	0	7	–	–	0	4	13
Cone Reduced Fat Vanilla	1 (3.7 oz)	170	5	15	3	–	–	0	0	20
Cookie Chocolate Chip	1 (1.2 oz)	160	8	10	4	–	–	0	1	15
Cookie Oatmeal Raisin	1 (1.1 oz)	150	6	10	3	–	–	0	1	13
Cookie Sugar	1 (1.1 oz)	160	7	5	3	–	–	0	0	11
McFlurry M&M's	1 (12 oz)	650	23	50	14	–	–	1	1	89
McFlurry Oreo Cookies	1 (12 oz)	510	17	45	9	–	–	1	1	64
Peanuts For Sundae	1 serv (0.3 oz)	45	4	0	1	–	–	0	1	0
Sundae Hot Caramel	1 (6.4 oz)	340	8	30	5	–	–	0	1	43
Sundae Hot Fudge	1 (6.3 oz)	330	9	25	7	–	–	0	1	48
Sundae Strawberry	1 (6.3 oz)	280	6	25	4	–	–	0	1	45
MAIN MENU SELECTIONS										
Angus Bacon & Cheese	1 (10.2 oz)	790	39	150	18	–	–	2	4	13
Angus Deluxe	1 (11.2 oz)	760	39	135	17	–	–	2	4	10
Angus Mushroom & Swiss	1 (10 oz)	770	40	135	17	–	–	2	4	8
Big Mac	1 (7.6 oz)	550	29	75	10	–	–	1	3	9
Cheeseburger	1 (4 oz)	300	12	40	6	–	–	1	2	7
Cheeseburger Double	1 (5.8 oz)	440	23	80	11	–	–	2	2	7
Chicken McNuggets	4 (2.3 oz)	190	12	25	2	–	–	0	1	0
Chicken Breast Strips	3 (4.4 oz)	380	23	55	4	–	–	0	1	0
Filet-O-Fish	1 (5 oz)	390	19	40	4	–	–	0	2	5
French Fries	1 sm (2.5 oz)	230	11	0	2	–	–	0	3	0
Grilled Onion Cheddar	1 (4.1 oz)	310	13	40	6	–	–	1	2	7
Hamburger	1 (3.5 oz)	250	9	25	4	–	–	1	2	6
McChicken	1 (5.1 oz)	360	16	35	3	–	–	0	2	5
McDouble	1 (5.3 oz)	390	19	65	8	–	–	1	2	7
McRib	1 (7.3 oz)	500	26	70	10	–	–	0	3	11
Quarter Pounder Double w/ Cheese	1 (10 oz)	750	43	160	19	–	–	3	3	10
Quarter Pounder w/ Cheese	1 (7.1 oz)	520	26	95	12	–	–	2	3	10
Sandwich Classic Chicken Crispy	1 (7.5 oz)	510	22	45	4	–	–	0	3	10
Sandwich Classic Chicken Grilled	1 (7 oz)	350	9	65	2	–	–	0	3	8
Sandwich Club Chicken Crispy	1 (8.4 oz)	620	29	70	7	–	–	0	3	11

FOOD	PORTION	CALS	TOTAL FAT	CHOL	SAT FAT	POLY FAT	MONO FAT	TRANS FAT	FIBER	SUGAR
Sandwich Club Chicken Grilled	1 (7.9 oz)	460	16	90	6	–	–	0	3	9
Sandwich Ranch BLT Chicken Crispy	1 (7.6 oz)	540	23	55	5	–	–	0	3	11
Sandwich Ranch BLT Chicken Grilled	1 (7.1 oz)	380	10	75	3	–	–	0	3	9
Sandwich Southern Style Crispy Chicken	1 (5.6 oz)	420	19	45	3	–	–	0	2	7
Snack Wrap Angus Bacon & Cheese	1 (5 oz)	390	21	75	10	–	–	1	1	4
Snack Wrap Angus Deluxe	1 (5.9 oz)	410	25	75	10	–	–	2	2	3
Snack Wrap Angus Mushroom & Swiss	1 (5.7 oz)	430	25	75	10	–	–	2	2	2
Snack Wrap Chipotle BBQ Crispy	1 (4.1 oz)	330	15	30	5	–	–	0	1	4
Snack Wrap Chipotle BBQ Grilled	1 (4.1 oz)	250	8	40	4	–	–	0	1	5
Snack Wrap Honey Mustard Crispy	1 (4.1 oz)	320	15	30	5	–	–	0	1	2
Snack Wrap Honey Mustard Grilled	1 (4.1 oz)	250	8	45	4	–	–	0	1	2
Snack Wrap Ranch Crispy	1 (4.2 oz)	350	19	35	5	–	–	0	1	2
Snack Wrap Ranch Grilled	1 (4.2 oz)	270	12	45	4	–	–	0	1	2
SALAD DRESSINGS AND SAUCES										
Dressing Newman's Own Creamy Caesar	1 pkg (2 oz)	190	18	20	4	–	–	0	0	2
Dressing Newman's Own Creamy Southwest	1 pkg (1.5 oz)	100	6	20	1	–	–	0	0	3
Dressing Newman's Own Low Fat Balsamic Vinaigrette	1 pkg (1.5 oz)	35	3	0	0	–	–	0	0	3
Dressing Newman's Own Low Fat Family Recipe Italian	1 pkg (1.5 oz)	50	3	0	1	–	–	0	0	2
Dressing Newman's Own Low Fat Sesame Ginger	1 pkg (1.5 oz)	90	3	0	0	–	–	0	1	9
Dressing Newman's Own Ranch	1 pkg (2 oz)	170	15	20	3	–	–	0	0	4
Honey	1 pkg (0.5 oz)	50	0	0	0	0	0	0	0	11
Ketchup	1 pkg (0.4 oz)	10	0	0	0	0	0	0	0	2
Sauce Chipotle Barbeque	1 pkg (1 oz)	50	0	0	0	0	0	0	0	10
Sauce Creamy Ranch	1 pkg (0.8 oz)	110	12	5	2	–	–	0	0	1

FOOD	PORTION	CALS	TOTAL FAT	CHOL	SAT FAT	POLY FAT	MONO FAT	TRANS FAT	FIBER	SUG
Sauce Honey Mustard	1 pkg (0.8 oz)	35	4	5	1	–	–	0	1	5
Sauce Hot Mustard	1 pkg (1 oz)	60	3	5	0	–	–	0	2	6
Sauce Spicy Buffalo	1 pkg (0.8 oz)	35	3	0	0	–	–	0	0	0
Sauce Sweet'N Sour	1 pkg (1 oz)	50	0	0	0	0	0	0	0	10
Sauce Tangy Barbecue	1 pkg (1 oz)	50	0	0	0	0	0	0	0	10
Sauce Tartar	1 serv (1 oz)	140	15	10	3	–	–	0	0	0
SALADS										
Bacon Ranch w/ Crispy Chicken	1 (11.3 oz)	390	22	70	6	–	–	0	4	7
Bacon Ranch w/ Grilled Chicken	1 (10.8 oz)	230	9	85	4	–	–	0	4	5
Bacon Ranch w/o Chicken	1 (7.9 oz)	140	7	25	4	–	–	0	3	4
Caesar w/ Crispy Chicken	1 (10.9 oz)	350	18	55	5	–	–	0	4	7
Caesar w/ Grilled Chicken	1 (10.4 oz)	190	5	70	3	–	–	0	4	5
Caesar w/o Chicken	1 (7.5 oz)	90	4	10	3	–	–	0	3	4
Croutons Butter Garlic	1 pkg (0.5 oz)	60	2	0	0	–	–	0	1	0
Fruit & Walnut Snack Size	1 pkg (5.7 oz)	210	8	5	2	–	–	0	2	25
Side Salad	1 (3.1 oz)	20	0	0	0	0	0	0	1	2
Southwest Grilled Chicken	1 (11.8 oz)	290	8	70	3	–	–	0	7	11
Southwest w/ Crispy Chicken	1 (12.3 oz)	450	21	50	5	–	–	0	7	13
Southwest w/o Chicken	1 (8.1 oz)	140	5	10	2	–	–	0	6	6

MRS. FIELDS

FOOD	PORTION	CALS	TOTAL FAT	CHOL	SAT FAT	POLY FAT	MONO FAT	TRANS FAT	FIBER	SUG
Bites Double Fudge	3 (1.6 oz)	200	10	45	5	–	–	0	1	21
Brownie Butterscotch Blondie	1 (2.1 oz)	260	10	50	6	–	–	0	0	28
Brownie Double Fudge	1 (2.1 oz)	260	13	60	8	–	–	0	1	27
Brownie Pecan Fudge	1 (2.1 oz)	270	15	55	7	–	–	0	2	25
Brownie Special Walnut Fudge & Blondie	1 (2.2 oz)	260	13	55	7	–	–	0	1	27
Brownie Toffee Fudge	1 (2.1 oz)	260	14	60	7	–	–	0	1	27
Brownie Walnut Fudge	1 (2.1 oz)	270	15	55	7	–	–	0	2	25
Cake Chocolate Chip	1 piece (2.9 oz)	350	17	50	8	–	–	0	tr	27
Coffee Cake Chocolate Chip	1 sm piece (2.2 oz)	240	11	30	4	–	–	0	1	16
Coffee Cake Chocolate Chip	1 lg (2.4 oz)	250	12	30	4	–	–	0	1	16
Cookie Butter	1 (1.5 oz)	200	8	20	5	–	–	0	tr	15
Cookie Chocolate Covered Peanut Butter	1 (2.5 oz)	340	19	20	10	–	–	0	1	26

FOOD	PORTION	CALS	TOTAL FAT	CHOL.	SAT FAT	POLY FAT	MONO FAT	TRANS FAT	FIBER	SUGAR
Cookie Chocolate Covered Semi-Sweet	1 (2.5 oz)	380	23	15	15	–	–	0	1	37
Cookie Chocolate Covered White Chunk Macadamia	1 (2.4 oz)	330	19	15	10	–	–	0	1	29
Cookie Cinnamon Sugar	1 (1.8 oz)	210	8	20	4	–	–	0	0	16
Cookie Cut Out	1 (2.4 oz)	280	11	2	5	–	–	1	0	28
Cookie Frosted Cinnamon Sugar	1 (2.1 oz)	270	11	20	5	–	–	1	0	25
Cookie Oatmeal Raisins & Walnuts	1 (1.7 oz)	200	9	15	3	–	–	0	1	16
Cookie Semi-Sweet Chocolate	1 (1.7 oz)	210	10	15	5	–	–	0	1	19
Cookie Semi-Sweet Chocolate w/ Walnuts	1 (1.7 oz)	220	11	15	5	–	–	0	1	17
Cookie Triple Chocolate	1 (1.7 oz)	210	10	15	6	–	–	0	1	19
Cookie White Chunk Macadamia	1 (1.7 oz)	230	12	15	6	–	–	0	0	19
Jelly Bellys	1 pkg (1.4 oz)	140	0	0	0	0	0	0	0	29
Mixed Nuts	1 pkg (2 oz)	350	32	0	5	–	–	0	3	2
Muffin Blueberry	1 (1.9 oz)	190	9	25	3	–	–	0	1	12
Muffin Chocolate Chip	1 (1.9 oz)	200	10	25	3	–	–	0	1	14
Nibbler Cinnamon Sugar	3 (1.4 oz)	180	8	10	3	–	–	0	0	12
Nibbler Debra's Special	3 (1.3 oz)	160	7	10	2	–	–	0	1	13
Nibbler Peanut Butter	3 (1.8 oz)	170	9	10	3	–	–	0	1	10
Nibbler Semi-Sweet Chocolate	3 (1.8 oz)	170	8	10	4	–	–	0	1	14
Nibbler Triple Chocolate	3 (1.8 oz)	160	8	10	4	–	–	0	1	15
Nibbler White Chunk Macadamia	3 (1.8 oz)	180	9	10	4	–	–	0	0	15
Taffy	1 pkg (2.4 oz)	160	2	0	2	–	–	0	0	23

NATHAN'S

FOOD	PORTION	CALS	TOTAL FAT	CHOL.	SAT FAT	POLY FAT	MONO FAT	TRANS FAT	FIBER	SUGAR
Apple Pie	1 (3.49 oz)	314	19	0	4	–	–	0	0	9
Bacon Cheeseburger	1 (10.7 oz)	783	50	136	20	–	–	0	2	10
Cheese Dog	1 (5.05 oz)	390	25	35	8	–	–	3	1	5
Cheese Fries	1 reg (8 oz)	564	42	0	7	–	–	2	4	5
Cheesesteak	1 (12.31 oz)	849	45	151	21	–	–	0	2	1
Cheesesteak Supreme	1 (16.29 oz)	879	45	151	20	–	–	0	3	3
Cheesesteak Supreme Chicken	1 (13.81 oz)	601	19	79	9	–	–	0	3	3

FOOD	PORTION	CALS	TOTAL FAT	CHOL	SAT FAT	POLY FAT	MONO FAT	TRANS FAT	FIBER	SUG
Chicken Tender Pita	1 (11.94 oz)	823	52	40	8	–	–	0	5	15
Chicken Tender Platter	1 (17.69 oz)	1245	90	44	14	–	–	0	10	31
Chicken Tenders	3 (6.19 oz)	526	39	30	6	–	–	0	3	8
Chicken Wings	5 (6.65 oz)	400	27	83	7	–	–	2	0	0
Chili Dog	1 (5.05 oz)	400	23	50	6	–	–	1	2	5
Corn Dog On A Stick	1 (2.89 oz)	380	21	15	5	–	–	0	1	13
Corn On The Cob w/ Butter	1 (5.05 oz)	140	2	0	0	–	–	0	2	6
Double Burger w/ Cheese	1 (15.61 oz)	1178	84	235	32	–	–	0	2	10
Famous Hot Dog	1 (3.53 oz)	297	18	34	7	–	–	tr	1	4
French Fries	1 reg (6.5 oz)	464	34	0	5	–	–	0	4	4
Funnel Cake	1 (4.21 oz)	580	29	30	5	–	–	3	1	43
Hot Dog Nuggets	6 (3.49 oz)	348	28	20	6	–	–	0	0	5
Mozzarella Sticks + Sauce	3 (5.64 oz)	390	28	32	8	–	–	0	1	6
Onion Rings	1 sm (5.6 oz)	544	45	0	6	–	–	0	1	4
Platter Grilled Chicken	1 (15 oz)	504	56	59	9	–	–	0	7	24
Pretzel Dog	1 (4.02 oz)	390	16	25	6	–	–	0	1	7
Pretzel King Size	1 (2.28 oz)	180	1	0	0	–	–	0	1	1
Sandwich Chicken Tender	1 (9.65 oz)	706	43	33	6	–	–	0	5	12
Sandwich Grilled Chicken	1 (9.03 oz)	554	32	65	5	–	–	0	3	3
Wrap Grilled Chicken Caesar	1 (10.34 oz)	700	34	75	11	–	–	0	1	2
Wrap Krispy Southwest Chipotle	1 (11.71 oz)	750	39	100	13	–	–	0	1	3

OLD SPAGHETTI FACTORY
BEVERAGES

FOOD	PORTION	CALS	TOTAL FAT	CHOL	SAT FAT	POLY FAT	MONO FAT	TRANS FAT	FIBER	SUG
Cherry Coke	1 (12 oz)	140	0	0	0	0	0	0	0	39
Coffee Black	1 (8 oz)	0	0	0	0	0	0	0	0	0
Coke	1 (12 oz)	130	0	0	0	0	0	0	0	37
Diet Coke	1 (12 oz)	0	0	0	0	0	0	0	0	0
Hot Tea	1 (8 oz)	0	0	0	0	0	0	0	0	0
Iced Tea Strawberry	1 (12 oz)	100	0	0	0	0	0	0	0	10
Italian Cream Soda	1 (7.5 oz)	140	3	10	2	–	–	0	0	24
Kid's Juice Bar	1 serv (2.4 oz)	60	0	0	0	0	0	0	0	14
Lemonade	1 (12 oz)	140	0	0	0	0	0	0	0	37
Lemonade Strawberry	1 (12 oz)	200	0	0	0	0	0	0	0	52
Masterpiece Shake	1 (8.5 oz)	700	39	85	21	–	–	0	1	63
Milk 2%	1 (13 oz)	180	7	30	5	–	–	0	0	17
Milk Skim	1 (13 oz)	130	1	5	0	–	–	0	0	18
Root Beer	1 (12 oz)	150	0	0	0	0	0	0	0	41
Sprite	1 (12 oz)	140	0	0	0	0	0	0	0	30

FOOD	PORTION	CALS	TOTAL FAT	CHOL	SAT FAT	POLY FAT	MONO FAT	TRANS FAT	FIBER	SUGAR
CHILDREN'S MENU SELECTIONS										
Fettuccine Alfredo	1 serv (10.3 oz)	770	48	145	30	–	–	2	3	3
Macaroni & Cheese	1 serv (8 oz)	390	10	25	6	–	–	0	2	5
Ravioli	1 serv (10 oz)	420	14	65	8	–	–	0	5	9
Ravioli Spinach & Cheese	1 serv (6.6 oz)	310	12	50	7	–	–	0	4	5
Sandwich Grilled Cheese	1 (4.5 oz)	480	30	45	15	–	–	0	2	2
Spaghetti Marinara w/ Sicilian Meatballs	1 serv (13 oz)	570	16	60	5	–	–	1	5	8
Spaghetti w/ Brown Butter & Mizithra Cheese	1 serv (8.7 oz)	660	37	100	22	–	–	1	3	3
Spaghetti w/ Clam Sauce	1 serv (10 oz)	440	9	75	5	–	–	0	3	3
Spaghetti w/ Marinara Sauce	1 serv (15 oz)	560	5	0	1	–	–	0	7	11
Spaghetti w/ Meat Sauce	1 serv (10 oz)	410	6	15	2	–	–	0	4	6
Spinach Tortellini w/ Alfredo Sauce	1 serv (6.8 oz)	530	30	110	17	–	–	1	3	3
DESSERTS										
Cake Chocolate Truffle Mousse	1 serv (9 oz)	850	41	80	25	–	–	1	5	89
Ice Cream Spumoni	1 serv (3 oz)	180	9	40	6	–	–	0	0	17
Ice Cream Vanilla	1 serv (3 oz)	170	9	35	6	–	–	0	0	14
Mud Pie	1 serv (6 oz)	490	20	25	12	–	–	0	1	52
MAIN MENU SELECTIONS										
Angel Hair	1 serv (8 oz)	420	2	0	0	–	–	0	2	4
Appetizer Bay Shrimp Crostini	1 serv (9.3 oz)	720	41	135	10	–	–	0	3	3
Appetizer Garlic Fries	1 serv (18.4 oz)	1410	107	10	17	–	–	1	10	7
Appetizer Portuguese Linguica	1 serv (17.5 oz)	1080	75	135	23	–	–	0	8	3
Baked Chicken	1 serv (18.3 oz)	1030	62	225	20	–	–	0	4	6
Baked Lasagna	1 serv (17.5 oz)	800	43	125	21	–	–	0	7	13
Bread Sicilian Garlic Cheese	4 serv (16 oz)	1310	76	120	33	–	–	1	6	10
Broccoli	1 sm (7.5 oz)	340	31	50	12	–	–	0	5	0
Burger Sliders	1 serv (23.6 oz)	1770	107	470	39	–	–	6	6	28

FOOD	PORTION	CALS	TOTAL FAT	CHOL	SAT FAT	POLY FAT	MONO FAT	TRANS FAT	FIBER	S
Cheese Manicotti w/ Marinara Sauce	1 serv (12 oz)	490	21	120	11	–	–	0	3	1
Chicken Marsala	1 serv (17.4 oz)	1050	57	200	26	–	–	1	3	7
Chicken Penne	1 serv (14.8 oz)	830	31	110	16	–	–	1	5	12
Dip Shrimp Spinach & Artichoke	4 serv (9.3 oz)	590	41	90	17	–	–	5	3	2
Factory Burger w/ Chips	1 serv (16.6 oz)	1370	84	245	26	–	–	3	4	12
Fettuccine Alfredo	1 serv (14.2 oz)	1080	70	215	44	–	–	2	4	5
Fettuccine or Penne	1 serv (8 oz)	420	2	0	0	–	–	2	4	3
Garlic Mizithra	1 serv (15 oz)	1240	77	175	38	–	–	2	4	7
Hearty Meal Clam Sauce	1 serv (25 oz)	1110	23	185	12	–	–	0	7	6
Hearty Meal Italian Sausage w/ Meat Sauce	1 serv (29 oz)	1350	42	110	15	–	–	1	12	14
Hearty Meal Marinara Sauce	1 serv (25 oz)	940	8	0	1	–	–	0	11	19
Hearty Meal Meat Sauce	1 serv (25 oz)	1020	15	40	5	–	–	1	11	14
Hearty Meal Mizithra Cheese & Brown Butter	1 serv (22.4 oz)	1750	101	275	62	–	–	3	7	8
Hearty Meal Pot Pourri	1 serv (26 oz)	1280	43	150	23	–	–	1	9	13
Hearty Meal Sauteed Mushroom Sauce	1 serv (30 oz)	1120	26	0	3	–	–	0	12	22
Hearty Meal Sicilian Meatballs	1 serv (31 oz)	1350	36	130	12	–	–	1	13	19
Lasagna Vegetariano	1 serv (20.6 oz)	830	48	120	25	–	–	0	9	15
Meatloaf Italian	1 serv (18.5 oz)	1180	68	230	32	–	–	2	6	8
Olive Tapenade	4 serv (7.4 oz)	800	66	0	7	–	–	0	2	1
Panini Chicken Smoked Mozzarella w/ Chips	1 serv (14.4 oz)	1280	68	105	16	–	–	0	18	11
Parmigiana Chicken	1 serv (19.2 oz)	810	30	105	7	–	–	0	5	10
Pasta Gluten Free	1 serv (9 oz)	470	1	0	0	–	–	0	2	0
Pasta Whole Wheat	1 serv (8 oz)	390	2	0	0	–	–	0	14	4
Platter #1 Lasagna & Chicken Marsala	1 (27.5 oz)	1090	66	225	26	–	–	1	7	17

FOOD	PORTION	CALS	TOTAL FAT	CHOL	SAT FAT	POLY FAT	MONO FAT	TRANS FAT	FIBER	SUGAR
Platter #2 Ravioli & Spaghetti w/ Meat Sauce	1 (21 oz)	880	22	95	10	–	–	0	10	15
Platter #3 Spaghetti w/ Meat Sauce Sausage & Meatballs	1 (25 oz)	1360	64	225	24	–	–	2	9	9
Ravioli Crab	1 serv (11 oz)	810	45	190	24	–	–	1	5	3
Ravioli Spinach & Cheese	1 serv (11 oz)	480	16	75	9	–	–	0	6	9
Ravioli Toasted Beef	4 serv (4 oz)	200	5	0	2	–	–	0	2	2
Ravioli Toasted Cheese	4 serv (4 oz)	210	6	0	4	–	–	0	2	3
Sandwich Sicilian Style Meatball w/ Chips	1 serv (16.4 oz)	1200	54	140	17	–	–	2	8	5
Sandwich Sicilian Style Sausage w/ Chips	1 serv (14.4 oz)	1140	55	90	19	–	–	0	9	4
Senior Meal Italian Sausage w/ Meat Sauce	1 serv (14 oz)	740	33	85	12	–	–	0	6	6
Senior Meal Pot Pourri	1 serv (10 oz)	520	19	60	10	–	–	0	4	5
Senior Meal Spaghetti Marinara	1 serv (10 oz)	370	4	0	0	–	–	0	5	8
Senior Meal Spaghetti Marinara w/ Sicilian Meatballs	1 serv (16 oz)	770	29	115	9	–	–	2	5	8
Senior Meal Spaghetti Mizithra & Brown Butter	1 serv (10 oz)	660	37	100	22	–	–	1	3	3
Senior Meal Spaghetti w/ Clam Sauce	1 serv (10 oz)	440	9	75	5	–	–	0	3	3
Senior Meal Spaghetti w/ Meat Sauce	1 serv (10 oz)	410	6	15	2	–	–	0	4	6
Senior Meal Spaghetti w/ Mushroom Sauce	1 serv (12 oz)	450	10	0	1	–	–	0	5	9
Side Alfredo Sauce	6 oz	640	67	210	42	–	–	2	0	0
Side Clam Sauce	6 oz	190	12	110	7	–	–	0	0	0
Side Marinara Sauce	6 oz	90	3	0	0	–	–	0	3	8
Side Marsala Sauce	6 oz	70	4	0	2	–	–	0	0	3
Side Meat Sauce	6 oz	140	7	25	2	–	–	0	2	5
Side Sausage	1 serv (4.5 oz)	340	27	70	11	–	–	0	2	0
Side Sauteed Mushroom Sauce	9 oz	200	14	0	2	–	–	0	3	10
Side Sicilian Meatballs	2 (6 oz)	420	27	130	10	–	–	1	1	0
Spaghetti	1 serv (9 oz)	460	3	0	1	–	–	0	4	4

FOOD	PORTION	CALS	TOTAL FAT	CHOL	SAT FAT	POLY FAT	MONO FAT	TRANS FAT	FIBER	SUG
Spaghetti Squash	1 serv (20.7 oz)	540	36	30	9	–	–	0	8	13
Spaghetti Vesuvius	1 serv (15 oz)	710	19	45	7	–	–	0	6	8
Spaghetti w/ Clam Sauce	1 serv (15 oz)	660	14	110	7	–	–	0	4	4
Spaghetti w/ Italian Sausage w/ Meat Sauce	1 serv (19 oz)	940	36	95	13	–	–	0	8	8
Spaghetti w/ Meat Sauce	1 serv (15 oz)	610	9	25	3	–	–	0	7	8
Spaghetti w/ Mizithra Cheese & Brown Butter	1 serv (13.4 oz)	1040	59	160	36	–	–	2	4	5
Spaghetti w/ Pot Pourri	1 serv (16 oz)	780	26	90	13	–	–	1	6	8
Spaghetti w/ Sauteed Mushroom Sauce	1 serv (18 oz)	670	16	0	2	–	–	0	7	13
Spaghetti w/ Sicilian Meatballs	1 serv (21 oz)	960	31	115	10	–	–	2	7	12
Spinach Tortellini w/ Alfredo Sauce	1 serv (12 oz)	930	55	200	32	–	–	2	5	5
SALADS										
BLT	1 (15.4 oz)	1000	85	115	21	–	–	0	9	5
Caesar Entree Chicken	1 (21.2 oz)	1130	90	160	18	–	–	0	6	5
Caesar Entree w/o Chicken	1 (14.5 oz)	820	72	70	16	–	–	0	6	5
Caesar Upgrade	1 (7 oz)	440	37	40	9	–	–	0	3	2
House w/ 1000 Island	1 (5 oz)	230	17	5	2	–	–	0	1	5
House w/ Balsamic	1 (4.5 oz)	260	21	0	2	–	–	0	1	2
House w/ Blue Cheese	1 (5 oz)	280	24	15	4	–	–	0	1	2
House w/ Caesar	1 (5 oz)	330	30	20	4	–	–	0	1	2
House w/ Creamy Pesto	1 (5 oz)	280	24	10	3	–	–	0	1	2
House w/ Fat Free Honey Mustard	1 (4.5 oz)	120	3	0	0	–	–	0	1	9
Senior Meal Caesar Chicken	1 serv (17 oz)	870	67	135	13	–	–	0	4	4
Senior Meal Caesar w/o Chicken	1 serv (10.2 oz)	560	48	50	11	–	–	0	4	4
SOUPS										
Chicken Mulligatawny	1 serv (9 oz)	260	19	60	9	–	–	0	1	6
Clam Chowder	1 serv (9 oz)	370	25	155	15	–	–	0	1	1
Cream Of Broccoli	1 serv (9 oz)	240	19	45	8	–	–	0	2	10
Minestrone	1 serv (9 oz)	60	2	0	0	–	–	0	2	2

ORANGE JULIUS
BEVERAGES

FOOD	PORTION	CALS	TOTAL FAT	CHOL	SAT FAT	POLY FAT	MONO FAT	TRANS FAT	FIBER	SUG
Barq's	1 sm (17 oz)	180	0	0	0	0	0	0	0	48

FOOD	PORTION	CALS	TOTAL FAT	CHOL	SAT FAT	POLY FAT	MONO FAT	TRANS FAT	FIBER	SUGAR
Coca-Cola	1 sm (17 oz)	160	0	0	0	0	0	0	0	43
Coffee Black	1 (12 oz)	0	0	0	0	0	0	0	0	0
Diet Coca-Cola	1 sm (17 oz)	0	0	0	0	0	0	0	0	0
Diet Pepsi	1 sm (17 oz)	0	0	0	0	0	0	0	0	0
Dr Pepper	1 sm (17 oz)	160	0	0	0	0	0	0	0	43
Julius Bananarilla	1 sm (16 oz)	350	6	0	6	–	–	0	3	58
Julius Blackberry	1 sm (16 oz)	380	6	0	5	–	–	0	4	67
Julius Cool Cappuccino	1 sm (16 oz)	430	11	5	10	–	–	0	2	63
Julius Cool Mocha	1 sm (16 oz)	700	14	10	11	–	–	0	3	105
Julius Eggnog	1 sm (16 oz)	330	8	25	7	–	–	0	2	55
Julius Lemon	1 sm (16 oz)	280	0	0	0	0	0	0	0	76
Julius Mango	1 sm (16 oz)	250	0	0	0	0	0	0	1	64
Julius Orange	1 sm (16 oz)	230	0	0	0	0	0	0	0	59
Julius Peach	1 sm (16 oz)	240	0	0	0	0	0	0	1	61
Julius Pina Colada	1 sm (16 oz)	330	5	0	5	–	–	0	2	64
Julius Pineapple	1 sm (16 oz)	230	0	0	0	0	0	0	1	59
Julius Pomegranate	1 sm (16 oz)	260	0	0	0	0	0	0	1	68
Julius Raspberry	1 sm (16 oz)	300	0	0	0	0	0	0	3	77
Julius Strawberry	1 sm (16 oz)	290	0	0	0	0	0	0	1	75
Julius Strawberry Banana	1 sm (16 oz)	380	6	0	5	–	–	0	3	69
Julius Tripleberry	1 sm (16 oz)	420	6	0	5	–	–	0	4	79
Julius Tropical	1 sm (16 oz)	370	6	0	6	–	–	0	3	63
Milk 2%	1 (8 oz)	110	5	15	3	–	–	0	0	11
Mountain Dew	1 sm (17 oz)	190	0	0	0	0	0	0	0	51
Mug	1 sm (17 oz)	160	0	0	0	0	0	0	0	47
Orange Juice	1 (12 oz)	170	0	0	0	0	0	0	0	36
Pepsi	1 sm (17 oz)	160	0	0	0	0	0	0	0	44
Sierra Mist	1 sm (17 oz)	170	0	0	0	0	0	0	0	43
Smoothie 3-Berry Blast	1 sm (12 oz)	310	1	5	0	–	–	0	4	61
Smoothie Banana Chill	1 sm (12 oz)	320	1	5	0	–	–	0	3	58
Smoothie Berry Banana Squeeze	1 sm (12 oz)	220	0	0	0	0	0	0	2	49
Smoothie Berry Lemon Lively	1 sm (12 oz)	290	1	5	0	–	–	0	3	56
Smoothie Blackberry Toner	1 sm (12 oz)	270	1	5	0	–	–	0	3	47
Smoothie Blackberry Storm	1 sm (12 oz)	360	4	5	3	–	–	0	3	64
Smoothie Cocoa Latte Swirl	1 sm (16 oz)	370	7	5	6	–	–	0	2	64
Smoothie Mango Passion	1 sm (12 oz)	230	0	5	0	–	–	0	1	46
Smoothie Orange Berry	1 sm (12 oz)	320	2	5	1	–	–	0	2	65
Smoothie Orange Swirl	1 sm (12 oz)	280	4	5	3	–	–	0	1	46

FOOD	PORTION	CALS	TOTAL FAT	CHOL	SAT FAT	POLY FAT	MONO FAT	TRANS FAT	FIBER	S
Smoothie Peaches & Cream	1 sm (12 oz)	240	0	5	0	–	–	0	1	4
Smoothie Pomegranate & Berries	1 sm (12 oz)	250	0	5	0	–	–	0	2	4
Smoothie Raspberry Creme	1 sm (12 oz)	330	3	5	3	–	–	0	2	6
Smoothie Raspberry Crush	1 sm (12 oz)	160	0	0	0	0	0	0	4	3
Smoothie Strawberry Sensation	1 sm (12 oz)	280	0	5	0	–	–	0	2	5
Smoothie Strawberry Xtreme	1 sm (12 oz)	270	0	5	0	–	–	0	2	5
Smoothie Tropical Tango	1 (12 oz)	240	2	5	1	–	–	0	2	4
Smoothie Tropi-Colada	1 (12 oz)	330	3	5	3	–	–	0	1	6
Smoothie Light Berry Pom Twlight	1 (12 oz)	140	0	5	0	–	–	0	3	2
Smoothie Light Pineapple Daylight	1 (12 oz)	110	0	5	0	–	–	0	1	2
Smoothie Light Strawberry Delight	1 (12 oz)	110	0	5	0	–	–	0	2	20
Smoothie Light Tropical Sunlight	1 (12 oz)	130	0	5	0	–	–	0	2	26
Sprite	1 sm (17 oz)	150	0	0	0	0	0	0	0	42
FOOD										
Dog Bacon Cheese	1 (5.6 oz)	490	33	75	14	–	–	1	1	3
Dog Cheese	1 (5.4 oz)	460	31	70	14	–	–	1	1	3
Dog Chicago	1 (9.4 oz)	430	27	55	11	–	–	1	3	6
Dog Chili Melt	1 (5.8 oz)	470	33	70	14	–	–	1	1	3
Dog Chili Slaw	1 (6.5 oz)	480	33	65	17	–	–	1	2	3
Dog Classic	1 (5 oz)	390	27	55	11	–	–	1	1	4
Dog Pepperoni Cheese	1 (5.7 oz)	460	31	65	13	–	–	1	2	3
Dog Relish	1 (5.5 oz)	420	27	55	11	–	–	1	1	7
Dog Reuben	1 (6.9 oz)	520	36	85	16	–	–	1	2	3
Dog Sauerkraut	1 (5.9 oz)	410	27	55	11	–	–	1	2	3
Dog Southwest Chili	1 (6.7 oz)	500	34	75	15	–	–	1	2	4
Dog Triple Cheese	1 (6.2 oz)	540	38	90	17	–	–	1	1	3
Pita Chicken Caesar	1 (6.6 oz)	450	22	35	4	–	–	0	6	2
Pita Chicken Fajita	1 (6.8 oz)	360	11	35	4	–	–	0	7	3
Pita Garden Veggie	1 (7.3 oz)	470	26	70	13	–	–	0	7	5
Pita Santa Fe Grilled Chicken	1 (6.8 oz)	450	21	40	6	–	–	0	7	2
Pita Steak Fajita	1 (8 oz)	410	14	40	5	–	–	0	7	3
Pita Turkey Club	1 (8 oz)	480	23	55	6	–	–	0	6	1
Sandwich Crispy Chicken	1 (7.4 oz)	600	30	55	5	–	–	0	7	8
Sandwich Grilled Chicken	1 (6.3 oz)	360	15	50	3	–	–	0	1	5

FOOD	PORTION	CALS	TOTAL FAT	CHOL	SAT FAT	POLY FAT	MONO FAT	TRANS FAT	FIBER	SUGAR
Sandwich Iron Grilled Classic Club	1 (9.4 oz)	600	24	85	8	–	–	0	3	4
Sandwich Iron Grilled Supreme BLT	1 (6 oz)	600	34	75	9	–	–	0	2	2
Sandwich Iron Grilled Turkey	1 (8.2 oz)	550	23	85	7	–	–	0	2	2

PANERA BREAD
BAKERY

FOOD	PORTION	CALS	TOTAL FAT	CHOL	SAT FAT	POLY FAT	MONO FAT	TRANS FAT	FIBER	SUGAR
Asiago Cheese Loaf	1 slice (2 oz)	160	4	10	3	–	–	0	1	0
Bagel Asiago Cheese	1	330	6	10	4	–	–	0	2	3
Bagel Blueberry	1	330	2	0	0	–	–	0	2	10
Bagel Chocolate Chip	1	370	6	0	4	–	–	0	2	14
Bagel Cinnamon Crunch	1	430	8	0	5	–	–	0	2	29
Bagel Cinnamon Swirl & Raisin	1	320	3	0	1	–	–	0	3	11
Bagel Everything	1	300	3	0	0	–	–	0	2	4
Bagel French Toast	1	350	5	0	3	–	–	0	2	15
Bagel Jalapeno & Cheddar	1	310	3	5	2	–	–	0	2	3
Bagel Plain	1	290	2	0	0	–	–	0	2	3
Bagel Sesame	1	310	3	0	0	–	–	0	2	3
Bagel Sweet Onion & Poppyseed	1	390	7	0	1	–	–	0	4	7
Bagel Whole Wheat	1	340	3	0	0	–	–	0	6	5
Baguette Whole Grain	1 slice (2 oz)	140	1	0	0	–	–	0	3	2
Bear Claw	1	550	28	65	12	–	–	1	3	32
Brownie Double Fudge w/ Icing	1	480	17	85	9	–	–	0	2	44
Cake Cinnamon Coffee Crumb	1 slice	470	25	105	9	–	–	0	1	30
Ciabatta	1 (6.25 oz)	460	6	0	1	–	–	0	3	3
Cinnamon Raisin	1 slice (2 oz)	180	3	10	2	–	–	0	1	11
Cinnamon Roll	1	620	24	100	14	–	–	1	3	33
Cobblestone	1	650	13	20	5	–	–	0	3	64
Cookie Candy	1	420	19	70	10	–	–	1	1	33
Cookie Chocolate Chipper	1	440	23	60	14	–	–	0	2	33
Cookie Chocolate Chipper	1 mini	110	6	15	4	–	–	0	1	8
Cookie Chocolate Duet w/ Walnuts	1	450	24	60	13	–	–	0	3	36
Cookie Easter Egg	1	480	22	55	13	–	–	1	1	38
Cookie Oatmeal Raisin	1	370	14	55	8	–	–	0	2	28

FOOD	PORTION	CALS	TOTAL FAT	CHOL	SAT FAT	POLY FAT	MONO FAT	TRANS FAT	FIBER	SU
Cookie Shortbread	1	350	21	55	12	–	–	1	1	11
Cookie Toffee Nut	1	460	19	80	13	–	–	0	1	29
Country Loaf	1 slice (2 oz)	140	1	0	0	–	–	0	1	0
Croissant French	1	310	18	60	11	–	–	1	1	4
Focaccia w/ Asiago Cheese	1 slice (2 oz)	160	5	5	2	–	–	0	1	1
French Baguette	1 slice (2 oz)	150	1	0	0	–	–	0	1	0
Honey Wheat Loaf	1 slice (2 oz)	170	3	0	2	–	–	0	2	4
Hot Cross Bun	1	220	5	35	3	–	–	0	1	19
Muffie Chocolate Chip	1	320	14	40	4	–	–	0	2	27
Muffie Pumpkin	1	290	11	15	2	–	–	0	1	26
Muffin Apple Crunch	1	450	12	60	3	–	–	0	2	49
Muffin Carrot Walnut	1	500	21	65	5	–	–	0	3	37
Muffin Pumpkin	1	580	22	30	4	–	–	0	2	51
Muffin Wild Blueberry	1	440	17	60	3	–	–	0	2	39
Pastry Cheese	1	400	22	65	14	–	–	1	1	15
Pastry Cherry	1	500	18	50	11	–	–	1	2	45
Pastry Chocolate	1	410	24	50	14	–	–	1	2	18
Pastry Fresh Apple	1	380	17	20	13	–	–	0	1	17
Pastry Ring Apple Cherry Cheese	1 slice	230	11	35	6	–	–	0	1	16
Pecan Braid	1	470	26	55	12	–	–	1	2	23
Pecan Roll	1	730	39	60	12	–	–	0	5	48
Scone Cinnamon Chip	1	600	31	125	19	–	–	1	2	34
Scone Orange	1 lg	470	11	45	7	–	–	0	3	62
Scone Orange	1 mini	160	4	15	3	–	–	0	1	21
Scone Strawberries & Cream	1	420	19	70	12	–	–	0	1	27
Scone Strawberries & Cream	1 mini	140	6	25	4	–	–	0	0	9
Scone Wild Blueberry	1 mini	160	6	25	4	–	–	–	1	8
Scone Wild Blueberry	1	440	18	75	12	–	–	0	2	25
Sesame Semolina Loaf	1 slice (2 oz)	140	1	0	0	–	–	0	1	1
Sourdough Roll	1 (2.5 oz)	200	1	0	0	–	–	0	1	0
Sourdough Round Loaf	1 slice(2 oz)	140	1	0	0	–	–	0	1	0
Sourdough Soup Bowl	1 (8 oz)	590	3	0	0	–	–	0	4	1
Spring Petites	1 mini	230	12	30	7	–	–	0	0	12
Stone Milled Rye Loaf	1 slice (2 oz)	140	1	0	0	–	–	0	2	0
Three Cheese Loaf	1 slice (2 oz)	140	2	5	1	–	–	0	1	1
Tomato Basil XL Loaf	1 slice (2 oz)	140	1	0	0	–	–	0	1	1
White Whole Grain Loaf	1 slice (2 oz)	140	3	0	1	–	–	0	2	1
Whole Grain Loaf	1 slice (2 oz)	130	1	0	0	–	–	0	3	2

FOOD	PORTION	CALS	TOTAL FAT	CHOL	SAT FAT	POLY FAT	MONO FAT	TRANS FAT	FIBER	SUGAR
BEVERAGES										
Apple Juice Organic	8 oz	120	0	0	0	0	0	0	0	29
Caffe Mocha	1 (11.5 oz)	380	16	40	11	–	–	0	2	42
Caramel Frozen	1 (16 oz)	600	33	60	15	–	–	1	0	82
Chocolate Milk Organic	8 oz	170	5	20	3	–	–	0	0	25
Hot Chocolate	1 (11 oz)	380	16	40	11	–	–	0	2	42
Iced Green Tea	1 (16 oz)	90	0	0	0	0	0	0	0	23
Iced Latte Chai Tea	1 (16 oz)	160	4	15	2	–	–	0	0	25
Latte Caffe	1 (8.5 oz)	120	5	20	3	–	–	0	0	11
Latte Caramel	1 (11.5 oz)	420	18	50	12	–	–	1	0	46
Latte Chai Tea	1 (10 oz)	200	5	15	3	–	–	0	0	32
Lemonade	1 (16 oz)	100	0	0	0	0	0	0	0	25
Mango Frozen	1 (16 oz)	330	10	20	7	–	–	0	2	56
Milk Organic	8 oz	120	5	20	3	–	–	0	0	12
Mocha Frozen	1 (16 oz)	570	20	50	14	–	–	1	2	78
Orange Juice	1 sm (8 oz)	110	0	0	0	0	0	0	1	26
Smoothie Black Cherry Low Fat	1 (16 oz)	290	2	5	1	–	–	0	2	53
Smoothie Mango Low Fat	1 (16 oz)	230	2	5	1	–	–	0	2	48
Smoothie Strawberry w/ Ginseng Low Fat	1 (16 oz)	260	2	5	1	–	–	0	2	53
Smoothie Wild Berry Low Fat	1 (16 oz)	290	2	5	1	–	–	0	1	65
CHILDREN'S MENU SELECTIONS										
Deli Sandwich Roast Beef	1	320	10	40	6	–	–	0	3	4
Deli Sandwich Smoked Ham	1	300	9	40	6	–	–	0	3	3
Deli Sandwich Smoked Turkey	1	290	8	30	5	–	–	0	3	3
Mac & Cheese	1 serv	490	30	55	13	–	–	1	1	7
Organic Yogurt All Flavors	1 tube	60	1	5	0	–	–	0	0	10
Sandwich Grilled Cheese	1	360	13	30	10	–	–	0	4	4
Sandwich Peanut Butter & Jelly	1	410	18	0	4	–	–	0	4	21
CREAM CHEESE										
Chive & Onion	1 oz	70	6	20	4	–	–	0	0	1
Hazelnut Reduced Fat	1 oz	80	6	15	4	–	–	0	0	3
Honey Walnut Reduced Fat	1 oz	80	6	15	4	–	–	0	0	4
Plain	1 oz	100	6	30	0	–	–	0	0	1
Plain Reduced Fat	1 oz	70	6	20	4	–	–	0	0	1
Raspberry Reduced Fat	1 oz	70	5	15	3	–	–	0	1	3
Veggie Reduced Fat	1 oz	60	5	15	3	–	–	0	1	1

FOOD	PORTION	CALS	TOTAL FAT	CHOL	SAT FAT	POLY FAT	MONO FAT	TRANS FAT	FIBER	SU
SALAD DRESSINGS										
BBQ Ranch	3 tbsp	140	12	10	2	–	–	0	0	7
Buttermilk Ranch Light	3 tbsp	80	4	0	1	–	–	0	1	3
Caesar	3 tbsp	150	16	35	3	–	–	0	0	1
Vinaigrette Asian Sesame Reduced Sugar	3 tbsp	90	8	0	1	–	–	0	0	4
Vinaigrette Balsamic Reduced Fat	3 tbsp	130	10	0	2	–	–	0	0	8
Vinaigrette Blue Cheese	3 tbsp	180	19	15	4	–	–	0	0	3
Vinaigrette Greek Herb	3 tbsp	220	24	0	4	–	–	0	0	0
Vinaigrette Thai Chili Low Fat	3 tbsp	60	2	0	0	–	–	0	0	7
Vinaigrette White Balsamic Apple	3 tbsp	150	12	0	2	–	–	0	0	10
SALADS										
Asian Sesame Chicken	1	410	20	60	4	–	–	0	3	6
BBQ Chopped Chicken	1	500	22	75	3	–	–	0	6	15
Caesar	1	390	27	50	8	–	–	1	3	2
Caesar Chicken	1	510	29	115	9	–	–	1	3	2
Chopped Chicken Cobb	1	500	36	140	9	–	–	1	3	2
Chopped Steak & Blue Cheese	1	850	64	130	21	–	–	2	4	9
Classic Cafe	1	170	11	0	2	–	–	0	4	12
Fruit Cup	1	60	0	0	0	0	0	0	1	12
Fuji Apple w/ Chicken	1	520	31	80	7	–	–	0	6	21
Greek	1	380	34	20	8	–	–	1	5	4
Thai Chopped Chicken	1	390	15	60	3	–	–	0	5	13
SANDWICHES										
Asiago Roast Beef On Asiago Cheese	1	700	27	100	14	–	–	1	4	5
Bacon Turkey Bravo On XL Tomato Basil	1	800	29	85	10	–	–	0	4	6
Breakfast Asiago Cheese Bagel w/ Bacon	1	610	28	245	13	–	–	1	2	4
Breakfast Asiago Cheese Bagel w/ Egg & Cheese	1	480	18	215	10	–	–	1	2	3
Breakfast Asiago Cheese Bagel w/ Sausage	1	640	32	260	15	–	–	1	2	4
Breakfast Bacon Egg & Cheese On Ciabatta	1	510	24	235	10	–	–	0	2	2

FOOD	PORTION	CALS	TOTAL FAT	CHOL	SAT FAT	POLY FAT	MONO FAT	TRANS FAT	FIBER	SUGAR
Breakfast Egg & Cheese On Ciabatta	1	390	15	205	7	–	–	0	2	2
Breakfast French Toast Bagel w/ Sausage	1	670	31	250	14	–	–	0	2	15
Breakfast Jalapeno & Cheddar Bagel w/ Bacon	1	590	25	240	11	–	–	0	3	4
Breakfast Jalapeno & Cheddar Bagel w/ Egg & Cheese	1	470	16	210	8	–	–	0	3	3
Breakfast Jalapeno & Cheddar Bagel w/ Sausage	1	630	29	255	12	–	–	0	3	4
Breakfast Power	1	340	14	220	7	–	–	1	4	2
Breakfast Sausage Egg & Cheese On Ciabatta	1	550	29	250	12	–	–	0	2	2
Breakfast Sweet Onion & Poppyseed Bagel w/ Steak	1	660	27	235	10	–	–	1	5	8
Chicken Caesar On Three Cheese	1	720	32	130	10	–	–	1	4	5
Italian Combo On Ciabatta	1	980	41	150	15	–	–	1	5	6
Jalapeno & Cheddar Bagel w/ Smoked Ham	1	500	16	225	8	–	–	1	3	3
Mediterranean Veggie On XL Tomato Basil	1	600	13	10	4	–	–	0	10	6
Napa Almond Chicken Salad On Sesame Semolina	1	690	26	60	5	–	–	0	5	12
Panini Chipotle Chicken On Artisan French	1	830	37	145	12	–	–	1	3	5
Panini Cuban Chicken	1	860	36	100	10	–	–	1	4	10
Panini Frontega Chicken On Focaccia	1	850	38	110	9	–	–	1	4	6
Panini Smokehouse Turkey On Three Cheese	1	690	25	100	12	–	–	1	4	4
Panini Steak & White Cheddar On French Baguette	1	950	35	95	15	–	–	1	5	3
Panini Tomato & Mozzarella On Ciabatta	1	770	10	35	1	–	–	1	6	10
Panini Turkey Artichoke On Focaccia	1	740	26	50	8	–	–	0	5	8

FOOD	PORTION	CALS	TOTAL FAT	CHOL	SAT FAT	POLY FAT	MONO FAT	TRANS FAT	FIBER	SU...
Sierra Turkey w/ Asiago Cheese On Focaccia	1	920	49	80	12	–	–	1	4	5
Smoked Ham & Swiss On Stone Milled Rye	1	590	17	90	8	–	–	1	5	3
Smoked Turkey Breast On Country	1	420	3	30	1	–	–	0	3	3
Tuna Salad On Honey Wheat	1	470	16	25	4	–	–	0	5	12
SOUPS										
Baked Potato	1 serv (12 oz)	350	13	70	1	–	–	1	3	7
Broccoli Cheddar	1 serv (12 oz)	290	16	30	9	–	–	1	7	0
Chicken Noodle Low Fat	1 serv (12 oz)	140	3	30	1	–	–	0	0	9
Cream Of Chicken & Wild Rice	1 serv (12 oz)	310	17	60	8	–	–	0	3	4
Creamy Tomato	1 serv (12 oz)	380	23	65	14	–	–	1	5	9
French Onion	1 serv (12 oz)	250	11	25	5	–	–	0	3	6
Garden Vegetable w/ Pesto Low Fat	1 serv (12 oz)	160	4	0	0	–	–	0	6	8
New England Clam Chowder	1 serv (12 oz)	450	34	50	20	–	–	2	3	6
Vegetarian Black Bean Low Fat	1 serv (12 oz)	170	4	0	2	–	–	0	5	4

PIZZA HUT
BEVERAGES

FOOD	PORTION	CALS	TOTAL FAT	CHOL	SAT FAT	POLY FAT	MONO FAT	TRANS FAT	FIBER	SU...
Diet Pepsi	1 (16 oz)	0	0	0	0	0	0	0	0	0
Mountain Dew	1 (16 oz)	220	0	0	0	0	0	0	0	58
Pepsi	1 (16 oz)	200	0	0	0	0	0	0	0	54
Sierra Mist	1 (16 oz)	200	0	0	0	0	0	0	0	54
OTHER MENU SELECTIONS										
Breadstick	1 (1.5 oz)	140	5	0	1	–	–	0	1	2
Breadstick Cheese	1 (2 oz)	170	6	15	3	–	–	0	1	2
Dipping Sauce Marinara	1 serv (3 oz)	60	0	0	0	0	0	0	2	9
Dipping Sauce Ranch	1 serv (1.5 oz)	220	23	10	4	–	–	0	0	1
Dipping Sauce Wing Blue Cheese	1 serv (1.5 oz)	230	24	20	5	–	–	0	0	2
Dipping Sauce Wing Ranch	1 serv (1.5 oz)	220	23	10	4	–	–	0	0	1
Fried Cheese Sticks	4 (4.2 oz)	380	24	40	9	–	–	2	2	3
Tuscani Pasta Chicken Alfredo	1 serv (10 oz)	580	32	50	9	–	–	1	4	4
Tuscani Pasta Meaty Marinara	1 serv (9.5 oz)	450	20	70	8	–	–	1	5	8

FOOD	PORTION	CALS	TOTAL FAT	CHOL	SAT FAT	POLY FAT	MONO FAT	TRANS FAT	FIBER	SUGAR
Wedge Fries	1 serv (4.3 oz)	320	18	0	4	–	–	0	3	0
Wings Crispy Bone In All American	2 (1.9 oz)	200	14	45	3	–	–	0	1	0
Wings Crispy Bone In Buffalo Burnin Hot	2 (2.6 oz)	230	15	45	3	–	–	0	1	2
Wings Crispy Bone In Buffalo Medium	2 (2.6 oz)	230	15	45	3	–	–	0	2	2
Wings Crispy Bone In Buffalo Mild	2 (2.6 oz)	230	15	45	3	–	–	0	1	2
Wings Crispy Bone In Garlic Parmesan	2 (2.5 oz)	300	25	45	5	–	–	0	1	1
Wings Crispy Bone In Honey BBQ	2 (2.9 oz)	260	14	45	3	–	–	0	1	12
Wings Crispy Bone In Lemon Pepper	2 (2.6 oz)	270	19	45	4	–	–	0	1	7
Wings Crispy Bone In Spicy Asian	2 (2.9 oz)	250	15	45	3	–	–	0	1	13
Wings Crispy Bone In Spicy BBQ	2 (2.9 oz)	240	14	50	3	–	–	0	1	11
Wings Traditional All American	2 (1.4 oz)	80	5	40	2	–	–	0	0	0
Wings Traditional Buffalo Medium	2 (2 oz)	110	6	40	2	–	–	0	1	2
Wings Traditional Buffalo Mild	2 (2 oz)	110	6	40	2	–	–	0	1	2
Wings Traditional Burnin Hot	2 (2 oz)	110	6	40	2	–	–	0	1	2
Wings Traditional Garlic Parmesan	2 (2 oz)	180	16	45	4	–	–	0	0	1
Wings Traditional Honey BBQ	2 (2.4 oz)	140	5	40	2	–	–	0	0	12
Wings Traditional Lemon Pepper	2 (2 oz)	150	10	40	2	–	–	0	0	7
Wings Traditional Spicy Asian	2 (2.3 oz)	130	5	40	2	–	–	0	0	13
Wings Traditional Spicy BBQ	2 (2.3 oz)	120	5	45	2	–	–	0	0	11
PIZZA										
Fit 'N Delicious 12 Inch Chicken Mushrooms & Jalapeno	1 slice (3.3 oz)	170	5	20	2	–	–	0	1	4

FOOD	PORTION	CALS	TOTAL FAT	CHOL	SAT FAT	POLY FAT	MONO FAT	TRANS FAT	FIBER	SUG
Fit 'N Delicious 12 Inch Chicken Red Onion & Green Pepper	1 slice (3.3 oz)	180	5	20	2	–	–	0	1	5
Fit 'N Delicious 12 Inch Diced Red Tomato Mushroom & Jalapeno	1 slice (3.1 oz)	150	4	10	2	–	–	0	2	4
Fit 'N Delicious 12 Inch Green Pepper Red Onion & Diced Red Tomato	1 slice (3.1 oz)	150	4	10	2	–	–	0	2	5
Fit 'N Delicious 12 Inch Ham Pineapple & Diced Red Tomato	1 slice (2.9 oz)	160	5	15	2	–	–	0	1	6
Fit 'N Delicious 12 Inch Ham Red Onion & Mushrooms	1 slice (2.9 oz)	160	5	15	2	–	–	0	1	4
Hand Tossed 12 Inch Cheese Only	1 slice (2.9 oz)	220	8	25	4	–	–	0	1	4
Hand Tossed 12 Inch Cheese Only Garlic Parmesan	1 slice (3 oz)	220	8	25	5	–	–	0	1	4
Hand Tossed 12 Inch Dan's Original	1 slice (3.6 oz)	260	12	30	5	–	–	0	1	4
Hand Tossed 12 Inch Ham & Pineapple	1 slice (3.2 oz)	200	6	20	3	–	–	0	1	5
Hand Tossed 12 Inch Hawaiian Luau	1 slice (3.5 oz)	240	9	25	4	–	–	0	1	5
Hand Tossed 12 Inch Italian Sausage & Red Onion	1 slice (3.5 oz)	240	10	25	5	–	–	0	1	4
Hand Tossed 12 Inch Meat Lover's	1 slice (3.7 oz)	300	16	40	7	–	–	0	1	4
Hand Tossed 12 Inch Pepperoni	1 slice (2.9 oz)	230	9	25	4	–	–	0	1	3
Hand Tossed 12 Inch Pepperoni Lover's	1 slice (3.3 oz)	270	13	35	6	–	–	0	1	4
Hand Tossed 12 Inch Pepperoni & Mushroom	1 slice (3.2 oz)	210	8	20	4	–	–	0	1	4
Hand Tossed 12 Inch Pepperoni Garlic Parmesan	1 slice (2.9 oz)	230	9	25	5	–	–	0	1	4
Hand Tossed 12 Inch Spicy Sicilian	1 slice (3.5 oz)	240	11	25	5	–	–	0	1	4
Hand Tossed 12 Inch Supreme	1 slice (3.7 oz)	260	12	30	5	–	–	0	1	4

FOOD	PORTION	CALS	TOTAL FAT	CHOL	SAT FAT	POLY FAT	MONO FAT	TRANS FAT	FIBER	SUGAR
Hand Tossed 12 Inch Triple Meat Italiano	1 slice (3.4 oz)	260	12	30	5	–	–	0	1	4
Hand Tossed 12 Inch Ultimate Cheese Lover's	1 slice (2.9 oz)	240	11	30	5	–	–	0	1	3
Hand Tossed 12 Inch Veggie Lover's	1 slice (3.6 oz)	200	6	15	3	–	–	0	2	4
Pan 12 Inch Cheese Only	1 slice (3.2 oz)	240	10	25	5	–	–	0	1	2
Pan 12 Inch Dan's Original	1 slice (3.9 oz)	280	14	30	5	–	–	0	1	2
Pan 12 Inch Ham & Pineapple	1 slice (3.4 oz)	230	9	20	4	–	–	0	1	3
Pan 12 Inch Hawaiian Luau	1 slice (3.6 oz)	260	12	25	5	–	–	0	1	3
Pan 12 Inch Italian Sausage & Red Onion	1 slice (3.7 oz)	270	13	25	5	–	–	0	1	3
Pan 12 Inch Meat Lover's	1 slice (4 oz)	330	19	40	7	–	–	0	1	2
Pan 12 Inch Pepperoni	1 slice (3.2 oz)	250	12	25	5	–	–	0	1	2
Pan 12 Inch Pepperoni Lover's	1 slice (3.5 oz)	290	14	35	6	–	–	0	1	2
Pan 12 Inch Pepperoni & Mushroom	1 slice (3.4 oz)	240	10	20	4	–	–	0	1	2
Pan 12 Inch Spicy Sicilian	1 slice (3.7 oz)	270	13	25	5	–	–	0	2	2
Pan 12 Inch Supreme	1 slice (3.9 oz)	290	14	30	5	–	–	0	2	2
Pan 12 Inch Triple Meat Italiano	1 slice (3.6 oz)	290	15	30	5	–	–	0	1	2
Pan 12 Inch Ultimate Cheese Lover's	1 slice (3.2 oz)	270	13	25	5	–	–	0	1	2
Pan 12 Inch Veggie Lover's	1 slice (3.8 oz)	230	9	15	4	–	–	0	2	3
PANormous 9 Inch Cheese Only	1 pie (13.4 oz)	1100	45	105	19	–	–	1	6	10
PANormous 9 Inch Dan's Original	1 pie (15.9 oz)	1270	62	125	23	–	–	1	7	10
PANormous 9 Inch Ham & Pineapple	1 pie (14 oz)	1020	37	80	14	–	–	1	6	14
PANormous 9 Inch Hawaiian Luau	1 pie (14.8 oz)	1150	49	105	18	–	–	1	6	14
PANormous 9 Inch Italian Sausage & Red Onion	1 pie (15.4 oz)	1210	56	110	21	–	–	1	7	12
PANormous 9 Inch Meat Lover's	1 pie (16.3 oz)	1470	80	175	30	–	–	2	6	10
PANormous 9 Inch Pepperoni	1 pie (12.9 oz)	1100	48	100	18	–	–	1	6	9

FOOD	PORTION	CALS	TOTAL FAT	CHOL	SAT FAT	POLY FAT	MONO FAT	TRANS FAT	FIBER	SUGA
PANormous 9 Inch Pepperoni Lover's	1 pie (16 oz)	1290	62	150	26	–	–	2	6	10
PANormous 9 Inch Pepperoni & Mushroom	1 pie (13.9 oz)	1050	42	85	16	–	–	1	7	10
PANormous 9 Inch Spicy Sicilian	1 pie (15.4 oz)	1220	57	115	22	–	–	2	7	11
PANormous 9 Inch Supreme	1 pie (16.2 oz)	1270	62	130	24	–	–	2	7	11
PANormous 9 Inch Triple Meat Lover's	1 pie (14.9 oz)	1280	62	135	23	–	–	1	6	9
PANormous 9 Inch Veggie Lover's	1 pie (15.4 oz)	1010	38	70	14	–	–	1	8	12
Personal Pan 6 Inch Cheese Only	1 (7.2 oz)	590	24	55	10	–	–	1	3	7
Personal Pan 6 Inch Dan's Original	1 (8.8 oz)	720	36	75	13	–	–	1	4	7
Personal Pan 6 Inch Ham & Pineapple	1 (7.5 oz)	550	20	45	8	–	–	0	3	9
Personal Pan 6 Inch Hawaiian Luau	1 (8 oz)	620	25	55	10	–	–	0	3	9
Personal Pan 6 Inch Italian Sausage & Red Onion	1 (8.6 oz)	690	32	65	12	–	–	0	4	8
Personal Pan 6 Inch Meat Lover's	1 (9.2 oz)	830	46	100	17	–	–	1	3	7
Personal Pan 6 Inch Pepperoni	1 (7.1 oz)	610	26	55	10	–	–	1	3	6
Personal Pan 6 Inch Pepperoni Lover's	1 (8.1 oz)	720	34	85	14	–	–	1	3	7
Personal Pan 6 Inch Pepperoni & Mushroom	1 (7.5 oz)	570	23	45	9	–	–	0	4	7
Personal Pan 6 Inch Spicy Sicilian	1 (8.6 oz)	680	32	70	12	–	–	1	4	7
Personal Pan 6 Inch Supreme	1 (9 oz)	720	36	70	14	–	–	1	4	7
Personal Pan 6 Inch Triple Meat Italiano	1 (8.4 oz)	730	36	80	13	–	–	1	3	6
Personal Pan 6 Inch Ultimate Cheese Lover's	1 (7.3 oz)	660	30	65	12	–	–	1	3	6
Personal Pan 6 Inch Veggie Lover's	1 (8.2 oz)	550	20	35	8	–	–	0	4	8

FOOD	PORTION	CALS	TOTAL FAT	CHOL	SAT FAT	POLY FAT	MONO FAT	TRANS FAT	FIBER	SUGAR
P'Zone Classic	½ serv (6.1 oz)	470	16	40	7	–	–	0	2	3
P'Zone Meaty	½ serv (6.6 oz)	550	23	55	10	–	–	1	2	2
P'Zone Pepperoni	½ serv (5.5 oz)	450	15	40	7	–	–	0	2	2
Stuffed Pizza Rollers	1 (2.7 oz)	220	10	25	5	–	–	0	1	3
Thin'N Crispy 12 Inch Cheese Only	1 slice (2.3 oz)	190	8	25	4	–	–	0	1	4
Thin'N Crispy 12 Inch Dan's Original	1 slice (3 oz)	240	12	30	5	–	–	0	1	4
Thin'N Crispy 12 Inch Ham & Pineapple	1 slice (2.6 oz)	180	6	20	3	–	–	0	1	5
Thin'N Crispy 12 Inch Hawaiian Luau	1 slice (2.8 oz)	220	10	25	4	–	–	0	1	5
Thin'N Crispy 12 Inch Italian Sausage & Red Onion	1 slice (2.8 oz)	220	10	25	4	–	–	0	1	4
Thin'N Crispy 12 Inch Meat Lover's	1 slice (3 oz)	280	16	40	6	–	–	0	1	4
Thin'N Crispy 12 Inch Pepperoni	1 slice (2.2 oz)	200	9	25	4	–	–	0	1	4
Thin'N Crispy 12 Inch Pepperoni Lover's	1 slice (2.6 oz)	250	13	35	6	–	–	0	1	4
Thin'N Crispy 12 Inch Pepperoni & Mushroom	1 slice (2.6 oz)	180	8	20	4	–	–	0	1	4
Thin'N Crispy 12 Inch Spicy Sicilian	1 slice (2.8 oz)	220	10	25	5	–	–	0	1	4
Thin'N Crispy 12 Inch Supreme	1 slice (3.1 oz)	240	12	30	5	–	–	0	1	4
Thin'N Crispy 12 Inch Triple Meat Italiano	1 slice (2.7 oz)	240	12	30	5	–	–	0	1	4
Thin'N Crispy 12 Inch Ultimate Cheese Lover's	1 slice (2.3 oz)	220	11	25	5	–	–	0	1	4
Thin'N Crispy 12 Inch Veggie Lover's	1 slice (3 oz)	180	6	15	3	–	–	0	1	4

POPEYE'S

BEVERAGES

FOOD	PORTION	CALS	TOTAL FAT	CHOL	SAT FAT	POLY FAT	MONO FAT	TRANS FAT	FIBER	SUGAR
Coffee Black	1 (16 oz)	0	0	0	0	0	0	0	0	0
Orange Juice	1 (10 oz)	140	0	0	0	0	0	0	0	30

FOOD	PORTION	CALS	TOTAL FAT	CHOL	SAT FAT	POLY FAT	MONO FAT	TRANS FAT	FIBER	SUG
BREAKFAST MENU SELECTIONS										
Biscuit Bacon	1 (5 oz)	400	25	5	12	–	–	0	3	2
Biscuit Chicken	1 (5.2 oz)	490	26	28	14	–	–	1	1	2
Biscuit Egg	1 (4.8 oz)	510	29	125	15	–	–	0	1	2
Biscuit Egg & Sausage	1 (6.5 oz)	690	45	157	22	–	–	0	1	2
Biscuit Sausage	1 (4.8 oz)	540	36	320	18	–	–	0	1	2
Biscuit Sausage & Gravy	1 (6.5 oz)	510	33	15	14	–	–	1	3	3
Grits	1 serv (5 oz)	370	5	0	1	–	–	0	7	0
Hashbrowns	1 serv (3.4 oz)	360	20	10	9	–	–	–	4	0
DESSERTS										
Apple Sauce	1 serv (4 oz)	50	0	0	0	0	0	0	2	8
Cheesecake Mardi Gras	1 serv (3 oz)	310	19	60	10	–	–	0	1	22
Pie Hot Sweet Potato	1 serv (3.5 oz)	350	19	15	8	–	–	0	2	10
Pie Mississippi Mud	1 serv (3 oz)	280	7	20	2	–	–	0	2	27
Pie Sliced Pecan	1 serv (3.3 oz)	410	21	70	6	–	–	0	1	22
MAIN MENU SELECTIONS										
Baguette	1 (1.3 oz)	90	2	0	0	–	–	0	1	1
Biscuit	1 (2.1 oz)	260	15	0	7	–	–	0	2	1
Butterfly Shrimp	8 (3.5 oz)	290	17	90	8	–	–	1	3	0
Cajun Fries	1 reg (3 oz)	260	14	10	5	–	–	1	2	0
Cajun Rice	1 reg (4.3 oz)	170	5	25	2	–	–	0	1	4
Catfish Fillets	2 (5.2 oz)	460	29	65	12	–	–	2	1	0
Cheddar Cheese Tortilla	1 (1.6 oz)	140	5	0	3	–	–	0	1	0
Chicken Livers	10 (10 oz)	1190	80	765	34	–	–	5	6	3
Chicken Wrap Loaded	1 (4.6 oz)	310	13	30	6	–	–	0	3	0
Chicken Wrap Naked	1 (3.4 oz)	200	6	25	4	–	–	0	1	0
Coleslaw	1 reg (4.8 oz)	220	15	10	3	–	–	0	2	15
Corn On The Cob	1 (10 oz)	190	2	0	1	–	–	0	4	0
Green Beans	1 serv (3.5 oz)	40	2	5	0	–	–	0	2	1
Jalapeno	1 (6 g)	0	0	0	0	0	0	0	1	0
Jambalaya Chicken & Sausage	1 serv (5.3 oz)	220	11	32	3	–	–	0	1	0
Macaroni & Cheese	1 serv (5.5 oz)	200	7	15	4	–	–	0	1	3
Mashed Potatoes Gravy	1 serv (5 oz)	110	4	5	2	–	–	0	1	1
Mild Breast	1 (5.5 oz)	440	27	110	11	–	–	1	2	0
Mild Leg	1 (2.4 oz)	160	9	40	4	–	–	0	1	0
Mild Tenders	3 (4.4 oz)	340	14	70	6	–	–	1	1	0
Mild Thigh	1 (2.8 oz)	280	21	50	8	–	–	0	1	0
Mild Wing	1 (2.2 oz)	210	14	60	4	–	–	0	1	0
Naked Tenders	3 (4 oz)	170	2	25	0	–	–	0	0	0

FOOD	PORTION	CALS	TOTAL FAT	CHOL	SAT FAT	POLY FAT	MONO FAT	TRANS FAT	FIBER	SUGAR
Nuggets	4 (1.8 oz)	150	9	25	4	–	–	1	1	0
Onion Rings	6 (2.6 oz)	280	19	10	8	–	–	1	2	2
Po'Boy Catfish	1 (11.2 oz)	800	50	75	16	–	–	2	3	3
Po'Boy Chicken	1 (22.3 oz)	660	34	75	9	–	–	1	3	3
Po'Boy Naked BBQ Chicken	1 (7.4 oz)	340	7	50	2	–	–	0	2	11
Po'Boy Shrimp	1 (9.5 oz)	690	42	75	13	–	–	1	5	3
Popcorn Shrimp	1 serv (3.5 oz)	330	9	65	9	–	–	1	3	0
Red Beans & Rice	1 reg (5.1 oz)	230	14	10	4	–	–	0	5	0
Spicy Breast	1 (5.5 oz)	420	27	110	9	–	–	1	3	0
Spicy Leg	1 (2.4 oz)	170	10	65	4	–	–	0	1	0
Spicy Thigh	1 (2.8 oz)	260	18	70	6	–	–	0	1	0
Spicy Wing	1 (2.2 oz)	210	14	55	6	–	–	0	1	0
Spicy Tenders	3 (4.4 oz)	310	15	80	6	–	–	1	2	0
SAUCES										
Cocktail	1 serv (1 oz)	30	0	0	0	0	0	0	0	6
Confetti Sauce	1 serv (1 oz)	65	0	0	0	0	0	0	0	10
Ranch	1 serv (1 oz)	150	15	10	3	–	–	0	0	1
Spicy BBQ	1 serv (1 oz)	45	0	0	0	0	0	0	0	8
Spicy Honey Mustard	1 serv (1 oz)	100	8	10	1	–	–	0	0	5
Tartar Sauce	1 serv (1 oz)	140	15	15	3	–	–	0	0	1

QUIZNOS
SALAD DRESSINGS

FOOD	PORTION	CALS	TOTAL FAT	CHOL	SAT FAT	POLY FAT	MONO FAT	TRANS FAT	FIBER	SUGAR
Acai Vinaigrette	1 reg	230	17	0	3	–	–	0	0	14
Balsamic Vinaigrette Fat Free	1 reg	130	0	0	0	0	0	0	0	20
Blue Cheese	1 reg	345	38	36	9	–	–	0	0	2
Honey Dijon	1 reg	450	44	35	7	–	–	1	0	13
Peppercorn Caesar	1 reg	480	50	34	9	–	–	0	0	3
Ranch	1 reg	350	36	24	5	–	–	0	0	3
Tzatziki	1 reg	450	46	48	9	–	–	0	0	2
SALADS										
Fresh Farmers Market Caprese Chicken w/o Dressing	1 reg	260	17	45	8	–	–	0	2	2
Fresh Farmers Market Chicken Caesar w/o Dressing	1 reg	130	5	46	3	–	–	1	2	3
Fresh Farmers Market Cobb w/o Dressing	1 reg	260	12	121	6	–	–	1	2	3

FOOD	PORTION	CALS	TOTAL FAT	CHOL	SAT FAT	POLY FAT	MONO FAT	TRANS FAT	FIBER	SUG
Fresh Farmers Market Harvest Chicken w/o Dressing	1 reg	220	6	20	2	–	–	0	4	25
Fresh Farmers Market Mediterranean Chicken w/o Dressing	1 reg	180	7	42	3	–	–	1	4	3
SANDWICHES										
Classic Sub Classic Club	1 sm	570	34	70	10	–	–	0	3	8
Classic Sub Classic Italian	1 sm	520	29	55	11	–	–	1	4	8
Classic Sub Honey Bacon Club	1 sm	480	21	45	5	–	–	0	3	15
Classic Sub Honey Bourbon Chicken	1 sm	320	6	20	3	–	–	0	4	14
Classic Sub Pork Cuban	1 sm	450	22	60	6	–	–	0	3	5
Classic Sub The Traditional	1 sm	430	20	45	7	–	–	0	4	8
Classic Sub Tuna Melt	1 sm	690	47	80	11	–	–	1	3	6
Classic Sub Turkey Bacon Guacamole	1 sm	540	28	45	8	–	–	0	5	9
Classic Sub Turkey Ranch & Swiss	1 sm	420	18	30	5	–	–	0	4	8
Classic Sub Ultimate Turkey Club	1 sm	560	34	70	10	–	–	0	3	7
Classic Sub Veggie	1 sm	510	28	25	9	–	–	0	6	9
Flatbread Sammies Bistro Steak Melt	1	410	23	50	6	–	–	0	1	6
Flatbread Sammies Cantina Chicken	1	280	7	20	2	–	–	0	2	12
Flatbread Sammies Chicken Bacon Ranch	1	380	19	40	5	–	–	0	1	4
Flatbread Sammies Italiano	1	420	25	55	8	–	–	0	1	4
Flatbread Sammies Roadhouse Steak	1	270	6	20	1	–	–	0	1	13
Flatbread Sammies Smoky Chipotle Turkey	1	390	23	45	6	–	–	0	1	4
Flatbread Sammies Veggie	1	340	20	15	5	–	–	0	3	5
Signature Sub Baja Chicken	1 sm	490	23	50	9	–	–	0	3	9
Signature Sub Black Angus On Rosemary Parmesan	1 sm	520	17	85	9	–	–	0	4	14
Signature Sub Buffalo Chicken	1 sm	470	22	50	8	–	–	0	3	7

FOOD	PORTION	CALS	TOTAL FAT	CHOL	SAT FAT	POLY FAT	MONO FAT	TRANS FAT	FIBER	SUGAR
Signature Sub Chicken Bacon Dipper	1 sm	630	38	95	14	–	–	1	3	8
Signature Sub Chicken Carbonara	1 sm	530	27	55	9	–	–	0	3	7
Signature Sub Chipotle Prime Rib	1 sm	600	34	85	10	–	–	1	3	7
Signature Sub Double Cheese Cheesesteak	1 sm	770	47	115	12	–	–	2	3	7
Signature Sub Harvest Chicken	1 sm	370	11	23	3	–	–	0	4	19
Signature Sub Honey Mustard Chicken	1 sm	520	26	45	8	–	–	0	3	10
Signature Sub Mesquite Chicken	1 sm	500	25	55	9	–	–	0	3	7
Signature Sub Peppercorn Steakhouse Dip	1 sm	630	37	91	10	–	–	1	3	7
Signature Sub Prime Rib & Blue	1 sm	570	29	90	11	–	–	1	3	7
Signature Sub Prime Rib & Peppercorn	1 sm	620	36	90	11	–	–	1	3	7
Signature Sub Prime Rib Mushroom & Swiss	1 sm	600	34	80	9	–	–	1	3	6
Signature Sub Southern BBQ Pulled Pork	1 sm	520	22	103	10	–	–	0	3	12
Toasty Bullets Beef Bacon & Cheddar	1	450	18	45	6	–	–	0	2	8
Toasty Bullets Italian	1	500	25	50	8	–	–	0	3	8
Toasty Bullets Pesto Turkey	1	380	13	25	3	–	–	0	3	8
Toasty Bullets Tuna Melt	1	510	31	50	6	–	–	0	2	6
Toasty Bullets Turkey Club	1	460	21	40	5	–	–	0	3	8
Toasty Favorites Honey Cured Ham	1 sm	490	28	60	8	–	–	0	3	7
Toasty Favorites Meatball	1 sm	450	21	60	8	–	–	0	6	10
Toasty Favorites Oven Roasted Turkey	1 sm	500	28	55	7	–	–	1	3	7
Toasty Favorites Roast Beef	1 sm	500	28	55	7	–	–	1	3	8
Toasty Favorites Turkey & Ham	1 sm	500	29	60	8	–	–	1	3	7
Toasty Favorites Veggie Caprese	1 sm	400	21	20	15	–	–	1	4	7

FOOD	PORTION	CALS	TOTAL FAT	CHOL	SAT FAT	POLY FAT	MONO FAT	TRANS FAT	FIBER	SUG
Toasty Torpedoes Beef Bacon & Cheddar	1	800	31	70	9	–	–	0	5	16
Toasty Torpedoes Italian	1	860	40	75	12	–	–	1	5	16
Toasty Torpedoes Pesto Turkey	1	690	22	40	5	–	–	0	5	15
Toasty Torpedoes Tuna Melt	1	980	56	85	11	–	–	0	4	12
Toasty Torpedoes Turkey Club	1	830	35	60	9	–	–	1	5	16

RED BURRITO

FOOD	PORTION	CALS	TOTAL FAT	CHOL	SAT FAT	POLY FAT	MONO FAT	TRANS FAT	FIBER	SUG
Burrito Bean & Cheese	1 serv (7.4 oz)	430	16	30	8	–	–	–	6	2
Burrito Beef Bean & Cheese	1 serv (9.8 oz)	560	24	65	11	–	–	–	6	4
Burrito Grilled Chicken	1 serv (9 oz)	480	17	60	8	–	–	–	6	3
Burrito Grilled Steak	1 serv (9 oz)	520	20	55	10	–	–	–	6	3
Chips & Salsa	1 serv (7.4 oz)	300	22	0	5	–	–	–	1	3
Chips Side	1 (1.3 oz)	100	8	0	2	–	–	–	0	0
Fresh Salsa	1 serv (4 oz)	30	0	0	0	0	0	–	1	3
Hard Taco Beef	1 serv (3.3 oz)	170	12	35	5	–	–	–	1	1
Hard Taco Chicken	1 serv (4 oz)	160	9	45	4	–	–	–	1	0
Hard Taco Steak	1 serv (3.8 oz)	200	13	45	5	–	–	–	1	1
Hot Sauce	1 serv (2 oz)	0	0	0	0	0	0	–	0	0
Jalapeno Coins	1 serv (1 oz)	5	0	0	0	0	0	–	1	0
Make It Wet	1 serv (3.6 oz)	140	10	30	6	–	–	–	1	1
Quesadilla	1 serv (5.7 oz)	560	33	85	19	–	–	–	2	1
Quesadilla Chicken	1 serv (8 oz)	720	45	125	21	–	–	–	2	1
Quesadilla Steak	1 serv (7.9 oz)	760	49	120	22	–	–	–	2	1
Queso	1 serv (3 oz)	110	8	10	3	–	–	–	0	2
Red Burrito Beef	1 serv (13.4 oz)	710	34	95	17	–	–	–	7	5
Red Burrito Chicken	1 serv (12.7 oz)	630	28	90	14	–	–	–	7	4
Red Burrito Steak	1 serv (12.6 oz)	660	31	85	16	–	–	–	7	4
Refried Bean In Tortilla Bowl	1 serv (4.8 oz)	360	18	5	5	–	–	–	7	1
Soft Taco Beef	1 serv (3.8 oz)	210	11	35	5	–	–	–	0	1
Soft Taco Chicken	1 serv (4.4 oz)	200	8	45	4	–	–	–	0	0
Soft Taco Southwest Chicken	1 serv (4 oz)	250	14	50	5	–	–	–	0	1
Soft Taco Steak	1 serv (4.3 oz)	240	12	45	5	–	–	–	0	1
Sour Cream	1 serv (1.4 oz)	50	4	15	2	–	–	–	0	3

FOOD	PORTION	CALS	TOTAL FAT	CHOL	SAT FAT	POLY FAT	MONO FAT	TRANS FAT	FIBER	SUGAR
Super Nachos	1 serv (10.7 oz)	690	29	20	8	–	–	–	5	5
Super Nachos Beef	1 serv (13 oz)	820	36	55	10	–	–	–	5	6
Super Nachos Chicken	1 serv (12.5 oz)	740	30	50	8	–	–	–	5	5
Super Nachos Steak	1 serv (12.4 oz)	740	38	45	11	–	–	–	14	6
Taco Salad Beef	1 (20.3 oz)	1080	64	110	21	–	–	–	8	11
Taco Salad Chicken	1 (19 oz)	920	51	100	15	–	–	–	8	9
Taco Salad Steak	1 (18.7 oz)	1000	58	95	18	–	–	–	8	9

ROBEKS
BAKED SELECTIONS

FOOD	PORTION	CALS	TOTAL FAT	CHOL	SAT FAT	POLY FAT	MONO FAT	TRANS FAT	FIBER	SUGAR
Gourmet Pretzels Apple Cinnamon	1	470	25	0	–	–	–	–	3	38
Gourmet Pretzels Spinach Feta	1	430	9	25	–	–	–	–	3	7
Gourmet Pretzels Tomato Parmesan	1	420	10	10	–	–	–	–	3	7
Muffin Banana	1	310	11	0	–	–	–	–	5	20
Muffin Blueberry	1	300	10	0	–	–	–	–	5	18
Muffin Chocolate	1	320	11	0	–	–	–	–	5	17
Power Cookie Breakfast Bar	1	230	10	21	–	–	–	–	1	18
Power Cookie Chocolate Chip w/ Walnuts	1	404	12	0	–	–	–	–	5	31
Power Cookie Lemon Poppyseed	1	371	7	0	–	–	–	–	4	30
Power Cookie Oatmeal Raisin Walnut	1	375	7	0	–	–	–	–	6	33
Power Cookie Peanut Butter	1	426	14	0	–	–	–	–	3	25

BEVERAGES

FOOD	PORTION	CALS	TOTAL FAT	CHOL	SAT FAT	POLY FAT	MONO FAT	TRANS FAT	FIBER	SUGAR
800 Lb Gorilla	1 (12 oz)	434	9	42	–	–	–	–	2	41
Freeze Lemon	1 (12 oz)	282	2	9	–	–	–	–	0	40
Freeze Orange	1 (12 oz)	290	1	3	–	–	–	–	0	47
Fresh Juice ABC	1 (12 oz)	150	0	0	0	0	0	0	2	19
Fresh Juice Apple	1 (12 oz)	180	0	0	0	0	0	0	0	45
Fresh Juice Carrot	1 (12 oz)	98	0	0	0	0	0	0	0	20
Fresh Juice Green-V	1 (12 oz)	96	1	0	–	–	–	–	2	11
Fresh Juice G-Snap	1 (12 oz)	120	1	0	–	–	–	–	3	14

FOOD	PORTION	CALS	TOTAL FAT	CHOL	SAT FAT	POLY FAT	MONO FAT	TRANS FAT	FIBER	SUG
Fresh Juice Lemonade Raspberry	1 (12 oz)	164	0	0	0	0	0	0	0	35
Fresh Juice Monkey C	1 (12 oz)	186	1	0	–	–	–	–	2	32
Fresh Juice Orange	1 (12 oz)	168	1	0	–	–	–	–	1	31
Naturally Light Banana Mango	1	162	0	0	0	0	0	0	3	36
Naturally Light Pineapple Mango	1	172	0	0	0	0	0	0	3	40
Naturally Light Raspberry Banana	1	161	0	0	0	0	0	0	3	33
Naturally Light Strawberry Pineapple	1	131	0	0	0	0	0	0	3	29
Shake Bananasplit	1 (12 oz)	274	0	0	0	0	0	0	2	39
Shake P-Nut Power	1 (12 oz)	362	16	0	–	–	–	–	4	23
Smoothie Acai Energizer	1 (12 oz)	161	1	3	–	–	–	–	2	26
Smoothie Awesome Acai	1 (12 oz)	146	1	0	–	–	–	–	1	26
Smoothie Banzai Blueberry	1 (12 oz)	172	2	0	–	–	–	–	2	–
Smoothie Berry Brilliance	1 (12 oz)	192	1	0	–	–	–	–	2	38
Smoothie Big Wednesday	1 (12 oz)	201	1	3	–	–	–	–	2	42
Smoothie Cardio Cooler	1 (12 oz)	244	1	3	–	–	–	–	3	45
Smoothie Citrus Stinger	1 (12 oz)	198	1	3	–	–	–	–	2	24
Smoothie Cranberry Quest	1 (12 oz)	208	1	0	–	–	–	–	1	44
Smoothie Dr. Robeks	1 (12 oz)	186	1	0	–	–	–	–	2	31
Smoothie Green Tea Sensation	1 (12 oz)	199	2	3	–	–	–	–	0	27
Smoothie Guava Lava	1 (12 oz)	206	1	3	–	–	–	–	2	42
Smoothie Hummingbird	1 (12 oz)	211	1	3	–	–	–	–	2	43
Smoothie Infinite Orange	1 (12 oz)	182	1	0	–	–	–	–	2	31
Smoothie Mahalo Mango	1 (12 oz)	201	1	3	–	–	–	–	2	45
Smoothie Malibu Peach	1 (12 oz)	181	0	0	0	0	0	0	1	38
Smoothie Outrageous Raspberry	1 (12 oz)	182	1	3	–	–	–	–	1	40
Smoothie Passionfruit Cove	1 (12 oz)	193	1	3	–	–	–	–	1	41
Smoothie Pina Koolada	1 (12 oz)	212	1	3	–	–	–	–	1	42
Smoothie Polar Pineapple	1 (12 oz)	183	1	3	–	–	–	–	1	40
Smoothie Pomegranate	1 (12 oz)	190	0	0	0	0	0	0	1	40
Smoothie Pomegranate Power	1 (12 oz)	217	1	0	–	–	–	–	3	42
Smoothie Pro Arobek	1 (12 oz)	260	1	0	··	–	–	–	2	40

FOOD	PORTION	CALS	TOTAL FAT	CHOL	SAT FAT	POLY FAT	MONO FAT	TRANS FAT	FIBER	SUGAR
Smoothie Raspberry Romance	1 (12 oz)	209	0	0	0	0	0	0	2	41
Smoothie Robeks Rejuvenator	1 (12 oz)	221	1	0	–	–	–	–	2	42
Smoothie South Pacific Squeeze	1 (12 oz)	200	1	3	–	–	–	–	2	36
Smoothie Strawnana Berry	1 (12 oz)	188	0	0	0	0	0	0	1	37
Smoothie Venice Burner	1 (12 oz)	227	1	3	–	–	–	–	3	33
Smoothie Zen Berry	1 (12 oz)	217	1	0	–	–	–	–	4	29

SKIPPERS
CHILDREN'S MENU SELECTIONS

FOOD	PORTION	CALS	TOTAL FAT	CHOL	SAT FAT	POLY FAT	MONO FAT	TRANS FAT	FIBER	SUGAR
Kids Catch Chicken Tenderloin + Chips & Kids Side	1 serv	560	11	30	4	–	–	–	1	24
Kids Catch Fish Bites + Chips & Kids Side	1 serv	490	15	0	8	–	–	–	3	26
Kids Catch Sandwich Grilled Cheese + Chips & Kids Side	1 serv	620	19	20	7	–	–	–	3	27
Kids Catch Shrimp + Chips & Kids Side	1 serv	520	11	50	3	–	–	–	2	25

MAIN MENU SELECTIONS

FOOD	PORTION	CALS	TOTAL FAT	CHOL	SAT FAT	POLY FAT	MONO FAT	TRANS FAT	FIBER	SUGAR
Baked Potato Plain	1	210	0	0	0	0	0	0	5	3
Basket Chicken & Fish + Chips & Slaw	1 serv	620	27	45	9	–	–	–	1	5
Basket Chicken & Shrimp + Chips & Slaw	1 serv	760	25	120	5	–	–	–	1	5
Basket Chicken + Chips & Slaw	2 pieces	730	25	70	7	–	–	–	0	4
Basket Clam Strips + Chips & Slaw	1 serv	890	34	75	6	–	–	–	12	4
Basket Clams & Fish + Chips & Slaw	1 serv	740	32	50	9	–	–	–	8	5
Basket Original Recipe Shrimp + Chips & Slaw	1 serv	800	25	165	4	–	–	–	3	6
Basket Popcorn Shrimp + Chips & Slaw	1 serv	750	25	180	5	–	–	–	2	5
Basket Prawn & Fish + Chips & Slaw	1 serv	730	41	235	10	–	–	–	2	5

FOOD	PORTION	CALS	TOTAL FAT	CHOL	SAT FAT	POLY FAT	MONO FAT	TRANS FAT	FIBER	SUGAR
Basket Prawn Seafood + Chips & Slaw	1 serv	720	40	280	7	–	–	–	tr	4
Basket Shrimp & Fish + Chips & Slaw	1 serv	650	27	90	8	–	–	–	2	6
Basket Shrimp Trio + Chips & Slaw	1 serv	1040	38	305	9	–	–	–	4	7
Clam Chowder	1 cup	120	8	5	0	–	–	–	tr	1
Clam Strips	1 serv	270	6	30	1	–	–	–	6	0
Coleslaw	1 sm	170	16	15	3	–	–	–	0	4
Fish Bites + Chips & Slaw	6 pieces	490	17	0	4	–	–	–	7	0
French Fries	1 reg	180	6	0	2	–	–	–	0	0
Grilled Veggies	1 serv	35	0	0	0	0	0	0	3	3
Halibut + Chips & Slaw	1 serv	580	30	45	5	–	–	–	0	4
Homestyle Chicken Tenderloin	1 piece	190	2	30	2	–	–	–	0	0
Hush Puppies	3 pieces	240	9	0	2	–	–	–	3	0
Original Fish Fillet	1 piece	80	4	0	4	–	–	–	1	1
Original Fish + Chips & Slaw	2 pieces	510	29	15	11	–	–	–	2	6
Original Shrimp	9 pieces	220	2	75	0	–	–	–	1	1
Sandwich Fish + Chips & Slaw	1 serv	800	34	20	9	–	–	–	4	14
Sandwich Fried Chicken + Chips & Slaw	1 serv	1260	49	105	15	–	–	–	3	12
Sandwich Grilled Chicken + Chips & Slaw	1 serv	1070	50	145	13	–	–	–	3	12
Skippers Platter + Chips & Slaw	1 serv	930	33	12	9	–	–	–	8	6
SALADS										
Caesar	1 sm	150	13	5	3	–	–	–	2	4
Caesar w/ Chicken	1 sm	340	17	100	4	–	–	–	2	4
Caesar w/ Salmon	1 sm	350	19	80	4	–	–	–	2	4
Green Salad w/o Dressing	1 sm	25	0	0	0	0	0	0	2	3
SMOOTHIE KING										
Acai Adventure	1 (20 oz)	435	5	6	1	–	–	–	4	74
Angel Food	1 (20 oz)	354	0	1	0	–	–	–	6	75
Banana Berry Treat	1 (20 oz)	364	0	6	0	0	0	0	5	75
Banana Boat	1 (20 oz)	524	12	51	6	–	–	–	6	77
Berry Punch	1 (20 oz)	360	0	0	0	0	0	0	4	84
Blackberry Dream	1 (20 oz)	365	1	0	0	–	–	–	2	68

FOOD	PORTION	CALS	TOTAL FAT	CHOL	SAT FAT	POLY FAT	MONO FAT	TRANS FAT	FIBER	SUGAR
Blueberry Heaven	1 (20 oz)	325	1	11	0	–	–	–	2	64
Caribbean Way	1 (20 oz)	395	0	0	0	0	0	0	6	89
Celestial Cherry High	1 (20 oz)	257	0	0	0	0	0	0	3	55
Cherry Picket	1 (20 oz)	273	1	6	0	–	–	–	2	54
Coconut Surprise	1 (20 oz)	460	7	3	6	–	–	–	3	83
Coffee Smoothie Caramel	1 (20 oz)	340	1	13	0	–	–	–	0	56
Coffee Smoothie Mocha	1 (20 oz)	260	2	18	0	–	–	–	1	36
Coffee Smoothie Vanilla	1 (20 oz)	347	1	8	0	–	–	–	0	65
Cranberry Cooler	1 (20 oz)	496	0	0	0	0	0	0	3	89
Cranberry Supreme	1 (20 oz)	554	1	0	0	–	–	–	3	96
Fruit Fusion	1 (20 oz)	355	1	12	0	–	–	–	0	66
Go Goji	1 (20 oz)	433	0	0	0	0	0	0	0	104
Grape Expectations	1 (20 oz)	398	0	0	0	0	0	0	3	90
Grape Expectations II	1 (20 oz)	548	0	0	0	0	0	0	6	125
Green Tea Tango	1 (20 oz)	282	3	16	2	–	–	–	2	40
Hearty Apple	1 (20 oz)	405	1	16	0	–	–	–	2	75
High Protein Almond Mocha	1 (20 oz)	366	9	51	1	–	–	–	2	37
High Protein Banana	1 (20 oz)	322	9	45	1	–	–	–	4	23
High Protein Chocolate	1 (20 oz)	366	9	51	1	–	–	–	2	37
High Protein Lemon	1 (20 oz)	372	9	45	1	–	–	–	1	40
High Protein Pineapple	1 (20 oz)	320	9	45	1	–	–	–	2	23
Immune Builder	1 (20 oz)	380	1	0	0	–	–	–	6	77
Instant Vigor	1 (20 oz)	366	0	6	0	–	–	–	4	72
Island Impact	1 (20 oz)	311	0	6	0	0	0	0	1	65
Island Treat	1 (20 oz)	333	0	0	0	0	0	0	6	70
Kids' Kup Berry Interesting	1 (12 oz)	277	0	0	0	0	0	0	3	62
Kids' Kup Choc-A-Laka	1 (12 oz)	245	3	28	1	–	–	–	2	32
Kids' Kup CW Jr.	1 (12 oz)	270	0	0	0	0	0	0	5	59
Kids' Kup Gimmie-Grape	1 (12 oz)	265	0	0	0	0	0	0	2	60
Kids' Kup Smarti Tarti	1 (12 oz)	200	0	0	0	0	0	0	0	46
Kiwi Island Treat	1 (20 oz)	498	1	6	0	–	–	–	0	96
Lemon Twist Banana	1 (20 oz)	358	0	0	0	0	0	0	3	82
Lemon Twist Strawberry	1 (20 oz)	438	0	0	0	0	0	0	3	104
Light & Fluffy	1 (20 oz)	395	0	0	0	0	0	0	6	89
Low Carb All Flavors	1 (20 oz)	268	9	3	4	–	–	–	1	3
Malts	1 (20 oz)	680	33	127	18	–	–	–	0	77
Mangofest	1 (20 oz)	285	0	0	0	0	0	0	1	69
Mangosteen Madness	1 (20 oz)	383	0	0	0	0	0	0	2	92
Mo'cuccino Caramel	1 (20 oz)	570	12	56	6	–	–	–	0	88
Mo'cuccino Mocha	1 (20 oz)	444	12	59	6	–	–	–	1	69

FOOD	PORTION	CALS	TOTAL FAT	CHOL	SAT FAT	POLY FAT	MONO FAT	TRANS FAT	FIBER	SUGAR
Mo'cuccino Vanilla	1 (20 oz)	525	12	51	6	–	–	–	0	85
Muscle Punch	1 (20 oz)	364	1	1	0	–	–	–	6	75
Muscle Punch Plus	1 (20 oz)	366	1	1	0	–	–	–	6	75
Orange Ka-Bam	1 (20 oz)	465	0	0	0	0	0	0	3	108
Organic Apple Acai	1 (20 oz)	353	5	0	1	–	–	–	4	58
Passion Passport	1 (20 oz)	395	0	0	0	0	0	0	2	93
Peach Slice	1 (20 oz)	314	0	1	0	–	–	–	1	55
Peach Slice Plus	1 (20 oz)	464	0	1	0	0	0	0	4	90
Peanut Power	1 (20 oz)	549	22	1	4	–	–	–	6	59
Peanut Power Plus Chocolate	1 (20 oz)	717	27	25	4	–	–	–	6	63
Peanut Power Plus Grape	1 (20 oz)	749	22	1	4	–	–	–	6	107
Peanut Power Plus Strawberry	1 (20 oz)	699	22	1	4	–	–	–	9	94
Pep Upper	1 (20 oz)	411	0	6	0	–	–	–	3	85
Pina Colada Island	1 (20 oz)	600	10	14	8	–	–	–	3	98
Pineapple Pleasure	1 (20 oz)	280	0	0	0	0	0	–	3	62
Pineapple Surf	1 (20 oz)	461	1	11	0	–	–	–	4	92
Pomegranate Punch	1 (20 oz)	464	0	0	0	0	0	0	1	108
Power Punch	1 (20 oz)	428	1	1	0	–	–	–	6	76
Power Punch Plus	1 (20 oz)	500	2	10	0	–	–	–	6	85
Raspberry Collider	1 (20 oz)	338	0	0	0	0	0	0	4	74
Raspberry Sunrise	1 (20 oz)	392	0	0	0	0	0	0	2	73
Shakes	1 (20 oz)	670	33	127	18	–	–	–	0	76
Slim-N-Trim Chocolate	1 (20 oz)	297	2	39	0	–	–	–	3	48
Slim-N-Trim Orange Vanilla	1 (20 oz)	215	1	11	0	–	–	–	0	38
Slim-N-Trim Strawberry	1 (20 oz)	375	1	11	0	–	–	–	5	72
Slim-N-Trim Vanilla	1 (20 oz)	253	1	11	0	–	–	–	3	42
Strawberry Kiwi Breeze	1 (20 oz)	376	0	6	0	0	0	0	3	84
Strawberry X-treme	1 (20 oz)	366	0	0	0	0	0	0	6	70
Super Punch	1 (20 oz)	395	0	0	0	0	0	0	6	90
Super Punch Plus	1 (20 oz)	459	0	0	0	0	0	0	6	91
The Activator Chocolate	1 (20 oz)	404	1	11	0	–	–	–	5	56
The Activator Strawberry	1 (20 oz)	556	1	7	0	–	–	–	8	89
The Activator Vanilla	1 (20 oz)	406	1	7	0	–	–	–	5	54
The Hulk Chocolate	1 (20 oz)	876	31	84	12	–	–	–	6	90
The Hulk Strawberry	1 (20 oz)	1035	32	87	13	–	–	–	8	125
The Hulk Vanilla	1 (20 oz)	872	32	89	13	–	–	–	5	88
The Shredder Chocolate	1 (20 oz)	311	3	45	0	–	–	–	1	19
The Shredder Strawberry	1 (20 oz)	356	1	11	0	–	–	–	3	41

FOOD	PORTION	CALS	TOTAL FAT	CHOL	SAT FAT	POLY FAT	MONO FAT	TRANS FAT	FIBER	SUGAR
The Shredder Vanilla	1 (20 oz)	283	2	22	0	–	–	–	0	12
Yerba Mate Mango	1 (20 oz)	372	0	0	0	0	0	0	1	76
Yerba Mate Mixed Berry	1 (20 oz)	348	0	1	0	–	–	0	3	81
Yerba Mate Pomegranate	1 (20 oz)	372	0	0	0	0	0	0	2	73
Yogurt D-Lite	1 (20 oz)	333	4	22	2	–	–	–	0	47
Youth Fountain	1 (20 oz)	253	0	0	0	0	0	0	3	54

SOUPLANTATION
BREAKFAST MENU SELECTIONS

FOOD	PORTION	CALS	TOTAL FAT	CHOL	SAT FAT	POLY FAT	MONO FAT	TRANS FAT	FIBER	SUGAR
Belgian Waffle	1	90	0	0	0	0	0	0	1	2
Biscuit Sweet Cinnamon w/ Frosting	1	270	13	10	7	–	–	0	0	14
Biscuit Sweet Maple Buttermilk	1	240	9	5	4	–	–	0	1	16
Biscuit Sweet Strawberry Buttermilk	1	250	9	5	4	–	–	0	1	19
Breakfast Burrito Country Ham & Egg	1	210	10	195	3	–	–	0	2	1
Breakfast Burrito Sweet Pepper Sausage Egg	1	210	11	195	3	–	–	0	2	1
Eggs Scrambled	½ cup	135	8	350	3	–	–	0	0	1
Focaccia Egg Scramble w/ Bacon	1 piece	180	8	70	3	–	–	0	1	1
French Toast	1 slice	150	4	85	2	–	–	0	1	4
Oatmeal Plain	¾ cup	110	2	0	0	–	–	0	3	0
Potatoes O'Brien	½ cup	140	6	0	0	–	–	0	2	3
Sticky Granola Clusters w/ Almonds	¼ cup	270	14	15	5	–	–	0	3	15
Sunrise Pasta Mediterranean	1 cup	210	12	75	4	–	–	0	2	3

DESSERTS

FOOD	PORTION	CALS	TOTAL FAT	CHOL	SAT FAT	POLY FAT	MONO FAT	TRANS FAT	FIBER	SUGAR
Apple Medley Fat Free	½ cup	70	0	0	0	0	0	0	1	12
Banana Royale Fat Free	½ cup	80	0	0	0	0	0	0	1	12
Cake Carrot & Cream Cheese Lava	1 piece	320	15	40	5	–	–	0	1	34
Cake Chocolate Lava	½ cup	330	8	5	4	–	–	0	0	47
Cobbler Apple	½ cup	360	10	5	5	–	–	0	1	10
Cobbler Caramel Apple	½ cup	390	12	5	5	–	–	0	2	50
Cobbler Cherry Apple	½ cup	330	10	0	5	–	–	0	2	29
Cookie Chocolate Chip	1 sm	75	3	5	2	–	–	0	0	6

FOOD	PORTION	CALS	TOTAL FAT	CHOL	SAT FAT	POLY FAT	MONO FAT	TRANS FAT	FIBER	SUG
Cookie Bar Chocolate Peanut Butter	1 piece	270	12	25	7	–	–	0	1	22
Frozen Yogurt Chocolate Nonfat	½ cup	110	0	0	0	0	0	0	1	17
Pudding Banana	½ cup	160	4	10	0	–	–	0	1	26
Pudding Butterscotch Low Fat	½ cup	140	3	10	0	–	–	0	0	24
Pudding Chocolate Low Fat	½ cup	150	3	10	1	–	–	0	0	24
Pudding Chocolate Low Fat No Sugar Added	½ cup	90	2	5	1	–	–	0	0	6

TACO CABANA
ADD-ONS

FOOD	PORTION	CALS	TOTAL FAT	CHOL	SAT FAT	POLY FAT	MONO FAT	TRANS FAT	FIBER	SUG
Dressing Southwest Ranch	1 serv (1 oz)	112	11	7	3	–	–	0	0	0
Guacamole	1 serv (3 oz)	110	9	0	1	–	–	0	4	1
Pico De Gallo	1 serv (1 oz)	5	0	0	0	0	0	0	0	1
Queso	1 serv (3 oz)	200	15	40	9	–	–	0	0	5
Salsa Black Bean & Corn	1 serv (1 oz)	30	0	0	0	0	0	0	1	1
Salsa Fuego	1 serv (1 oz)	5	0	0	0	0	0	0	0	1
Salsa Pineapple	1 serv (1 oz)	20	0	0	0	0	0	0	0	5
Salsa Ranch	1 serv (1 oz)	35	4	5	1	–	–	0	0	1
Salsa Roja	1 serv (1 oz)	5	0	0	0	0	0	0	0	1
Salsa Verde	1 serv (1 oz)	10	0	9	0	0	0	0	0	1
Shredded Cheese	1 serv (1 oz)	110	9	30	5	–	–	0	0	0
Sour Cream	1 serv (3 oz)	160	14	55	10	–	–	0	0	3

BREAKFAST MENU SELECTIONS

FOOD	PORTION	CALS	TOTAL FAT	CHOL	SAT FAT	POLY FAT	MONO FAT	TRANS FAT	FIBER	SUG
Breakfast Burrito Bacon & Egg	1	410	18	350	7	–	–	0	2	2
Breakfast Burrito Barbacoa	1	510	25	110	14	–	–	0	2	2
Breakfast Burrito Chorizo & Egg	1	400	18	310	7	–	–	0	2	2
Breakfast Burrito Potato & Egg	1	440	21	250	7	–	–	0	2	2
Breakfast Taco Bacon & Egg	1	230	10	250	4	–	–	0	1	0
Breakfast Taco Barbacoa	1	250	12	55	7	–	–	0	1	0
Breakfast Taco Chorizo & Egg	1	200	9	160	4	–	–	0	1	0
Breakfast Taco Potato & Egg	1	210	10	140	3	–	–	0	1	0
Plates Huevos Rancheros	1 serv	770	38	515	14	–	–	0	9	1

FOOD	PORTION	CALS	TOTAL FAT	CHOL	SAT FAT	POLY FAT	MONO FAT	TRANS FAT	FIBER	SUGAR
Plates Steak Fajitas & Scrambled Eggs	1 serv	800	37	515	14	–	–	0	9	2
Platter Eggs Mexicana	1 serv	920	52	480	20	–	–	0	9	6
MAIN MENU SELECTIONS										
Black Beans	1 serv	80	0	0	0	0	0	0	2	2
Borracho Beans	1 serv	140	3	5	1	–	–	0	7	1
Burrito Bean & Cheese	1	730	35	50	16	–	–	0	11	3
Burrito Beef Ground	1	710	30	85	14	–	–	0	6	5
Burrito Beef Ultimo Ground	1	800	38	105	18	–	–	0	7	6
Burrito Black Bean	1	450	8	0	4	–	–	0	5	6
Burrito Chicken Breast Fajita	1	630	24	95	12	–	–	0	3	5
Burrito Chicken Stewed	1	660	25	100	11	–	–	0	7	5
Burrito Chicken Ultimo Stewed	1	760	33	120	15	–	–	0	8	6
Burrito Steak Fajita	1	650	27	70	14	–	–	0	2	4
Chips	1 serv (2.5 oz)	180	16	0	4	–	–	0	5	1
Fajitas Chicken Personal	1 serv	740	20	70	9	–	–	0	13	8
Fajitas Chicken Platter	1 serv	1670	52	160	23	–	–	0	26	15
Fajitas Steak Personal	1 serv	760	24	45	10	–	–	0	12	7
Flautas Chicken	1	100	4	15	1	–	–	0	1	0
Refried Beans	1 serv	250	13	10	5	–	–	0	6	1
Taco Beef Ground	1	230	9	30	5	–	–	0	1	1
Taco Chicken Breast Fajita	1	190	4	30	2	–	–	0	1	0
Taco Crispy Chicken Stewed	1	160	7	40	3	–	–	0	2	1
Taco Crispy Ground Beef	1	180	10	30	4	–	–	0	2	1
Taco Soft Bean & Cheese	1	300	14	20	7	–	–	0	4	0
Taco Soft Black Bean	1	200	4	0	2	–	–	0	2	2
Taco Soft Carne Guisada	1	190	6	30	2	–	–	0	1	0
Taco Soft Chicken Stewed	1	210	7	40	3	–	–	0	2	1
Taco Steak Fajita	1	200	6	10	3	–	–	0	1	0
Tortilla Corn	1	70	1	0	0	–	–	0	2	0
Tortilla Flour	1	120	3	0	2	–	–	0	1	0
TASTI D-LITE										
Acai	4 oz	70	2	5	1	–	–	0	0	11
Banana	4 oz	70	1	5	1	–	–	0	0	11
Banana 'N Peanut Butter	4 oz	90	3	5	1	–	–	0	0	11
Bananas Foster	4 oz	70	1	5	1	–	–	0	0	11
Burnt Sugar	4 oz	70	1	0	1	–	–	0	0	14
Buttercrunch	4 oz	80	3	0	1	–	–	0	0	11

FOOD	PORTION	CALS	TOTAL FAT	CHOL	SAT FAT	POLY FAT	MONO FAT	TRANS FAT	FIBER	SUGAR
Cappuccino	4 oz	70	2	5	1	–	–	0	0	10
Cherry Cake	4 oz	70	2	5	1	–	–	0	0	12
Chocoleche	4 oz	80	2	5	1	–	–	0	0	13
Cinnamon Crunch	4 oz	70	1	5	1	–	–	0	0	11
Coffee Liqueur	4 oz	70	2	5	1	–	–	0	0	10
Creme Brulee	4 oz	70	2	5	1	–	–	0	0	12
Egg Nog	4 oz	70	2	10	1	–	–	0	0	11
German Chocolate Cake	4 oz	80	2	0	1	–	–	0	0	13
Latte	4 oz	70	2	5	1	–	–	0	0	11
Mud Pie	4 oz	80	2	0	1	–	–	0	0	14
Nutella	4 oz	90	3	5	2	–	–	0	0	13
Peanut Butter Batter	4 oz	90	3	0	1	–	–	0	1	11
Peanut Cluster	4 oz	90	3	5	1	–	–	0	0	12
Pecan Praline	4 oz	70	2	5	1	–	–	0	0	12
Pina Colada	4 oz	80	2	5	1	–	–	0	0	12
Raspberry	4 oz	70	2	5	1	–	–	0	0	12
Rice Pudding	4 oz	80	1	5	1	–	–	0	0	12
Tapioca Pudding	4 oz	70	2	5	1	–	–	0	0	12
Tart 'N Tasti	4 oz	100	1	5	1	–	–	0	0	21
Tart 'N Tasti Acai	4 oz	100	2	5	1	–	–	0	0	18
Tart 'N Tasti Mango	4 oz	100	1	5	1	–	–	0	0	19
Tiramisu	4 oz	70	1	0	1	–	–	0	0	11
Toasted Almond Fudge	4 oz	80	1	0	1	–	–	0	0	14
Toffee Crunch	4 oz	90	3	0	2	–	–	0	0	14

WENDY'S
BEVERAGES

FOOD	PORTION	CALS	TOTAL FAT	CHOL	SAT FAT	POLY FAT	MONO FAT	TRANS FAT	FIBER	SUGAR
Barq's Root Beer	1 sm	180	0	0	0	0	0	0	0	50
Coca-Cola	1 sm	160	0	0	0	0	0	0	0	44
Diet Coke	1 sm	0	0	0	0	0	0	0	0	0
Frosty Chocolate	1 sm	300	8	30	5	–	–	0	0	42
Frosty Vanilla	1 sm	280	7	30	5	–	–	0	0	40
Frosty Shake Caramel	1 sm	650	14	50	9	–	–	1	0	97
Frosty Shake Chocolate	1 sm	580	13	45	8	–	–	1	2	93
Frosty Shake Strawberry	1 sm	550	13	45	8	–	–	1	1	90
Frosty Shake Wild Berry	1 sm	520	13	45	8	–	–	1	1	79
Lemonade Light Minute Maid	1 sm	5	0	0	0	0	0	0	0	0
Sprite	1 sm	160	0	0	0	0	0	0	0	43

FOOD	PORTION	CALS	TOTAL FAT	CHOL	SAT FAT	POLY FAT	MONO FAT	TRANS FAT	FIBER	SUGAR
TruMoo Lowfat Chocolate Milk	1	140	3	10	2	–	–	0	0	20
TruMoo Lowfat Milk	1	100	3	10	2	–	–	0	0	11
Water Nestle Pure Life	1 serv	0	0	0	0	0	0	0	0	0
CHILDREN'S MENU SELECTIONS										
Kid's Meal Cheeseburger	1	290	13	45	6	–	–	1	1	5
Kid's Meal Chicken Nuggets	1 serv	180	11	25	3	–	–	0	1	1
Kid's Meal Hamburger	1	250	10	35	4	–	–	1	1	5
Sandwich Crispy Chicken	1	330	14	30	3	–	–	0	2	4
SALAD DRESSINGS AND TOPPINGS	–									
Buttery Best Spread	1 serv	50	5	0	1	–	–	0	0	0
Cheddar Cheese Shredded	1 serv	70	6	15	4	–	–	0	0	0
Croutons Gourmet	1 serv	80	3	0	0	–	–	0	0	0
Dipping Sauce Heartland Ranch	1 serv	120	12	10	2	–	–	0	0	2
Dressing Avocado Ranch	1 serv	100	10	10	2	–	–	0	0	1
Dressing Classic Ranch	1 serv	100	10	10	2	–	–	0	0	1
Dressing Classic Ranch Light	1 serv	50	5	10	1	–	–	0	0	1
Dressing Creamy Red Jalapeno	1 serv	100	10	10	2	–	–	0	0	1
Dressing French Fat Free	1 serv	40	0	0	0	0	0	0	0	8
Dressing Italian Vinaigrette	1 serv	70	6	0	1	–	–	0	0	3
Dressing Lemon Garlic Caesar	1 serv	110	11	10	2	–	–	0	0	1
Dressing Thousand Island	1 serv	160	15	15	3	–	–	0	0	4
Dressing Vinaigrette Pomegranate	1 serv	60	3	0	0	–	–	0	0	7
Hot Chili Seasoning	1 pkg	5	0	0	0	0	0	0	0	1
Ketchup	1 pkg	10	0	0	0	0	0	0	0	2
Nugget Sauce Barbecue	1 serv	45	0	0	0	0	0	0	0	4
Nugget Sauce Honey Mustard	1 serv	80	6	10	1	–	–	0	0	3
Nugget Sauce Sweet & Sour	1 serv	50	0	0	0	0	0	0	0	11
Saltine Crackers	1 serv	25	1	0	0	–	–	0	0	0
Seasoned Tortilla Strips	1 serv	80	5	0	2	–	–	0	1	0
SALADS										
Apple Pecan Chicken	1 serv	340	11	105	7	–	–	0	5	20
Baja	1 serv	540	32	90	14	–	–	1	12	10
BLT Cobb w/o Dressing	1 serv	450	25	275	11	–	–	0	3	5

FOOD	PORTION	CALS	TOTAL FAT	CHOL	SAT FAT	POLY FAT	MONO FAT	TRANS FAT	FIBER	SUG
Caesar Side w/o Dressing & Croutons	1 serv	60	4	10	3	–	–	0	2	2
Garden Salad w/o Dressing & Croutons	1 serv	25	0	0	0	0	0	0	2	3
Spicy Chicken Caesar w/o Dressing & Croutons	1 serv	470	25	90	12	–	–	1	5	3
SANDWICHES AND SIDES										
Bacon Deluxe Double	1	890	56	195	24	–	–	3	3	10
Bacon Deluxe Single	1	670	40	120	17	–	–	2	3	10
Baconator Double	1	970	63	210	27	–	–	3	2	10
Baconator Single	1	660	40	120	17	–	–	2	2	9
Baked Potato Plain	1 (10 oz)	270	0	0	0	0	0	0	7	3
Baked Potato w/ Sour Cream & Chives	1	320	4	10	2	–	–	0	7	4
Cheesy Cheddarburger	1	300	15	55	7	–	–	1	1	4
Chicken Nuggets	5	220	14	35	3	–	–	0	0	1
Chili	1 sm	210	6	40	3	–	–	0	6	6
Club Asiago Ranch w/ Homestyle Chicken	1	690	36	95	12	–	–	0	4	9
Club Asiago Ranch w/ Spicy Chicken	1	710	37	110	12	–	–	0	3	9
Club Asiago Ranch w/ Ultimate Chicken Grill	1	570	27	125	10	–	–	0	3	9
Double ½ Lb	1	800	48	175	21	–	–	3	3	10
Double Stack	1	400	21	85	9	–	–	2	1	5
Fries	1 med	420	21	0	4	–	–	0	6	0
Go Wrap Grilled Chicken	1	260	10	50	4	–	–	0	1	3
Go Wrap Homestyle Chicken	1	320	16	35	5	–	–	0	1	1
Go Wrap Spicy Chicken	1	340	16	45	5	–	–	0	1	1
Jr. Bacon Cheeseburger	1	400	24	65	9	–	–	1	2	5
Jr. Cheeseburger	1	290	13	45	6	–	–	1	1	5
Jr. Cheeseburger Deluxe	1	350	19	55	7	–	–	1	2	6
Jr. Hamburger	1	250	10	35	4	–	–	1	1	5
Sandwich Crispy Chicken	1	380	20	35	4	–	–	0	2	4
Sandwich Homestyle Chicken Fillet	1	510	21	60	6	–	–	0	4	8
Sandwich Monterey Crispy Chicken	1	400	20	45	6	–	–	0	2	4
Sandwich Spicy Chicken Fillet	1	530	22	75	6	–	–	0	3	8

FOOD	PORTION	CALS	TOTAL FAT	CHOL	SAT FAT	POLY FAT	MONO FAT	TRANS FAT	FIBER	SUGAR
Sandwich Ultimate Chicken Grill	1	390	10	90	4	–	–	0	3	10
Single ¼ Lb	1	580	33	105	14	–	–	2	3	10
The "W"	1	580	33	105	14	–	–	2	3	9
Triple ¾ Lb	1	1060	67	255	30	–	–	4	3	10
Wrap Crispy Chicken Caesar	1	430	25	45	7	–	–	0	2	1

INDEX